Current Progress in Hematology

Current Progress in Hematology

Editor: Martha Roper

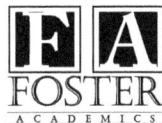

FA
FOSTER
ACADEMICS

www.fosteracademics.com

www.fosteracademics.com

FOSTER
ACADEMICS

Cataloging-in-Publication Data

Current progress in hematology / edited by Martha Roper.
    p. cm.
Includes bibliographical references and index.
ISBN 978-1-63242-480-8
1. Hematology. 2. Hematology--Technique. 3. Blood--Diseases. 4. Hematological oncology. I. Roper, Martha.
RC633 .C87 2017
616.15--dc23

Foster Academics,
118-35 Queens Blvd., Suite 400,
Forest Hills, NY 11375, USA

ISBN 978-1-63242-480-8 (Hardback)

Contents

Preface

This book on hematology provides significant information about blood cells to help develop a good understanding of this subject and related fields. Blood cells or haematopoietic cells are the cells found in blood and are produced by hematopoiesis. The three main types of blood cells are white blood cells, red blood cells and platelets. Together with plasma, these blood cells form blood in our body. This book unfolds the innovative aspects of hematology which will be crucial for the progress of this field in the future. This text includes some of the vital pieces of work being conducted across the world, on various topics related to blood cells. Students, researchers, hematologists and all associated with this subject will benefit alike from this book.

After months of intensive research and writing, this book is the end result of all who devoted their time and efforts in the initiation and progress of this book. It will surely be a source of reference in enhancing the required knowledge of the new developments in the area. During the course of developing this book, certain measures such as accuracy, authenticity and research focused analytical studies were given preference in order to produce a comprehensive book in the area of study.

This book would not have been possible without the efforts of the authors and the publisher. I extend my sincere thanks to them. Secondly, I express my gratitude to my family and well-wishers. And most importantly, I thank my students for constantly expressing their willingness and curiosity in enhancing their knowledge in the field, which encourages me to take up further research projects for the advancement of the area.

Editor

Limited Density of an Antigen Presented by RMA-S Cells Requires B7-1/CD28 Signaling to Enhance T-Cell Immunity at the Effector Phase

Xiao-Lin Li[1], Marjolein Sluijter[2], Elien M. Doorduijn[2], Shubha P. Kale[1], Harris McFerrin[1], Yong-Yu Liu[3], Yan Li[4,1], Madhusoodanan Mottamal[1], Xin Yao[1], Fengkun Du[1], Baihan Gu[1], Kim Hoang[1], Yen H. Nguyen[1], Nichelle Taylor[1], Chelsea R. Stephens[1], Thorbald van Hall[2], Qian-Jin Zhang[1]*

1 Department of Biology, Xavier University of Louisiana, New Orleans, Louisiana, United States of America, 2 Clinical Oncology, K1-P, Leiden University Medical Center, Leiden, the Netherlands, 3 Department of Basic Pharmaceutical Sciences, University of Louisiana at Monroe, Monroe, Louisiana, United States of America, 4 College of Chemistry & Environmental Science, Hebei University, Hebei Province, Baoding, China

Abstract

The association of B7-1/CD28 between antigen presenting cells (APCs) and T-cells provides a second signal to proliferate and activate T-cell immunity at the induction phase. Many reports indicate that tumor cells transfected with B7-1 induced augmented antitumor immunity at the induction phase by mimicking APC function; however, the function of B7-1 on antitumor immunity at the effector phase is unknown. Here, we report direct evidence of enhanced T-cell antitumor immunity at the effector phase by the B7-1 molecule. Our experiments *in vivo* and *in vitro* indicated that reactivity of antigen-specific monoclonal and polyclonal T-cell effectors against a Lass5 epitope presented by RMA-S cells is increased when the cells expressed B7-1. Use of either anti-B7-1 or anti-CD28 antibodies to block the B7-1/CD28 association reduced reactivity of the T effectors against B7-1 positive RMA-S cells. Transfection of Lass5 cDNA into or pulse of Lass5 peptide onto B7-1 positive RMA-S cells overcomes the requirement of the B7-1/CD28 signal for T effector response. To our knowledge, the data offers, for the first time, strong evidence that supports the requirement of B7-1/CD28 secondary signal at the effector phase of antitumor T-cell immunity being dependent on the density of an antigenic peptide.

Editor: Xue-feng Bai, Ohio State University, United States of America

Funding: This study was supported by funding from NIH (RCMI, 8G12MD007595), Louisiana Cancer Research Consortium (LCRC) and Xavier University's Center for Undergraduate Research (CUR) to Dr. Qian-Jin Zhang. Dr. Thorbald van Hallwas supported by Dutch Cancer Society (UL2010-4785). Dr. Harris McFerrin was supported by funding from the NIGMS (P20GM103424). This study was also supported by funding from Louisiana Board of Regents Eminent Alumni Scholars Program, Kellogg Professorship IV in the Arts and Sciences to Dr. Shubha P. Kale. The funders had no role in study design, data collection and analysis, decision to publish, or preparation of the manuscript.

Competing Interests: The authors have declared that no competing interests exist.

* Email: qzhang2@xula.edu

Introduction

It is well established that in the induction phase of CD8$^+$ T-cell responses, T cells require two signals through cell-cell interactions with antigen presenting cells (APCs) for their activation and proliferation [1,2]. Major Histocompatibility Complex class I (MHC-I) presentation of antigen to the T-Cell Receptor (TCR) serves as the first signal, while association of B7-1 (or CD80) with the CD28 molecule expressed on T cells triggers the second signal. B7-1 is not expressed on most tumor cells; therefore, if tumors express MHC-I and trigger the first signal, they may not fully activate anti-tumor specific T cells [3]; however, transfecting the B7-1 gene into tumor cells can render them capable of effectively stimulating antitumor T-cell activation, leading to cancer eradication *in vivo* [4–8]. The augmented antitumor T-cell responses by B7-1 expressing tumor cells occur in the induction phase of immunity.

Transporter associated with antigen processing (TAP)-deficient tumors represent immune-escape variants [9]. Presentation of MHC-I-restricted antigen in these tumors is insufficient; therefore, the induction of the T-cell responses is either difficult [10] or less

efficient [11]. Introduction of the B7-1 gene into TAP-deficient tumor cells stimulates immune system to generate stronger T-cell mediated immune responses against B7-1 negative parental counterparts [10–12], suggesting that the induction phase of T-cell immunity is augmented by B7-1. Recent evidence indicates that CD8$^+$ T cells generated by B7-1 expressing tumor cells recognized a panel of the TAP independent antigens [13]. One of the antigens, Lass5, derived from the ceramide synthase Lass5 (or Trh4/CerS5) protein, located in the endoplasmic reticulum (ER) lumen, associates with H-2D^b and is presented by many TAP-deficient, but not TAP-proficient, mouse cells [11,13]. Although both TAP-proficient and TAP-deficient mouse cells express Lass5 protein, peptide/D^b complexes are selectively presented on TAP-deficient counterparts, most likely due to competition of TAP-mediated peptide antigens [14].

In this study, we have addressed whether expression of B7-1 on TAP-deficient tumor cells can functionally enhance T-cell immunities at the effector phase. We have confirmed that B7-1/CD28 signaling at the effector phase of immunity is required to enhance T-cell based immune response against Lass5 antigen secretion assays, either T cells or target RMA-S/B7-1-culture was added with 10 microgram/ml relevant mAbs against either mouse CD28 (for CTL-culture) or mouse B7-1 (for RMA-S/B7-1-culture) for 1 hour at room temperature. The relevant purified Hamster IgG-isotype control antibody was used as an experimental control. The antibody-containing cultures were then used for ^{51}Cr-release assays (for bulk-cultured CTLs) or intracellular IFN-gamma secretion assays (for LnB5 T-cells).

In Vivo Tumor Growth

C57BL/6 mice were treated with three alternate procedures before tumor cell challenge. 1) The mice were immunized i.p with PBS; 2) The mice were immunized i.p. with Lass5-peptide-pulsed and mitomycin-c-treated RMA-S/pUB cells or RMA-S/B7-1 cells at 5×10^6 cells/mouse; and 3) After one week of immunization with 5×10^6 cells/mouse Lass5-peptide-pulsed and mitomycin-c-treated RMA-S/pUB cells, the mice were depleted of NK effectors by using concentrated NK1.1 mAb (clone 16-10A1, 0.5 mg/mouse injection). The mAb treatment was performed every other day for the first one and half weeks and once a week for the following weeks. Twenty three days post-immunization, the mice were challenged s.c. with 5×10^6 live RMA-S/pUB or RMA-S/B7-1 cells per mouse. Tumor growth was initially detected by palpation daily, and once tumor were palpable, tumor volume was measured by a caliper and calculated by the formula $V = \pi \times abc/6$ (where a, b, and c are the orthogonal diameters). The experimental mice were terminated at animal facility by CO2 inhalation when the tumor size reached a volume 30×10^2 (mm^3). Each experimental group contained 4 to 5 mice described in table 1.

Results

Inhibition of RMA-S/B7-1 cell growth in immunized syngeneic mice

B7-1 molecule expression on tumor cells can elicit anti-tumor immunity at the induction phase [11,12,20,21]; however, there has been no direct evidence to support the enhancement of anti-tumor immunity at the effector phase by B7-1. To test this possibility, RMA-S cells were transfected with the B7-1 gene (designated as RMA-S/B7-1) or a relevant vector (designated as RMA-S/pUB). B7-1 expression on RMA-S/B7-1 but not RMA-S/pUB cells was confirmed by FACS assay (Fig. 1A-a).

To test if B7-1 enhanced T-cell based antitumor immunity at the effector phase, we conducted an *in vivo* tumor-growth inhibition experiment. Since RMA–S cells present a well-known H-2D^b-restricted Lass5 peptide, we immunized mice with Lass5-peptide-pulsed and mitomycin-c-treated RMA-S/pUB and RMA-S/B7-1 cells, respectively. PBS-immunization was used as control.

Twenty-three-days after immunization, each group was divided into two sub-groups that were challenged with 5×10^6 cells/mouse of live RMA-S/B7-1 or RMA-S/pUB cells, respectively. Tumor sizes were measured twice a week after challenge with live tumor cells. The tumors appeared in all mice during the initial week in control PBS-immunized groups while the tumors appeared in most mice at 1.5 weeks in tumor-immunized groups (table 2, Fig. 1B-e insert), suggesting that antitumor immunity was established in tumor-immunized groups. This established immunity dramatically inhibited the growth of B7-1 expressing tumors at 1.5 weeks (table 2). During this time point, both RMA-S/pUB- or RMA-S/B7-1-immunized mice challenged with RMA-S/B7-1 cells had tumors that were much smaller in size, and tumors were found in only two out of nine mice, compared to those challenged with the RMA-S/pUB cells in which larger tumors grew quickly in all mice. The difference in tumor sizes between RMA-S/pUB- and RMA-S/B7-1-cell challenged groups at 1.5 week time point was statistically significant (P<0.05). Results suggested that anti-tumor immunity at the effector phase played an important role in inhibiting B7-1 expressing tumor growth. After the initial two weeks of tumor growth, the RMA-S/pUB tumors continued to grow quickly in both RMA-S/pUB and RMA-S/B7-1 immunized mice while no tumors could be detected in the immunized mice challenged with RMA-S/B7-1 cells (Fig. 1B-e and 1C). In PBS-immunized mice, RMA-S/pUB and RMA-S/B7-1 tumors continued to grow dramatically except in one mouse in which the RMA-S/B7-1 tumor had regressed during initial 1.5 weeks (data not shown). Our results suggested that a major component of the anti-B7-1 expressing tumor immunity is T effectors but not NK effectors because: 1) the RMA-S/B7-1 tumors grew quickly in PBS-immunized mice while no RMA-S/B7-1 tumors appeared in tumor-immunized mice at initial week and 2) NK activity could only inhibit less than 1×10^6 challenged B7-1 expressing RMA-S cells per mouse [22]. In our experiment, 5×10^6 tumor cells per mouse were injected. To further confirm T effectors provided anti-RMA-S/B7-1 tumor protective immunity, we treated the peptide-pulsed RMA-S/pUB-immunized mice with anti NK1.1 mAb before live cell challenge. Figure 1A (b, c and d) indicated that anti-NK1.1 mAb treatment depleted NK cells in the mice. These mice challenged with RMA-S/pUB or RMA-S/B7-1 cells displayed tumor growth patterns (Fig. 1B-f) similar to the peptide-pulsed RMA-S/pUB-immunized mice without anti-NK1.1 mAb treatment (see Fig. 1B-e insert). The RMA-S/B7-1 cells in the mAb-treated mice grew and formed small tumors that disappeared at week 2 after tumor cell challenge while the RMA-S/pUB cells continuously grew to form large tumors in the mAb-treated mice (Fig. 1B-f). Statistical analysis of tumor sizes indicated significant differences between the two mouse groups during the initial week and 1.5 week time points (P<0.05 and<0.01

Table 1. C57/BL6 mice used in each different experimental group.

number of mice	RMA-S/pUB -challenge*	RMA-S/B7-1-challenge*
RMA-S/pUB-immunized	4	5
RMA-S/B7-1-immunized	4	5
PBS-immunized	4	4
NK depletion and RMA-S/pUB-immunized	4	4

*indicates the number of mice per group.
Results of statistical analysis for mouse tumor sizes at specific time points were obtained using Paired Student *t* test, and differences were considered significant at P<0.05.

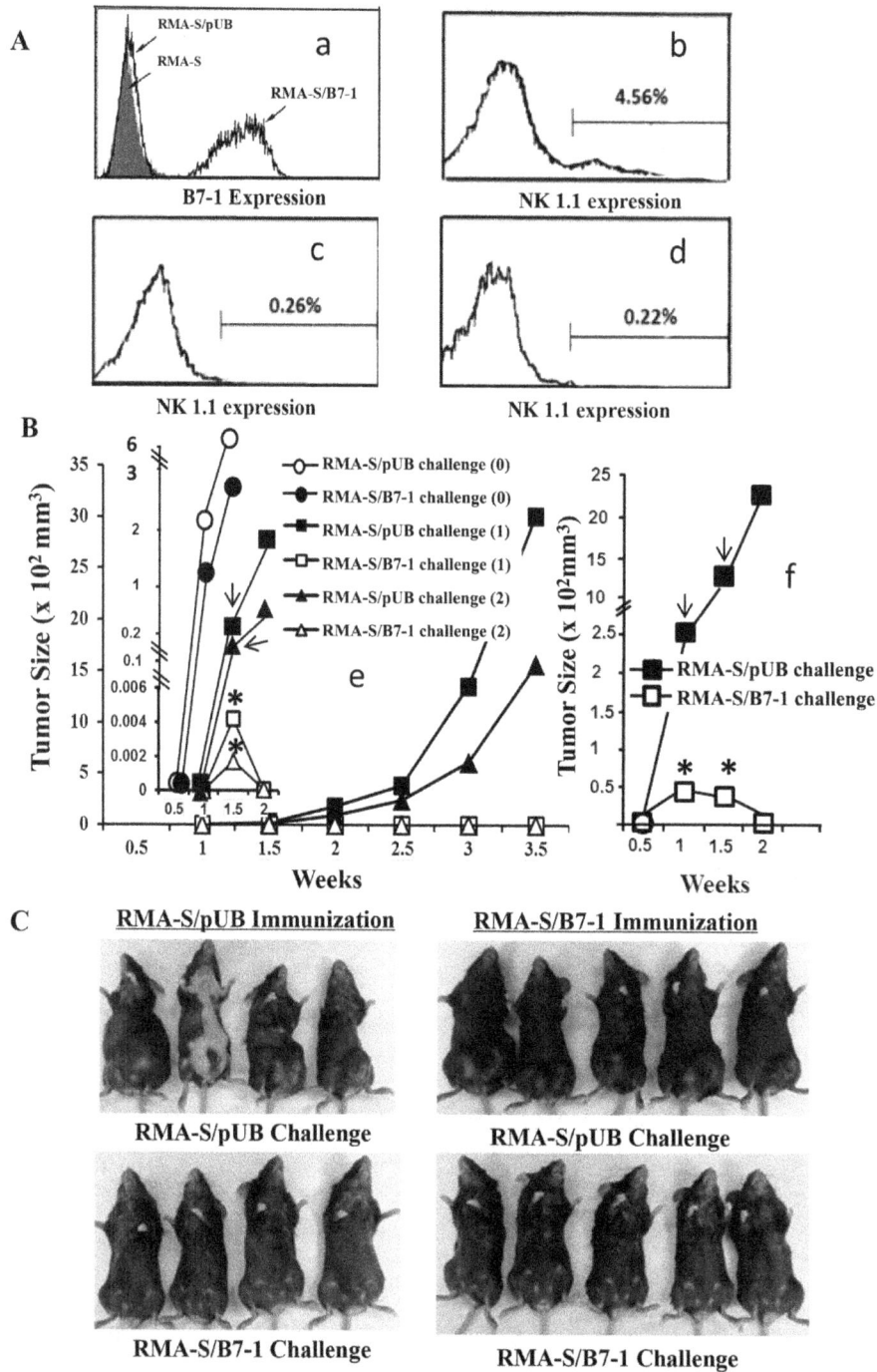

Figure 1. Inhibition of B7-1 expressing RMA-S tumor growth in Lass5-antigen immunized mice. A: a) B7-1 expression in the transfectants. B7-1 expression was determined by FACS assay using FITC-conjugated anti-mouse CD80 mAb; b, c and d) NK1.1 population in mouse splenocytes were detected by anti-NK1.1 mAb. b) Normal mouse splenocytes, c) and d) the splenocytes from tumor-immunized and anti-NK1.1 mAb treated mouse (c: on the tumor cell challenge time and d: end of experiment). B and C: *In vivo* tumor growth assays. B: e) mice immunized with PBS (0), Lass5-peptide-pulsed and mitomycin-c-treated RMA-S/pUB (1) or RMA-S/B7-1 (2) cells. After immunization, the mice were challenged s.c with RMA-S/pUB or RMA-S/B7-1 cells. The insert indicates tumor growth during the time point of the initial tumor cell injection through two weeks. f) Mice immunized with Lass5-peptide-pulsed and mitomycin-c-treated RMA-S/pUB cells and followed by anti-NK1.1 mAb treatment. Afterwards, the mice were challenged s.c with RMA-S/pUB or RMA-S/B7-1 cells. Statistical analysis of tumor sizes indicated significant differences between RMA-S/pUB '↓' and RMA-S/B7-1 '*' cell challenge groups at relevant time points (P value≤0.05 or 0.01). C: Tumor sizes at the endpoint were shown in the mice immunized with Lass5-peptide-pulsed and mitomycin-c-treated RMA-S/pUB or RMA-S/B7-1 cells and followed by challenge with live RMA-S/pUB or RMA-S/B7-1 cells.

Table 2. Tumor formation in the mouse groups during the initial time points.

Mice immunized With or without Tumor cells	Challenge of live tumor cells	
	RMA-S/pUB Number of mice with tumor	RMA-S/B7-1 Number of mice with tumor
RMA-S/pUB-immunized group	4*	1*
RMA-S/B7-1-immunized group	4*	1*
PBS immunized group	4#	4#
RMA-S/pUB- and mAb treated group	4#	4#

#indicates that tumors appear at initial week after the inoculation.
*indicates that tumors appear at initial 1.5 weeks after the inoculation. Total mice per group were shown in the Material and Method Section.

respectively). NK activities could play an auxiliary function in controlling RMA-S/B7-1 tumor growth. In the NK depleted and tumor-immunized mice, RMA-S/B7-1 tumors appeared at initial week and disappeared at week 2 (table 2; Fig. 1A-f), while in the tumor-immunized mice RMA-S/B7-1 tumors appeared at 1.5 weeks and disappeared at week 2 (Fig. 1A-e insert). These results indicated that NK activity could only control early or late appearance of RMA-S/B7-1 tumors and could not inhibit tumor growth.

Bulk-culture T cells more efficiently kill RMA-S/B7-1 cells, and the killing activities require the B7-1/CD28 axis

To confirm *in vivo* experiments, *in vitro* ^{51}Cr-release assays were performed. Two T-cell bulk cultures generated by immunization of mice with Lass5-peptide-pulsed and mitomycin-C-treated RMA-S/pUB or RMA-S/B7-1 cells were used to determine if the B7-1/CD28 axis could enhance T-cell killing activity. Figure 2 showed that two T-cell bulk cultures killed B7-1-expressing RMA-S/B7-1 targets more efficiently than RMA-S/pUB targets (Fig. 2A and B). These results suggested that the role of B7-1 molecule in increasing immune response at the effector phase could occur in Lass5-peptide-stimulated T-cell bulk cultures.

To confirm enhanced T-cell killing activity was associated with the B7-1/CD28 axis, blocking antibodies against B7-1 and CD28 molecules were used. We first performed assays to block the B7-1/CD28 axis using a mAb against mouse B7-1, and an IgG isotype antibody was used as a control. After incubation of RMA-S/B7-1 targets with the mAb or the isotype antibody at room temperature for 1 hour, the targets were mixed with effectors, and the effector killing activities were determined. Results showed that T-cell killing activities against the antibody-incubated RMA-S/B7-1 targets were reduced to a level similar to those observed in RMA-S/pUB cells incubated with isotype-control antibody while isotype-blocked RMA-S/B7-1 cell killing remained at higher levels (Fig. 3A and B). In addition, blocking of the B7-1/CD28 axis by using a mAb against mouse CD28 displayed similar results (Fig. 3C and D). These assays suggested that enhanced killing activities of T effectors required B7-1/CD28 binding.

It has been reported that NK activity can be triggered *in vitro* by B7-1, and this occurred even in the absence of CD28 and could not be blocked by anti-CD28 mAb [23]. Our preparation of T-cell bulk-cultures displayed killing activities for RMA-S/B7-1 targets being reduced by anti-CD28 mAb, suggesting that the role of NK cells was negligible.

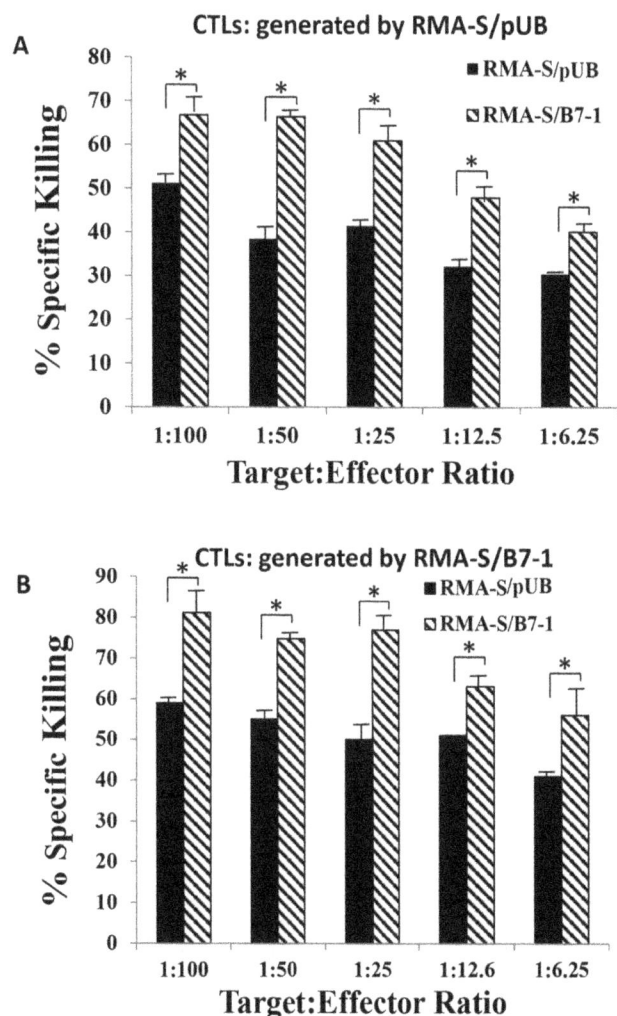

Figure 2. Efficient killing of B7-1 expressing tumor cells by bulk culture T cells. *In vitro* ^{51}Cr-release assays were conducted. (A): Bulk-culture T effectors were generated by immunizing mice with Lass5 peptide-pulsed mitomycin-c-treated RMA-S/pUB cells. (B): Bulk-culture T effectors were generated by immunizing mice with Lass5 peptide-pulsed mitomycin-c-treated RMA-S/B7-1 cells. One out of three experiments with similar results was shown. * indicated that P-values were less than 0.05.

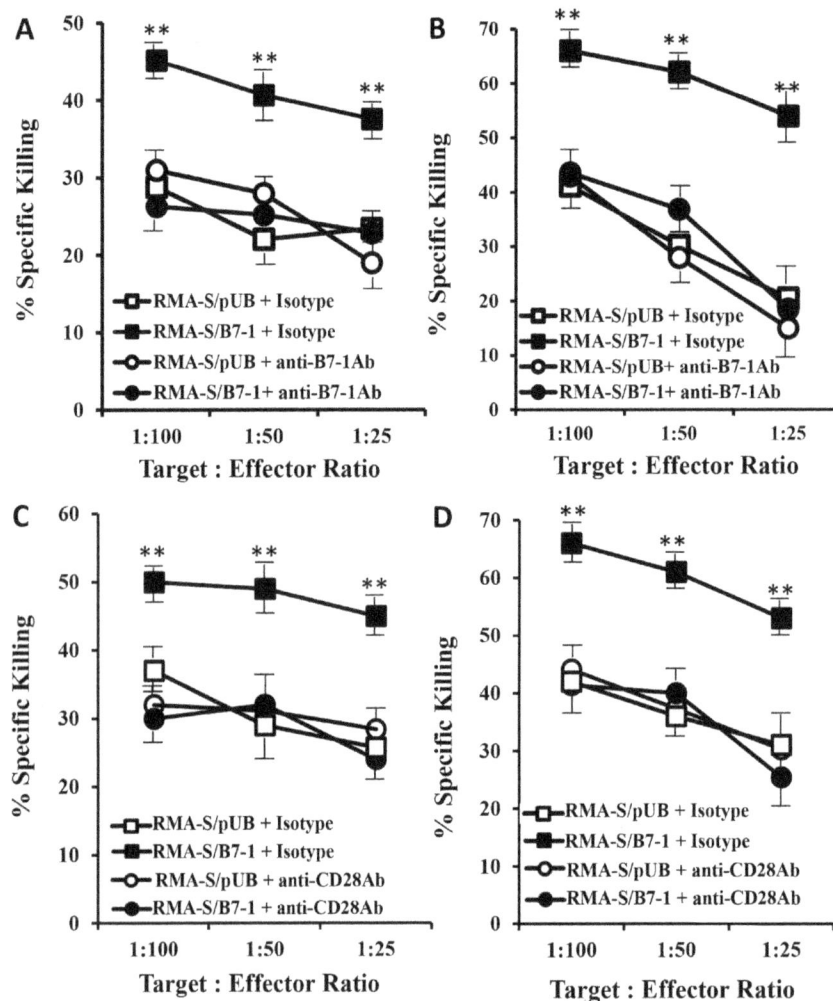

Figure 3. Effects of anti-CD80 and CD28 antibodies on reducing killing activities of bulk culture T effectors against RMA-S/B7-1 cells. Lift-panel (A and C): The cytolytic T effectors were generated by immunization of mice with mitomycin-c-treated RMA-S/pUB cells pulsed with Lass5 peptide. Right-panel (B and D): The cytolytic T effectors were generated by immunization of mice with mitomycin-c-treated RMA-S/B7-1 cells pulsed with Lass5 peptide. Up-panel (A and B): ^{51}Cr-labeled RMA-S/B7-1 and RMA-S/pUB target cells were incubated with either anti-mouse B7-1 mAb or relevant IgG-control. After incubation, the cells were then incubated with antigen-specific bulk culture T effectors for *in vitro* ^{51}Cr-release assays. Bottom-panel (C and D): Cytolytic bulk culture T effectors were incubated with either anti-mouse CD28 mAb or relevant IgG-control. After incubation, the T-cells were then incubated with ^{51}Cr-labeled RMA-S/B7-1 and RMA-S/pUB target cells for *in vitro* ^{51}Cr-release assays. ** indicated that P-values were less than 0.05 among 'RMA-S/B7-1+ Isotype' and other targets at each 'Target: Effector' ratio.

B7-1/CD28 axis plays a major role in increasing LnB5 T-cell activation

To confirm that the role of the B7-1/CD28 axis in delivering a signal into and activating the T-cells at the effector phase was not due simply to binding, the LnB5 T-cell clone specific for the Lass5 peptide [13] was employed. We incubated the LnB5 cells with different amount of either RMA-S/B7-1 or RMA-S/pUB cells and measured the concentration of IFN-gamma secretion by the LnB5 T-cells. Results clearly showed that RMA-S/B7-1 cells stimulated T-cell activation more efficiently than the RMA-S/pUB cells as indicated by more IFN-gamma secretion (Fig. 4A). Enhanced T-cell activation was confirmed to be due to the B7-1/CD28 axis because blocking B7-1/CD28 binding between RMA-S/B7-1 targets and LnB5 effectors by either anti-B7-1 or anti-CD28 antibodies or both reduced IFN-gamma secretion to the levels similar to that of LnB5 T-cells incubated with RMA-S/pUB cells (Fig. 4B, C and D). These results indicate that the B7-1/

CD28 axis provides a second signal, triggering enhancement of Lass5 antigen specific T-cell activation at the effector phase.

Requirement of B7-1/CD28 signaling at the effector phase of immunity is overcome by Lass5-overexpressing targets

Why does enhanced response to Lass5 antigen require the secondary signal at the effector phase? The possible reasons are 1) the Lass5 peptide has a low affinity for H-2D^b binding and/or 2) the Lass5 peptide is generated at a limited level. Both of these possibilities would reduce antigenic peptide surface stability or expression. These situations may reduce the strength of the first signal and therefore require help by the secondary signal to efficiently activate function of T effectors. We have previously performed peptide-binding and peptide-stability assays demonstrating binding and stability of the Lass5 peptide to H-2D^b at levels comparable to the levels of high affinity binders such as the

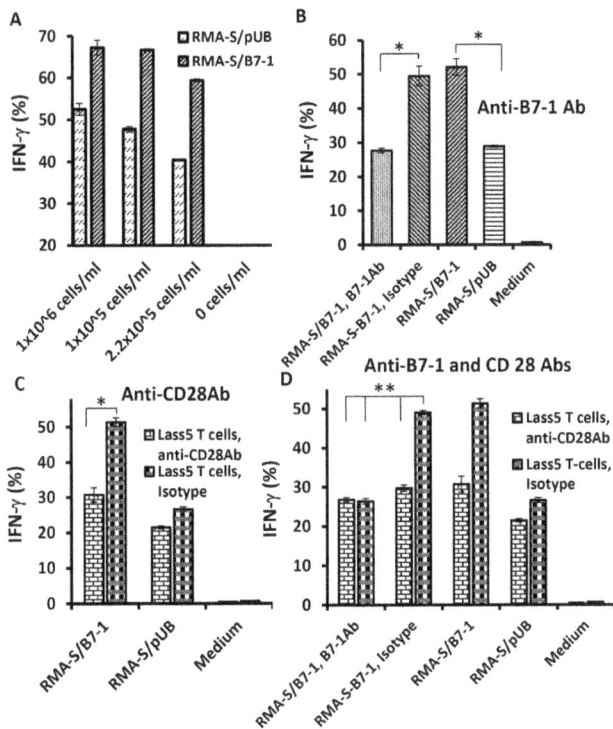

Figure 4. Importance of B7-1:CD28 axis in enhancing a Lass5 specific LnB5 T-cell clone activation. The RMA-S/pUB and RMA-S/B7-1 transfectants were used as targets recognized by a Lass5 specific LnB5 T-cell clone. Lass5 specific T-cell clone activation detected by the intracellular IFN-gamma release assays were conducted with stimulators RMA-S/pUB and RMA-S/B7-1 cells in (A) to (D). (A): 8×10^3 T-cells were incubated with indicated amounts of RMA-S/pUB and RMA-S/B7-1 cells. (B): 8×10^3 T-cells were incubated with 1×10^5 stimulators that previously incubated with either anti-B7-1 mAb or isotype control (for RMA-S/B7-1). (C): 8×10^3 T cells were incubated with either anti-CD28 mAb or isotype control before co-culture with 1×10^5 stimulators (RMA-S/pUB or RMA-S/B7-1). (D): Before co-culture of the T-cells and stimulators, 8×10^3 T-cells were incubated with either anti-CD28 mAb or Isotype control and 1×10^5 RMA-S/B7-1 stimulator cells were incubated with either anti-B7-1 mAb or Isotype control. One out of at least two experiments with similar results was shown. * and ** indicated that P-values were less than 0.05.

viral gp33 epitope (KAVYNFATM) from LCMV [14]. Computer modeling analysis of Lass5 peptide and two immunodominant viral epitopes, ASNENMETM from the influenza-A virus and KAVYNFATM from LCMV virus, demonstrated that the relative binding capacity of the Lass5 peptide is weaker than influenza-A viral peptide but stronger than LCMV viral peptide (data not shown). These results suggested that binding capacity of the Lass5 epitope to the H-2D^b molecule is similar to immunodominant viral epitopes.

To test if increased Lass5 expression could overcome the requirement of the B7-1/CD28 axis for enhancing immune response, RMA-S/B7-1 and RMA-S/puB cells were further transfected with a Lass5 (Trh4) cDNA-carrying LZRS retroviral vector. Lass5 mRNA over-expression in the transfectants was detected by quantitative PCR (no antibody available). Long and short Lass5 transcripts were detected, and only the long transcript contained a Lass5 coding sequence [13]. Table 3 shows that both RMA-S/B7-1.Trh4 and RMA-S/pUB.Trh4 cells expressed higher levels of Lass5 mRNA compared to that detected in RMA-S

cells. The levels of the increased Lass5 transcripts in RMA-S/B7-1.Trh4 and RMA-S/pUB.Trh4 cells were about 822 and 535 respectively.

Overexpression of Lass5 mRNA in transfectants enhanced LnB5 T-cell recognition. Both RMA-S/B7-1.Trh4 and RMA-S/pUB.Trh4 cells stimulated LnB5 effectors to secrete IFN-gamma at levels higher than that found in Trh4-untransfected counterparts (Fig. 5A), suggesting that higher IFN-gamma secretion in the T-effectors was induced by the recognition of increased number of D^b/Lass5 complexes on the surface of the transfectants. In addition, LnB5 T-effectors stimulated by RMA-S/B7-1.Trh4 or RMA-S/pUB.Trh4 cells secreted similar levels of IFN-gamma (Fig. 5A). Apparently, B7-1 expression on the RMA-S/B7-1.Trh4 cells provided a negligible role in serving as a secondary signal for T-cell activation. This was further confirmed by antibody blocking assays in which both anti-B7-1 and/or anti-CD28 antibodies could not reduce T-effector activation (Fig. 5A). The results might indicate that the transfectants expressed an increased number of D^b/Lass5 complexes which provided a stronger first signal for T effector activation and thus overcame the requirement for the B7-1/CD28 signal. To further confirm the increased number of D^b/Lass5 complexes being a critical factor for providing enhanced T-cell killing activity that bypass the requirement of B7-1/CD28 signaling, RMA-S/B7-1 and RMA-S/pUB cells were pulsed with Lass5 peptide as targets in polyclonal T-cell based ^{51}Cr-release assays. The peptide-pulsed targets should express much more surface D^b/Lass5 complexes, and they displayed higher responses for T-cell killing, compared to RMA-S/B7-1 and RMA-S/pUB cells (Fig. 5B). The blockage of the B7-1/CD28 axis by the antibodies did not reduce T-cell killing activities on the peptide-pulsed RNA-S/B7-1 targets (Fig. 5B).

Taken together, the results indicated that naturally expressed Lass5 epitope provides a relatively weak first signal for T-effector response and thus the secondary signal is required. Increasing the number of Lass5 epitopes on the cell surface compensates for the inadequate first signal and bypasses the requirement for the B7-1/CD28 secondary signal for T-effector responses.

Discussion

We have demonstrated that, in comparison with RMA-S/pUB cells, RMA-S/B7-1 cells are more efficiently recognized by Lass5 specific T-cell clones or bulk-cultures of T effectors. The enhanced T-cell based immune response against RMA-S/B7-1 cells occurs at the effector phase of the immunity and requires binding of B7-1 on tumor cells to CD28 on antigen specific T effectors. This requirement can be overcome by an increase in Lass5 expression in tumor cells.

In antitumor immunity, B7-1-transfected tumor cells are potent immunogens which provoke robust T-cell-based antitumor immune reactions [10,11]. The existence of the enhanced immunity may reflect the involvement of tumor-direct priming for antitumor-specific T-cell generation [12]. Although numerous accumulated data support the importance of B7-1 in the induction phase of antiviral and antitumor immunity, the involvement of this molecule in the effector phase has emerged recently. There is a report indicating that in influenza-infected mice, B7-expressing dendritic cells (DCs) trigger both CTL cytotoxicity and release of inflammatory mediators while B7-negative epithelial cells trigger only CTL cytotoxicity [24]. Furthermore, the authors show that inhibiting B7/CD28 interactions significantly decreases the release of inflammatory mediators and that this decrease coincides with a corresponding reduction in mediator-producing CD8$^+$ T cells [24]. Another report indicates that absence of costimulation by

Table 3. Lass5 mRNA expression in RMA-S transfectants.

Lass5 mRNA	RMA-S		RMA-S/pUB.Trh4		RMA-S/B7-1.Trh4	
	Mean	StDev	Mean	StDev	Mean	StDev
Long	1.00	0.12	534.84	26.09	821.84	33.01
Short	3.86	0.32	12.21	1.25	8.27	1.19

Note: Lass5 mRNA expression was determined by quantitative PCR using specific primers. Levels of Lass5 mRNA expression of two natural splice variants (long and short) were normalized with mRNA of the GAPDH housekeeping gene. Only long transcript is coding for the Lass5 peptide MCLRMTAVM.

B7/CD28 association at the effector phase leads to reduced survival of influenza virus specific effector cells [25]. Apparently, B7/CD28 association at the effector phase was associated with an increase in the number of virus specific CD8[+] T cells. In antitumor

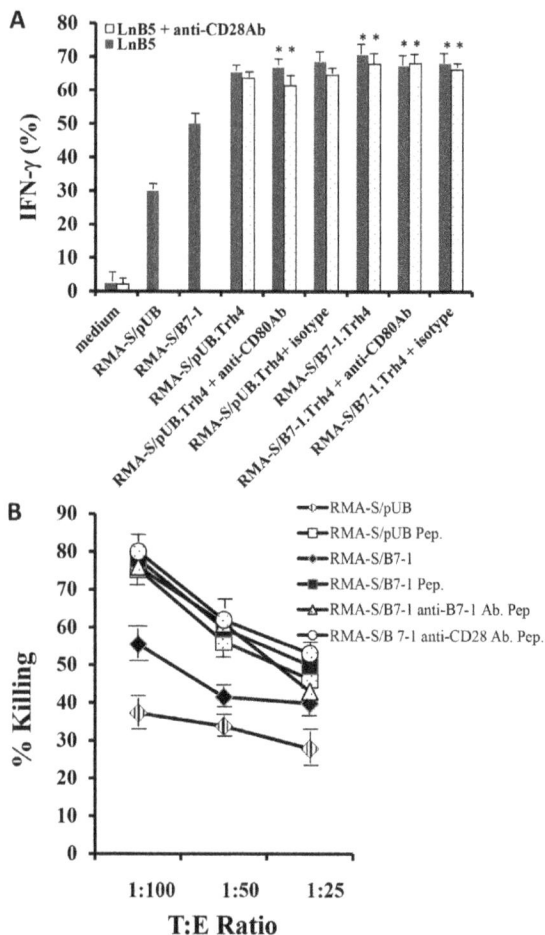

immunity, one report suggested that B7-1 was involved in enhanced antitumor immunity at the effector phase. Bai et al [26], by determining the sizes of murine B7-1 positive and negative tumors in tumor-carrying RAG$-/-$ mice that were administered tumor-antigen specific CTLs, found that the CTLs inhibited growth of the B7-1 positive tumors more efficiently than the B7-1 negative counterparts. These results are very similar to our *in vivo* results (Fig. 1B-e insert). Our work *in vitro* expands upon these *in vivo* findings by removing confounding factors *in vivo* to further confirm that B7-1/CD28 signaling is involved at the effector phase of antitumor immunity. Specifically, our results of CTL activation and killing assays provide important information that directly indicates the association of B7/CD28 signaling with the effector phase of antitumor immunity because our *in vitro* working system contains only cloned or bulk-cultured CTLs with B7-1 positive or negative targets and thus this system eliminates possible confounding factors. Our results from *in vitro* experiments also indicate that the same number of CTLs provide higher activation/killing activities against B7-1 positive than B7-1 negative tumor cells. This differs from that reported by other research groups [24,25] who demonstrated that the influenza viral specific immune responses at the effector phase with or without B7/CD28 association were influenced by the numbers of the CTLs. Of particular note, the enhanced CTL activities in our experiments cannot be attributed simply to B7-1/CD28 association leading to target/T-cell close binding, because the association activates the T effectors to secrete more IFN-gamma suggesting that a signal is delivered into the T effectors (Fig. 4).

Others have demonstrated that NK activities were involved in B7-1 expressing RMA-S cells *in vitro* and *in vivo* [22,23]. In *in vitro* assays, the report [23] indicated that NK activities were independent of B7-1/CD28 association, since an anti-CD28 mAb was unable to block NK reactivity. In our experiments, the enhanced activity of the polyclonal T effectors can be blocked by an anti-CD28 mAb (Fig. 3C and D), suggesting negligible NK activities in the T-cell bulk-cultures. In *in vivo* assays, NK activities were reported [22] to control B7-1 expressing RMA-S tumor growth, and this control was dependent on initial cell numbers in the inoculate. In the case of inoculation with more than 1×10^6 B7-1 expressing tumor cells per mouse, NK activities only temporally inhibited but did not block tumor formation and growth [22]. Our results support this point of view (Fig. 1B-e insert). In PBS-immunized mice, all RMA-S/B7-1-inoculated mice grew tumors during the first week and the growth rate of the tumors was decreased 2.34-fold, compared to growth rate of the RMA-S/pUB tumors. However, both B7-1 positive and negative tumors grew quickly in the following weeks with one exception in which one RMA-S/B7-1 tumor was regressed.

T-cell-based immunity but not NK activity plays a major role in controlling B7-1 expressing RMA-S tumor growth at the effector phase. Our *in vivo* tumor immunization and NK depletion

Figure 5. Increase in Lass5 expression Bypasses B7-1/CD28 requirement for T effectors' response. Lass5 specific LnB5 T-cell clone (A) and T-cell bulk culture (B) were used to determine B7-1/CD28 requirement. (A): Lass5 high expressing RMA-S/pUB.Trh4 and RMA-S/B7-1.Trh4 cells were used as targets that were recognized by LnB5 T-cell clone. The antibodies against CD80 (B7-1) or CD28 molecules were used to block B7-1/CD28 axis. The isotype Ig was used as a control. (B): Lass5-peptide (50 micromole) pulsed RMA-S/pUB and RMA-S/B7-1 cells were used as targets that were recognized by T-cell bulk culture for ^{51}Cr-release assays. Pep means Lass5 peptide. One out of two experiments with similar results for each assay was shown. * * and *** indicated no statistical significance.

experiment (Fig. 1B-f) demonstrates this issue. Without NK activity, antigen specific T effectors inhibited growth of B7-1 positive RMA-S tumors more efficiently than growth of B7-1 negative counterparts. At least, the results at the initial week reflect inhibitive function of T effectors at the effector phase. The following weeks may suggest both the induction and effector phase of T cell immunity being activated by challenged B7-1 positive tumor stimulation.

Lass5 peptide is a suitable H-2D^b binder, similar to immuno-dominant viral epitopes [14] (and unpublished data). Its expression at a limited level on the surface of RMA-S cells was suggested by the evidence indicating that it cannot be presented by TAP-proficient RMA cells [13] (because of other TAP-dependent peptides' competition) and can be presented by Lass5-transfected RMA cells [14]. Transfection of Trh4 (Lass5) gene into or Lass5 peptide-pulse on RMA-S/B7-1 and RMA-S/pUB cells enhances T-cell responsiveness and bypasses the requirement for B7-1/CD28 signaling at the effector phase (Fig. 5A and B). Reports showed that the association between MHC-I/peptide complexes on targets and T-cell receptors (TCRs) on T cells served as first signal for T-cell responsiveness and this signal requires clustering of the TCRs with the MHC-I/peptide complexes at the interface [27–29]. Recent report indicated that the density of the MHC-I/peptide complexes can regulate TCR signaling [30]. Our results indicating enhanced T-cell responsiveness and decreased B7-1/CD28 requirement (Fig. 5A and B) may be ascribed to increased Lass5 peptide densities on target cells associated with relative larger TCR clusters on the effectors that provide a stronger first signal for T-cell responses without requirement of B7-1/CD28 signaling.

Besides B7-1/CD28 signaling, association of B7-1 with cyto-toxic T lymphocyte-associated antigen 4 (CTLA-4) provides another signal to T-cells. This B7-1/CTLA-4 signal, unlike the B7-1/CD28 signal, terminates T effector activation [31]. Blocking B7-1/CD28 association by anti-CD28 mAb reduced T effector activation and killing activity (Fig. 3C–D and 4C–D). The reduction in T-effector function cannot be attributed to blockage of B7-1/CD28 positive signal thereby activating the B7-1/CTLA-4 negative signal, because blocking both signals by combinations of anti-CD28 and anti-CTLA-4 (clone: 9H10) mAbs did not recover T-effector killing activity against RMA-S/B7-1 targets (data not shown). In Trh4-transfected or Lass5 peptide-pulsed RMA-S/B7-1 target system (Fig. 5), blockage of B7-1/CD28 association by anti-CD28 mAb did not activate the B7-1/CTLA-4 negative signaling because reduction of T-effector activities was not observed. It is not clear that why CTLA-4 does not promote a negative signal to inhibit T-effector function in our working system. Some reports have provided an opposite evidence in which CTLA-4 played active signal for T-cell activation [5,32]. In our current work, the results of B7-1/CTLA-4 signaling are limited but we are interested in investigating further.

TAP2-deficient RMA-S cells can present many different TAP-independent antigens, as demonstrated by different T-cell clones being generated [13]. In future studies, we will investigate if the results observed with Lass5 antigenic peptide presentation can be expanded to other TAP-independent antigens. If these antigens display similar results, it suggests that 1) T-cell responses to TAP-independent antigens require B7-1/CD28 signaling at the effector phase and 2) a potential mechanism in which the first signal strength regulates the requirement of secondary B7-1/CD28 signaling shown in Lass5 antigen presentation can be confirmed to be an important role for T-cell response to TAP-independent antigens at the effector phase. Since many types of human cancers down-regulate TAP molecules [33,34], understanding how T-cells respond to these types of cancers may provide useful information for cancer immunotherapy.

Acknowledgments

We would like to thank Dr. Ian Davenport (Xavier University) for reviewing the manuscript and to thank Mr. Reginald Starks (Xavier University) for taking care of the animals used in the study. We would also like to thank RCMI and LCRC Core Facility for supporting this study.

Author Contributions

Contributed reagents/materials/analysis tools: QJZ TvH SPK YYL HM. Wrote the paper: QJZ. Designed T cell clone experiments: TvH. Designed all other experiments: QJZ. Conducted most of the experiments: XLL. Conducted the T cell clone experiments: MS ED TvH. Analyzed data and participated in the many discussions on the findings and follow up experiments: SPK YYL HM. Did computer modeling analysis: MM. Performed animal experiments: XY YL FD. Performed animal experiments: BG. Undergraduate students, supported by Xavier's Center for Undergraduate Research, who participated in and assisted with the experiments: KH YHN NT CRS.

References

1. Robey E, Allison JP (1995) T-cell activation: integration of signals from the antigen receptor and costimulatory molecules. Immunol Today 16: 306–310.
2. Van Gool SW, Vandenberghe P, de Boer M, Ceuppens JL (1996) CD80, CD86 and CD40 provide accessory signals in a multiple-step T-cell activation model. Immunol Rev 153: 47–83.
3. Zang X, Allison JP (2007) The B7 family and cancer therapy: costimulation and coinhibition. Clin Cancer Res 13: 5271–5279.
4. Townsend SE, Allison JP (1993) Tumor rejection after direct costimulation of CD8+ T cells by B7-transfected melanoma cells. Science 259: 368–370.
5. Chen L, Ashe S, Brady WA, Hellstrom I, Hellstrom KE, et al. (1992) Costimulation of antitumor immunity by the B7 counterreceptor for the T lymphocyte molecules CD28 and CTLA-4. Cell 71: 1093–1102.
6. Bixby DL, Yannelli JR (1998) CD80 expression in an HLA-A2-positive human non-small cell lung cancer cell line enhances tumor-specific cytotoxicity of HLA-A2-positive T cells derived from a normal donor and a patient with non-small cell lung cancer. Int J Cancer 78: 685–694.
7. Boyerinas B, Park SM, Murmann AE, Gwin K, Montag AG, et al. (2012) Let-7 modulates acquired resistance of ovarian cancer to Taxanes via IMP-1-mediated stabilization of multidrug resistance 1. Int J Cancer 130: 1787–1797.
8. Bueler H, Mulligan RC (1996) Induction of antigen-specific tumor immunity by genetic and cellular vaccines against MAGE: enhanced tumor protection by coexpression of granulocyte-macrophage colony-stimulating factor and B7-1. Mol Med 2: 545–555.
9. Dunn GP, Bruce AT, Ikeda H, Old LJ, Schreiber RD (2002) Cancer immunoediting: from immunosurveillance to tumor escape. Nat Immunol 3: 991–998.
10. Wolpert EZ, Petersson M, Chambers BJ, Sandberg JK, Kiessling R, et al. (1997) Generation of CD8+ T cells specific for transporter associated with antigen processing deficient cells. Proc Natl Acad Sci U S A 94: 11496–11501.
11. Li XL, Liu YY, Knight D, Odaka Y, Mathis JM, et al. (2009) Effect of B7.1 costimulation on T-cell based immunity against TAP-negative cancer can be facilitated by TAP1 expression. PLoS One 4: e6385.
12. Li XL, Zhang D, Knight D, Odaka Y, Glass J, et al. (2009) Priming of immune responses against transporter associated with antigen processing (TAP)-deficient tumours: tumour direct priming. Immunology 128: 420–428.
13. van Hall T, Wolpert EZ, van Veelen P, Laban S, van der Veer M, et al. (2006) Selective cytotoxic T-lymphocyte targeting of tumor immune escape variants. Nat Med 12: 417–424.
14. Oliveira CC, Querido B, Sluijter M, Derbinski J, van der Burg SH, et al. (2011) Peptide transporter TAP mediates between competing antigen sources generating distinct surface MHC class I peptide repertoires. Eur J Immunol 41: 3114–3124.
15. Levitsky HI, Lazenby A, Hayashi RJ, Pardoll DM (1994) In vivo priming of two distinct antitumor effector populations: the role of MHC class I expression. J Exp Med 179: 1215–1224.
16. van Hall T, Sijts A, Camps M, Offringa R, Melief C, et al. (2000) Differential influence on cytotoxic T lymphocyte epitope presentation by controlled

expressed by TAP-deficient tumor cells, and this requirement can be overcome when the targets express high levels of the Lass5 antigen.

Materials and Methods

Ethics Statement

The Xavier University of Louisiana Institutional Animal Care and Use Committee (IACUC) approved animal protocol (012711-001BI) used in this study. C57BL/6 mice (6-week-old females) were purchased from Charles River Laboratories and were maintained in pathogen-free animal facilities at Xavier University of Louisiana. Each ventilated and sealed cage contained 5 mice with bedding materials of aspen shavings or shreds. All mice were treated in accordance with the Institute of Laboratory Animal Research (NIH, Bethesda, MD) Guide for the Care and Use of Laboratory Animals. In *in vivo* experiments, the tumor size reached a volume 30×10^2 (mm^3) or the mice were sacrificed by CO_2 upon observed distress.

Peptide

H-2D^b restricted peptide Lass5 (MCLRMTAVM) at 98% purification was purchased from GL Biochem Ltd (Shanghai, China) and used for this study. The peptide was dissolved in pure DMSO at a stock concentration of 10 mg/ml and stored at −20°C.

Cell Lines and Cell Culture

Mouse TAP2-deficient RMA-S cells were transfected with either pUB6-vector or pUB6-based B7-1 cDNA [11]. The transfectants were designated as RMA-S/pUB and RMA-S/B7-1 cells and were maintained in RPMI 1640 (Mediatech Inc., Manassas, VA., USA) supplemented with 10% FCS, 2 mM L-glutamine, 100 IU/ml penicillin, 100 microgram/ml streptomycin and 20 mM HEPES and supplemented with 10 microgram/ml Blasticidin. In addition, both cell lines were further transfected with Lass5 (Trh4/CerS5) expressing LZRS-retroviral vector [14]. The Lass5-vector transfectants were designated as RMA-S/B7-1.Trh4 and RMA-S/pUB.Trh4 cells respectively.

Hybridoma

Hybridoma producing anti-mouse NK1.1 monoclonal antibody (mAb), clone PK 136 was obtained from ATCC (Manassas, VA). Culture of the hybridoma and purification of the NK1.1 mAb was performed using a published protocol [15] with slight modification. The mAb was concentrated and purified using the ammonium sulfate method and purified mAb was obtained at a concentration of about 100 mg per milliliter and used for *in vivo* depletion of mouse NK cells.

FACS Assays

FACS assays were performed to detect B7-1 on transfected cells and to detect the NK1.1 cell population in mouse splenocytes. B7-1 expressed on RMA-S/pUB and RMA-s/B7-1 transfectants was labeled with a FITC-conjugated anti-mouse CD80 mAb (clone 16-10A1, Biolegend, San Diego, CA, USA). The NK cell population was detected in mouse splenocytes by labeling with anti-mouse CD16/32 (Fc-receptor) mAb (clone 93, Biolegend, San Diego, CA, USA), followed by labeling with FITC-conjugated anti-mouse NK1.1 mAb (clone PK136, Biolegend, San Diego, CA, USA). After extensively washing, the cell pellets were suspended in PBS at 1×10^6 cells/ml concentration. Expression of cell surface B7-1 molecule and NK1.1 protein was determined by using a BD FACScalibur.

Quantitative PCR analysis of Lass5 expressing transfectants

Total RNA isolation and cDNA preparation from RMA-S/B7-1.Trh4 and RMA-S Trh4/pUB cells were performed using an RNeasy Mini Kit (Qiagen, MD, USA). Five hundred nanograms of purified total RNA were used to synthesize cDNA using a High Capacity RNA-to-cDNA Kit (Applied Biosystems, Foster City, USA). Quantitative PCR on short and long transcripts of Trh4 was done as described previously [13]. SensiMix SYBR No-ROX kit from GC Biotech Bioline (Alphen aan den Rijn, NL) was used in a C1000 Thermal Cycler (Bio-Rad, Hercules, CA, USA) and results were analyzed using Bio-Rad CFX manager software. Long Trh4 (Lass5) transcripts were amplified with Power SYBR Green Master Mix (Applied Biosystems) on a GeneAmp 7300 System (Applied Biosystems).

Generation of Cytolytic T Lymphocytes (CTL) and ^{51}Cr-release Assays

Antigens used for CTL generation were prepared using the following procedures: RMA-S/B7-1 or RMA-S/pUB cells were incubated at 26°C overnight with 100 micromole D^b-restricted and TAP-independent Lass5 peptide [13]. Afterwards, the cells were treated with 30 microgram/ml mitomycin-c for 3-hours at 26°C and washed extensively. The peptide-pulsed RMA-S/B7-1 or RMA-S/pUB cells were then injected i.p. into C57BL/6 mice (5×10^6 cells/mouse). After a 9-day immunization, the RMA-S/pUB- or RMA-S/B7-1-immunized mice were killed by CO_2. The immunized spleens were re-stimulated with mitomycin-c treated, 100 micromole Lass5-pulsed RMA-S/pUB or RMA-S/B7-1 cells (1×10^7 cells/1×10^8 splenocytes). ^{51}Cr-release assays were conducted by using target cells indicated in each figures. Percentage data were converted to logarithmic data before statistical analysis. Two-way ANOVA followed by Dunnett's Multiple Comparison test or Unpaired Student's t-test were performed. Results were considered significant if P value ≤ 0.05.

T-cell activation assays

Lass5-specific T cell clone LnB5 was generated as previously described [13]. T-cell activities were measured by intracellular IFN-gamma staining of T-cells conducted as previously described [16,17]. In brief, 8×10^3 Lass5-specific LnB5 cells were incubated with indicated amounts of stimulator cells for 4-h in the presence of 1 microgram/ml GolgiPlug (BD Biosciences). After incubation the cells were fixed, permeabilized and stained with PE-conjugated IFN-gamma-specific mAb, using an intracellular cytokine staining starter kit (BD Biosciences). Afterwards, the cells were stained with FITC-conjugated anti-mouse CD8a mAb and washed extensively. The cell samples were then analyzed using a FACS Calibur flow cytometer (BD Biosciences). Percentage data were converted to logarithmic data before statistical analysis. Two-way ANOVA followed by Dunnett's Multiple Comparison test or Student's t-test were performed. Results were considered significant if P value ≤ 0.05.

Reduction of CTL Killing Activity by Blocking of B7-1/CD28 Binding

mAbs against mouse B7-1 (Clone 16-10A1; Armenian Hamster IgG), CD28 (Clone 37.51; Golden Syrian Hamster IgG), and relevant purified Hamster IgG-isotype controls were purchased (eBioscience, San Diego, CA). Both mAbs were reported to functionally block B7-1/CD28 binding [18,19]. Before adding bulk-cultured CTLs or the LnB5 T-cell clone into target cell cultures for ^{51}Cr- release assays or intracellular IFN-gamma expression of either proteasome immunosubunits or PA28. J Exp Med 192: 483–494.

17. Ly LV, Sluijter M, van der Burg SH, Jager MJ, van Hall T (2013) Effective cooperation of monoclonal antibody and peptide vaccine for the treatment of mouse melanoma. J Immunol 190: 489–496.

18. Razi-Wolf Z, Freeman GJ, Galvin F, Benacerraf B, Nadler L, et al. (1992) Expression and function of the murine B7 antigen, the major costimulatory molecule expressed by peritoneal exudate cells. Proc Natl Acad Sci U S A 89: 4210–4214.

19. Yu XZ, Bidwell SJ, Martin PJ, Anasetti C (2000) CD28-specific antibody prevents graft-versus-host disease in mice. J Immunol 164: 4564–4568.

20. Boussiotis VA, Freeman GJ, Gribben JG, Nadler LM (1996) The role of B7-1/B7-2:CD28/CLTA-4 pathways in the prevention of anergy, induction of productive immunity and down-regulation of the immune response. Immunol Rev 153: 5–26.

21. Kaufmann AM, Gissmann L, Schreckenberger C, Qiao L (1997) Cervical carcinoma cells transfected with the CD80 gene elicit a primary cytotoxic T lymphocyte response specific for HPV 16 E7 antigens. Cancer Gene Ther 4: 377–382.

22. Kelly JM, Takeda K, Darcy PK, Yagita H, Smyth MJ (2002) A role for IFN-gamma in primary and secondary immunity generated by NK cell-sensitive tumor-expressing CD80 in vivo. J Immunol 168: 4472–4479.

23. Chambers BJ, Salcedo M, Ljunggren HG (1996) Triggering of natural killer cells by the costimulatory molecule CD80 (B7-1). Immunity 5: 311–317.

24. Hufford MM, Kim TS, Sun J, Braciale TJ (2011) Antiviral CD8+ T cell effector activities in situ are regulated by target cell type. J Exp Med 208: 167–180.

25. Dolfi DV, Duttagupta PA, Boesteanu AC, Mueller YM, Oliai CH, et al. (2011) Dendritic cells and CD28 costimulation are required to sustain virus-specific CD8+ T cell responses during the effector phase in vivo. J Immunol 186: 4599–4608.

26. Bai XF, Bender J, Liu J, Zhang H, Wang Y, et al. (2001) Local costimulation reinvigorates tumor-specific cytolytic T lymphocytes for experimental therapy in mice with large tumor burdens. J Immunol 167: 3936–3943.

27. Germain RN (1997) T-cell signaling: the importance of receptor clustering. Curr Biol 7: R640–644.

28. Boniface JJ, Rabinowitz JD, Wulfing C, Hampl J, Reich Z, et al. (1998) Initiation of signal transduction through the T cell receptor requires the multivalent engagement of peptide/MHC ligands [corrected]. Immunity 9: 459–466.

29. Cochran JR, Aivazian D, Cameron TO, Stern LJ (2001) Receptor clustering and transmembrane signaling in T cells. Trends Biochem Sci 26: 304–310.

30. Anikeeva N, Gakamsky D, Scholler J, Sykulev Y (2012) Evidence that the density of self peptide-MHC ligands regulates T-cell receptor signaling. PLoS One 7: e41466.

31. Teft WA, Kirchhof MG, Madrenas J (2006) A molecular perspective of CTLA-4 function. Annu Rev Immunol 24: 65–97.

32. Wu Y, Guo Y, Huang A, Zheng P, Liu Y (1997) CTLA-4-B7 interaction is sufficient to costimulate T cell clonal expansion. J Exp Med 185: 1327–1335.

33. Seliger B, Maeurer MJ, Ferrone S (1997) TAP off–tumors on. Immunol Today 18: 292–299.

34. Ritz U, Seliger B (2001) The transporter associated with antigen processing (TAP): structural integrity, expression, function, and its clinical relevance. Mol Med 7: 149–158.

Impaired Clearance of Early Apoptotic Cells Mediated by Inhibitory IgG Antibodies in Patients with Primary Sjögren's Syndrome

Menelaos N. Manoussakis[1,2]*, **George E. Fragoulis**[1], **Aigli G. Vakrakou**[1], **Haralampos M. Moutsopoulos**[1]

1 Department of Pathophysiology, School of Medicine, University of Athens, Athens, Greece, **2** Hellenic Pasteur Institute, Athens, Greece

Abstract

Objectives: Deficient efferocytosis (i.e. phagocytic clearance of apoptotic cells) has been frequently reported in systemic lupus erythematosus (SLE). Todate, patients with primary Sjögren's syndrome (SS) have not been assessed for phagocytosis of apoptotic cells (ApoCell-phagocytosis) and of particulate targets (microbeads, MB-phagocytosis).

Design: ApoCell-phagocytosis and MB-phagocytosis were comparatively assessed by flow cytometry in peripheral blood specimens and monocyte-derived macrophage (MDM) preparations from healthy blood donors (HBD) and consecutive SS, SLE and rheumatoid arthritis (RA) patients. Cross-admixture ApoCell-phagocytosis experiments were also performed using phagocytes from HBD or patients, and apoptotic cells pretreated with whole sera or purified serum IgG derived from patients or HBD.

Results: Compared to HBD, approximately half of SS and SLE patients studied (but not RA) manifested significantly reduced ApoCell-phagocytosis ($p<0.001$) and MB-phagocytosis ($p<0.003$) by blood-borne phagocytes that correlated inversely with disease activity ($p\leq0.004$). In cross-admixture assays, healthy monocytes showed significantly reduced ApoCell-phagocytosis when fed with apoptotic cells that were pretreated with sera or purified serum IgG preparations from SS and SLE patients ($p<0.0001$, compared to those from HBD or RA). Such aberrant effect of the SS and SLE sera and IgG preparations correlated linearly with their content of IgG antibodies against apoptotic cells ($p\leq0.0001$). Phagocytic dysfunction maybe also present in certain SS and SLE patients, as supported by deficient capacity of MDM for ApoCell-phagocytosis and MB-phagocytosis under patients' serum-free conditions.

Conclusion: Similarly to SLE, efferocytosis is frequently impaired in SS and is primarily due to the presence of inhibitory IgG anti-ApoCell antibodies and secondarily to phagocytes' dysfunction.

Editor: Masataka Kuwana, Keio University School of Medicine, Japan

Funding: The study was supported by grants from the Hellenic Rheumatology Society (ERE141/10 to M.N.M), the Propondis Foundation (to A.G.V.) and the Lillian Voudouri Foundation. The funders had no role in study design, data collection and analysis, decision to publish, or preparation of the manuscript.

Competing Interests: The authors have declared that no competing interests exist.

* Email: menman@med.uoa.gr

Introduction

Apoptosis represents a major mechanism of programmed cell death that is essential for the regulation of tissue growth and homeostasis [1]. Normally, cells dying by apoptosis undergo specific changes that target them for rapid clearance by professional phagocytes, such as macrophages. This process leads to the active production of anti-inflammatory mediators by phagocytes and thus facilitates the "immunologically silent" removal of apoptotic cells [2]. The prompt elimination of apoptotic cells (also termed "efferocytosis") [3] is a very crucial biological process, since lingering apoptotic cells eventually proceed to the state of "late apoptosis" or "secondary necrosis" wherein they may contribute to inflammatory reactions via the release of immunogenic intracellular components, including modified autoantigens and "danger signals" [4]. In fact, apoptosis and efferocytosis act in concert to regulate various processes, such

as embryogenesis, tissue homeostasis, tolerance the elimination of damaged cells, and the resolution of inflammation [5–7].

The occurrence of defective efferocytosis in certain inflammatory diseases is thought to have pathogenetic significance, based on the pro-inflammatory potential of secondary necrotic cells [8] Among them, systemic lupus erythematosus (SLE) is regarded as the archetypical disease model where the impaired clearance of apoptotic cells by macrophages represents a possible mechanism for the development of chronic autoimmune reactions and organ damage [9–11]. Apart from defective efferocytosis, various in vitro clearance defects of macrophages have been described in SLE, including aberrant Fc-gamma receptor-mediated uptake of IgG ligand-coated erythrocytes [12] and decreased phagocytosis of yeast cells [13] and particulate targets [10]. These aberrations have been attributed to intrinsic defects of patients' phagocytes [9], to the decreased density of circulating macrophages [14], as well as to the effect of serum components [11,15–17].

Primary Sjögren's syndrome (SS), which is characterized by mononuclear cell infiltrates in exocrine glands and parenchymal organs, shares several immunologic manifestations with SLE. These include various features of B-cell hyperactivity, such as the profound hypergammaglobulinemia, multiple autoantibodies, circulating immune complexes and evidence of complement consumption [18]. In this context, we presently sought to comparatively investigate the capacity of peripheral blood monocytes and monocyte-derived macrophages (MDM) of SS and SLE patients for phagocytosis of apoptotic cells and of particulate targets. For this purpose, we established ex-vivo phagocytosis assays and assessed patients with SLE, SS and RA, as well as healthy individuals. Our findings indicate that considerable proportions of SS and SLE patients (but not RA) manifest deficient phagocytosis of apoptotic cells and of particulate targets that correlate with the activity of these diseases, and apparently owes primarily to inhibitory IgG anti-ApoCell antibodies and secondarily to the dysfunction of phagocytes.

Patients and Methods

Patients

Specimens of peripheral blood were obtained after informed consent from 43 consecutive unselected Greek Caucasian patients with primary-SS, 27 with SLE and 14 with RA [19–21] (**Table 1**), as well as from Greek Caucasian healthy blood donors (2 groups; HBD-1 and HBD-2, 17 each, age- and sex-matched to the SS and SLE groups, respectively). In all assays, HBD-1 and HBD-2 groups exhibited similar results, without statistical difference to each other. Thus, they were subsequently considered as a single group (HBD) in the comparative analyses. The study was approved by the Medical council of "Laikon" University Hospital (Research Ethics Committee). Written informed consent was given by all individuals for their participation in the study, as well as for the usage of their clinical records. Patients' medical records were retrospectively analyzed for demographic variables, clinical and laboratory features. At the time of the study, patients studied were assessed for disease activity by calculation of ESSDAI (for SS) [22], SLEDAI (for SLE), DAS28 (for RA) and for disease severity by SSDDI (for SS) [23], SLICC-ACR (for SLE) [24] and by global disease severity index (for RA). None of the SLE or RA patients studied manifested any evidence of secondary or associated Sjögren's syndrome. SS patients were also analyzed for the presence of extraglandular manifestations and of type-I disease, as previously [25]. At the time of investigation, none of the patients or controls studied displayed evidence of infection or had history of infection with hepatitis viruses or HIV. Sera were tested for anti-Ro/SSA, anti-La/SSB by counter-immunoelectrophoresis, for anti-C1q, anti-native histone and anti-chromatin antibodies by ELISA (QuantaLite), for C3 and C4 complement levels by radial immunodiffusion and for C1q levels by nephelometry. Total immunoglobulin IgG was isolated from serum samples of patients and HBD using the Melon Gel purification Kit (Pierce), according to the manufacturer's protocol, aliquoted and stored at $-20°C$. Protein yields were quantified spectrophotometrically and purification was routinely found to be more than 95% by SDS-PAGE electrophoresis.

Generation of early apoptotic cells

The Jurkat cell line (ATCC) was grown in RPMI-1640 medium (Gibco) supplemented with 10% heat-inactivated human AB-serum and 0.1% gentamicin. Apoptosis was induced in Jurkat cells by exposure to Ultraviolet-B irradiation (800 mJ/cm^2) at room temperature using Stratalinker-1800 (Stratagene), as previously [26]. Subsequently, cells were washed twice with PBS, seeded into Petri dishes 60×15 mm in the above culture medium (0.7×10^7 cells/mL) and incubated for 4-hrs at $37°C$. The percentage of apoptotic cells was determined by flow cytometry (Facscalibur, BD) using annexin-V/propidium iodide staining (R&D). As determined in extensive preliminary experiments and verified at each preparation, after the 4-hrs incubation, approximately 60% of Jurkat cells were early apoptotic (annexin-V-positive/propidium iodide-negative, mean $\pm$SEM: $61.2\pm5.0\%$, n = 10 experiments), with the remaining of cells being viable (negative for both annexin-V and propidium iodide, $37.5\pm4.3\%$). In such preparations, late apoptotic cells (positive for both annexin-V and propidium iodide) were typically <2% of cells ($1.9\pm0.2\%$).

Assessment of serum IgM and IgG immunoglobulin binding to apoptotic cells

The levels of IgM and IgG antibodies to early apoptotic cells (anti-ApoCell) were assayed in serum specimens (diluted to 20% and 5% v/v, respectively) by flow cytometry as previously [16], using early apoptotic Jurkat cells prepared as above and FITC-labeled rabbit antisera to human IgM or IgG immunoglobulin as secondary antibody (Dako), respectively. In each experiment, the reproducibility and inter-assay variation was evaluated by testing two standard specimens (aliquoted and stored at $20°C$) in duplicates consisted of pooled sera from 3 healthy donors (negative control) and 3 SLE patients (positive control), respectively. For the estimation of ApoCell-specific serum IgM or IgG antibody binding, the non-specific binding of the secondary antibody was considered as baseline, the values obtained were normalized to the standard negative control specimen and the results were expressed as binding index (percent gated by mean fluorescence intensity). Coefficient variation for standard specimens was less than 12.5% between different experiments. The occurrence of anti-ApoCell antibodies in purified IgG preparations (50 µg/mL) of patients and controls was also assessed by flow cytometry as above.

Assessment of phagocytosis of apoptotic cells (ApoCell-phagocytosis) by peripheral blood monocytes

For the assessment of ApoCell-phagocytosis by peripheral blood phagocytes, freshly prepared early apoptotic Jurkat cells were labeled with the fluorescent dye carboxylfluorescein diaceteate-succinimidylester (CFSE, Molecular Probes) and were added (1×10^6 cells) in duplicate samples (100 µl) of freshly drawn heparinized peripheral blood. Mixtures were incubated for 90-min at $37°C$ and subsequently, erythrocytes were destroyed with a lysis buffer (Pharmingen). In preliminary experiments, using fluorescence microscopy, normal peripheral blood monocytes and polymorphonuclear cells were found to ingest appreciable amounts of CFSE-stained apoptotic cells, but not viable cells. ApoCell-phagocytosis by monocytes was quantitatively assessed in peripheral blood samples from HBD and patients by flow cytometry, using the appropriate forward/side scatter pattern gate and confirmation by staining with CD14 monoclonal antibody (Santa Cruz). Monocytes were electronically gated, and the uptake of fluorescent CFSE-stained apoptotic Jurkat cells by these cells was estimated as ApoCell-phagocytosis index (ApoCell-PhI), which was calculated as the product of the percentage of gated fluorescent-positive cells by their mean fluorescence intensity. The localization of apoptotic Jurkat cells in the gate of granulocytes had precluded the assessment of ApoCell-phagocytosis by the latter type of cells.

Table 1. Selected anthropometric, clinical and laboratory features of the patients studied.

Disease Features	SS (n = 43)	SLE (n = 27)	RA (n = 14)
Age, years, median (range)	52.5 (33–67)	37.5 (19–45)	60.0 (38–75)
Sex, female:male	43:0	25:2	7:7
Disease duration, years, median (range)	11 (2–23)	11 (1–20)	10 (1–17)
Sicca man manifestations, no. positive (%)	43 (100)	0 (0.0)	0 (0.0)
Disease activity, median (range) [a]	9 (0–41)	4 (0–16)	5.2 (3.5–7.0)
Disease severity, median (range) [a]	2 (2–11)	2 (0–6)	2.9 (1.3–5.4)
Type-I SS disease, no. positive (%) [a]	25 (58.1)	NA	NA
ANA, titer^{-1}, median (range)	320 (0–2560)	640 (0–2560)	0
Anti-Ro/SSA, no. positive (%)	29 (67.4)	15 (40.5)	0 (0.0)
Anti-La/SSB, no. positive (%)	13 (30.2)	0 (0.0)	0 (0.0)
Anti-dsDNA, no. positive (%)	0 (0.0)	18 (47.4)	0 (0.0)
Anti-chromatin, no. positive (%)	0/27 (0.0)	4/19 (21.1)	0 (0.0)
Anti-histone, no. positive (%)	0/27 (0.0)	5/19 (26.3)	0 (0.0)
Low serum C3 and/or C4, no. positive (%) [b]	18 (41.9)	23 (60.5)	0 (0.0)
Low serum C1q, no. positive (%) [c]	5/17 (29.4)	5/15 (33.3)	ND
Rheumatoid factor, no. positive (%)	20 (46.5)	ND	11 (78.6)

a: disease activity, disease severity and Type-I SS disease were defined as described in Patients and Methods,
b: low serum C3<90 mg/dl and C4<20 mg/dl,
c: low serum C1q<15 mg/dl, NA: not applicable, ND: not done.

ApoCell-phagocytosis by monocyte-derived macrophages (MDM)

For the preparation of MDM, mononuclear cells were isolated from peripheral blood of patients and healthy donors by density-gradient centrifugation (BD-Vacutainer), washed thrice with HBSS (Gibco) and plated onto 24-well plates (Corning, 4×10^6 cells/well) in DMEM (Gibco) supplemented with 10% heat-inactivated FBS. Following 1-hour incubation at 37°C, 5% CO_2, non-adherent cells were removed by washing with HBSS and the adherent monocytes were allowed to mature to macrophages by cultivation for 8-days in X-VIVO-10 medium (Lonza) containing 10% heat-inactivated AB human serum, as previously [26]. Culture medium was changed at day-3, and following an additional 5-day culture, the supernatant was aspirated and fresh preparations of early apoptotic cells were added in each well, in X-VIVO-10 (3×10^6 cells/ml). MDM were washed thrice with cold PBS to remove the non-ingested apoptotic cells, were detached with EDTA-lidocaine solution and ApoCell-phagocytosis was analyzed by flow cytometry, as above. MDM preparations were typically 50-65% CD14-positive.

Cross-admixture experiments for the assessment of the influence of serum factors in ApoCell-phagocytosis

To assess the influence of serum components in ApoCell-phagocytosis, apoptotic cells were pre-treated (for 15-min at 37°C) with DMEM culture medium alone, with whole serum or with purified IgG preparations (50 µg/ml) derived from autoimmune patients or HBD. Apoptotic cells were washed and incubated (1×10^6 cells) with preparations of isolated peripheral blood mononuclear cells (1×10^6 cells) or MDM (1×10^5 cells) derived from a healthy donor, and the samples were analyzed for ApoCell-phagocytosis, as above. In separate experiments, prior the addition to mixtures, serum samples from HBD were heat-inactivated (56°C, 30-min) to destroy complement. The rates of ApoCell-phagocytosis by healthy MDM of apoptotic cells pretreated with purified IgG preparations (50 µg/ml) derived from either autoimmune patients or HBD were also comparatively investigated by two-color flow cytometry analyses of healthy MDM stained with CD14-PE (BD-Pharmingen) and CFSE-labelled IgG-pretreated apoptotic cells, as well as by single-color flow cytometry using apoptotic cells labelled with the pH-sensitive fluorescent dye pHrodo succinimidyl ester (pHrodo-SE, Life Technologies, 20 ng/ml at room temperature for 30-min), which allows the actual detection of ingested apoptotic cells owing to increased light emission in the acidic environment of the phagosomes of phagocytes [27].

Phagocytosis assay of fluorescent microbeads (MB-phagocytosis) by peripheral blood phagocytes and MDM

Fluorescent monodisperse polystyrene microbeads (MB) with 1-µm diameter (Fluoresbrite YG, Polysciences) were used. The experimental conditions were optimized in preliminary experiments, where the ingestion of MB was verified by fluorescent microscopy. In such experiments, the application of uncoated microbeads or microbeads coated with human immunoglobulin or human serum albumin had yielded equivalent results, whereas no discernible uptake was observed upon incubation of blood samples with microbeads at 4°C. In brief, duplicate samples of heparinized peripheral blood (200 µl) were mixed with MB (4×10^7 beads/ml) and were incubated for 30-min at 37°C. Erythrocytes were lysed as above, and following three washings with cold PBS to remove the non-ingested MB, the samples were analyzed by flow cytometry. Typical laser scatter properties were used to determine separate acquisition gates for granulocytes and monocytes. MB-phagocytosis index (MB-PhI) was calculated as the product of the percentage of gated fluorescence-positive cells by their mean fluorescence intensity. MB-phagocytosis by MDM preparations was also assessed as above.

Statistical analyses

Correlations were calculated using the Spearman's rank correlation coefficient. Group comparisons were performed by Mann-Whitney rank sum test. For paired comparisons, Wilcoxon signed-rank test and one-way analysis of variance were used, when appropriate. Analyses were conducted using SPSS 15.0 and Graph Pad 5.0 softwares. The results were expressed as median and range, and correlations with two-tailed p-values less than 0.05 were considered statistically significant.

Results

Serological aberrations in SS and SLE patients studied

Serological analyses had revealed several aberrations, including the presence of various anti-nuclear autoantibodies in the serum samples from the SS and SLE patients studied, but not in those from RA (**Table 1**).

Significantly impaired ApoCell-phagocytosis by peripheral blood monocytes of SS and SLE patients

The study of ApoCell-phagocytosis had yielded similar results between RA patients and HBD, but significantly decreased ApoCell-PhI values in both SS and SLE patient groups, compared to HBD (p = 0.0002 and p<0.0001, respectively) and to RA patients (p = 0.0009 and p = 0.0004, respectively) (**Figure 1A**). Conversely, ApoCell-PhI values were not statistically different between SS and SLE patients. Decreased ApoCell-phagocytosis was observed in approximately half of SS and SLE patients, compared to none of RA patients studied (**Figure 1A**).

Among SS patients, ApoCell-phagocytosis by monocytes (ApoCell-PhI values) was found to correlate inversely with ESSDAI scores (r = −0.559, p = 0.004, **Figure 1B**) and to be significantly impaired among patients with type-I disease (in type-I disease; median: 168, range: 119–206, in type-II disease; median: 221, range: 130–338, p = 0.04) or with anti-Ro/SSA autoantibodies (in anti-Ro/SSA-positive; median: 164, range: 119–227, in anti-Ro/SSA-negative; median: 190, range: 142–338, p = 0.03). In SLE patients, ApoCell-phagocytosis by monocytes (ApoCell-PhI values) correlated inversely with SLEDAI scores (r = −0.627, p = 0.0008, **Figure 1C**) and to be significantly impaired among patients with serum anti-Ro/SSA antibodies (in anti-Ro/SSA-positive; median: 149, range: 47–191, in anti-Ro/SSA-negative; median: 194, range: 136–308, p = 0.002), anti-dsDNA antibodies (in anti-dsDNA-positive; median: 154, range: 110–213, in anti-dsDNA-negative; median: 194, range: 47–308, p = 0.02) and low C3 complement levels (in those with low C3; median: 162, range: 47–212, in those with normal C3; median: 193, range: 123–308, p = 0.03).

Impaired ApoCell-phagocytosis by MDM preparations of SS and SLE patients

The in-vitro differentiation of monocytes to macrophages (MDM) represents a surrogate for tissue macrophages [28] and a convenient means for the study of ApoCell-phagocytosis in the absence of direct influence of serum factors. In this context, ApoCell-phagocytosis was comparatively investigated in preparations of MDM derived from HBD and from SS and SLE patients. All HBD studied manifested substantial ApoCell-phagocytosis by MDM, whereas a significant number of SS and SLE cases showed impaired ApoCell-phagocytosis (ApoCell-PhI values less than two SD below the mean of HBD; in 4/9 of SS and in 7/10 of SLE) (**Figure 1D**). Parallel ApoCell-phagocytosis assays of peripheral blood monocytes from these individuals revealed significant

agreement with those of MDM, being normal in all HBD (10/10), but impaired in the majority of patients (in 9/9 of SS and in 8/10 of SLE). In these patients, the occurrence of deficient ApoCell-phagocytosis by MDM always (in 11/11 of cases) correlated with decreased ApoCell-phagocytosis by peripheral blood monocytes. However, in 6 MDM preparations from patients (5 with SS and 1 with SLE), normal ApoCell-phagocytosis was associated with defective uptake by peripheral blood monocytes, a fact which likely suggests the influence of serum factors that operated only in the peripheral blood assays.

ApoCell-phagocytosis by healthy monocytes is inefficiently supported by sera from SS and SLE patients

In preliminary experiments, the addition of serum specimens from healthy individuals was found to promote the ApoCell-phagocytosis by healthy peripheral blood monocytes. In fact, the replacement of healthy serum by DMEM resulted in significantly lower uptake of apoptotic cells (n = 13; median reduction: 48.0%, range: 34.2–56.9%, p = 0.001). In addition, the heat-treatment of HBD sera (n = 6) was also found to result in considerable reduction of ApoCell-phagocytosis by healthy monocytes (median reduction: 22.9%, range: 18.9–45.8%, p = 0.004), indicating the physiologic participation of heat-labile serum factors in the ingestion of apoptotic cells by monocytes.

In cross-admixture experiments, the application of apoptotic cells pre-treated with sera from SS and SLE patients (but not RA patients) resulted in significantly reduced ApoCell-phagocytosis by healthy peripheral blood monocytes (both for p<0.0001), compared to pretreatment with sera from HBD (**Figure 1E**). In those experiments, ApoCell-PhI values obtained following the pretreatments with SS and SLE sera showed positive correlations with C3 and C4 complement levels (for SS sera; r = 0.510, p = 0.007 and r = 0.447, p = 0.02, respectively, for SLE sera; r = 0.467, p = 0.03 and r = 0.546, p = 0.008, respectively). Among SS and SLE sera used, those with reactivity to Ro/SSA and to native histones, respectively, showed significantly decreased ApoCell-phagocytosis (among SS sera: the anti-Ro/SSA-positive; median: 206, range: 118–320, the anti-Ro/SSA-negative; median: 356, range: 289–462, p = 0.0008, among SLE sera: the anti-histone-positive; median: 255, range: 209–300, the anti-histone-negative; median: 327, range: 245–450, p = 0.02).

Additional cross-admixture ApoCell-phagocytosis assays were also performed using peripheral blood monocytes obtained from selected SS and SLE patients with deficient ApoCell-phagocytosis (6 from SS and 3 from SLE patients) and apoptotic cells pre-treated with either the autologous serum or serum from a HBD. In these experiments, the pre-treatment of apoptotic cells with HBD serum was found to increase significantly ApoCell-phagocytosis values over those obtained with the autologous sera (median increase: 21.8%, range: 18.7–79.9%, p = 0.02). In fact, the incubation of apoptotic cells with HBD serum was found to confer normal ApoCell-phagocytosis values to the monocytes of 4/6 SS patients and of 1/3 SLE patients studied, a finding which suggests the key contribution of serum factor(s) in the aberrations observed, in a loss-of-function and/or a gain-of-function mode.

Purified serum IgG from SS and SLE patients display inhibitory activity against ApoCell-phagocytosis that correlates with its binding to apoptotic cells

Sera from autoimmune patients (SS; n = 20, SLE; n = 14, RA; n = 5) and HBD (n = 12) were screened by flow cytometry for IgM and IgG immunoglobulin reactivity to early apoptotic cells. Such analyses had revealed that the levels of IgM anti-ApoCell

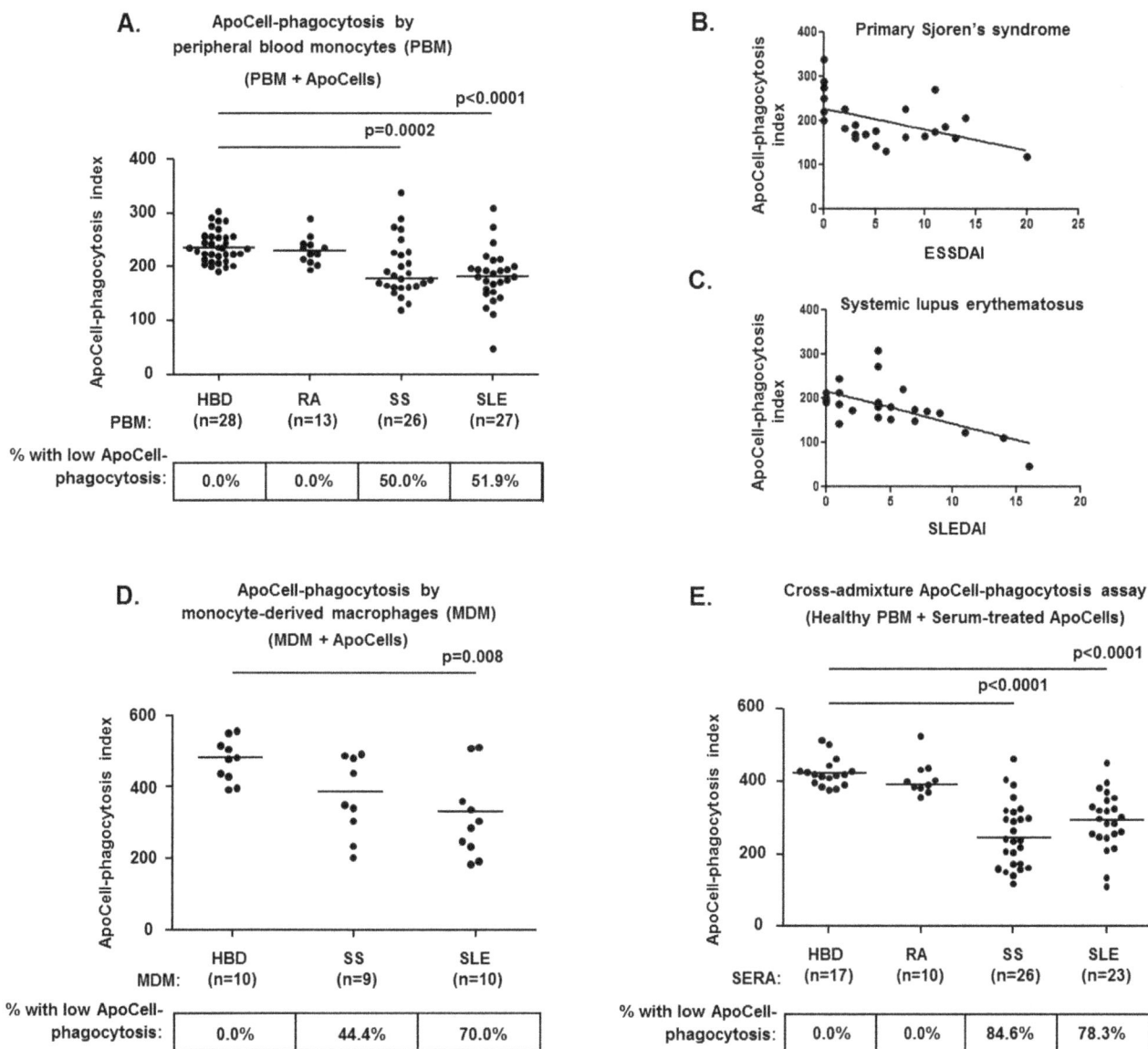

Figure 1. The peripheral blood (PB) monocytes and monocyte-derived macrophages (MDM) of SS and SLE patients manifest significantly impaired ApoCell-phagocytosis. The aberrant uptake of apoptotic cells by blood-borne phagocytes largely resides in the patients' sera. **A.** Significantly decreased ApoCell-phagocytosis by PB monocytes in SS and SLE patients, but not in RA. **B–C.** The ApoCell-phagocytosis index values observed in SS and SLE patients correlated inversely with the disease activity indices of these diseases. **D.** Decreased ApoCell-phagocytosis by MDM in SS and SLE patients. **E.** Cross-admixture experiments illustrating the significantly reduced capacity of sera from SS and SLE patients to support ApoCell-phagocytosis by normal peripheral blood (PB) monocytes, in contrast to sera from HBD and from RA patients. In panels A, C and D the horizontal lines indicate the median levels in each group, whereas the numbers in boxes indicate the percentages of individuals with decreased ApoCell-phagocytosis, as defined by the presence of ApoCell-PhI values that were two standard deviations below the corresponding mean of HBD. Statistically significant comparisons of patient groups to HBD are shown. In panel B, the mean ApoCell-PhI values of SS-derived MDM were marginally different compared to MDM (p = 0.06).

antibodies were significantly decreased in the sera of SS patients (median IgM anti-ApoCell binding index [range]: 1.34 [0.22–5.05]) compared to HBD (3.26 [1.44–5.97], p = 0.0079), but not in those from SLE and RA patients (SLE: 4.91 [0.60–8.50], RA: 2.48 [1.58–3.28], differences not significant). In direct contrast, significantly increased levels of IgG anti-ApoCell antibodies were observed in the sera of SS and SLE patients (median IgG anti-ApoCell binding index [range]; SS: 1.70 [0.33–6.63], SLE: 1.57 [0.41–5.13], compared to HBD (0.54 [0.38–0.73], for p = 0.035 and p = 0.001, respectively), but not in those from RA patients (0.70 [0.55–1.17], difference not significant). Rheumatoid factor

positivity was not found to influence the IgG or IgM anti-ApoCell binding assay results (data not shown).

The rates of ApoCell-phagocytosis that were observed in the cross-admixture experiments presented above (application of healthy peripheral blood monocytes and sera-pretreated apoptotic cells) correlated inversely and highly significantly with the levels of IgG anti-ApoCell antibodies in those sera, (r = −0.631, p = 0.0009), but not those of IgM (r = 0.284, difference not significant). Therefore, to address whether the IgG anti-ApoCell antibodies that were present in the sera of SS and SLE patients may interfere adversely with the ingestion of apoptotic cells, serum

IgG immunoglobulins were purified from the sera of autoimmune patients and controls and subsequently analyzed for anti-ApoCell reactivity, as well as in cross-admixture ApoCell-phagocytosis assays. The levels of anti-ApoCell antibodies were significantly increased in the IgG preparations derived from SS and SLE patients (both for $p<0.0001$, compared to HBD), but in not those from RA (**Figure 2A**). In addition, anti-ApoCell levels were significantly higher among anti-Ro/SSA antibody-positive patients (median: 1.833, range: 0.426-5.500) compared to antibody-negative ones, (median: 1.030, range: 0.445–2.020, $p = 0.019$). In cross-admixture ApoCell-phagocytosis assays, the application of healthy MDM and purified IgG-pretreated early apoptotic cells had revealed significantly reduced ApoCell-phagocytosis upon the application of IgG preparations derived from SS and SLE patients (for $p<0.0001$ and $p = 0.0002$, respectively, compared to HBD) but not from RA (**Figure 2B & 2C**) suggesting the inhibitory effect of IgG anti-ApoCell antibodies in SS and SLE on ApoCell-phagocytosis. The significantly impaired engulfment of apoptotic cells following their pretreatment with purified IgG from SS and SLE patients compared to that from HBD, was also demonstrated by comparative ApoCell-phagocytosis assays using pHrodo-SE-labelled apoptotic cells (**Figure 2D**). Importantly, highly significant inverse correlation was found between the rate of ApoCell-phagocytosis obtained by the various IgG preparations used and the levels of anti-ApoCell antibodies in those preparations ($r = -0.661$, $p<0.0001$, **Figure 2E**). Similar inverse correlation was observed between the ApoCell-PhI values obtained with the application of whole sera in the cross-admixture experiments described earlier, and the anti-ApoCell levels that were detected in purified IgG preparations from the respective sera used (in 25 sera; 8 from SS, 7 from SLE, 4 from RA patients and 6 from HBD, $r = -0.595$, $p = 0.0017$).

Significantly impaired MB-phagocytosis by peripheral blood monocytes of SS and SLE patients

RA patients displayed similar MB-phagocytosis indices to those of HBD. In direct contrast, both SS and SLE groups were found to manifest highly significantly decreased levels of MB-phagocytosis by granulocytes and by monocytes compared to HBD, as well as to RA (**Figure 3A & 3B**). Conversely, there were no differences of MB-phagocytosis indices between SS and SLE patients for either granulocytes or monocytes (**Figure 3A & 3B**). The overall analysis of phagocytosis index values had revealed a highly significant correlation between the levels of MB-phagocytosis and ApoCell-phagocytosis by monocytes in the various groups studied ($r = 0.432$, $p = 0.001$).

Among the various clinical and serological parameters examined, the degree of MB-phagocytosis by monocytes was found to positively correlate with the C4 serum complement levels in both SS and SLE patients (SS; $r = 0.377$, $p = 0.03$, SLE; $r = 0.520$, $p = 0.03$). Furthermore, in SS patients, the occurrence of extraglandular disease correlated with significantly lower levels of MB-phagocytosis by granulocytes (glandular SS; median = 41, range: 5–84, extraglandular SS; median = 14, range: 3–63, $p = 0.003$), as well as by monocytes (glandular SS; median = 58, range: 11–132, extraglandular SS; median = 24, range: 1–87, $p = 0.002$). Finally, MB-phagocytosis indices in SS patients also inversely correlated with ESSDAI (for granulocytes; $r = -0.432$, $p = 0.01$, for monocytes; $r = -0.520$, $p = 0.002$) and SSDDI (for granulocytes; $r = -0.355$, $p = 0.02$, for monocytes; $r = -0.475$, $p = 0.006$).

Impaired MB-phagocytosis by MDM preparations of SS and SLE patients

The study of MB-phagocytosis by MDM had yielded similar results between RA patients and HBD, whereas significantly decreased MB-phagocytosis was observed in both SS and SLE patient groups, compared to HBD ($p = 0.01$ and $p = 0.004$, respectively), as well as to RA patients (**Figure 3C**). The overall analysis of MB-PhI values had revealed a significant correlation of the levels of MB-phagocytosis by MDM with those obtained by peripheral blood monocytes in the various groups studied ($r = 0.552$, $p = 0.01$). In SS patients, MB-phagocytosis by MDM was marginally lower among patients with extraglandular disease (median = 184, range: 34–312), compared to those with disease confined in glands (median = 282, range: 252–468, $p = 0.07$), as well as among patients with type-I SS (median = 183, range: 34–312), compared to those without (median = 281, range: 252–468, $p = 0.06$). Among the SLE patients studied, the occurrence of decreased MB-phagocytosis by MDM was not found to correlate significantly with any of the clinical and serological parameters examined.

Discussion

Several previous studies had documented that the monocytes of SLE patients manifest reduced clearance of various targets [29], including defective efferocytosis [9,11,17,26]. In fact, the accumulation of apoptotic cells in lymph node and skin biopsies of SLE patients is thought to signify the deficient phagocytic clearance of apoptotic cells in vivo [30]. These data had provided a mechanistic explanation for the development of chronic inflammatory and autoimmune reactions in SLE patients, via the progression of uncleared apoptotic cells to the state of secondary necrosis and the release thereof of alarmins and modified self antigens that activate innate and acquired immune system [31]. In fact, experimental mice that are deficient for molecules involved in the phagocytosis of apoptotic cells display defective efferocytosis, as well as features of SLE, such as the development of antinuclear antibodies and glomerulonephritis [32]. In the same context, lupus-prone strains of mice are reported to display decreased phagocytosis of apoptotic cells by macrophages [33].

SLE and SS are immunologically similar disorders in several respects [18], therefore in this study we sought to evaluate directly the capacity of the peripheral blood monocytes of SS and SLE patients for uptake of early apoptotic cells, employing simple and reproducible ex-vivo ApoCell-phagocytosis assays. In addition, several lines of experimental evidence from mice and human studies indicate that apoptosis plays a crucial role in the pathophysiology of SS [34–36], whereas SS-related autoantigens, such as Ro(SSA) and La(SSB), have been shown to be clustered at the surface of apoptotic cells [37].

In good concordance with previous studies [9,26], our findings indicate that compared to healthy individuals, approximately half of the SLE patients tested manifested significantly impaired ApoCell-phagocytosis by monocytes. In addition, this study provides first evidence that, in a manner similar to SLE, deficient uptake of early apoptotic cells by monocytes also characterizes a significant proportion of SS patients, whereas such aberration is not apparently present among RA patients. Interestingly, previous studies of experimental animal models had indicated decreased ApoCell-phagocytosis by macrophages not only in lupus-prone strains of mice [33] but also in mice susceptible to SS-like sialadenitis [38]. In addition, defective efferocytosis has been described to occur in the heart of fetuses of certain SS and SLE patients owing to aberrant opsonization of apoptotic cells by

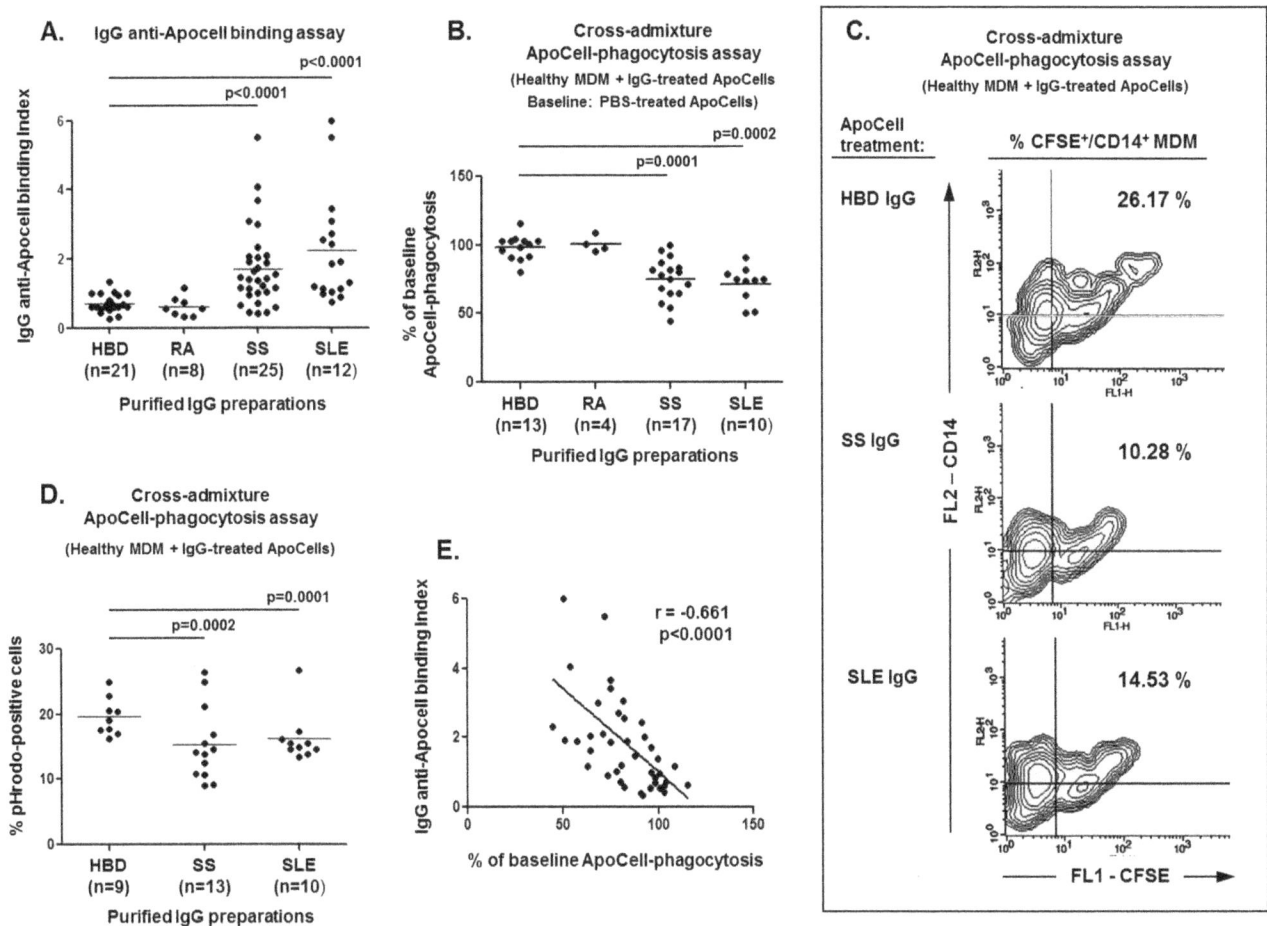

Figure 2. Inhibitory effect of IgG on ApoCell-phagocytosis. Purified serum IgG preparations from SS and SLE patients display inhibitory activity on ApoCell-phagocytosis by healthy MDM that correlates with its binding activity to early apoptotic cells. **A.** Purified serum IgG preparations from SS and SLE patients (but not RA) display significantly increased binding to early apoptotic cells. Binding index was normalized and expressed as fold increase over the binding of a purified IgG preparation from a HBD used in all experiments. **B–D.** Cross-admixture ApoCell-phagocytosis experiments demonstrating that the pretreatment of early apoptotic cells with purified serum IgG preparations derived from SS and SLE (but not from RA) results in decreased ApoCell-phagocytosis by healthy MDM, as compared to treatment with IgG from HBD. In **B**, data are expressed as percent of baseline ApoCell-phagocytosis values (e.g. treatment of apoptotic cells with PBS only, considered as 100%). Similar results were obtained by slightly different experimental setups assaying the ingestion of CFSE-labelled IgG-pretreated apoptotic cells by electronically gated CD14-stained MDM in dual-color flow cytometry (**C**; representative results from 3 independent experiments) or the uptake of pHrodo-SE-labelled apoptotic cells in single-color flow cytometry (**D**). **E.** Highly significant inverse correlation between the rates of ApoCell-phagocytosis obtained by the various purified serum IgG preparations used (shown in A) and the levels of anti-ApoCell antibodies in those preparations (shown in A).

maternal IgG anti-Ro/SSA and anti-La/SSB antibodies [39]. Furthermore, in the present study the rates of ApoCell-phagocytosis in SS and SLE patients correlated inversely and highly significantly with the activity indices of these disorders. Although larger cohort studies with a wide sampling of patients are needed, our findings support aberrant efferocytosis as an important pathogenetic mechanism for both SS and SLE and as a promising field of search for novel biomarkers for these diseases. In fact, the inverse correlation between deficient ApoCell-phagocytosis and disease activity has been also previously observed in SLE patients [11].

The underlying cause of defective efferocytosis in SLE has been attributed to the presence of intrinsic functional defects in patients' phagocytes [9,11,17,26] and/or aberrant serum factors [16,17]. Our findings mainly indicate that serum factors in SS and SLE patients are mostly responsible for the observed impairment of ApoCell-phagocytosis; however, certain lines of evidence may be also supportive to the notion of disordered function of patients'

phagocytes per se. First, in line with previous reports in SLE patients [9], [26], our data indicate that ApoCell-phagocytosis is deficient in several MDM preparations that were derived from SS and SLE patients by cultivation in the absence of patients' sera, a fact that may at least partly support a model of intrinsically defective monocyte in these disorders. Alternatively, the impaired capacity of phagocytes of SS and SLE patients for uptake of prey may be viewed as a result of cellular activation taking place in vivo, a notion probably also implied by the significant correlation between the findings in the various phagocytosis assays and the activity indices of these diseases. Finally, the notably low capacity of SS and SLE patients for phagocytosis of particulate targets by blood-borne monocytes and MDM that was observed may reflect an overall dysfunction of phagocytes in the proper engulfment of certain preys in these disorders. Interestingly, deficient phagocytosis of particulate targets is also reported in primary biliary cirrhosis [40], a disease with striking clinicopathologic similarities to SS [41]. On the other hand, it should be noticed that in sharp

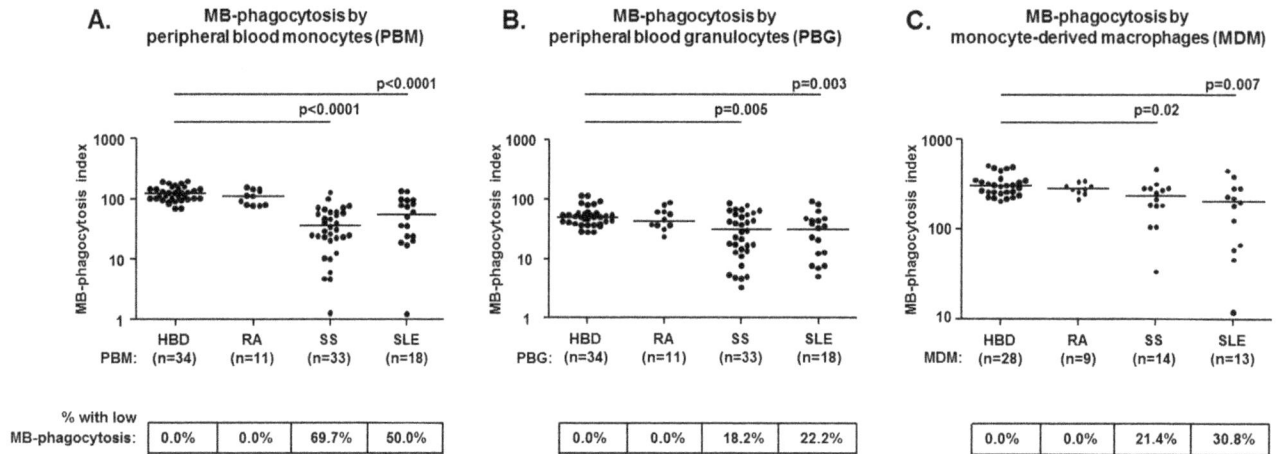

Figure 3. Impaired MB-phagocytosis by peripheral blood (PB) phagocytes (A; monocytes B; granulocytes) and by monocyte-derived macrophages (MDM, C) obtained from SS and SLE patients, but not from RA patients. The horizontal lines indicate the median levels in each group, whereas the numbers in boxes indicate the percentages of individuals with decreased MB-phagocytosis, as defined by the presence of MB-PhI values that were two standard deviations below the corresponding mean of HBD. Statistically significant comparisons of patient groups to HBD are shown.

contrast to the above deficient phagocytic capacities, the blood-borne monocytes of SS and SLE were found remarkably hyperfunctional in the phagocytosis of necrotic cell debris [42].

The addition of healthy serum was found to facilitate significantly the ingestion of apoptotic cells by blood-borne monocytes derived from healthy individuals, as well as from SLE or SS patients. These findings are in good agreement with the previously observed capacity of sera from healthy individuals to restore the phagocytic ability of macrophages from SLE patients [11]. In addition, ApoCell-phagocytosis by healthy monocytes was presently shown to be severely impaired following the substitution of HBD sera by sera derived from SS and SLE patients. Consistent with previous observations [17], the sera from approximately 80% of SLE patients studied were not as efficient as healthy sera in supporting of ApoCell-phagocytosis by normal blood-borne monocytes. In this study, we present first evidence that such incapacity is also manifested by the vast majority of sera from SS patients studied. The precise nature of this aberration in SS and SLE patients is unclear. Normally, several serum proteins (such as complement C1q, IgM, C-reactive protein, serum amyloid protein, milk fat globule-EGF factor 8 protein [MFG-e8] and mannose-binding lectin) attach to apoptotic cells and induce the deposition of C3 and its degradation products C3b and iC3b, thus enhancing efferocytosis by phagocytes via recognition by complement receptors CR3 and CR4 [43]. In this context, mice lacking such bridging molecules, such as MFG-e8, Mer or C1q are reported to develop lupus-like manifestations associated with inefficient removal of apoptotic cells [32]. In line to these observations, several quantitative and functional aberrations of the above opsonins have been described in SLE and SS patients, including hypocomplementemia, which is considered as one of the major immunological markers and of key clinical importance for both disorders [44,45]. In fact, an intact classical complement pathway is essential for the phagocytic removal of apoptotic cells [46], whereas the deficient ApoCell-phagocytosis in SLE patients has been previously attributed to defective opsonization of apoptotic cells by aberrantly low levels of C1q, C3, and C4 complement proteins [17]. Our results from the cross-admixture experiments also implicate the role of aberrant serum complement function in SS and SLE patients in the observed defect of

ApoCell-phagocytosis. The capacity of the SS and SLE patients' sera to assist ApoCell-phagocytosis by healthy monocytes was found to inversely correlate with C3 and C4 complement levels in these sera. In line with these observations, the decomplementation of normal sera by heat-inactivation largely diminished their capacity to support ApoCell-phagocytosis by healthy monocytes.

Most remarkably however, our results had indicated that the inhibitory component of SS and SLE sera to ApoCell-phagocytosis largely resides in the IgG immunoglobulin fraction. Serum IgG preparations from SS and SLE patients (but not from controls) were very frequently found to possess significant inhibitory activity on ApoCell-phagocytosis by normal monocytes, as well as enhanced binding capacity for the surface of early apoptotic cells. Moreover, the rate of ApoCell-phagocytosis obtained by the various IgG preparations used in cross-admixture experiments was presently found to correlate significantly in an inverse manner with the levels of anti-ApoCell antibodies in those preparations. In fact, serum antibodies against late, but not against early apoptotic cells, have been previously reported in the serum of SLE patients and to prevent the uptake of opsonized late apoptotic cells by phagocytes [16].

The nature of IgG antibodies to early apoptotic cells that we have detected in the sera of SS and SLE patients is presently unclear. In the recent years, growing evidence indicates that various types of serum autoantibodies may interfere with the clearance of apoptotic cells by phagocytes. Such autoantibody responses may involve reactivities against surface membranous molecules of the apoptotic cells and/or the phagocytes [16,47], as well as against bridging molecules that normally facilitate ApoCell-phagocytosis [48]. Recently, the occurrence of anti-C3 complement autoantibodies in SLE patients has been shown to react to C3 bound on apoptotic cells and thus to interfere with the proper C3-mediated recognition and clearance of apoptotic cells by phagocytes [49]. Anti-nuclear antibodies, which are a hallmark feature of SLE and SS, may also hamper the uptake of apoptotic cells by phagocytes. In fact, autoantibodies from SLE and SS patients are reported to opsonize late apoptotic cells and to inhibit their uptake by macrophages via an Fc-gamma receptor-dependent mechanism [16]. In line with these observations, our results from cross-admixture experiments had also indicated that the occurrence of specific anti-nuclear antibodies in the sera of SLE (anti-histones) and SS patients (anti-Ro/SSA) is associated with failure to support the ApoCell-phagocytosis by healthy monocytes, whereas we have found increased IgG binding activity to early apoptotic cells among anti-Ro/SSA-positive sera. Notably, apoptotic cells are reportedly characterized by surface translocation of various nuclear constituents, including the ribonucleoproteins Ro/SSA and La/SSB [37], which represent the major targets of autoimmune responses in SS. Importantly also, IgG anti-Ro/SSA and anti-La/SSB antibodies have been previously shown to opsonize in-vitro apoptotic cardiocytes and thus to inhibit their clearance by phagocytes [39]. To this end, detailed autoantibody depletion and antigen inhibition experiments are in progress in this laboratory to delineate the characteristics and role of particular antibody specificities in the clearance of apoptotic cells. On the other hand, loss-of-function processes involving the natural IgM immunoglobulins of SS patients may also have a role, as indicated by the occurrence of significantly decreased IgM anti-ApoCell levels that we observed in the SS patients, compared to healthy individuals. In fact, the important role of natural IgM antibodies for the clearance of apoptotic cells, microbes and various small particles is well-described [50].

In conclusion, this study demonstrates that in a manner similar and comparable to SLE, a significant portion of SS patients is characterized by impaired uptake of early apoptotic cells, as well as of particulate targets by blood-borne phagocytes and macrophages that apparently involves both loss-of-function and gain-of-function processes. Importantly, these aberrations were found to correlate with various clinico-serologic disease indices of SS and SLE, and thus may represent promising areas of search for novel biomarkers for these disorders. The defective clearance of apoptotic cells in SS and SLE appears primarily to depend on serologic aberrations, such as the occurrence of inhibitory IgG anti-ApoCell antibodies and hypocomplementemia, and secondarily on the dysfunction of phagocytes. Such failure of efferocytosis may lead to the accumulation of immunogenic and inflammagenic secondary necrotic cells and debris and the perpetuation thereof of a vicious cycle of inflammatory and autoimmune reactions. In fact, we have recently demonstrated that, SS and SLE patients also manifest impaired serum-mediated degradation of necrotic cell debris that leads to increased amounts of circulating nuclear material and their massive uptake by blood-borne phagocytes [42]. Altogether, these aberrations may represent major causes of the inflammatory and autoimmune reactions that characterize SS and SLE, and may thus hold key roles in the pathogenesis of these disorders.

Author Contributions

Conceived and designed the experiments: MNM. Performed the experiments: GEF AGV. Analyzed the data: MNM GEF AGV HMM. Wrote the paper: MNM GEF AGV HMM.

References

1. Majno G, Joris I (1995) Apoptosis, oncosis, and necrosis. An overview of cell death. Am J Pathol 146: 3–15.
2. Voll RE, Herrmann M, Roth EA, Stach C, Kalden JR, et al. (1997) Immunosuppressive effects of apoptotic cells. Nature 390: 350–351.
3. Vandivier RW, Henson PM, Douglas IS (2006) Burying the dead: the impact of failed apoptotic cell removal (efferocytosis) on chronic inflammatory lung disease. Chest 129: 1673–1682.
4. Munoz LE, van Bavel C, Franz S, Berden J, Herrmann M, et al. (2008) Apoptosis in the pathogenesis of systemic lupus erythematosus. Lupus 17: 371–375.
5. Cohen JJ, Duke RC, Fadok VA, Sellins KS (1992) Apoptosis and programmed cell death in immunity. Annu Rev Immunol 10: 267–293.
6. Han H, Iwanaga T, Uchiyama Y, Fujita T (1993) Aggregation of macrophages in the tips of intestinal villi in guinea pigs: their possible role in the phagocytosis of effete epithelial cells. Cell Tissue Res 271: 407–416.
7. Hopkinson-Woolley J, Hughes D, Gordon S, Martin P (1994) Macrophage recruitment during limb development and wound healing in the embryonic and foetal mouse. J Cell Sci 107 (Pt 5): 1159–1167.
8. Munoz LE, Janko C, Grossmayer GE, Frey B, Voll RE, et al. (2009) Remnants of secondarily necrotic cells fuel inflammation in systemic lupus erythematosus. Arthritis Rheum 60: 1733–1742.
9. Herrmann M, Voll RE, Zoller OM, Hagenhofer M, Ponner BB, et al. (1998) Impaired phagocytosis of apoptotic cell material by monocyte-derived macrophages from patients with systemic lupus erythematosus. Arthritis Rheum 41: 1241–1250.
10. Gaipl US, Munoz LE, Grossmayer G, Lauber K, Franz S, et al. (2007) Clearance deficiency and systemic lupus erythematosus (SLE). J Autoimmun 28: 114–121.
11. Ren Y, Tang J, Mok MY, Chan AW, Wu A, et al. (2003) Increased apoptotic neutrophils and macrophages and impaired macrophage phagocytic clearance of apoptotic neutrophils in systemic lupus erythematosus. Arthritis Rheum 48: 2888–2897.
12. Kimberly RP, Salmon JE, Edberg JC, Gibofsky A (1989) The role of Fc gamma receptors in mononuclear phagocyte system function. Clin Exp Rheumatol 7 Suppl 3: S103–108.
13. Svensson BO (1975) Serum factors causing impaired macrophage function in systemic lupus erythematosus. Scand J Immunol 4: 145–150.
14. Shoshan Y, Shapira I, Toubi E, Frolkis I, Yaron M, et al. (2001) Accelerated Fas-mediated apoptosis of monocytes and maturing macrophages from patients with systemic lupus erythematosus: relevance to in vitro impairment of interaction with iC3b-opsonized apoptotic cells. J Immunol 167: 5963–5969.
15. Sarmiento LF, Munoz LE, Chirinos P, Bianco NE, Zabaleta-Lanz ME (2007) Opsonization by anti-dsDNA antibodies of apoptotic cells in systemic lupus erythematosus. Autoimmunity 40: 337–339.
16. Reefman E, Horst G, Nijk MT, Limburg PC, Kallenberg CG, et al. (2007) Opsonization of late apoptotic cells by systemic lupus erythematosus autoantibodies inhibits their uptake via an Fcgamma receptor-dependent mechanism. Arthritis Rheum 56: 3399–3411.
17. Bijl M, Reefman E, Horst G, Limburg PC, Kallenberg CG (2006) Reduced uptake of apoptotic cells by macrophages in systemic lupus erythematosus: correlates with decreased serum levels of complement. Ann Rheum Dis 65: 57–63.
18. Manoussakis MN, Georgopoulou C, Zintzaras E, Spyropoulou M, Stavropoulou A, et al. (2004) Sjogren's syndrome associated with systemic lupus erythematosus: clinical and laboratory profiles and comparison with primary Sjogren's syndrome. Arthritis Rheum 50: 882–891.
19. Vitali C, Bombardieri S, Jonsson R, Moutsopoulos HM, Alexander EL, et al. (2002) Classification criteria for Sjogren's syndrome: a revised version of the European criteria proposed by the American-European Consensus Group. Ann Rheum Dis 61: 554–558.
20. Tan EM, Cohen AS, Fries JF, Masi AT, McShane DJ, et al. (1982) The 1982 revised criteria for the classification of systemic lupus erythematosus. Arthritis Rheum 25: 1271–1277.
21. Aletaha D, Neogi T, Silman AJ, Funovits J, Felson DT, et al. (2010) 2010 Rheumatoid arthritis classification criteria: an American College of Rheumatology/European League Against Rheumatism collaborative initiative. Arthritis Rheum 62: 2569–2581.
22. Seror R, Ravaud P, Bowman SJ, Baron G, Tzioufas A, et al. (2010) EULAR Sjogren's syndrome disease activity index: development of a consensus systemic disease activity index for primary Sjogren's syndrome. Ann Rheum Dis 69: 1103–1109.
23. Vitali C, Palombi G, Baldini C, Benucci M, Bombardieri S, et al. (2007) Sjogren's Syndrome Disease Damage Index and disease activity index: scoring systems for the assessment of disease damage and disease activity in Sjogren's syndrome, derived from an analysis of a cohort of Italian patients. Arthritis Rheum 56: 2223–2231.
24. Gladman D, Ginzler E, Goldsmith C, Fortin P, Liang M, et al. (1996) The development and initial validation of the Systemic Lupus International Collaborating Clinics/American College of Rheumatology damage index for systemic lupus erythematosus. Arthritis Rheum 39: 363–369.
25. Ioannidis JP, Vassiliou VA, Moutsopoulos HM (2002) Long-term risk of mortality and lymphoproliferative disease and predictive classification of primary Sjogren's syndrome. Arthritis Rheum 46: 741–747.
26. Tas SW, Quartier P, Botto M, Fossati-Jimack L (2006) Macrophages from patients with SLE and rheumatoid arthritis have defective adhesion in vitro, while only SLE macrophages have impaired uptake of apoptotic cells. Ann Rheum Dis 65: 216–221.
27. Esmann L, Idel C, Sarkar A, Hellberg L, Behnen M, et al. (2010) Phagocytosis of apoptotic cells by neutrophil granulocytes: diminished proinflammatory neutrophil functions in the presence of apoptotic cells. J Immunol 184: 391–400.
28. Gantner F, Kupferschmidt R, Schudt C, Wendel A, Hatzelmann A (1997) In vitro differentiation of human monocytes to macrophages: change of PDE

profile and its relationship to suppression of tumour necrosis factor-alpha release by PDE inhibitors. Br J Pharmacol 121: 221–231.

29. Katsiari CG, Liossis SN, Sfikakis PP (2010) The pathophysiologic role of monocytes and macrophages in systemic lupus erythematosus: a reappraisal. Semin Arthritis Rheum 39: 491–503.

30. Baumann I, Kolowos W, Voll RE, Manger B, Gaipl U, et al. (2002) Impaired uptake of apoptotic cells into tingible body macrophages in germinal centers of patients with systemic lupus erythematosus. Arthritis Rheum 46: 191–201.

31. Urbonaviciute V, Furnrohr BG, Meister S, Munoz L, Heyder P, et al. (2008) Induction of inflammatory and immune responses by HMGB1-nucleosome complexes: implications for the pathogenesis of SLE. J Exp Med 205: 3007–3018.

32. Viorritto IC, Nikolov NP, Siegel RM (2007) Autoimmunity versus tolerance: can dying cells tip the balance? Clin Immunol 122: 125–134.

33. Licht R, Dieker JW, Jacobs CW, Tax WJ, Berden JH (2004) Decreased phagocytosis of apoptotic cells in diseased SLE mice. J Autoimmun 22: 139–145.

34. Manoussakis MN, Spachidou MP, Maratheftis CI (2010) Salivary epithelial cells from Sjogren's syndrome patients are highly sensitive to anoikis induced by TLR-3 ligation. J Autoimmun 35: 212–218.

35. Salomonsson S, Jonsson MV, Skarstein K, Brokstad KA, Hjelmstrom P, et al. (2003) Cellular basis of ectopic germinal center formation and autoantibody production in the target organ of patients with Sjogren's syndrome. Arthritis Rheum 48: 3187–3201.

36. Okuma A, Hoshino K, Ohba T, Fukushi S, Aiba S, et al. (2013) Enhanced apoptosis by disruption of the STAT3-IkappaB-zeta signaling pathway in epithelial cells induces Sjogren's syndrome-like autoimmune disease. Immunity 38: 450–460.

37. Casciola-Rosen LA, Anhalt G, Rosen A (1994) Autoantigens targeted in systemic lupus erythematosus are clustered in two populations of surface structures on apoptotic keratinocytes. J Exp Med 179: 1317–1330.

38. O'Brien BA, Geng X, Orteu CH, Huang Y, Ghoreishi M, et al. (2006) A deficiency in the in vivo clearance of apoptotic cells is a feature of the NOD mouse. J Autoimmun 26: 104–115.

39. Clancy RM, Neufing PJ, Zheng P, O'Mahony M, Nimmerjahn F, et al. (2006) Impaired clearance of apoptotic cardiocytes is linked to anti-SSA/Ro and -SSB/La antibodies in the pathogenesis of congenital heart block. J Clin Invest 116: 2413–2422.

40. Allina J, Stanca CM, Garber J, Hu B, Sautes-Fridman C, et al. (2008) Anti-CD16 autoantibodies and delayed phagocytosis of apoptotic cells in primary biliary cirrhosis. J Autoimmun 30: 238–245.

41. Selmi C, Meroni PL, Gershwin ME (2012) Primary biliary cirrhosis and Sjogren's syndrome: Autoimmune epithelitis. J Autoimmun 39: 34–42.

42. Fragoulis GE, Vakrakou AG, Papadopoulou A, Germenis A, Kanavakis E, et al. (2014) Impaired degradation and aberrant phagocytosis of necrotic cell debris in the peripheral blood of patients with primary Sjogren's syndrome. J Autoimmun http://dx.doi.org/10.1016/j.jaut.2014.08.004 [Epub ahead of print].

43. Ogden CA, Elkon KB (2006) Role of complement and other innate immune mechanisms in the removal of apoptotic cells. Curr Dir Autoimmun 9: 120–142.

44. Gaipl US, Kuhn A, Sheriff A, Munoz LE, Franz S, et al. (2006) Clearance of apoptotic cells in human SLE. Curr Dir Autoimmun 9: 173–187.

45. Ramos-Casals M, Brito-Zeron P, Soria N, Nardi N, Vargas A, et al. (2009) Mannose-binding lectin-low genotypes are associated with milder systemic and immunological disease expression in primary Sjogren's syndrome. Rheumatology (Oxford) 48: 65–69.

46. Gullstrand B, Martensson U, Sturfelt G, Bengtsson AA, Truedsson L (2009) Complement classical pathway components are all important in clearance of apoptotic and secondary necrotic cells. Clin Exp Immunol 156: 303–311.

47. Chen XW, Shen Y, Sun CY, Wu FX, Chen Y, et al. (2011) Anti-class a scavenger receptor autoantibodies from systemic lupus erythematosus patients impair phagocytic clearance of apoptotic cells by macrophages in vitro. Arthritis Res Ther 13: R9.

48. Shoenfeld Y, Szyper-Kravitz M, Witte T, Doria A, Tsutsumi A, et al. (2007) Autoantibodies against protective molecules–C1q, C-reactive protein, serum amyloid P, mannose-binding lectin, and apolipoprotein A1: prevalence in systemic lupus erythematosus. Ann N Y Acad Sci 1108: 227–239.

49. Kenyon KD, Cole C, Crawford F, Kappler JW, Thurman JM, et al. (2011) IgG autoantibodies against deposited C3 inhibit macrophage-mediated apoptotic cell engulfment in systemic autoimmunity. J Immunol 187: 2101–2111.

50. Litvack ML, Post M, Palaniyar N (2011) IgM promotes the clearance of small particles and apoptotic microparticles by macrophages. PLoS One 6: e17223.

3

Biospecimen Long-Chain N-3 PUFA and Risk of Colorectal Cancer: A Meta-Analysis of Data from 60,627 Individuals

Bo Yang[1,2], Feng-Lei Wang[1], Xiao-Li Ren[3], Duo Li[1]*

1 Department of Food Science and Nutrition, Zhejiang University, Hangzhou, China, **2** Department of Preventive Medicine, Wenzhou Medical University, Wenzhou, China, **3** Medical Laboratory Animal Center, Wenzhou Medical University, Wenzhou, China

Abstract

Background: Several prospective cohort and case-control studies reported the inconsistent association between biospecimen composition of C20 and C22 long-chain (LC) n-3 polyunsaturated fatty acid (PUFA) and colorectal cancer (CRC) risk. The aim of the present study was to investigate the association of biospecimen LC n-3 PUFA with CRC risk based on prospective cohort and case-control studies.

Methods and Results: Cochrane Library, PubMed, and EMBASE database were searched up to February 2014 for eligible studies. Risk ratios (RRs) or odds ratios (ORs) from prospective and case-control studies were combined using a random-effects model in the highest vs. lowest categorical analysis. Nonlinear dose-response relationships were assessed using restricted cubic spline regression models. Difference in tissue composition of LC n-3 PUFA between cases and noncases was analyzed as standardized mean difference (SMD). Three prospective cohort studies and 8 case-control studies were included in the present study, comprising 60,627 participants (1,499 CRC cases and 59,128 noncases). Higher biospecimen LC n-3 PUFA was significantly associated with a lower risk of CRC in case-control (pooled OR: 0.76; 95% CI: 0.59, 0.97; $I^2 = 10.00\%$) and prospective cohort studies (pooled RR: 0.70; 95% CI: 0.55, 0.88; $I^2 = 0.00\%$), respectively. A significant dose-response association was found of biospecimen C20:5n-3 (P for nonlinearity $= 0.02$) and C22:6n-3 (P for trend $= 0.01$) with CRC risk, respectively. Subjects without CRC have significantly higher biospecimen compositions of C20:5n-3 (SMD: 0.27; 95%: 0.13, 0.41), C22:6n-3 (SMD: 0.23; 95%: 0.11, 0.34) and total LC n-3 PUFA (SMD: 0.22; 95% CI: 0.07, 0.37) compared with those with CRC.

Conclusions: The present evidence suggests human tissue compositions of LC n-3 PUFA may be an independent predictive factor for CRC risk, especially C20:5n-3 and C22:6n-3. This needs to be confirmed with more large-scale prospective cohort studies.

Editor: Antonio Moschetta, IRCCS Istituto Oncologico Giovanni Paolo II, Italy

Funding: This was an independent study; the study subsidies of postgraduate students were paid from grants from the National Natural Science Foundation of China (No: 81273054) and the PhD Programs Foundation of Ministry of Education of China (No: 20120101110107). The funders had no role in study design, data collection and analysis, decision to publish, or preparation of the manuscript.

Competing Interests: The authors have declared that no competing interests exist.

* Email: duoli@zju.edu.cn

Introduction

Colorectal cancer (CRC) is the most frequently diagnosed, and has a higher incidence or mortality in both women and men in developed countries than in developing countries [1–3]. Dietary factors were postulated to play an important role in the prevention of CRC [4]. Data from human studies suggested that dietary fatty acids, as subtypes of fat in most foods, were closely associated with the development of CRC [5,6]. Recently, a meta-analysis of 13 prospective cohort studies [7] assessed the impact of total dietary fat on the risk of CRC, and indicated that dietary polyunsaturated fatty acid (PUFA) was not associated with the increased risk of CRC. One of the explains was that the true associations might be modified by the different effects of PUFA (omega-3 and omega-6) on the development of CRC. Seafood-derived long-chain (LC) omega-3 polyunsaturated fatty acid (n-3 PUFA), including

C20:5n-3, C22:5n-3 and C22:6n-3, is suggested to reduce the risk of CRC in many epidemiological studies [8,9]. However, dietary data from meta-analyses of prospective cohort studies provided an insufficient evidence of protective effects of dietary LC n-3 PUFA on CRC risk [10,11], which may be due to inaccuracy in dietary assessment and an insufficient amount or variety of intake. Taking into account the difficulty in measuring dietary fatty acids accurately, more comprehensive attentions should be paid to a biomarker as a helpful tool that has been used to reflect intake closely to act as objective indices of true dietary intake. The most common biomarkers for dietary intake of LC n-3 PUFA from marine food or fish oil are C20:5n-3 and C22:6n-3, which can be determined in a variety of human biospecimens such as blood (serum/plasma/erythrocytes), adipose tissue (AT) and hair.

Accumulating evidences from in vitro and in vivo studies [12–14] indicate that LC n-3 PUFA as constituents of membrane phospholipids can work through several actions to protect against the initiation and early stages of CRC, including activating protein kinase C, enhancing CRC cell apoptosis, reducing inflammation and decreasing fecal bile acids as well as neutral sterol excretion. Nevertheless, results from prospective and case-control studies revealed inconsistent associations of human tissue LC n-3 PUFA with CRC risk. Most of case-control studies [15–17] reported that tissue composition of LC n-3 PUFA was inversely associated with CRC risk, whereas prospective cohort studies showed inverse [18] or null associations [19,20] between tissue LC n-3 PUFA and CRC risk. Tissue compositions of LC n-3 PUFA were reported to be significantly lower in subjects with CRC (cases) compared with control subjects without CRC (noncases) in some case-control studies [21,22], whereas inconsistent results were reported in other case-control studies [16,17,23–25].

The aim of the present study was to examine the relationship between LC n-3 PUFA compositions in human biospecimens and CRC risk based on prospective cohort and case-control studies. Additionally, the differences in biospecimens (plasma/serum/erythrocytes/whole blood/AT) compositions of LC n-3 PUFA between cases and noncases were also investigated based on case-control studies. We therefore conducted a meta-analysis to clarify the role of tissue compositions of LC n-3 PUFA in the etiology of CRC.

Methods

Literature research

We identified prospective and case-control studies which reported the association between LC n-3 PUFA composition in biospecimen and CRC risk from PubMed, EMBASE and Cochrane Library database up to February 2014. Search strategy was ("Fatty Acids, omega-3" AND "Colorectal Neoplasms") for PubMed, ("Colorectal tumor" AND "omega 3 fatty acid") for EMBASE and ("Fatty Acids, Omega-3" AND "Colorectal Neoplasms") for Cochrane Library databases. We also searched systematic reviews from the above-mentioned database, and check the reference lists to identify studies that might have been missed. We followed MOOSE guidelines of observational studies [26] for conducting and reporting meta-analyses (Checklist S1).

Eligibility criteria

To examine the associations of human biospecimen LC n-3 PUFA with risk of CRC, the inclusion criteria were: 1) Participants: Any aged adults from the same population; 2) Exposure: LC n-3 PUFA compositions in human biospecimen (serum/plasma/whole blood/erythrocytes/AT); 3) Outcomes: evaluating CRC incidence as outcome variable and providing risk ratio (RR) or odds ratio (OR) with the corresponding 95% confidence interval (CI) of CRC for all categories of LC n-3 PUFA compositions; 4) Study design: prospective studies (cohort, nested case-control and case-cohort study) and case-control study.

To investigate the differences in human biospecimens LC n-3 PUFA compositions between cases and noncases, the inclusion criteria were: 1) Participants: both the cases and noncases in each study were from the same population; 2) Outcomes: human biospecimen compositions of $C22{:}6n{-}3$, $C22{:}5n{-}3$, $C20{:}5n{-}3$ or total LC n-3 PUFA in cases and noncases; 3) Study design: case-control study.

Definition of exposure

In the present meta-analysis, biospecimen LC n-3 PUFA composition was defined as the sum of $C22{:}6n{-}3$, $C22{:}5n{-}3$, $C20{:}5n{-}3$ compositions in human biospecimens (serum/plasma/whole blood/erythrocytes/AT). Blood LC n-3 PUFA composition was defined as the sum of $C22{:}6n{-}3$, $C22{:}5n{-}3$, $C20{:}5n{-}3$ compositions in human blood (plasma/serum/erythrocytes/whole blood).

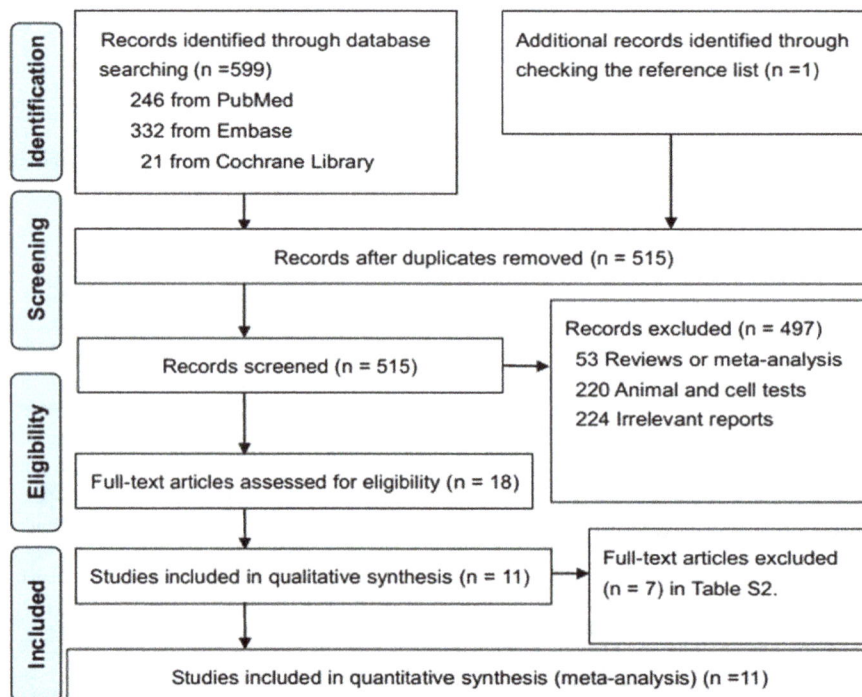

Figure 1. PRISMA Flow Diagram for included prospective cohort and case-control studies.

Table 1. Characteristics of included prospective and case-control studies in the meta-analysis of association between biospecimen long-chain n-3 PUFA and the risk of colorectal cancer.

Author (year)	Design (Nation)	Population (case/participants)	Gender (Age)	Exposure of interest — Measurement	Range (H vs. L)	Outcomes RR/OR (95%CI)	Covariates adjusted
Cottet (2013)	Cohort (France)	Subjects from E3N-EPIC cohort (328/19934)	F 40–65 y	Erythrocyte GLC (% tFC)	EPA:>1.18 vs. <0.89	0.88 (0.62–1.25)	BMI, physical activity, energy intake, alcohol consumption, smoking, educational level, menopausal status, and family history
					DHA:>7.21 vs. <6.10	0.83 (0.57–1.22)	
Pot (2008)	Case-control (Netherlands)	Subjects from the POLIEP study (498/861)	Both 18–75 y	Serum GLC (% tFC)	EPA:>1.00 vs. <0.70	0.79 (0.55–1.15)	Family history, BMI, indication for endoscopy, physical activity, smoking regular use of drugs, hormone replacement therapy, diet change due to gastrointestinal complaints, and daily intake of energy, alcohol, fat, fiber, red meat, vegetables and legumes and cholesterol.
					DHA:>0.60 vs. <0.50	0.71 (0.49–1.02)	
Ghadimi (2008)	Case-control (Japan)	Subjects form study on dietary, lifestyle factors and colon cancer (203/382)	F and M 35–75 y	Serum GLC (% tFC)	F:		Age, BMI, history of CRC, history of diabetes; smoking, alcohol consumption, vigorous exercise and season of data collection.
					EPA:>10.48 vs. <5.50	0.62 (0.22–1.80)	
					DPA:>1.80 vs. <1.00	1.60 (0.35–7.31)	
					DHA:>20.2 vs. <13.8	0.43 (0.14–1.38)	
					LC n-3:>32.8 vs. <21.3	0.54 (0.19–1.54)	
					M:		
					EPA:>9.50 vs. <5.70	1.22 (0.48–3.54)	
					DPA:>1.70 vs. <1.10	0.40 (0.15–1.09)	
					DHA:>19.2 vs. <14.2	2.30 (0.675–7.35)	
					LC n-3:>29.5 vs. <21.8	0.86 (0.28–2.21)	
Hall (2007)	Cohort (USA)	Subjects from the primary prevention of cancer and CVD disease (178/14916)	M 40–84 y	Whole blood GLC (% tFC)	EPA: 2.21–4.07 vs. 0.89–1.55	0.60 (0.29–1.23)	BMI, multivitamin use, history of diabetes, useof drugs, vigorous exercise, alcohol intake, and quartile of red meat intake.
					DHA: 2.83–6.22 vs. 0.69–1.87	0.69 (0.39–1.23)	
					LC n-3: 6.06–11.41 vs. 2.43–4.43	0.60 (0.32–1.11)	

Table 1. Cont.

Author (year)	Design (Nation)	Population (case/participants)	Gender (Age)	Exposure of interest Measurement	Range (H vs. L)	Outcomes RR/OR (95%CI)	Covariates adjusted
Kuriki (2006)	Case-control (Japan)	Subjects form Hospital-based Epidemiologic Research Program; (74/295)	Both 20–80 y	EM; GLC (% tFC)	EPA:>1.70 vs. <1.18	0.69 (0.32–1.50)	BMI, habitual exercise, drinking and smoking status, green-yellow vegetable intake, and family history.
					DPA:>1.50 vs. <1.24	0.83 (0.34–2.05)	
					DHA:>6.10 vs. <5.06	0.36 (0.14–0.93)	
Kojima (2005)	Cohort (Japan)	Subjects from Collaborative Cohort Study for the Evaluation of Cancer Risk (JACC Study); 169/23863;	F and M 20–81y	Serum; GLC (% tFC)	F:		Family history, BMI, education, smoking and alcohol drinking, green leafy vegetable intake, and physical exercise
					F-EPA:>3.33 vs. <1.73	0.83 (0.39–1.80)	
					DPA:>0.94 vs. <0.66	0.64 (0.30–1.39)	
					DHA:>5.92 vs. <4.20	0.80 (0.33–1.93)	
					M:		
					EPA:>3.84 vs. <1.91	0.44 (0.18–1.08)	
					DPA:>1.02 vs. <0.68	0.30 (0.11–0.80)	
					DHA:>6.25 vs. <4.23	0.23 (0.07–0.76)	
Busstra (2003)	Case-control (Netherlands)	Subjects from colorectal adenomas study; 52/109;	Both <75 y	Adipose; GLC (% tFC)	LC n-3:>0.27 vs. <0.20	0.30 (0.10–1.10)	Age, family background, energy intake and gender

Abbreviations: H: the highest category; L: the lowest category; F: females; M: males; GLC: Gas liquid chromatography; tFC: total fatty acid; EPA: eicosapentaenoic acid (C20: 5n-3); DPA: docosapentaenoic acid (C22: 5n-3); DHA: docosahexaenoic acid (C22: 6n-3); LC n-3: long-chain n-3 polyunsaturated fatty acid (C20: 5n-3+C22: 5n-3+C22: 6n-3).

Table 2. Characteristics of included case-control studies in the mea-analysis of different long-chain n-3 PUFA compositions between subjects with and without colorectal cancer.

Author (year)	Design (Nation)	Gender (F or M)	Mean age (years)	Cases	Controls	Biospecimen	Subtypes	Case vs. Control (Mean ±SD) (% total fatty acids)	P^a value
Okuno (2013)	Case-control (Japan)	Both	60.5	41	61	Plasma	C20:5n-3	2.27±1.14 vs 3.04±1.65	0.006
						Plasma	C22:5n-3	0.99±0.26 vs1.00±0.22	0.80
						Plasma	C22:6n-3	7.63±1.43 vs 7.84±1.59	0.49
						Erythrocyte	C20:5n-3	1.86±0.71 vs 2.23±0.85	0.02
						Erythrocyte	C22:5n-3	2.11±0.30 vs 2.12±0.27	0.93
						Erythrocyte	C22:6n-3	7.81±0.90 vs 7.90±1.06	0.64
						Adipose	C20:5n-3	0.12±0.19 vs 0.10±0.07	0.62
						Adipose	C22:5n-3	0.28±0.18 vs 0.25±0.22	0.37
						Adipose	C22:6n-3	0.58±0.32 vs 0.66±0.39	0.28
Giuliani (2013)	Case-control (Italy)	Both	60.0	52	50	Adipose	C20:5n-3	0.02 ± 0.03 vs 0.02±0.03	NS
						Adipose	C22:5n-3	0.16±0.10 vs 0.15±0.12	NS
						Adipose	C22:6n-3	0.16±0.12 vs 0.14±0.12	NS
Pot (2008)	Case-control (Netherlands)	Both	46.5	363	498	Serum	C22:5n-3	0.80±0.50 vs 0.80±0.60	NS
						Serum	C22:6n-3	0.60±0.30 vs 0.60±0.30	NS
Ghadimi (2008)	Case-control (Japan)	F	58.0	55	112	Serum	C20:5n-3	0.24±0.13 vs 0.27±0.15	0.12
						Serum	C22:5n-3	0.07±0.03 vs 0.05±0.04	0.001
						Serum	C22:6n-3	0.48±0.16 vs 0.56±0.31	0.02
						Serum	LC n-3	0.79±0.27 vs 0.88±0.54	0.18
		M	60.0	148	67	Serum	C20:5n-3	0.24±0.10 vs 0.26±0.12	0.220.
						Serum	22:5n-3	0.07±0.04 vs 0.06±0.05	001
						Serum	C22:6n-3	0.50±0.25 vs 0.57±0.20	0.06
						Serum	LC n-3	0.80±0.34 vs 0.89±0.37	0.53
Kuriki (2006)	Case-control (Japan)	Both	50.0	74	221	Erythrocyte	C20:5n-3	1.40±0.50 vs 1.50±0.60	NS
						Erythrocyte	C22:5n-3	1.40±0.40 vs 1.40±0.30	NS
						Erythrocyte	C22:6n-3	5.30±1.00 vs 5.50±1.30	NS
						Erythrocyte	LC n-3	8.10±1.60 vs 8.40±2.00	NS
Busstra (2003)	Case-control (Netherlands)	F	46.5	52	57	Adipose	LC n-3	1.10±0.09 vs 1.14±0.10	NS
Baro (1998)	Case-control (Spain)	Both	58.5	17	29	Plasma	C20:5n-3	0.96±0.19 vs 0.79±0.21	NS
						Plasma	C22:5n-3	0.70±0.05 vs 0.65±0.09	NS
						Plasma	C22:6n-3	3.02±0.18 vs 2.91±0.28	NS
						Erythrocyte	C22:6n-3	6.25±0.20 vs 6.34±0.33	NS
Fernandez-Banares (1996)	Case-control (Spain)	Both	62.0	22	12	Plasma	C20:5n-3	0.46± 0.03 vs 0.70±0.07	0.001

Table 2. Cont.

Author (year)	Design (Nation)	Gender (F or M)	Mean age (years)	No. of subjects		Biospecimen LC n-3 PUFA compositions (% total fatty acids)			
				Cases	Controls	Biospecimen	Subtypes	Case vs. Control (Mean ±SD)	P^a value
						Plasma	C22:5n-3	0.58± 0.06 vs 0.47±0.05	NS
						Plasma	C22:6n-3	3.42± 0.19 vs 3.45±0.15	NS

Abbreviations: F: females; M: males; NO.: Number; NS: no significance; LC n-3: long-chain n-3 polyunsaturated fatty acid (C20: 5n-3+C22: 5n-3+C22: 6n-3).
^{a}P value for different LC n-3 PUFA compositions between cases and controls.

Data extraction

Data extraction was finished independently and performed twice by two reviewers (XLR and FLW), and disagreements were reconciled by consensus. The following data were extracted form each original study: participant characteristics (e.g., nationality, age, gender and number of participants), biospecimen LC n-3 composition as exposure of interest (e.g., measurement method, exposure source, and exposure range), biospecimen compositions of C22:6n-3, C22:5n-3, C20:5n-3 and total LC n-3 PUFA in cases and noncases, adjusted covariates and RR (OR) including 95% CI for all categories of LC n-3 PUFA composition. Our search was restricted to human studies, and we did not contact authors for the detailed information of primary studies and unpublished studies.

Statistic analysis

We conducted two types of meta-analysis. Firstly, we performed a meta-analysis for the highest category vs. lowest. Multivariate adjusted RR (OR) for the highest vs lowest category to assess the association of biospecimen LC n-3 with CRC risk from each original study was firstly transformed to their logarithm (logRR or logOR), and the corresponding 95% CIs were used to calculate corresponding standard errors (selogRR or selogOR). Summary RR (SRR) including corresponding 95% CI as the summary risk estimate for all prospective and case-control studies was estimated using a random-effects model [27], which considers both within-study and between-study variability. The second meta-analysis was that the differences in biospecimen compositions of C22:6n-3, C22:5n-3, C20:5n-3 and total LC n-3 compositions between cases and noncases were also analyzed as standardized mean difference (SMD) by pooling the data from case-control studies, respectively. Heterogeneity among studies was assessed with the Q test and I^2 statistic. I^2 statistic describes the proportion of total variation attributable to between-study heterogeneity as opposed to random error or chance. We defined the low, moderate and high degrees of heterogeneity by I^2 values of 25%, 50% and 75% as cut-off points [28], and considered an I^2 value greater than 50% as indicative of heterogeneity according to Cochrane Handbook. In the presence of substantial heterogeneity, stratified analysis was conducted to identify the possible sources of heterogeneity by study design (case-control and prospective study), different regions (Asia and West (Europe and USA)), gender (women and men) and biospecimen types (blood and adipose tissue). Meta-regression with restricted maximum likelihood (REML) estimation was conducted to assess the potentially important covariates exerting substantial impact on between-study heterogeneity. Sensitivity analysis was performed to evaluate possible influence of individual study with potential bias on overall risk. Publication bias was quantitatively examined by Begg's test and Egger's regression test [29].

Furthermore, the dose-response association of biospecimen LC n-3 PUFA with CRC risk was performed in the present study. Original studies with 3 or more categories were included in the dose-response analysis. Midpoint of upper and lower boundaries was taken as the dose of the quantile if the study only reported the range; if the highest quantile was open-ended, its dose was regarded as 1.2-fold the highest boundary [30]; if the lowest quantile or reference category was open-ended, the midpoint of lowest boundary and zero was taken as the dose of lowest quantile. A nonlinear (curvilinear) trend was tested by using a 2-stage random-effects dose-response meta-analysis [31,32]. The compositionof LC n-3 PUFA in biospecimen was modeled by using restricted cubic splines with 3 knots (2 spline transformations) at percentiles (25%, 50%, and 75%) of the distribution [33]. A P-value for nonlinearity was calculated by testing the null hypothesis that the coefficient of the second spline is equal to zero [34]. In the

Study	Biospecimen		RR/OR (95% CI)	Weight (%)
Prospective cohort study				
Cottet, 2013	Erythrocyte		0.86 (0.66, 1.11)	38.04
Hall, 2007	Whole blood		0.60 (0.32, 1.12)	6.55
Kojima, 2005	Serum		0.59 (0.34, 1.02)	8.39
Subtotal (I-squared = 10.0%, p = 0.329)			0.76 (0.59, 0.97)	52.98
Case-control study				
Pot, 2008	Serum		0.75 (0.58, 0.97)	37.38
Ghadimi, 2008	Serum		0.68 (0.33, 1.42)	4.69
Kuriki, 2006	Erythrocyte		0.51 (0.21, 1.24)	3.18
Busstra, 2003	Adipose		0.30 (0.09, 0.99)	1.76
Subtotal (I-squared = 0.0%, p = 0.444)			0.70 (0.55, 0.88)	47.02
Overall (I-squared = 0.0%, p = 0.506)			0.74 (0.63, 0.87)	100.00

NOTE: Weights are from random effects analysis

.04   1   5

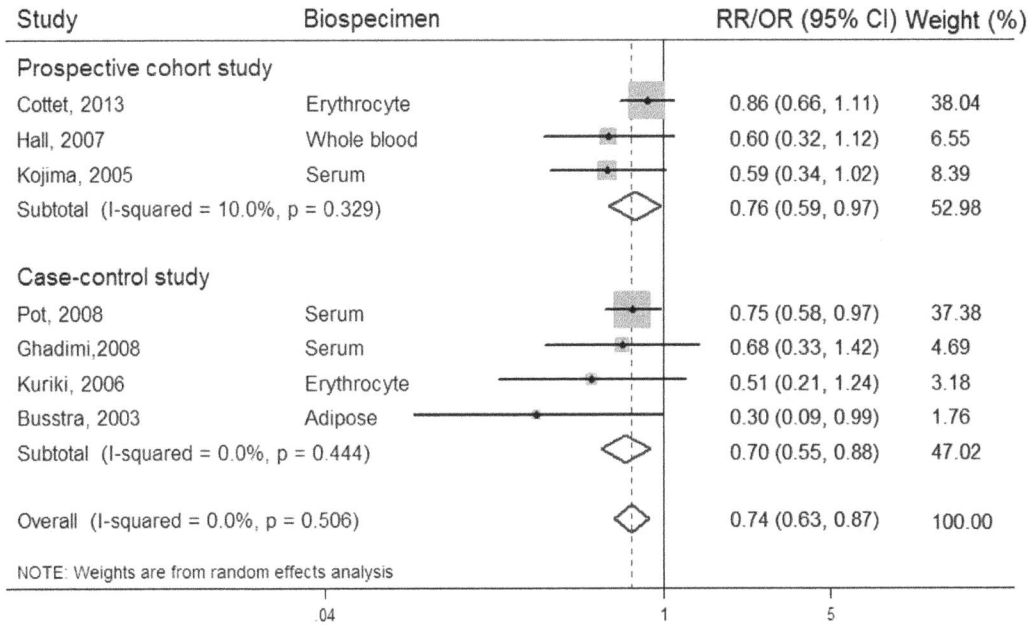

Figure 2. Forest plot corresponding to the random-effects meta-analysis quantifying the relationship between LC n-3 PUFA composition and CRC risk for the highest vs. lowest category. Relative risks (RRs) or odds ratios (ORs) compared the highest vs. lowest category of biospecimen LC n-3 PUFA composition and were grouped by study designs. The size of the gray box representing each risk estimate was proportional to the weight that the risk estimate contributed to the summary risk estimate. The diamonds denoted summary risk estimate.

presence of substantial linear trends (P-value for nonlinearity >0.05), a linear dose-response analysis [32] was conducted to examine the association between every 1% increment of LC n-3 PUFA composition in biospecimens and the risk of CRC. Statistical analyses of the combined data were performed by STATA version 11.0 (Stata CORP, College Station, TX). P-value less than 0.05 were considered statistically significant in the present study.

Results

Study characteristics

We identified 599 potential studies from electronic search, and 515 studies were left after removing duplicates. Eleven relevant studies were eligible for the present study after full text review (Figure 1; Table S1). A total of 1,499 CRC cases among 60,627 participants were included in the present study, separately from 3 prospective cohort [18–20] and 8 case-control studies [15–17,21–25]. Of the 3 cohort studies, 2 studies were conducted in West (Europe [19] and USA [20]), and 1 study was conducted in Japan [18]. Of the 8 case-control studies, 5 studies were conducted in Europe [15,16,22,24,25], and 3 studies were conducted in Japan [17,21,23]. Of the 11 included studies, 6 studies assessed serum (plasma) biomarker of LC n-3 composition [15,18,20,21,23–25], 4 studies assessed RBC biomarker [17,19,21,24], 1 study [20] assessed whole blood biomarker and 3 studies assessed AT biomarker [16,21,22]. LC n-3 PUFA compositions in biospecimens were quantified by gas liquid chromatography (GLC), and measurement unit was percentage of total fatty acids (% tFC) except for 1 study (mg/dL) [23]. Two studies separately provided data of males (M) and females (F) [18,23], 1 study only provided data of females [19], and 1 study only provided data of males [20]. For the analysis on association between biospecimen LC n-3 PUFA and CRC risk, the characteristics of included 3 prospective cohort and 4 case-control studies were summarized in Table 1.

For the analysis of different biospecimen LC n-3 PUFA compositions between subjects with CRC (cases) and control subjects without CRC (noncases), the characteristics of included 8 case-control studies were summarized in Table 2.

Highest vs lowest category

Overall, 3 prospective cohort [18–20] and 4 case-control studies [15–17,23] were eligible for the meta-analysis on the association of LC n-3 PUFA composition in biospecimens with CRC risk, comprising 60,360 participants. A significantly inverse association between biospecimens LC n-3 PUFA and CRC risk was observed in 60,360 participants (summary RR = 0.74; 95% CI: 0.63, 0.87), with no between-study heterogeneity ($I^2 = 0.00\%$) (Figure 2). Biospecimen C20:5n-3 and C22:6n-3 were both inversely associated with the risk of CRC, and the summary RR was 0.78 (95% CI: 0.64, 0.96; $I^2 = 0.00\%$) and 0.68 (95% CI: 0.54, 0.84; $I^2 = 0.00\%$), respectively (Table 3). However, no significant association was found of biospecimen C22:5n-3 with CRC risk in 15,593 participants from 1 prospective and case-control studies (summary OR = 0.80; 95% CI: 0.42, 1.52; $I^2 = 47.60\%$).

In stratified analysis (Table 3), there was no evidence that the estimated summary RR differed significantly by sex (P for meta-regression = 0.14). We further focused on the difference in pooled association estimate between prospective cohort and case-control study. In 3 cohort studies, biospecimen C20:5n-3, C22:6n-3 and LC n-3 PUFA was all significantly associated with the lower risk of CRC, and the pooled RR was 0.77 (95% CI: 0.58, 1.00; $I^2 = 0.00\%$), 0.76 (95% CI: 0.56, 1.01; $I^2 = 0.00\%$), and 0.76 (95% CI: 0.59, 0.97; $I^2 = 10.00\%$), respectively. However, only one prospective cohort study separately reported an association between serum C22:5n-3 and CRC risk in Japan males and females [18], and the pooled RR is 0.47 (95% CI: 0.23, 0.97; $I^2 = 28.60\%$). In 4 case-control studies, higher biospecimen LC n-3 composition was also significantly associated with a lower risk of CRC (pooled OR = 0.70; 95% CI: 0.55, 0.88; $I^2 = 0.00\%$),

Table 3. Subgroup analysis for association between biospecimen long-chain n-3 PUFA and risk of colorectal cancer.

Factors stratified	C20:5n-3					C22:6n-3					LC n-3 PUFA				
	N[a]	SRR (95% CI)	I² (%)	P[b]	P[c]	N	SRR (95% CI)	I² (%)	P	P	N	SRR (95% CI)	I² (%)	P	P
Overall analysis	6	0.78 (0.64, 0.96)	0.00	0.89		6	0.68 (0.54, 0.84)	0.00	0.42		7	0.74 (0.63, 0.87)	0.00	0.50	
Study design					0.93					0.37					0.63
PC	3	0.77 (0.58, 1.00)	0.00	0.49		3	0.76 (0.56, 1.01)	0.00	0.30		3	0.76 (0.59, 0.97)	10.00	0.33	
CC	3	0.79 (0.58, 1.05)	0.00	0.89		3	0.55 (0.36, 0.85)	30.60	0.00		4	0.70 (0.55, 0.88)	0.00	0.45	
Regions					0.65					0.10					0.30
West (USA and Europe)	4	0.81 (0.63, 1.02)	0.00	0.64		3	0.75 (0.59, 0.96)	0.00	0.80		4	0.76 (0.61, 0.93)	19.70	0.29	
Asia	2	0.72 (0.48, 1.07)	0.00	0.77		3	0.34 (0.13, 0.85)	43.00	0.17		3	0.60 (0.40, 0.89)	0.00	0.88	
Gender					0.42					0.24					0.14
Female	3	0.85 (0.62, 1.15)	0.00	0.82		2	0.78 (0.56, 1.09)	0.00	0.56		3	0.83 (0.66, 1.05)	0.00	0.70	
Male	3	0.65 (0.19,1.11)	13.00	0.32		5	0.47 (0.26, 0.88)	33.00	0.22		3	0.53 (0.33, 0.84)	13.70	0.32	
Biospecimens					0.68					0.58					0.73
Serum	3	0.77 (0.57, 1.02)	0.00	0.57		3	0.63 (0.45, 0.86)	0.00	0.38		3	0.71 (0.57, 0.89)	0.00	0.73	
Erythrocytes	2	0.80 (0.60, 1.06)	0.00	0.74		2	0.70 (0.48, 1.01)	23.50	0.27		2	0.79 (0.55, 1.15)	17.80	0.27	
Whole blood	1	0.80 (0.60, 1.06)				1	0.69 (0.39, 1.23)				1	0.60 (0.32, 1.12)			

Abbreviations: LC n-3: long-chain n-3 polyunsaturated fatty acid (C20: 5n-3+C22: 5n-3+C22: 6n-3); SRR: summary risk ratio; PC: prospective cohort study; CC: case-control study.
[a]N, number of included studies.
[b]P value for heterogeneity within subgroup.
[c]P value for heterogeneity between subgroups with meta-regression analysis.

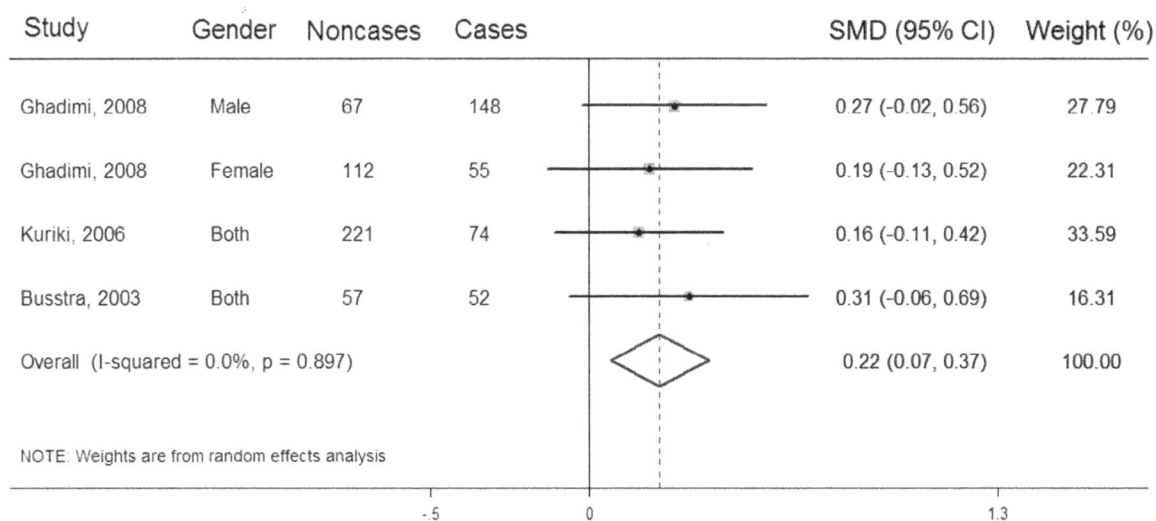

Study	Gender	Noncases	Cases		SMD (95% CI)	Weight (%)
Ghadimi, 2008	Male	67	148		0.27 (-0.02, 0.56)	27.79
Ghadimi, 2008	Female	112	55		0.19 (-0.13, 0.52)	22.31
Kuriki, 2006	Both	221	74		0.16 (-0.11, 0.42)	33.59
Busstra, 2003	Both	57	52		0.31 (-0.06, 0.69)	16.31
Overall (I-squared = 0.0%, p = 0.897)					0.22 (0.07, 0.37)	100.00

NOTE: Weights are from random effects analysis

-.5   0   1.3

Figure 3. Forest plot corresponding to the random-effects meta-analysis analysis on difference in biospecimen compositions of LC n-3 PUFA between cases and noncases. Case-control studies are referred to by first author, year of publication, gender and biospecimen types. The combined standardized mean difference (SMD) was achieved using random-effects model. Grey square represents SMD in each study, with square size reflecting the study-specific weight and the 95% CI represented by horizontal bars. SMD from individual study were pooled by random effect model. The diamond indicates summary SMD.

especially biospecimen C22:6n-3 (pooled OR = 0.55; 95% CI: 0.36, 0.85; I^2 = 30.60%), whereas biospecimen C20:5n-3 exhibited no significant association (pooled OR = 0.79; 95% CI: 0.58, 1.05; I^2 = 0.00%). There were 2 case-control studies reported the association of biospecimen C22:5n-3 with CRC risk [17,23], and the pooled OR is 1.25 (95% CI: 0.65, 2.41; I^2 = 0.00%). However, the results of the meta-regression did not show the significant difference between the two study designs. No evidence of significant difference was found between other subgroups with meta-regression (Table 3).

In a sensitivity analysis, we sequentially omitted 1 study at a time and reanalyzed the remaining data. We found that exclusion of any individual study did not substantially change the overall association. In publication bias analysis, there was also no indication of publication bias as suggested by visual inspection of Begg's funnel plot (P for bias = 0.452) and Egger's regression test (P for bias = 0.175).

Difference in LC n-3 PUFA compositions between cases and noncases

There were 4 case-control studies eligible for the analysis of different biospecimen total LC n-3 PUFA composition between cases and noncases [15–17,23]. Compared with 329 cases, 457 noncases have a significantly higher LC n-3 PUFA composition in biospecimens (SMD: 0.22; 95% CI: 0.07, 0.37), with no between-study heterogeneity (I^2 = 0.00%) (Figure 3). Similarly, there were 7 case-control studies eligible for analyses on different biospecimen C20:5n-3 and C22:6n-3 composition between cases and noncases [15,17,21–25], respectively. Compared with 623 CRC cases, 1315 noncases have significantly higher biospecimen C20:5n-3 (SMD: 0.27; 95% CI: 0.13, 0.41; I^2 = 36.20%) and C22:6n-3 composition (SMD: 0.23; 95% CI: 0.11, 0.34; I^2 = 0.00%) (Table 4). However, no significant difference was found in biospecimen C22:5n-3 composition between 587 cases and 817 noncases from 6 case-control studies (SMD: −0.08; 95% CI: −0.22, 0.06; I^2 = 17.60%) (Table 4).

Stratified analysis indicated that there was a significantly higher blood C20:5n-3 and C22:6n-3 compositions in noncases com-pared with cases, whereas adipose tissue C20:5n-3 and C22:6n-3 compositions exhibited no significant difference between cases and noncases (Table 4). Results from meta-regression only showed a significant difference in C20:5n-3 composition between the two biospecimens (P value = 0.05). Furthermore, biospecimen compositions of C20:5n-3 and C22:6n-3 were both significantly higher in Asian noncases compared with cases, whereas no significant difference was observed in Western noncases compared with cases. There was no significant difference between the two populations with meta-regression (Table 4).

Dose-response analysis

Four eligible studies were available to evaluate the dose-response association of biospecimen LC n-3 PUFA with CRC risk [16,17,20,23], and there was a significantly nonlinear trend in 15,593 participants (P for nonlinearity = 0.01; P for trend = 0.01) (Figure 4D). Six eligible studies were available to evaluate the dose-response analysis on relationship of biospecimen C20:5n-3 and C22:6n-3 with CRC risk in 60,291 participants [15,17–20,23], respectively (Figure 4 A and C). A significantly nonlinear dose-response association was observed between biospecimen C20:5n-3 and CRC risk (P for nonlinearity = 0.021; P for trend = 0.001). The nonlinear association between biospecimen C22:6n-3 and CRC risk was not significant (P for nonlinearity = 0.10), but the overall association in the linear dose-response model was significant (P for trend = 0.012), with a 1% increment of biospecimen C22:6n-3 composition associated with 5% reduced risk of CRC (pooled RR = 0.95; 95% CI: 0.92, 0.98; I^2 = 15.00%). Likewise, three relevant studies were available to evaluate the dose-response relationship between biospecimen C22:5n-3 and CRC risk [17,18,23], but no significant nonlinear and linear trend was observed in 24,540 individuals, respectively (P for nonlinearity = 0.10; P for trend = 0.38) (Figure 4B).

Discussion

To our knowledge, this is the first meta-analysis evaluating an association between biospecimen LC n-3 PUFA and CRC risk.

Table 4. Subgroup analysis for different biospecimen long-chain n-3 PUFA compositions between subjects with and without CRC.

Factors stratified	C20:5n-3					C22:5n-3					C22:6n-3				
	N[a]	SMD (95% CI)	Heterogeneity I² (%)	P[b]	P[c]	N	SMD (95% CI)	Heterogeneity I² (%)	P	P	N	SMD (95% CI)	Heterogeneity I² (%)	P
Overall analysis	7	0.27 (0.13, 0.41)	36.20	0.18		6	−0.08 (−0.22, 0.06)	17.60	0.17		7	0.23 (0.11, 0.34)	0.00	0.38
Region					0.74					0.12				0.45
West	4	0.29 (−0.10, 0.67)	56.00	0.07		3	−0.33 (−0.64, 0.00)	0.00	0.43		4	0.30 (−0.06, 0.67)	51.00	0.08
East	3	0.24 (0.08, 0.40)	27.90	0.23		3	−0.02 (−0.16, 0.11)	0.00	0.44		3	0.24 (0.11, 0.38)	0.00	0.94
Gender					0.90					0.22				0.25
Female	1	0.22 (−0.10, 0.55)	.	.		1	−0.28 (−0.61, 0.04)	.	.		1	0.29 (−0.04, 0.61)	.	.
Male	1	0.34 (0.14, 0.55)	.	.		1	0.05 (−0.15, 0.25)	.	.		1	0.37 (0.21, 0.52)	.	.
Both	5	0.26 (0.05, 0.46)	50.10	0.05		5	−0.03 (−0.28, 0.05)	12.60	0.33		5	0.18 (0.03, 0.33)	10.80	0.34
Biospecimens					0.05					0.54				0.55
Blood	5	0.30 (0.15, 0.44)	17.60	0.27		4	−0.04 (−0.20, 0.11)	26.70	0.12		5	0.24 (0.10, 0.40)	18.0	0.25
Adipose	2	−0.07 (−0.35, 0.20)	0.00	0.59		2	−0.02 (−0.35, 0.30)	28.10	0.24		2	0.19 (−0.09, 0.47)	0.00	0.84

Abbreviations: CRC, colorectal cancer; N: number of included case-control studies; PC: prospective cohort study; CC: case-control study; SMD: standard mean difference compared with colorectal cancer subjects.

[a] N, number of included studies.

[b] P value for heterogeneity within each subgroup.

[c] P value for heterogeneity between subgroups with meta-regression analysis.

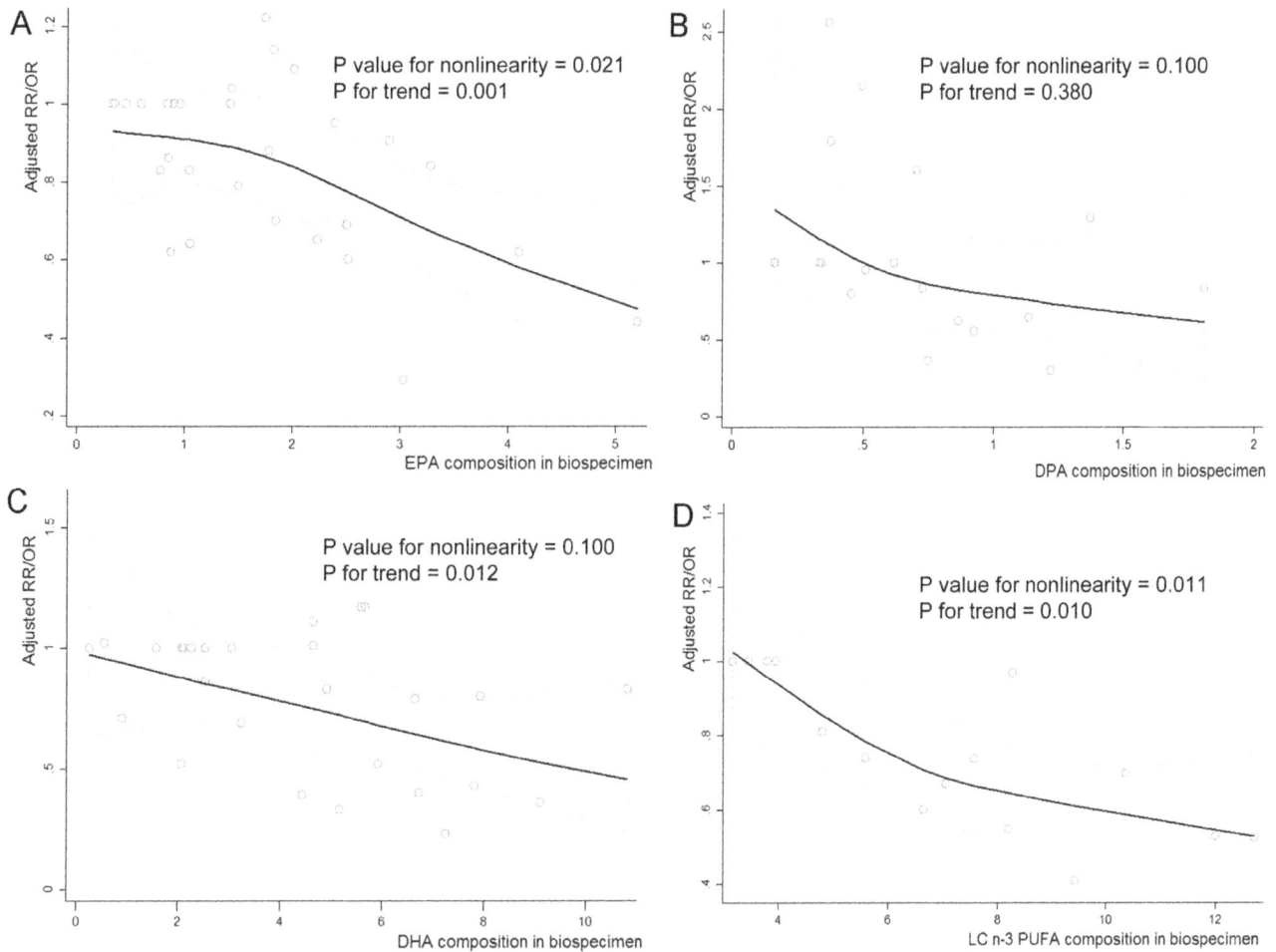

Figure 4. Nonlinear dose-response trend analysis assessed by restricted cubic spline model with three knots. Adjusted ORs (RRs) from all category of biospecimen C20:5n-3, C22:5n-3, C22:6n-3 and total LC n-3 PUFA in each study were separately represented by the small gray circle in the figure A, B, C and D, and corresponding nonlinear dose-response relationship was represented by the black solid line shown in figure A, B, C, and D by using restricted cubic splines functional model with three knots at percentiles 25%, 50%, and 75% of the distribution, respectively.

Overall, our findings suggested that biospecimen composition of LC n-3 PUFA was inversely associated with CRC risk, especially C20:5n-3 and C22:6n-3. Tissue compositions of C20:5n-3, C22:6n-3 and total LC n-3 PUFA were all significantly lower in CRC subjects compared with controls without CRC.

There are several hypothesized mechanisms explaining the possible protective role of tissue LC n-3 PUFA in the etiology of CRC carcinogenesis. The lower composition of LC n-3 PUFA in cases was observed in the present study, suggesting that the characteristic LC n-3 PUFA composition in biospecimen may be involved in the mechanism of CRC progression. Firstly, LC n-3 PUFA existing in biomembrane phospholipids has been found to be involved in the regulation of downstream receptor activity, cell proliferation and apoptosis process by alternation of the fluidity, structure and/or function of lipid rafts or caveolae located in cell surface [13,35,36]. In addition, LC n-3 PUFA, especially C20:5n-3, can may modulate cyclooxygenases (COX) activity, leading to the reduction of n-6 family derived 2-series PG (e.g., PGE_2) with promoting tumor growth effects [37] in favor of n-3 family derived 3-series PG (e.g., PGE_3) with suppressive effects in several cell types including CRC cells [38,39]. Lastly, LC n-3 PUFA may have an antineoplastic effect through alteration in the cellular redox state and increased oxidative stress. The evidence from experi-

mental studies indicated that the oxidative stress and colonocyte apoptosis induced by the fermentation product short-chain fatty acid butyrate might be potentiated by both intrinsic and extrinsic apoptosis pathways medicated by C22:6n-3 [36,40].

In subgroup analyses by study design for the highest category vs lowest, the pooled association estimates of LC n-3 PUFA including the specific subtypes were all significant in prospective cohort studies, although the pooled estimate of C20:5n-3 and C22:5n-3 from case-control studies did not reach statistical significance. Prospective cohort studies greatly decreased the possibility of recall bias and selection biases, which are always inherent in retrospective case-control studies, in view of exposure information was collected before suffering from the disease. Thus, prospective cohort designs are warranted to elucidate causal relationships. In addition, the difference in the number and types of the potential covariates adjusted in multivariable statistic models probably resulted in the discrepant results between cohort and case-control studies. Therefore, we cannot exclude the possibility that the true associations might be distorted in case-control studies adjusting for few confounding factors. For the stratified analysis of LC n-3 PUFA composition between cases and noncases by biospecimen types, blood (serum/plasma/erythrocytes) compositions of LC n-3 PUFA revealed that a statistically significant difference between cases and noncases, but not AT. The heterogeneity between the two biospecimens may be partially explained by different metabolic characteristics of these human biospecimens (serum/plasma/erythrocyte/AT) as biomarkers. Plasma (serum) biomarker represents a combination of triacylglycerol, cholesterol esters and phospholipids found in lipoproteins, and reflects dietary intakes of the past few hours or days [41]. Determination of LC n-3 PUFA composition in erythrocytes provides a biomarker for over several weeks, considering that the half-life of erythrocytes is 120 days [42]. Conversely, AT biomarker represents mostly triacylglycerol, and reflects long-term dietary intake of fatty acids, mainly because of its slow turnover and lack of response to acute diseases. However, given that concentrations of PUFA are very low in AT [43], this tissue does not seem to be a perfect biomarker of LC n-3 PUFA. Furthermore, although biospecimen compositions of fatty acids were mainly determined by GLC in these observational studies, all measurement steps may be accomplished by different methodological procedures, chemicals, and equipments. Hence, the difference between blood and AT biomarker of LC n-3 PUFA may be partly attributed to no agreed standard procedures.

Several strengths could be highlighted in our study. Firstly, our present study showed a characteristic biospecimen compositions of LC n-3 PUFA associated with CRC risk, and further analyzed the difference in the compositions of biospecimen LC n-3 PUFA between CRC cases and noncases. In addition, a biomarker as an indicator of some biological state or condition can closely reflect an integrated measurement of diet over time, thus recall bias might not occur in case-control studies. Finally, no evidence of potential publication bias was observed in the present study, though publication bias could be of concern because small studies with null results tend not to be published. In addition, there are also several potential limitations in the present study. Firstly, meta-analyses of observational studies are susceptible to inherent biases (e.g., report biases and unknown residual confoundings), which might have affected the summarized results. Secondly, selection bias might be unavoidable, due to inclusion of case-control studies with regards to elucidating causal relationships. Thirdly, data on association of tissue biomarker with colon or rectal cancer risk was

not provided by the original studies, respectively. Given that therapeutic strategy for colon cancer and rectal cancer may differ [2,44], future epidemiological studies should further investigate whether LC n-3 PUFA in human tissues could be beneficial for colon or rectal cancer, respectively. Fourthly, the limited numbers of cohort studies included in this meta-analysis might diminish the statistical power to detect the association between biospecimen LC n-3 PUFA and CRC risk. Therefore, care must be exercised in the extrapolation of our findings to larger populations of CRC individuals.

In conclusion, this meta-analysis provided a sufficient evidence that human biospecimen LC n-3 composition was inversely associated with the risk of CRC, especially C20:5n-3 and C22:6n-3. Populations without CRC have higher tissue compositions of C20:5n-3, C22:6n-3 and total LC n-3 PUFA than those with CRC. These evidences have important public health implications for CRC prevention. LC n-3 PUFA profile in human tissues may be an independent predictive factor for CRC risk. Future epidemiological studies should focus on whether the risk of colon or rectal cancer could be modified by increasing LC n-3 PUFA composition in human tissues, respectively. Nevertheless, the protective effect of human tissue LC n-3 PUFA on CRC risk needs to be replicated by further large-scale prospective studies.

Supporting Information

Checklist S1 MOOSE Checklist of the Present Meta-Analysis.
(DOC)

Table S1 Observational studies Excluded from Meta-Analysis.
(DOC)

Author Contributions

Wrote the paper: BY DL. Study conception and design: DL BY. Acquisition of data: FLW XLR. Analysis and interpretation of data: BY FLW.

References

1. Butler LM, Wang R, Koh WP, Yu MC (2008) Prospective study of dietary patterns and colorectal cancer among Singapore Chinese. Br J Cancer 99: 1511–1516.
2. Cai F, Dupertuis YM, Pichard C (2012) Role of polyunsaturated fatty acids and lipid peroxidation on colorectal cancer risk and treatments. Curr Opin Clin Nutr Metab Care 15: 99–106.
3. Ji BT, Devesa SS, Chow WH, Jin F, Gao YT (1998) Colorectal cancer incidence trends by subsite in urban Shanghai, 1972–1994. Cancer Epidemiol Biomarkers Prev 7: 661–666.
4. Penkov A, Popov B (2011) Diet and colorectal cancer. Annals of Nutrition and Metabolism 58: 375–376.
5. Zhong X, Fang YJ, Pan ZZ, Li B, Wang L, et al. (2013) Dietary fat, fatty acid intakes and colorectal cancer risk in Chinese adults: A case-control study. European Journal of Cancer Prevention 22: 438–447.
6. Murff HJ, Shrubsole MJ, Cai Q, Smalley WE, Dai Q, et al. (2012) Dietary intake of PUFAs and colorectal polyp risk. Am J Clin Nutr 95: 703–712.
7. Liu L, Zhuang W, Wang RQ, Mukherjee R, Xiao SM, et al. (2011) Is dietary fat associated with the risk of colorectal cancer? A meta-analysis of 13 prospective cohort studies. Eur J Nutr 50: 173–184.
8. Song M, Chan AT, Fuchs CS, Ogino S, Hu FB, et al. (2014) Dietary intake of fish, omega-3 and omega-6 fatty acids and risk of colorectal cancer: A prospective study in U.S. men and women. Int J Cancer.
9. Pham NM, Mizoue T, Tanaka K, Tsuji I, Tamakoshi A, et al. (2013) Fish consumption and colorectal cancer risk: an evaluation based on a systematic review of epidemiologic evidence among the Japanese population. Jpn J Clin Oncol 43: 935–941.
10. Shen XJ, Zhou JD, Dong JY, Ding WQ, Wu JC (2012) Dietary intake of n-3 fatty acids and colorectal cancer risk: A meta-analysis of data from 489000 individuals. British Journal of Nutrition 108: 1550–1556.
11. Geelen A, Schouten JM, Kamphuis C, Stam BE, Burema J, et al. (2007) Fish consumption, n-3 fatty acids, and colorectal cancer: A meta-analysis of prospective cohort studies. American Journal of Epidemiology 166: 1116–1125.
12. Yang T, Fang S, Zhang HX, Xu LX, Zhang ZQ, et al. (2013) N-3 PUFAs have antiproliferative and apoptotic effects on human colorectal cancer stem-like cells in vitro. J Nutr Biochem 24: 744–753.
13. Turk HF, Chapkin RS (2013) Membrane lipid raft organization is uniquely modified by n-3 polyunsaturated fatty acids. Prostaglandins Leukot Essent Fatty Acids 88: 43–47.
14. Kansal S, Bhatnagar A, Agnihotri N (2014) Fish oil suppresses cell growth and metastatic potential by regulating PTEN and NF-kappaB signaling in colorectal cancer. PLoS One 9: e84627.
15. Pot GK, Geelen A, van Heijningen EM, Siezen CL, van Kranen HJ, et al. (2008) Opposing associations of serum n-3 and n-6 polyunsaturated fatty acids with colorectal adenoma risk: an endoscopy-based case-control study. Int J Cancer 123: 1974–1977.
16. Busstra MC, Siezen CLE, Grubben MJAL, Van Kranen HJ, Nagengast FM, et al. (2003) Tissue levels of fish fatty acids and risk of colorectal adenomas: A case-control study (Netherlands). Cancer Causes and Control 14: 269–276.
17. Kuriki K, Wakai K, Hirose K, Matsuo K, Ito H, et al. (2006) Risk of colorectal cancer is linked to erythrocyte compositions of fatty acids as biomarkers for dietary intakes of fish, fat, and fatty acids. Cancer Epidemiol Biomarkers Prev 15: 1791–1798.
18. Kojima M, Wakai K, Tokudome S, Suzuki K, Tamakoshi K, et al. (2005) Serum levels of polyunsaturated fatty acids and risk of colorectal cancer: A prospective study. American Journal of Epidemiology 161: 462–471.
19. Cottet V, Collin M, Gross AS, Boutron-Ruault MC, Morois S, et al. (2013) Erythrocyte membrane phospholipid fatty acid concentrations and risk of colorectal adenomas: a case-control nested in the French E3N-EPIC cohort study. Cancer Epidemiol Biomarkers Prev 22: 1417–1427.

20. Hall MN, Campos H, Li H, Sesso HD, Stampfer MJ, et al. (2007) Blood levels of long-chain polyunsaturated fatty acids, aspirin, and the risk of colorectal cancer. Cancer Epidemiol Biomarkers Prev 16: 314–321.

21. Okuno M, Hamazaki K, Ogura T, Kitade H, Matsuura T, et al. (2013) Abnormalities in fatty acids in plasma, erythrocytes and adipose tissue in Japanese patients with colorectal cancer. In Vivo 27: 203–210.

22. Giuliani A, Ferrara F, Scimo M, Angelico F, Olivieri L, et al. (2013) Adipose tissue fatty acid composition and colon cancer: a case-control study. Eur J Nutr.

23. Ghadimi R, Kuriki K, Tsuge S, Takeda E, Imaeda N, et al. (2008) Serum concentrations of fatty acids and colorectal adenoma risk: a case-control study in Japan. Asian Pac J Cancer Prev 9: 111–118.

24. Baro L, Hermoso JC, Nunez MC, Jimenez-Rios JA, Gil A (1998) Abnormalities in plasma and red blood cell fatty acid profiles of patients with colorectal cancer. Br J Cancer 77: 1978–1983.

25. Fernandez-Banares F, Esteve M, Navarro E, Cabre E, Boix J, et al. (1996) Changes of the mucosal n3 and n6 fatty acid status occur early in the colorectal adenoma-carcinoma sequence. Gut 38: 254–259.

26. Stroup DF, Berlin JA, Morton SC, Olkin I, Williamson GD, et al. (2000) Meta-analysis of observational studies in epidemiology: a proposal for reporting. Meta-analysis Of Observational Studies in Epidemiology (MOOSE) group. JAMA 283: 2008–2012.

27. DerSimonian R, Laird N (1986) Meta-analysis in clinical trials. Control Clin Trials 7: 177–188.

28. Higgins JP, Thompson SG, Deeks JJ, Altman DG (2003) Measuring inconsistency in meta-analyses. BMJ 327: 557–560.

29. Egger M, Davey Smith G, Schneider M, Minder C (1997) Bias in meta-analysis detected by a simple, graphical test. BMJ 315: 629–634.

30. Liu Q, Cook NR, Bergström A, Hsieh CC (2009) A two-stage hierarchical regression model for meta-analysis of epidemiologic nonlinear dose–response data. Computational Statistics & Data Analysis 53: 4157–4167.

31. Jackson D, White IR, Thompson SG (2010) Extending DerSimonian and Laird's methodology to perform multivariate random effects meta-analyses. Stat Med 29: 1282–1297.

32. Orsini N, Bellocco R, Greenland S (2006) Generalized least squares for trend estimation of summarized dose-response data. Stata Journal 6: 40–57.

33. Harrell FE Jr, Lee KL, Pollock BG (1988) Regression models in clinical studies: determining relationships between predictors and response. J Natl Cancer Inst 80: 1198–1202.

34. Orsini N, Li R, Wolk A, Khudyakov P, Spiegelman D (2012) Meta-analysis for linear and nonlinear dose-response relations: examples, an evaluation of approximations, and software. Am J Epidemiol 175: 66–73.

35. Rogers KR, Kikawa KD, Mouradian M, Hernandez K, McKinnon KM, et al. (2010) Docosahexaenoic acid alters epidermal growth factor receptor-related signaling by disrupting its lipid raft association. Carcinogenesis 31: 1523–1530.

36. Hull MA (2011) Omega-3 polyunsaturated fatty acids. Best Pract Res Clin Gastroenterol 25: 547–554.

37. Hawcroft G, Loadman PM, Belluzzi A, Hull MA (2010) Effect of eicosapentae-noic acid on E-type prostaglandin synthesis and EP4 receptor signaling in human colorectal cancer cells. Neoplasia 12: 618–627.

38. Hopkins GJ, Kennedy TG, Carroll KK (1981) Polyunsaturated fatty acids as promoters of mammary carcinogenesis induced in Sprague-Dawley rats by 7,12-dimethylbenz[a]anthracene. J Natl Cancer Inst 66: 517–522.

39. Poole EM, Bigler J, Whitton J, Sibert JG, Kulmacz RJ, et al. (2007) Genetic variability in prostaglandin synthesis, fish intake and risk of colorectal polyps. Carcinogenesis 28: 1259–1263.

40. Kolar SS, Barhoumi R, Callaway ES, Fan YY, Wang N, et al. (2007) Synergy between docosahexaenoic acid and butyrate elicits p53-independent apoptosis via mitochondrial Ca(2+) accumulation in colonocytes. Am J Physiol Gastro-intest Liver Physiol 293: G935–943.

41. Kohlmeier L (1995) Future of dietary exposure assessment. Am J Clin Nutr 61: 702S–709S.

42. Theret N, Bard JM, Nuttens MC, Lecerf JM, Delbart C, et al. (1993) The relationship between the phospholipid fatty acid composition of red blood cells, plasma lipids, and apolipoproteins. Metabolism 42: 562–568.

43. Hirsch J, Farquhar JW, Ahrens EH Jr, Peterson ML, Stoffel W (1960) Studies of adipose tissue in man. A microtechnic for sampling and analysis. Am J Clin Nutr 8: 499–511.

44. Cockbain AJ, Toogood GJ, Hull MA (2012) Omega-3 polyunsaturated fatty acids for the treatment and prevention of colorectal cancer. Gut 61: 135–149.

4

Fluorescently Activated Cell Sorting Followed by Microarray Profiling of Helper T Cell Subtypes from Human Peripheral Blood

Chiaki Ono[1,2], Zhiqian Yu[1,2], Yoshiyuki Kasahara[1,2], Yoshie Kikuchi[1,2], Naoto Ishii[3,4], Hiroaki Tomita[1,2,4]*

1 Department of Disaster Psychiatry, Internal Research Institute of Disaster Science, Tohoku University, Sendai, Japan, **2** Department of Biological Psychiatry, Tohoku University Graduate School of Medicine, Sendai, Japan, **3** Department of Microbiology and Immunology, Tohoku University Graduate School of Medicine, Sendai, Japan, **4** Tohoku Medical Megabank Organization, Tohoku University, Sendai, Japan

Abstract

Background: Peripheral blood samples have been subjected to comprehensive gene expression profiling to identify biomarkers for a wide range of diseases. However, blood samples include red blood cells, white blood cells, and platelets. White blood cells comprise polymorphonuclear leukocytes, monocytes, and various types of lymphocytes. Blood is not distinguishable, irrespective of whether the expression profiles reflect alterations in (a) gene expression patterns in each cell type or (b) the proportion of cell types in blood. $CD4^+$ Th cells are classified into two functionally distinct subclasses, namely Th1 and Th2 cells, on the basis of the unique characteristics of their secreted cytokines and their roles in the immune system. Th1 and Th2 cells play an important role not only in the pathogenesis of human inflammatory, allergic, and autoimmune diseases, but also in diseases that are not considered to be immune or inflammatory disorders. However, analyses of minor cellular components such as $CD4^+$ cell subpopulations have not been performed, partly because of the limited number of these cells in collected samples.

Methodology/Principal Findings: We describe fluorescently activated cell sorting followed by microarray (FACS–array) technology as a useful experimental strategy for characterizing the expression profiles of specific immune cells in the circulation. We performed reproducible gene expression profiling of Th1 and Th2, respectively. Our data suggest that this procedure provides reliable information on the gene expression profiles of certain small immune cell populations. Moreover, our data suggest that GZMK, GZMH, EOMES, IGFBP3, and STOM may be novel markers for distinguishing Th1 cells from Th2 cells, whereas IL17RB and CNTNAP1 can be Th2-specific markers.

Conclusions/Significance: Our approach may help in identifying aberrations and novel therapeutic or diagnostic targets for diseases that affect Th1 or Th2 responses and elucidating the involvement of a subpopulation of immune cells in some diseases.

Editor: Hiroshi Shiku, Mie University Graduate School of Medicine, Japan

Funding: This work was supported by a grant-in-aid for scientific research on innovative areas (No. 24116007), Health and Labour Sciences Research Grants research on psychiatric and neurological diseases and mental health (H19-kokoro-ippan-001), a grant-in-aid from the Japan Research Foundation for Clinical Pharmacology, and an Intramural Research Grant (No. 21-9) for Neurological and Psychiatric Disorders from the National Center of Neurology and Psychiatry. The funders had no role in study design, data collection and analysis, decision to publish, or preparation of the manuscript.

Competing Interests: The authors have declared that no competing interests exist.

* Email: htomita@med.tohoku.ac.jp

Introduction

Comprehensive gene expression analyses of peripheral blood samples have been performed to identify biomarkers for a wide range of diseases such as leukemia [1,2], autoimmune diseases [3,4], graft-versus-host disease [5], and inflammatory [6] and allergic disorders [7,8], which primarily affect peripheral blood cells. Expression profiling of blood samples has also been applied to diseases that primarily affect the brain (e.g., demyelinating diseases [9], neurodegenerative diseases [10,11], and psychiatric disorders [12,13]) or peripheral organs other than blood (e.g., cancers [14,15] and diabetes mellitus [16]). There are several reasons for researches to identify molecules dysregulated in peripheral blood samples from patients with these diseases

primarily unrelated to peripheral blood. (1) Immune cells in the affected organ and peripheral blood interact. Dysregulated molecules in immune cells circulating in peripheral blood may directly or indirectly influence the pathogenesis in the affected organ or reflect immunological conditions related to the affected organ. (2) The affected organ and peripheral blood from the same individual share exactly the same genomic coding information and may therefore have similar transcriptional regulation patterns. A part of the dysregulated transcriptional activities in the affected organ can also be observed in peripheral blood in the same manner. (3) Blood samples are relatively easy to obtain compared to other organ tissues or cells.

In addition to the lack of complete knowledge about the mechanisms linking aberrations in peripheral blood with the pathogenesis of the affected organ, there is another limitation to comprehensive gene expression studies of peripheral blood samples. A blood sample comprises red blood cells, white blood cells, and platelets. White blood cells consist of polymorphonuclear leukocytes, monocytes, and various types of lymphocytes. Because blood samples utilized for gene expression studies are heterogeneous mixtures of various types of cells, it is difficult to determine with certainty of whether an expression profile reflects alterations in (a) gene expression patterns in each cell type or (b) the proportion of cell types in blood. Moreover, alterations in a gene expression pattern in a certain cell type can be offset by changes in the expression profiles of the other cell types in a blood sample. In this context, the expression profiles of major components of blood samples, such as CD11$^+$ monocytes or CD4$^+$ helper T (Th) cells, have been evaluated using magnetic cell separation [17,18]. However, analyses of minor cellular components, such as CD4$^+$ cell subpopulations, have not been performed in part because of the limited number of these cells in the collected samples.

To solve these problems, we developed a protocol of fluorescently activated cell sorting followed by microarray (FACS–array) suitable for characterizing the gene expression profiles of specific immune cells in blood samples. The FACS-array approach has been applied to various kinds of cells and tissues, including neuronal and blood cells [19,20,21]. Several studies used the FACS–array approach to isolate subpopulations of leukocytes, including CD4$^+$ T cells, CD8$^+$ T cells, B cells, monocytes, and granulocytes [21]. However, these subpopulations are themselves heterogeneous. For example, CD4$^+$ T cells consist of subclasses, including type 1 and type 2 T helper cells (Th1 and Th2, respectively). The comprehensive gene expression profiling of these minor subpopulations of human blood cells remains unevaluated, probably due to technical difficulties with analysis of very small number of cells

In this study, we used the FACS–array procedure to characterize the expression profiles of type 1 and type 2 Th cells (Th1 and Th2, respectively). CD4$^+$ Th cells are classified into two functionally distinct subclasses, Th1 and Th2 cells, on the basis of the unique characteristics of their secreted cytokines and roles in the immune system. Th1 cells synthesize interleukin-2 (IL-2), interferon-γ(IFN-γ), and tumor necrosis factor-β and induce a phagocytic cell-mediated immune response and proinflammatory effects, whereas Th2 cells synthesize IL-4, IL-5, IL-6, and IL-10 and induce a nonphagocytic humoral immune response and anti-inflammatory effects [22]. Th1 and Th2 cells have been shown to play an important role not only in the pathogenesis of human inflammatory, allergic, and autoimmune diseases [23,24] but also in diseases that are not considered immune or inflammatory disorders [25,26]. For example, the ratio of functional activities of Th2 cells to those of Th1 cells is elevated in blood samples from patients with schizophrenia [27], mood disorders [28], trauma-related mental health conditions [29,30], and lupus erythematosus. This ratio is lowered in patients with rheumatoid arthritis [31]. In these previous studies, the Th1/Th2 imbalance was analyzed on the basis of the levels of serum cytokines, which are presumably secreted by Th1 and Th2 cells.

In contrast to this indirect evidence suggestive of dysfunction of Th1 and/or Th2 cells, our FACS–array procedure provides exact and comprehensive information on the molecules dysregulated in Th1 and Th2 cells in blood samples from patients, along with the exact ratio of Th1 and Th2 cell numbers. To date, there have been no studies aimed at evaluating the expression profiles of specific immune cells, except for microarray analysis of artificially differentiated Th1 and Th2 cells, which were derived from CD4$^+$ cells *in vitro* by stimulation with IL-12 and IL-4, respectively [32].

Microarray studies of intrinsic Th1 and Th2 cells in blood samples should provide useful information for understanding the immune cell-relevant pathophysiology of various types of diseases. This article describes the FACS–array procedure as a useful experimental strategy that is useful for characterizing the expression profiles of specific immune cells from blood samples under unstimulated conditions. We here performed the reproducible gene expression profiling of Th1 and Th2 cells.

Materials and Methods

PBMC Isolation

Blood samples (20 ml) were drawn from 23 healthy individuals after obtaining written informed consent. Subjects who were affected by health conditions, including allergic or infectious diseases, or who took medication for such conditions were excluded from the study. To isolate peripheral blood mononuclear cells (PBMCs), each blood sample was diluted with an equal amount of phosphate-buffered saline (PBS; Gibco BRL/Invitrogen Technologies, Carlsbad, CA, USA) and overlaid onto Ficoll-Paque PLUS separation medium (GE Healthcare, Buckinghamshire, England). The cells at the plasma/Ficoll interface were collected and washed with PBS containing 10 mM EDTA and 2% fetal bovine serum (FBS), followed by a wash with RPMI 1640 medium containing 10% FBS. The total number of PBMCs was counted using a C-chip cell counter (NanoEnTek, Seoul, Korea). The cells were then cryopreserved at a concentration of approximately 1×10^7 cells/mL in RPMI 1640 medium containing 10% FBS and 10% dimethyl sulfoxide (Wako, Osaka, Japan). Immediately after isolation, the cells were frozen at −80°C for 24 h. Subsequently, the cells were kept in liquid nitrogen until they were subjected to cell sorting. All experimental procedures described in this article were carried out according to a protocol approved by the Ethics Committee of Tohoku University Graduate School of Medicine.

Antibodies and Flow Cytometry

The following monoclonal antibodies were used to isolate subpopulations of Th cells from human blood samples using a FACS system: FITC-conjugated anti-human CD4 antibody (clone PRA-T4, BD Biosciences Pharmingen, San Jose, CA, USA) for labeling CD4$^+$ Th cells, APC-conjugated anti-human CXCR3 (CD183) antibody (clone 1C6, BD Biosciences Pharmingen) for labeling CXCR3$^+$ Th1 cells, and PE-conjugated anti-human CCR4 antibody (clone 1G1, BD Biosciences Pharmingen) for labeling CCR4$^+$ Th2 cells. A nonpermeating red fluorescent dye, propidium iodide (PI), was used to stain dead cells. To isolate Th1 and Th2 cells, the frozen PBMCs were thawed rapidly, washed with PBS, and stained with fluorophore-conjugated monoclonal antibodies specific to the surface markers, and separated on a FACS system, Aria (Becton, Dickinson and Company, Franklin Lakes, NJ, USA) as follows. (1) The lymphocytic subpopulation of PBMCs was selected on the basis of their unique forward and side scatter properties on fluorocytometry. (2) Among the lymphocytes, PI-negative (viable) cells were selected. (3) Among the viable lymphocytes, CD4$^+$ Th cells were selected. (4) On the basis of the signal intensity of fluorostaining for the CXCR3 and CCR4 markers, viable Th cells were separated into four subgroups, CXCR3$^+$/CCR4$^-$ Th1 cells, CXCR3$^-$/CCR4$^+$ Th2 cells, CXCR3$^+$/CCR4$^+$ double-positive cells, and CXCR3$^-$/CCR4$^-$ double-negative cells. Data was analyzed using FACS Diva software (version 4.0.1.2; Becton, Dickinson and Company). (Figure 1A).

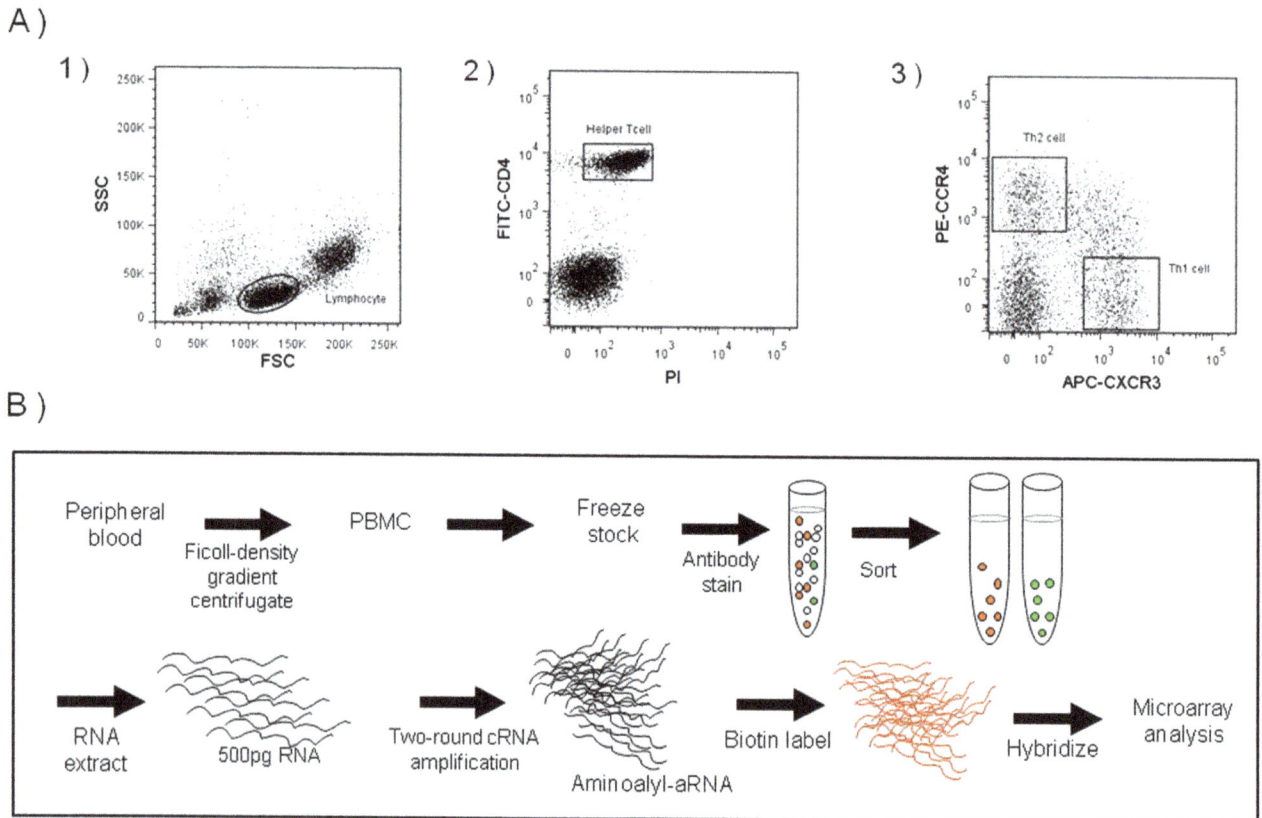

Figure 1. Schematic of the FACS–array procedure for peripheral blood cells. (A) Schematic of analysis of helper T (Th) cells using the FACS–array procedure for peripheral blood cells, where PBMCs are isolated on a density gradient centrifuge and stained with fluorescence-labeled antibodies (CD4-FITC, CXCR3-APC, and CCR4-PE) and PI for FACS. Total RNA was extracted from each subclass of lymphocytes and subjected to two rounds of cRNA amplification. Synthesized aminoallyl-aRNA samples were labeled with biotin and subjected to microarray analysis. (B) Dot plot imaging of FACS isolation of Th1 and Th2 cells. (1) Lymphocytic subpopulation of PBMCs was selected on the basis of their unique forward and side scatter properties on fluorocytometry. (2) Among the lymphocytes, PI-negative (viable) CD4$^+$ Th cells were selected. (3) On the basis of the signal intensity of fluorostaining for the CXCR3 and CCR4 markers, the viable Th cells were separated into two subgroups: CXCR3$^+$/CCR4$^-$ as Th1 cells and CXCR3$^-$/CCR4$^+$ as Th2 cells.

RNA Isolation

Total RNA was isolated from each cell sample using the RNeasy Mini or Micro RNA isolation kit (Qiagen, Valencia, CA, USA). The RNeasy Mini kit was used with samples 1–6 in Table 1, which were collected from 2008/10/27 to 2008/12/24. The RNeasy kit was replaced with the Micro kit after 2009/2/19 to obtain highly concentrated RNA samples and applied to samples 7–23. Genomic DNA in the RNA samples was digested with RNase-free DNase I (Qiagen). The total RNA was eluted with 30 μl (from the RNeasy Mini columns) or 15 μl (from the RNeasy MinElute Spin Columns of the Micro kit) of RNase-free water. The concentration, 28S/18S ribosomal RNA (rRNA) ratio, and RNA integrity number (RIN) of the purified RNA samples were measured using the 2100 Bioanalyzer (Agilent, Santa Clara, CA, USA) with the RNA 6000 Pico Chip kit (Agilent). The RNA samples were then stored at −80°C until use.

Evaluation of the Effects of Freezing of Cells on the Quantity and Quality of RNA Extracted from PBMCs

Each PBMC sample was divided in two, and one of these PBMC aliquots was immediately subjected to 0.4% trypan blue staining and total RNA extraction procedures, as described above. The remaining half of the PBMC aliquots was stored in liquid nitrogen, as described above, for 4 days and subjected to 0.4%

trypan blue staining and total RNA extraction. In both cases, the RNA samples were frozen at −80°C immediately after extraction. The quality and quantity of the RNA samples were measured using the Agilent Bioanalyzer 2100, as described above.

Evaluation of Amplification Systems with Small Amounts of RNA for Microarray Analysis

There are at least three commercially available kits for amplifying several hundred picograms of total RNA to a certain amount of biotinylated cRNA that would be sufficient for the Illumina BeadChip–based microarray experiments: (1) TargetAmp 2-Round Aminoallyl aRNA amplification kit 1.0 (Epicentre Biotechnologies, Madison, WI, USA) with biotin-X-X-NHS (Epicentre Biotechnologies), (2) MessageAmp II aRNA amplification kit with biotin-11-CTP and biotin-16-UTP (Ambion, Austin, TX, USA), and (3) WT-Ovation FFPE RNA amplification system V2 (NuGEN, San Carlos, CA, USA). Six small aliquots (100 pg) of total RNA samples extracted from human peripheral blood leukocytes (Clontech Laboratories, Palo Alto, CA, USA) were amplified and biotinylated using each of the three kits in duplicates and applied to the Illumina Human-6v2 Expression BeadChips (Illumina, San Diego, CA, USA), according to the manufacturer's instructions. As a control, two standard amounts of aliquots (500 ng) of the same total RNA samples were subjected to

Table 1. Characteristics of the samples and demographics of the subjects.

Sample ID	Gender	Age	Date	PBMCs (10^7)	% of CD4+ Th1	% of CD4+ Th2	WP	WN	Th1 Cell count	Th1 Total RNA [pg]	Th1 rRNA ratio	Th1 RIN	Th2 Cell count	Th2 Total RNA [pg]	Th2 rRNA ratio	Th2 RIN	Exclusion
1	M	29	2008/10/27	2.3	13.4	12.8	4.0	60.0	135,950	39,046	1.05	6.6	125,129	28,099	2.58	9.8	
2	M	33	2008/10/27	2.4	2.7	10.1	0.2	79.6	27,508	181	0.00	0.0	118,257	19,591	2.14	9.6	○
3	M	45	2008/10/27	2.6	13.6	13	4.8	49.5	224,169	29,106	1.57	9.5	195,447	53,970	2.80	9.7	
4	M	35	2008/10/27	2.5					45,724	1,899	1.67	8.4	79,310	15,866	1.38	9.2	
5	F	24	2008/12/24	2.3	22.4	9.9	1.8	50.2	402,727	33,177	1.81	9.8	169,925	20,788	2.25	9.5	
6	M	31	2008/12/24	1.7	15.1	24.7	2.2	50.9	90,545	1,225	1.25	9.2	156,472	8,437	1.82	9.9	
7	M	29	2009/2/19	1.3	20.3	7.1	2.8	60.6	100,127	31,412	1.64	9.2	38,771	8,921	2.29	7.2	
8	F	25	2009/2/19	1.3	21.5	11.6	3.0	56.0	228,225	126,966	1.75	9.7	138,596	22,862	2.12	9.7	
9	F	40	2009/2/19	2.3	9.8	4.8	0.9	79.4	110,375	22,104	1.07	5.1	52,798	17,552	1.27	6.6	○
10	F	40	2009/2/19	2.4	23	7.1	3.0	59.8	300,216	253,100	1.76	9.7	103,144	38,941	2.06	9.4	
11	F	31	2009/2/25	2.3	13.9	15.6	2.1	52.8	137,250	60,538	2.03	9.7	180,248	112,817	2.58	9.9	
12	F	45	2009/2/25	3.5	21.3	15.4	3.1	46.7	277,014	140,393	2.44	9.9	202,758	70,557	1.34	9.7	
13	F	24	2009/2/25	2.9	7.4	6.0	1.1	80.3	329,185	228,191	2.12	9.8	311,759	109,503	2.41	9.9	
14	F	41	2009/3/18	1.5	29.5	12.9	8.2	39.0	471,293	79,309	0.85	6.8	256,889	43,138	1.58	9.0	○
15	F	58	2009/11/5														○
16	M	64	2009/11/5	1.5	9.2	10.6	6.4	57.3	68,056	8,820	1.60	9.0	235,539	53,617	1.64	8.7	
17	M	33	2009/12/8	1.5	4.8	13.2	0.6	72.9	53,624	22,593	0.00	2.7	120,117	18,036	2.41	8.1	○
18	F	42	2009/12/8	1.6	9.1	18.7	2.2	56.1	75,100	14,538	1.58	8.3	136,106	36,742	1.00	7.3	○
19	F	27	2009/12/8	2.3	4.3	14.6	0.8	69.7	48,775	15,117	1.40	3.5	145,623	22,727	1.69	9.6	○
20	F	61	2009/12/8	1.9	20.7	12.8	13.5	36.4	100,929	3,452	0.00	2.4	90,503	22,277	1.60	8.8	○
21	M	43	2009/12/8	2.8	34.3	17.1	8.8	24.9	120,054	3,215	0.00	1.8	127,457	24,263	1.16	7.3	○
22	F	58	2009/12/8	1.8	17.8	13.3	4.2	57.2	73,052	19,272	1.68	6.6	68,117	34,239	1.21	7.1	
23	M	47	2009/12/15	2.2	17.2	6.9	4.1	61.0	39,779	2,778	0.20	5.4		7,609	1.70	9.3	○
Av		39.4		2.1	15.8	12.3	3.7	57.2	157,258	51,656	1.25	7.3	143,378	35,934	1.86	8.9	
SD		12.0		0.6	8.3	4.7	3.2	14.2	126,384	72,241	0.76	2.8	67,308	29,113	0.53	1.1	

The table shows gender and age, the number of PBMCs from each subject, the cell count and extracted RNA quality indicators of each sorted type 1 and type 2 helper T (Th1 and Th2, respectively) cell sample, and the proportion of each subclass among the CD4+ cells. As the proportion of each subclass among the CD4+ cells, percentages of Th1, Th2, CXCR3+/CCR4+ double-positive population (WP), and CXCR3-/CCR4- double-negative population (WN) in the CD4+ Th cells are shown in "% of CD4+" columns. RNA quality of each Th1 and Th2 sample is indicated as a 28S/18S ribosomal RNA (rRNA) ratio and an RNA integrity number (RIN) of total RNA measured using the Agilent Bioanalyzer 2100. The "Exclusion" column indicates whether a sample met the exclusion criteria: 28S/18S rRNA ratio of <1.0 or RIN of <6.5.

biotinylated cRNA synthesis in duplicates following the standard protocol using the Illumina TotalPrep RNA amplification kit (Ambion) and applied to the same BeadChip microarray. We assessed the amplification efficiency of each kit, congruence between the duplicated microarray data, and linearity of the small amount- and standard amount-based microarray data.

Microarray Analysis of Th1 and Th2 Cells

Total RNA (300–500 pg) extracted from each isolated cell sample was subjected to aminoallyl-aRNA amplification using the TargetAmp Round Aminoallyl aRNA amplification kit 1.0 and the MinElute cleanup kit (Qiagen). The aminoallyl-aRNA was labeled with biotin-X-X-NHS (Epicentre Biotechnologies) and processed again using the MinElute cleanup kit (Qiagen). After determination of the concentration using NanoDrop 2000 (Thermo Fisher Scientific, Waltham, MA, USA), 1.0–1.5 μg of biotin-labeled aRNA was hybridized to the Illumina Human-6v2 Expression BeadChips, according to the manufacturer's instructions. Each BeadChip was labeled with streptavidin–Cy3 (GE Healthcare), washed, and scanned on the Illumina Bead Station 500X (Illumina). Signal intensity of each BeadChip was measured and normalized using BeadStudio software (Illumina).

Expression data

RNA expression data have been submitted to the Gene Expression Omnibus (GEO; http://www.ncbi.nlm.nih.gov/geo) with the series accession number GSE59295.

Flow Cytometric validation of Th1- and Th2-specific genes detected in FACS–array experiments

Some of the genes detected as Th1-dominant genes in Th1 and Th2 microarray data are known to be expressed in natural killer (NK) cells. Therefore, we performed flow cytometric analysis with PE-labeled anti-human CD56 antibody. Similarly, we analyzed the expression of IL17RB, detected among Th2-dominant genes in the microarray data, using APC–Cy7-labeled anti-human IL17RB antibody in a flow cytometric experiment.

Immunohistochemical validation of Th1- and Th2-Dominant genes detected in FACS–array experiments

To confirm the validity of the FACS–array procedure, representative Th1- and Th2-specific genes were selected from the top five on the basis of the microarray data, and coexpression of the protein product with the Th1-specific transcription factor T-bet and the Th2-specific transcription factor GATA3 was analyzed in human CD4$^+$ T cells. Human CD14$^-$/CD4$^+$ Th cells were isolated from PBMCs using the CD14 and CD4 microbeads (Miltenyi Biotec, Bergisch Gladbach, Germany) and magnetic-activated cell sorting column technology (Miltenyi Biotec). Subsequently, the cells were spread on BioCoat collagen I 8-well culture slides (Becton, Dickinson and Company). The cells were incubated at room temperature for 20 min and fixed with 4% paraformaldehyde. After overnight incubation at 4°C with primary antibodies, the cells were rinsed in PBS and then incubated at room temperature in the dark with secondary antibodies. The primary antibodies used for immunostaining were as follows: anti-human T-bet (1:200 dilution, RabMAb), anti-human GATA3 (1:100 dilution, Novus Biologicals or Abcam), anti-Tbr-2 (EOMES; 1:100 dilution, Millipore), anti-IL17RB (1:100 dilution, Sigma), and anti-CNTNAP1 (1:100 dilution, Sigma-Aldrich). The corresponding secondary antibodies were as follows: Alexa Fluor 488 or 594 -conjugated anti-rabbit IgG (1:500

dilution, Invitrogen) for anti-Tbet; Alexa Fluor 488-conjugated anti-rabbit or mouse IgG (1:500 dilution, Invitrogen) for anti-CNTNAP1; Alexa Fluor 594- conjugated anti-rabbit or mouse IgG (1:500 dilution, Invitrogen) for anti-GATA3; and Alexa Fluor 488-conjugated anti-chicken IgG (1:500 dilution, Invitrogen) for anti-Tbr2. After incubation with the secondary antibodies, the tissues were rinsed in PBS and subjected to nuclear staining with 4,6-diamidino-2-phenylindole (Invitrogen). Microscopic images were captured using a BIOREVO Bz9000 (KEYENCE, Osaka, Japan).

The numbers of cells that co-expressed EOMES and T-bet among EOMES-positive cells and among T-bet-positive cells were counted and used to calculate specificity and sensitivity of EOMES as a Th1 cell marker. Likewise, the numbers of cells that co-expressed CNTNAP1 and GATA-3 among CNTNAP1-positive cells and among GATA-3-positive cells were counted and used to calculate specificity and sensitivity of CNTNAP1 as a Th2 cell marker.

Results

FACS and RNA Extraction

Of 2.1 ± 0.6 (mean $\pm$ SD) $\times10^7$ PBMCs, $13.6\pm5.5\%$ were PI$^-$/CD4$^+$ cells, which are thought to be viable Th cells. Among the PI$^-$/CD4$^+$ cells, $15.8\pm8.3\%$ were CXCR3$^+$/CCR4$^-$ cells, which are believed to be Th1 cells, whereas $12.3\pm4.7\%$ were CXCR3$^-$/CCR4$^+$ cells, which are thought to be Th2 cells. More than half of the PI$^-$/CD4$^+$ cells ($57.2\pm14.2\%$) were CXCR3$^-$/CCR4$^-$ double-negative cells and $3.7\pm3.2\%$ were CXCR3$^+$/CCR4$^+$ double-positive cells. The ratio of the Th1 cell number to the Th2 cell number varied widely among individuals (1.1 ± 0.8).

The amount of total RNA extracted from 10^4 each of the Th1 and Th2 cells was 0.07–8.43 ng and 0.54–6.3 ng, respectively (0.01–15.3 ng and 0.46–6.7 ng, respectively, from 1 ml of whole blood samples). The 28S/18S rRNA ratio of the Th1 and Th2 samples was 0.0–2.4 and 1.0–2.8, respectively, and RIN of the samples was 0–9.9 and 6.6–9.9, respectively. The samples with a 28S/18S rRNA ratio of <1.0 or RIN of <6.5 were excluded from further analysis (Table 1). Cell viability, calculated as a cell count per milliliter, after the freeze–thaw procedure was approximately 88%. There was no decrease in quantity or quality of RNA samples extracted from frozen stocks of PBMCs compared with fresh PBMCs.

Evaluation of RNA Amplification Systems

The TargetAmp aRNA amplification kit, MessageAmp II aRNA amplification kit, and WT-Ovation FFPE RNA amplification kit amplified 100 pg of human leukocyte total RNA to 4.4 ± 0.6 μg (43,500-fold), 0.45 ± 0.05 μg (4500-fold), and 2.1 ± 0.9 μg (21,000-fold) of biotinylated aRNA, respectively. The amplification efficiency of each of these three systems was much higher than that of the standard amplification protocol using the Illumina TotalPrep RNA amplification kit, which amplified 500 ng of the same total RNA to 53 μg of biotinylated cRNA (106-fold; Figure 2A). Because the amount of aRNA obtained using the MessageAmp II kit was not sufficient for a microarray experiment, biotinylated aRNA samples obtained using the TargetAmp and WT-Ovation kits were used in the Illumina Human-6v2 Expression BeadChip-based microarray experiment. TargetAmp kit-amplified human leukocyte total RNA (100 pg each) showed 8044 and 8260 transcripts in duplicated measurements with signal intensities of >50 and a detection p value of < 0.05, among 48,701 transcripts. WT-Ovation kit-amplified human leukocyte total RNA samples showed 9306 and 9168 transcripts,

A)

	Total Prep RNA Amplificaton Kit	TargetAmp 2-Round Aminoallyl-aRNA Amplification kit 1.0	Messageamp II aRNA Amplification Kit	NuGEN WT-Ovation FFRE RNA Amplification System V2
	One round	Two round	Two round	One round
System	dsDNA synthesis	dsDNA synthesis	dsDNA synthesis	dsDNA synthesis
		IVT	IVT	
		dsDNA synthesis	dsDNA synthesis	SPIA™ Amplification
	IVT	IVT	IVT	
Input RNA	500ng	100pg	100pg	100pg
Amplified RNA	53.1±1mg	4.35±0.55mg	0.45±0.05mg	2.1±0.9 mg
Amplified fold	106	4.35×10^4	4×10^3	2.1×10^4

B)

C)

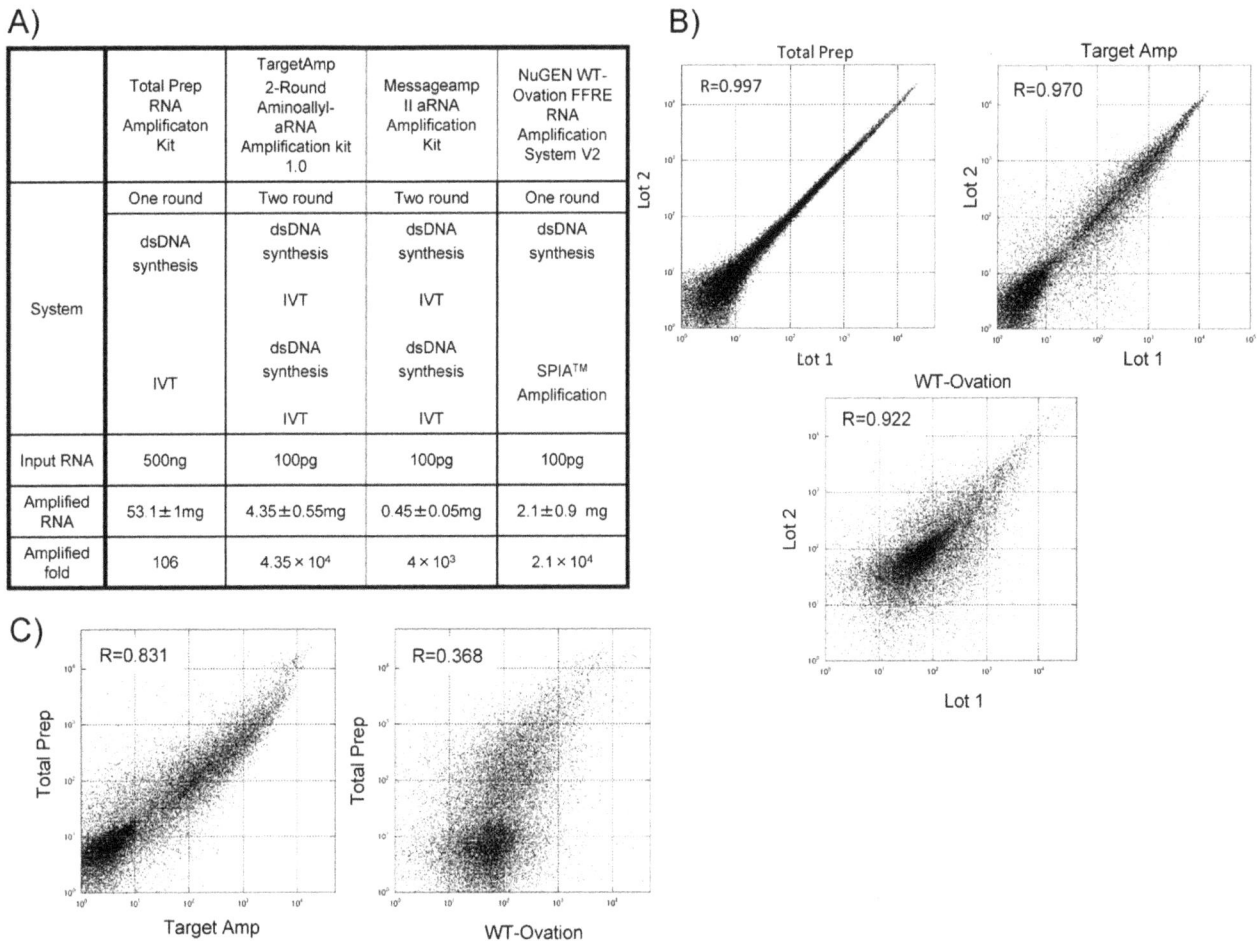

Figure 2. Evaluation of RNA amplification systems for the FACS-array procedure. (**A**) A summary of principles of the four RNA amplification systems and efficacy of amplification. Some data are shown as mean ± SD. (**B**) Scatter plots showing correlations between the gene expression profiles of duplicated batches of amplified RNA from the same small amount of human lymphocyte RNA using three RNA amplification systems. TotalPrep: amplified using the Total Prep RNA amplification kit (Illumina), Target Amp: amplified using the TargetAmp 2-round aminoallyl-aRNA amplification kit 1.0, and WT-Ovation: amplified using the WT-Ovation FFRE RNA amplification system V2 (NuGEN). (**C**) Scatter plots showing correlations between the gene expression profiles of amplified RNA from the same small amount of human lymphocyte RNA using TargetAmp/WT-Ovation and conventional TotalPrep.

which met the same criteria. These numbers were comparable to the number of transcripts, 9270 and 9393 observed in microarray data of the standard TotalPrep protocol-amplified human leukocyte total RNA samples.

Spearman's rank correlation coefficient of the duplicated microarray expression profiles of the samples amplified using the TargetAmp and MessageAmp II kits were 0.95 and 0.92, respectively, whereas this coefficient for the samples amplified using the standard TotalPrep kit was approximately 1.00 (Figure 2B). Spearman's correlation between the expression profiles of the samples amplified using the TargetAmp kit and standard TotalPrep protocol was 0.83, whereas that between the expression profiles of the samples amplified using the WT-Ovation kit and standard TotalPrep protocol was 0.37 (Figure 2C). The above data suggest that the TargetAmp kit yielded better reproducibility and linearity than the WT-Ovation kit. Accordingly, the TargetAmp kit was used for the rest of the FACS–array experiments.

Overview of Th1–Th2 Microarray Expression Profiles

Spearman's correlation of signal intensities of total probes between individuals among the 13 Th1 and Th2 aRNA samples was higher than 0.89 and 0.87, respectively, except for 1 outlier sample (Sample 3). Among 48,701 transcripts, 5891 transcripts passed the criteria (signal intensity, >50; detection p value, <0.05) in all 12 Th1 microarray data, whereas 5704 transcripts passed the same criteria in all 12 Th2 microarray data, and 5351 transcripts were overlapped between the Th1 and Th2 data sets. Signal intensities of representative Th1- and Th2-specific cytokines are shown in Figure 3A.

The Th1 marker *CXCR3* was expressed in all Th1 samples, and the average signal intensity of *CXCR3* was 17.4-fold higher in the Th1 samples than in the Th2 samples. The average signal intensity of other Th1 markers, *IFNG* and *IL12RB*, in the Th1 samples was 7.5- and 6.3-fold higher than that in the Th2 samples, respectively. On the other hand, the average signal intensity of other Th2 markers, *CCR4*, *GPR44 (CRTH2)*, and *CCR3*, in the Th2 samples was 5.2-, 15.8-, and 24.6-fold higher than that in the Th1 samples, respectively. (Figure 3A).

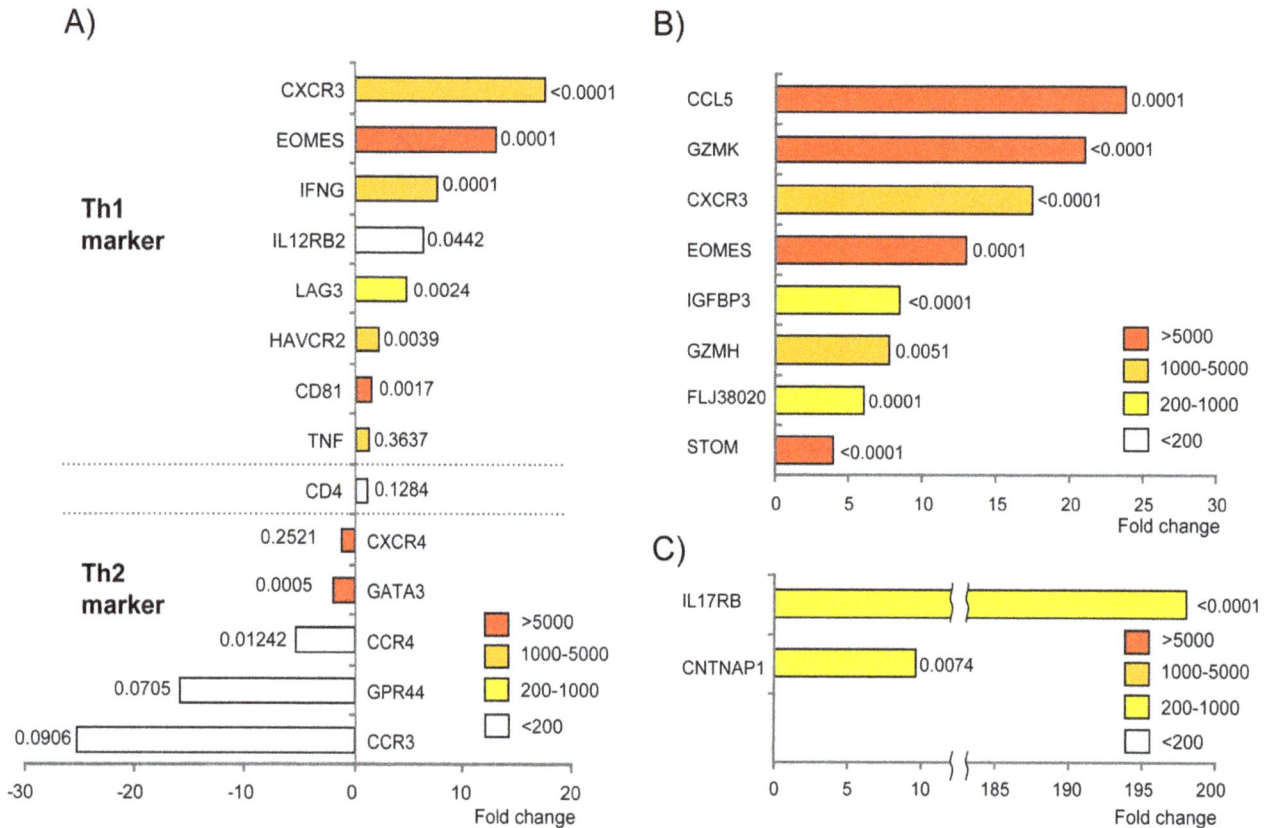

Figure 3. Differences in expression levels of representative genes between human Th1 and Th2 cells. Gene expression profiles of human Th1 and Th2 cells isolated from blood samples of 12 healthy individuals were analyzed using Illumina Human-6v2 Expression BeadChips arrays. Each bar represents a fold change of averaged signal intensity each gene in the Th1 microarray data divided by averaged signal intensity of the same gene in Th2 microarray data. Indicated next to each bar diagram is the *p* value obtained from a paired *t* test to evaluate a difference in signal intensity for each gene between the Th1 and Th2 microarray data from the 12 donors. Colors indicate the signal intensity of genes. Red: a very high expression level (>5000), orange: high level of expression (1000–5000), yellow: medium expression level (200–1000), and white: low expression level (<200). (**A**) Fold changes of well-established Th1 and Th2 genes in the comparison between human Th1 and Th2 microarray data. Positive fold changes mean that transcripts are more abundant in Th1 microarray data than in Th2 data, and negative values indicate the opposite. (**B**) Fold changes of the most prominent Th1-specific genes, which showed a signal intensity of >200 and a fold change of >2 in Th1 microarray data compared with that in Th2 data. (**C**) Fold changes of the most prominent Th2-specific genes, which showed a signal intensity of >200 and a fold change of >2 in Th2 microarray data compared with that in Th1 data.

As novel candidate Th1-specific marker genes, 82 transcripts met the criteria (average signal intensity of >200 in the Th1 samples and >2-fold higher average signal intensity in the Th1 samples than in the Th2 samples analyzed in this study), which are shown in Table S1. Among them, eight genes (*CCL5*, *GZMK*, *CXCR3*, *EOMES*, *IGFBP3*, *GZMH* and *STOM*) showed >2-fold higher signal intensity in the Th1 samples than in the Th2 samples for all individuals (Figure 3A). As for candidate Th2-specific marker genes, 38 transcripts met the criteria (average signal intensity of >200 in the Th2 samples and >2-fold higher average signal intensity in the Th2 samples than in the Th1 samples analyzed in this study), which are shown in Table S2. Among them, two genes [*IL17RB* and (*contactin-associated protein 1 CNTNAP1*] showed >2-fold higher signal intensity in the Th2 samples than in the Th1 samples for all individuals (Figure 3C). Over-representation analysis indicated that genes relevant to the "disulfide bond" category ($p = 7.61E-05$, $p = 0.012$ after Bonferroni correction) and "zymogen" category ($p = 1.23E-04$, $p = 0.018$ after Bonferroni correction) were significantly overrepresented among the 82 Th1-dominant genes, whereas no specific gene category was overrepresented among the 38 Th2-dominant genes (Figure S1).

Immunohistochemical Validation of Th1- and Th2-Dominant Genes Detected in FACS–array Experiments

To evaluate cell type-specific expression at the protein level, we performed immunohistochemical analysis of the protein expression of the novel candidate Th1 and Th2 markers and the coexpression of EOMES, IL17RB, and CNTNAP1 with the Th1-specific transcription factor T-bet (TBX21) and the Th2-specific transcription factor GATA3 (Figure 4A). After confirmation of distinct expression patterns between T-bet and GATA3 (Figure 4A), the coexpression of EOMES with T-bet (Figure 4B) and the coexpression of CNTNAP1 with GATA3 (Figure 4C) were observed among human CD4+ cells. Immunostaining with two specific antibodies to IL17RB failed to produce a signal in any of the human CD4+ cells, which suggests the expression of *IL17RB* mRNA, but not protein, in Th2 cells (data not shown).

The number of total EOMES-positive cells, total T-bet-positive cells, and cells that co-expressed EOMES and T-bet were 103, 93,

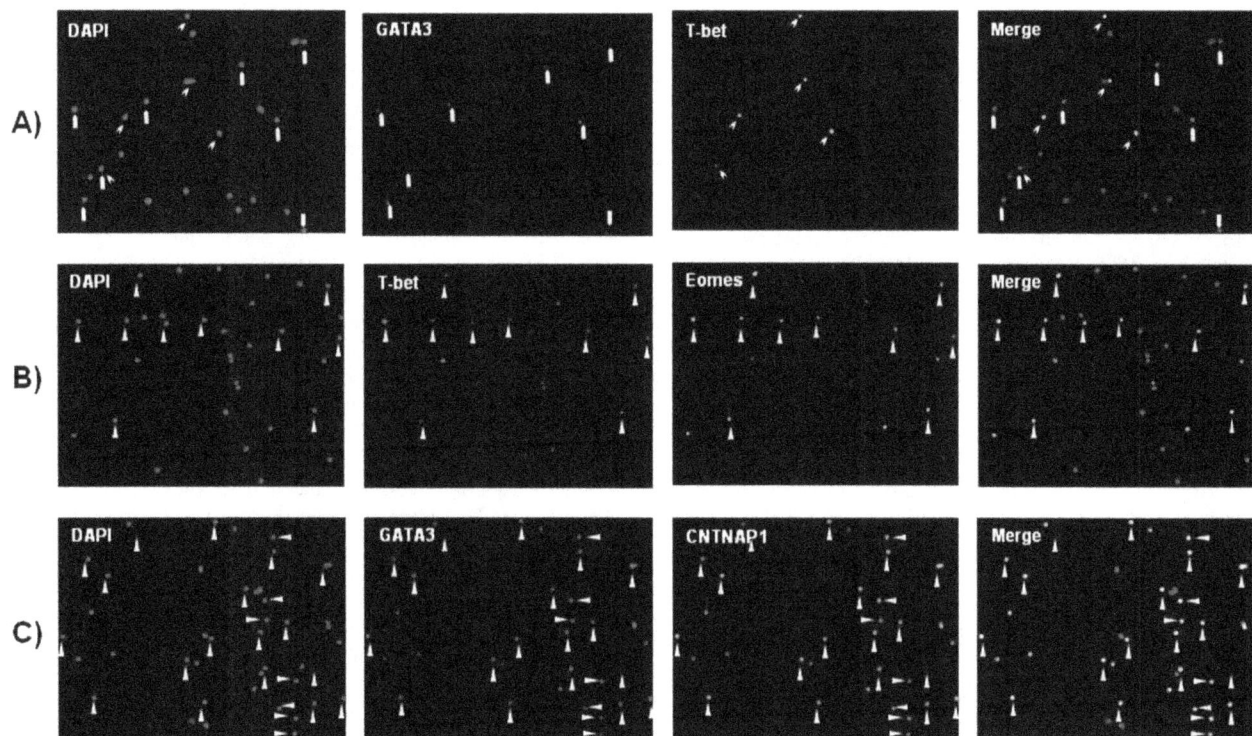

Figure 4. Coexpression of T-bet, GATA-3, and Th1- and Th2-dominant markers in CD4$^+$ cells. (**A**) Costaining of CD4$^+$ cells with antibodies to the Th1-specific transcription factor T-bet (red) and the Th2-specific transcription factor GATA-3 (green) indicated that T-bet$^+$ cells and GATA-3$^+$ cells were distinct cell populations among the CD4$^+$ cells. Cell nuclei were stained with 4,6-diamidino-2-phenylindole (DAPI) (blue). (**B**) Costaining of CD4$^+$ T cells with antibodies to T-bet (red) and EOMES (green) showed that T-bet and EOMES were coexpressed in the CD4$^+$ cells. Cell nuclei were stained with DAPI (blue). (**C**) Costaining of CD4$^+$ cells with antibodies to GATA-3 (red) and CNTNAP1 (green) showed that GATA-3 and CNTNAP1 were coexpressed in the CD4$^+$ cells. Cell nuclei were stained with DAPI (blue).

and 75, respectively. The number of total CNTNAP1-positive cells, total GATA-3-positive cells, and cells that co-expressed CNTNAP1 and GATA-3 were 234, 236, and 234, respectively. Accordingly, the specificity and sensitivity of EOMES as a Th1 cell marker were 73% and 87.2%, respectively, whereas the specificity and sensitivity of CNTNAP1 as a Th2 cell marker were 100% and 99.2%, respectively.

Discussion

Here we established a FACS–array protocol for assessing the gene expression profiles of minor cellular components of blood samples by validating each of the following processes (Figure 1B).

Validity of RNA Extraction Procedures

The amount of RNA in the Th1 (0.26±0.26 pg/cell) and Th2 cells (0.24±0.12 pg/cell) was comparable to that extracted from leukocytes (0.25 pg/cell) in the Biology Data Book [33]. According to the book, the amount of RNA extracted from leukocytes is smaller than that extracted from other tissues, such as liver (2.5 pg/cell), kidney (1.1 pg/cell), and brain (2.6 pg/cell). These data suggest that the gene expression profiling of small populations of leukocytes is difficult. RIN, a widely accepted RNA quality indicator, of the Th1 and Th2 samples was 7.3±2.8 and 8.9±1.1, respectively. The 28S/18S rRNA ratio of the Th1 and Th2 samples was 1.2±0.8 and 1.9±0.5, respectively. Although most of the cells showed high RIN, 34.8% and 8.7% of the Th1 and Th2 cells, respectively, showed RIN of <6.5 or a 28S/18S rRNA ratio of <1.0. Low RIN may be because of damage caused to cells

during sorting (Table 1). Our gene expression profile-based evaluation suggested that samples with RIN of <6.5 or a 28S/18S rRNA ratio of <1.0 should be excluded from the subsequent experiments, an approach that is consistent with previous reports [34].

After exclusion of these samples, the correlation coefficient of any combinations of the remaining samples was >0.95 and inclusion/exclusion of further samples did not significantly affect the gene expression profiling data.

Evaluation of the Amplification System

The amount of total RNA extracted from Th1 and Th2 cells is approximately 30–50 ng/10 ml of a blood sample. On the other hand, the widely used Affymetrix microarray system requires 10 μg of total RNA (www.affymetrix.com), whereas even Illumina BeadChip system, which is one of the microarray systems that uses small amounts of RNA, recommends at least 500 ng of RNA. Therefore, to evaluate the gene expression profiles of minor cellular components, it is essential to amplify total RNA. To date, at least three RNA amplification systems are commercially available: TargetAmp, MessageAmp II, and WT-Ovation. In our study using 100 pg of high-quality total RNA from human lymphocytes, the TargetAmp and WT-Ovation kits, but not the MessageAmp II kit, produced the amount of amplified RNA sufficient for Illumina-based microarray experiments. According to the instruction manuals or comments from technical support of each vendor, the minimum required starting amount of total RNA samples for the TargetAmp or WT-Ovation kit is 10 pg. Nevertheless, the minimum amount for the MessageAmp II kit is 100 pg, which suggests that the first two systems above are suitable for smaller amounts of RNA samples.

The correlation coefficient of the duplicated microarray expression profiles of the samples amplified using the TargetAmp kit was 0.97, and the correlation of gene expression profiles developed using TargetAmp two round-amplified RNA and the standard one round-amplified (TotalPrep) RNA was 0.83. The correlation coefficient of duplicates of WT-Ovation kit-amplified DNA was 0.92. On the other hand, the correlation of gene expression profiles developed using WT-Ovation kit-amplified DNA and the standard one round-amplified RNA was only 0.37, which suggests that TargetAmp is the most reliable two-round amplification system (Figure 2C). The correlation of gene expression profiles developed using TargetAmp and the standard method was higher than that of gene expression profiles developed using WT-Ovation and the standard method. This may indicate that the mode of action of WT-Ovation is different from that of TargetAmp and the standard method, both of which are based on *in vitro* transcription amplification (Figure 2A). WT-Ovation is based on single primer isothermal amplification.

Validity of the FACS–array Procedure, Which is Based on the Measurement of Established Th1 and Th2 Cell Markers

Among Th1 markers, *CXCR3* and *IFNG* showed signal intensities of >1000. On the other hand, the signal intensities of *IL-2* and *T-bet* were below reliably detectable levels in Th1 microarray data, although TBX21 protein expression in CD4$^+$ cells was confirmed using immunohistochemistry (Figure 4). Both of the microarray-detectable genes, *CXCR3* and *IFNG*, showed 5.7- to 139.5-fold and 1.7- to 83.6-fold higher signal intensity, respectively, in Th1 cells than in Th2 cells from the same individuals.

Th2 markers *CCR3*, *CCR4*, and *GPR44* (*CRTH2*) were exclusively expressed in the Th2 cells, while these genes were not expressed in the Th1 cells. Signal intensities of the other major Th2 cytokines, *IL-4*, *IL-5*, and *IL-13*, were below reliably detectable levels in microarray data. Taken together, our data suggest that the FACS–array procedure provides reliable information on the gene expression profiles of certain small populations of immune cells.

Caution is needed when interpreting previous reports indicating that CCR4 is expressed not only on Th2 cells but also on CD25$^+$/CD4$^+$/FOXP3$^+$ regulatory T cells (T$_{reg}$ cells) [35,36]. Although the population of CD4$^+$/CXCR3$^-$/CCR4$^+$ cells constitutes 12.3±4.7% among CD4$^+$ cells in the present study, previous studies indicated that the proportion of CCR4$^+$/CD25$^+$/CD4$^+$/FOXP3$^+$ T$_{reg}$ cells is up to 5% among peripheral CD4$^+$ cells [37]. In addition, average signal intensity for Gata-3 staining of CD4$^+$/CXCR3$^-$/CCR4$^+$ cells is 6550, whereas average signal intensity for FOXP3 is 40. Thus, CD4$^+$/CXCR3$^-$/CCR4$^+$ cells in the present study may include T$_{reg}$ cells to some extent, but the majority of this CD4$^+$CXCR3$^-$CCR4$^+$ population is likely to be Th2 cells.

Novel Th1 and Th2 Marker Genes

In this study, *CCL5*, *GZMK*, *CXCR3*, *EOMES*, *IGFBP3*, *GZMH*, and *STOM* were found to be the most prominent marker genes for distinguishing Th1 cells from Th2 cells. Among them, *CCL5* and *CXCR3* are well-established Th1-specific markers [38,39]. *EOMES* was recently recognized as a transcription factor that participates in T cell differentiation into Th1 cells [40]. Our data show sustained *EOMES* expression in mature Th1 cells,

suggesting that it could serve as a Th1 cell marker in blood samples. Previous reports have indicated that human granzymes, including *GZMK* and *GZMH*, are predominantly expressed in NK cells and CD8$^+$ T cells, whereas the expression levels of these genes are low in CD4$^+$ T cells [41,42]. In our study, in addition to granzymes, NK cell-related genes, *LRG1* and *NKG1*, were exclusively expressed in Th1 cells (Table S1). The Th1-specific transcription factor T-bet, as well as IFN-γ, are also expressed in NK cells [43], which supports the notion that among CD4$^+$ T cells, Th1 cells may have gene expression profiles similar to those of NK cells. To our knowledge, previous findings never linked the expression of *IGFBP3*, and *STOM* with Th1 cells, and our data suggest that these molecules are novel Th1 cell markers.

Our data also indicate that two genes, *IL17RB* and *CNTNAP1*, are Th2 cell markers. IL17RB is the receptor for IL-17B and IL-17E (IL-25), which has been shown to induce Th2 responses. Recent studies revealed that IL17RB is highly expressed on the surface of a subset of naive and activated CD4$^+$ invariant NK T cells. In addition, among CD4$^+$ T cell subpopulations, IL17RB is expressed in activated Th2 central memory cells but not in activated T cells [44,45,46]. Our data show that IL17RB mRNA, but not protein, is expressed in mature Th2 cells. CNTNAP1 is known as neurexin IV. Neurexins are a large family of proteins that act as neuronal cell surface receptors. The function and localization of neurexins, however, have not been elucidated in immune cells. To our knowledge, CNTNAP1 has never been shown to be involved in Th2-specific cellular functions.

To date, Th1 and Th2 cells have been identified using a small number of cell surface markers. There should be heterogeneity among the Th1 and Th2 cells; therefore, there may be additional markers that can be used to identify Th1 and Th2 cell subpopulations. Our data indicate that there are genes that show more pronounced Th1- and Th2-specific gene expression patterns than the established markers. These markers should be tested for the detection of Th1 and Th2 cells or for the classification of T cell populations.

Among them, EOMES and CNTNAP1 were subjected to the protein expression analysis along with T-bet and GATA3 as Th1- and Th2-specific markers, respectively. At the beginning, we decided to validate the findings using cell sorting analysis of CD4$^+$ cells double-stained with antibodies to EOMES and T-bet (or antibodies to CNTNAP1 and GATA-3); however, we could not detect specific signals of these double-stained cells probably because of difficulties with sorting of cells labeled with nuclear protein-specific markers. Therefore, we utilized the immunostaining approach, which is a well-established method for the analysis of nuclear proteins to confirm the coexpression of EOMES and T-bet (or CNTNAP1 and GATA-3). Our data suggest that EOMES and CNTNAP1 may be candidate markers for Th1 and Th2 cells, respectively, at least in immunostaining experiments.

In summary, we developed a FACS–array protocol to characterize the gene expression profiles of specific immune cells in blood samples and successfully applied this protocol to the characterization of the expression profiles of Th1 and Th2 cell populations. Our approach may help to identify aberrations and novel therapeutic or diagnostic targets for the diseases that affect Th1 or Th2 responses.

Supporting Information

Figure S1 Fold change of Th1-dominant genes which belong to significantly over-represented functional categories. Over-representation analysis of Th1 dominant genes indicated that genes relevant to the "disulfide bond" category

$(p = 7.61E-05, \ p = 0.012$ after Bonferroni correction) and "zymogen" category $(p = 1.23E-04, \ p = 0.018$ after Bonferroni correction) were significantly overrepresented. Figure S1 A and B indicate fold changed of Th1 which belong to "disulfide bond" and "zymogen" categories respectively. Th1 cell dominant genes Each bar represents a fold change of averaged signal intensity each gene in the Th1 microarray data divided by averaged signal intensity of the same gene in Th2 microarray data. Colors indicate the signal intensity of genes. Red: a very high expression level ($>$ 5000), orange: high level of expression (1000–5000), yellow: medium expression level (200–1000).
(TIF)

Table S1 Th1-dominant genes. These genes met the following criteria: average signal intensity of $>$200 in Th1 samples, signal intensity is $>$2-fold higher in Th1 samples than in Th2 samples, and the p value of paired Student's t test is $<$0.05

in the comparison of signal intensity between the Th1 and Th2 cells.
(XLSX)

Table S2 Th2-dominant genes. These genes met the following criteria: average signal intensity of $>$200 in Th2 samples, signal intensity is $>$2-fold higher in Th2 cells than in Th1 cells, and the p value of paired Student's t test is $<$0.05 in the comparison of signal intensity between the Th1 and Th2 cells.
(XLSX)

Author Contributions

Performed the experiments: CO. Analyzed the data: CO HT. Wrote the paper: CO HT. Conceived the general study design and organized and supervised all experiments: HT. Designed each experiment and interpreted the results: CO ZY. Advisory for FACS sorting: NI. Assisted with immunohistochemical validation: Y. Kasahara. Assisted with microarray experiments: Y. Kikuchi.

References

1. Haouas H, Haouas S, Uzan G, Hafsia A (2010) Identification of new markers discriminating between myeloid and lymphoid acute leukemia. Hematology 15: 193–203.

2. Staratschek-Jox A, Classen S, Gaarz A, Debey-Pascher S, Schultze JL (2009) Blood-based transcriptomics: leukemias and beyond. Expert Rev Mol Diagn 9: 271–280.

3. Arasappan D, Tong W, Mummaneni P, Fang H, Amur S (2011) Meta-analysis of microarray data using a pathway-based approach identifies a 37-gene expression signature for systemic lupus erythematosus in human peripheral blood mononuclear cells. BMC Med 9: 65.

4. Bansard C, Lequerre T, Derambure C, Vittecoq O, Hiron M, et al. (2011) Gene profiling predicts rheumatoid arthritis responsiveness to IL-1Ra (anakinra). Rheumatology 50: 283–292.

5. Takahashi N, Sato N, Takahashi S, Tojo A (2008) Gene-expression profiles of peripheral blood mononuclear cell subpopulations in acute graft-vs-host disease following cord blood transplantation. Experimental Hematology 36: 1760–1770.

6. Burczynski ME, Peterson RL, Twine NC, Zuberek KA, Brodeur BJ, et al. (2006) Molecular classification of Crohn's disease and ulcerative colitis patients using transcriptional profiles in peripheral blood mononuclear cells. J Mol Diagn 8: 51–61.

7. Dorsam GP, Hoselton SA, Sandy AR, Samarasinghe AE, Vomhof-Dekrey EE, et al. (2010) Gene expression profiling and network analysis of peripheral blood monocytes in a chronic model of allergic asthma. Microbiology and Immunology 54: 558–563.

8. Liu Z, Yelverton RW, Kraft B, Tanner SB, Olsen NJ, et al. (2005) Highly conserved gene expression profiles in humans with allergic rhinitis altered by immunotherapy. Clinical and Experimental Allergy 35: 1581–1590.

9. Gurevich M, Tuller T, Rubinstein U, Or-Bach R, Achiron A (2009) Prediction of acute multiple sclerosis relapses by transcription levels of peripheral blood cells. BMC Med Genomics 2: 46.

10. Chen KD, Chang PT, Ping YH, Lee HC, Yeh CW, et al. (2011) Gene expression profiling of peripheral blood leukocytes identifies and validates ABCB1 as a novel biomarker for Alzheimer's disease. Neurobiology of Disease 43: 698–705.

11. Shehadeh LA, Yu K, Wang L, Guevara A, Singer C, et al. (2010) SRRM2, a potential blood biomarker revealing high alternative splicing in Parkinson's disease. PLoS One 5: e9104.

12. Gardiner E, Beveridge NJ, Wu JQ, Carr V, Scott RJ, et al. (2011) Imprinted DLK1-DIO3 region of 14q32 defines a schizophrenia-associated miRNA signature in peripheral blood mononuclear cells. Molecular Psychiatry.

13. Takahashi M, Hayashi H, Watanabe Y, Sawamura K, Fukui N, et al. (2010) Diagnostic classification of schizophrenia by neural network analysis of blood-based gene expression signatures. Schizophrenia Research 119: 210–218.

14. Suzuki K, Kachala SS, Kadota K, Shen R, Mo Q, et al. (2011) Prognostic immune markers in non-small cell lung cancer. Clinical Cancer Research 17: 5247–5256.

15. Baine MJ, Chakraborty S, Smith LM, Mallya K, Sasson AR, et al. (2011) Transcriptional profiling of peripheral blood mononuclear cells in pancreatic cancer patients identifies novel genes with potential diagnostic utility. PLoS One 6: e17014.

16. Grayson BL, Wang L, Aune TM (2011) Peripheral blood gene expression profiles in metabolic syndrome, coronary artery disease and type 2 diabetes. Genes Immun 12: 341–351.

17. Martinez FO, Gordon S, Locati M, Mantovani A (2006) Transcriptional profiling of the human monocyte-to-macrophage differentiation and polarization: new molecules and patterns of gene expression. J Immunol 177: 7303–7311.

18. Saldanha-Araujo F, Haddad R, Malmegrim de Farias KC, Alves Souza AD, Palma PV, et al. (2011) Mesenchymal stem cells promote the sustained expression of CD69 on activated T-lymphocytes: roles of canonical and non-canonical NF-kappaB signaling. J Cell Mol Med.

19. Lobo MK, Karsten SL, Gray M, Geschwind DH, Yang XW (2006) FACS-array profiling of striatal projection neuron subtypes in juvenile and adult mouse brains. Nat Neurosci 9: 443–452.

20. Marsh ED, Minarcik J, Campbell K, Brooks-Kayal AR, Golden JA (2008) FACS-array gene expression analysis during early development of mouse telencephalic interneurons. Dev Neurobiol 68: 434–445.

21. Beliakova-Bethell N, Massanella M, White C, Lada SM, Du P, et al. (2014) The effect of cell subset isolation method on gene expression in leukocytes. Cytometry A 85: 94–104.

22. Liles WC, Van Voorhis WC (1995) Review: nomenclature and biologic significance of cytokines involved in inflammation and the host immune response. J Infect Dis 172: 1573–1580.

23. Romagnani S (2004) Immunologic influences on allergy and the TH1/TH2 balance. J Allergy Clin Immunol 113: 395–400.

24. Romagnani S (1994) Lymphokine production by human T cells in disease states. Annu Rev Immunol 12: 227–257.

25. Myint AM, Leonard BE, Steinbusch HW, Kim YK (2005) Th1, Th2, and Th3 cytokine alterations in major depression. J Affect Disord 88: 167–173.

26. Elenkov IJ, Chrousos GP (1999) Stress Hormones, Th1/Th2 patterns, Pro/Anti-inflammatory Cytokines and Susceptibility to Disease. Trends Endocrinol Metab 10: 359–368.

27. Riedel M, Spellmann I, Schwarz MJ, Strassnig M, Sikorski C, et al. (2007) Decreased T cellular immune response in schizophrenic patients. J Psychiatr Res 41: 3–7.

28. Pavon L, Sandoval-Lopez G, Eugenia Hernandez M, Loria F, Estrada I, et al. (2006) Th2 cytokine response in Major Depressive Disorder patients before treatment. J Neuroimmunol 172: 156–165.

29. Rook GA, Zumla A (1997) Gulf War syndrome: is it due to a systemic shift in cytokine balance towards a Th2 profile? Lancet 349: 1831–1833.

30. Heizmann O, Koeller M, Muhr G, Oertli D, Schinkel C (2008) Th1- and Th2-type cytokines in plasma after major trauma. J Trauma 65: 1374–1378.

31. Kidd P (2003) Th1/Th2 balance: the hypothesis, its limitations, and implications for health and disease. Altern Med Rev 8: 223–246.

32. Hamalainen H, Zhou H, Chou W, Hashizume H, Heller R, et al. (2001) Distinct gene expression profiles of human type 1 and type 2 T helper cells. Genome Biol 2: RESEARCH0022.

33. Altman PL, Dittmer DS (1972) Biology Data Book Federation of American Societies for Experimental Biology.

34. Giusti B, Rossi L, Lapini I, Magi A, Pratesi G, et al. (2009) Gene expression profiling of peripheral blood in patients with abdominal aortic aneurysm. Eur J Vasc Endovasc Surg 38: 104–112.

35. Hirahara K, Liu L, Clark RA, Yamanaka K, Fuhlbrigge RC, et al. (2006) The majority of human peripheral blood CD4+CD25highFoxp3+ regulatory T cells bear functional skin-homing receptors. J Immunol 177: 4488–4494.

36. Baatar D, Olkhanud P, Sumitomo K, Taub D, Gress R, et al. (2007) Human peripheral blood T regulatory cells (Tregs), functionally primed CCR4+ Tregs and unprimed CCR4- Tregs, regulate effector T cells using FasL. J Immunol 178: 4891–4900.

37. Takahashi R, Kano Y, Yamazaki Y, Kimishima M, Mizukawa Y, et al. (2009) Defective regulatory T cells in patients with severe drug eruptions: timing of the dysfunction is associated with the pathological phenotype and outcome. J Immunol 182: 8071–8079.

38. Kondo T, Nakazawa H, Ito F, Hashimoto Y, Osaka Y, et al. (2006) Favorable prognosis of renal cell carcinoma with increased expression of chemokines associated with a Th1-type immune response. Cancer Sci 97: 780–786.

39. Dorner BG, Scheffold A, Rolph MS, Huser MB, Kaufmann SH, et al. (2002) MIP-1alpha, MIP-1beta, RANTES, and ATAC/lymphotactin function together with IFN-gamma as type 1 cytokines. Proc Natl Acad Sci U S A 99: 6181–6186.

40. Suto A, Wurster AL, Reiner SL, Grusby MJ (2006) IL-21 inhibits IFN-gamma production in developing Th1 cells through the repression of Eomesodermin expression. J Immunol 177: 3721–3727.

41. Sedelies KA, Sayers TJ, Edwards KM, Chen W, Pellicci DG, et al. (2004) Discordant regulation of granzyme H and granzyme B expression in human lymphocytes. J Biol Chem 279: 26581–26587.

42. Bade B, Boettcher HE, Lohrmann J, Hink-Schauer C, Bratke K, et al. (2005) Differential expression of the granzymes A, K and M and perforin in human peripheral blood lymphocytes. Int Immunol 17: 1419–1428.

43. Szabo SJ, Kim ST, Costa GL, Zhang X, Fathman CG, et al. (2000) A novel transcription factor, T-bet, directs Th1 lineage commitment. Cell 100: 655–669.

44. Chtanova T, Tangye SG, Newton R, Frank N, Hodge MR, et al. (2004) T follicular helper cells express a distinctive transcriptional profile, reflecting their role as non-Th1/Th2 effector cells that provide help for B cells. J Immunol 173: 68–78.

45. Wang H, Mobini R, Fang Y, Barrenas F, Zhang H, et al. Allergen challenge of peripheral blood mononuclear cells from patients with seasonal allergic rhinitis increases IL-17RB, which regulates basophil apoptosis and degranulation. Clin Exp Allergy.

46. Stock P, Lombardi V, Kohlrautz V, Akbari O (2009) Induction of airway hyperreactivity by IL-25 is dependent on a subset of invariant NKT cells expressing IL-17RB. J Immunol 182: 5116–5122.

5

25-Hydroxyvitamin D3-Deficiency Enhances Oxidative Stress and Corticosteroid Resistance in Severe Asthma Exacerbation

Nan Ian[1]❂, Guangyan Luo[2]❂, Xiaoqiong Yang[1], Yuanyuan Cheng[1], Yun zhang[1], Xiaoyun Wang[1], Xing Wang[1], Tao Xie[1], Guoping Li[1,3]*, Zhigang Liu[3]*, Nanshan Zhong[4]*

1 Inflammations & Allergic Diseases Research Unit, Affiliated Hospital of Luzhou Medical College, Luzhou, 646000, Sichuan, China, 2 Hygiene Section, Luzhou Medical College, Luzhou, 646000, Sichuan, China, 3 State Key Laboratory of Respiratory Disease for Allergy at Shengzhen University, School of Medicine, Shenzhen University, Nanhai Ave 3688, Shenzhen, Guangdong, 518060, PR China, 4 State Key Laboratory of Respiratory Disease, Guangzhou Medical University, Guangdong, 510120, PR China

Abstract

Oxidative stress plays a significant role in exacerbation of asthma. The role of vitamin D in oxidative stress and asthma exacerbation remains unclear. We aimed to determine the relationship between vitamin D status and oxidative stress in asthma exacerbation. Severe asthma exacerbation patients with 25-hydroxyvitamin D3-deficiency (V-D deficiency) or 25-hydroxyvitamin D-sufficiency (V-D sufficiency) were enrolled. Severe asthma exacerbation with V-D-deficiency showed lower forced expiratory volume in one second (FEV1) compared to that with V-D-sufficiency. V-D-deficiency intensified ROS release and DNA damage and increased TNF-α, OGG1 and NFκB expression and NFκB phosphorylation in severe asthma exacerbation. Supplemental vitamin D3 significantly increased the rates of FEV1 change and decreased ROS and DNA damage in V-D-deficiency. Vitamin D3 inhibited LPS-induced ROS and DNA damage and were associated with a decline in TNF-α and NFκB in epithelial cells. H_2O_2 reduces nuclear translocation of glucocorticoid receptors in airway epithelial cell lines. V-D pretreatment enhanced the dexamethasone-induced nuclear translocation of glucocorticoid receptors in airway epithelial cell lines and monocytes from 25-hydroxyvitamin D3-deficiency asthma patients. These findings indicate that V-D deficiency aggravates oxidative stress and DNA damage, suggesting a possible mechanism for corticosteroid resistance in severe asthma exacerbation.

Editor: Anil Kumar, University of Missouri-Kansas City, United States of America

Funding: This project was supported by Chinese National Science Foundation Grant 81170032. The funders had no role in study design, data collection and analysis, decision to publish, or preparation of the manuscript.

Competing Interests: The authors have declared that no competing interests exist.

* Email: lzlgp@163.com (G. Li); lzg195910@126.com (ZL); nanshan@vip.163.com (NZ)

❂ These authors contributed equally to this work.

Background

Severe asthma is unresponsive to treatment, including systemically administered corticosteroids [1]. Asthma exacerbation results in oral steroid use, an emergency room visit, or hospitalization [2]. Severe asthma is defined as asthma that requires treatment with high dose inhaled corticosteroids plus a second controller and/or systemic corticosteroids to prevent it from becoming "uncontrolled" or that remains "uncontrolled" despite this therapy [3]. The multiple risk factors for asthma exacerbation include a complex mix of environmental, immunological and host genetic factors. Epidemiological studies have shown that low serum 25-hydroxyvitamin D3 levels are associated with a higher risk of upper and lower respiratory infections [4]. Vitamin D status has a linear relationship with respiratory infections and lung function [5], and V-D deficiency (a serum 25 (OH) D3 <30 ng/ml) has been associated with severe asthma exacerbation [6].

An endotoxin is a common environmental contaminant that causes asthma exacerbation [7]. Environmental endotoxins modulate the exacerbation of asthma. High levels of endotoxins are associated with asthma symptoms and current use of asthma medication. Endotoxins augment atopic inflammation and induce cellular steroid resistance [8,9]. Corticosteroid-resistant asthma demonstrates the airway expansion of specific gram-negative bacteria [10]. The underlying mechanisms by which endotoxins modulate asthma are not completely understood. Oxidative stress is an important aspect of the host innate immune response to foreign pathogens such as bacterial lipopolysaccharides (LPS). Excessive activation of redox signaling might lead to pathologic endothelial cell (EC) activation and barrier dysfunction [11]. Invading pathogens might result in overwhelming lung production of reactive oxygen species (ROS). Oxidants initiate inflammation of the airways, which might contribute to the pathogenesis and/or exacerbation of airway diseases [12]. Oxidative stress is associated with DNA damage, which is frequently induced by ROS released from neutrophils or respiratory tract epithelial cells [13].

It has recently been shown that an imbalance between oxidants and antioxidants is associated with oxidative stress, which plays a key role in the severity of asthma [14]. One study shows that Vitamin D supplementation could replenish blood levels and lower oxidative stress and cardiovascular disease [15]. Vitamin D exhibited therapeutic and preventive effects against oxidative stress, hepatic, pancreatic and renal injury in alloxan-induced diabetes in rats [16]. Vitamin D played a role against cellular stress in breast epithelial cells [17]. However, whether oxidative stress and DNA damage are associated with asthma exacerbation and the vitamin D status is unknown. To address this question, we studied the effect of the vitamin D status on oxidative stress and DNA damage in patients with severe asthma exacerbation and in LPS-stimulated cells.

Methods

Subjects

Asthma patients with acute exacerbation were admitted to the respiratory department of the affiliated hospital of Luzhou medical college (a 3000-bed hospital in Luzhou City, Sichuan, China), Luzhou, China, between September 2011 and December 2012. Acute exacerbation of asthma was defined as a worsening of asthma symptoms including shortness of breath, cough, wheezing, chest tightness, or a combination of these symptoms. Severe asthma exacerbations were defined as those that required treatment with systemic corticosteroids [18]. Patients with a radiological diagnosis of pneumonia, impaired consciousness on admission or smoking history >10 packs/year were excluded from the study. The serum levels of 25-hydroxyvitamin D3 (vitamin D3) were measured at the beginning of the study. We categorized this measurement into deficiency ($\leq$30 ng/mL) and sufficiency (>30 ng/mL) categories based on a previous report [19]. The forced expiratory volume in one second (FEV1) was measured with a Jaeger Lung Function Analyzer (Jaeger Co., H chberg, Germany).

Ethics statement

The study was approved by the Ethics Committee of the Affiliated Hospital of Luzhou Medical College (KY2013014). The participants provided their written informed consent to participate in this study. The Ethics Committee of the Affiliated Hospital of Luzhou Medical College approved the use of written consent.

Therapy of asthma exacerbations

Asthmatic patients with severe asthma exacerbation were treated with 80 mg/day of methylprednisolone for 7 days [18]. The asthma patients with V-D-deficiency were randomly divided into V-D-supplement group and no V-D-supplement group. The asthma patients with V-D-deficiency in V-D-supplement group were intramuscularly injected with 7.5 mg vitamin of D3 at day 1 and 4.

Measurement of vitamin D3, TNF-α and SOD in serum

The serum vitamin D3 and tumor necrosis factor-α (TNF-αwere determined in triplicate samples from each patient by enzyme-linked immunosorbent assay (ELISA). The ELISA kits for TNF-α were purchased from R&D Systems (Minneapolis, MN). The ELISA kits for vitamin D3 were purchased from IBL (Germany). The superoxide dismutases (SOD) activity in serum was measured using the SOD assay kit WST (Nanjing Jiancheng Bioengineering Institute, China).

Mononuclear cell separation

The peripheral blood obtained from the asthma patients and normal donors was processed for separation of mononuclear cells. Peripheral blood was diluted 1:1 with sterile phosphate-buffered saline (PBS), layered over Ficoll-Hypaque (GE Healthcare Bio-Sciences AB, Stockholm, Sweden) and centrifuged at 1500 rpm for 15 min at room temperature. Peripheral blood mononuclear cells (PBMC) were collected from the interphase layer and washed with PBS. PBMC were resuspended with RPMI-1640 medium.

Airway epithelial cells culture

After the human airway epithelial cells (16HBE) had grown to 85% confluence in 6-well plastic plates containing DMEM/F12 culture medium with 10% of foetal calf serum (FCS), the medium was replaced with a serum-free DMEM/F12 culture medium. The cells were then treated with LPS and/or 100 nM 1, 25(OH) 2 D3 (CAT. # 083M4033V, Sigma) in a serum-free culture medium.

Measurement of ROS in PBMC and cultured epithelial cells

The cells were loaded with 10 μM H2DCF-DA (Invitrogen, Molecular Probes, USA) or 10 μM dihydroethidium (DHE) at 37°C for 30 minutes according to the manufacturer's instructions. After removing the excess probes, the cells were kept at 37°C with 5% CO_2. The fluorescence intensity was detected by a flow cytometer (Beckman Coulter, US) and a Leica TCS SP5 confocal microscope (Leica, Germany). For each sample, 10,000 events were collected.

Measurement of DNA damage in PBMC and cultured epithelial cells

A comet assay was used to detect the DNA damage and was performed as previously described [20]. A total of 10 μl of cell suspension containing 20,000 cells was mixed with 90 μl of low-melting-point agarose (LMA) (Sigma) in PBS at 37°C and layered onto slides, which had been coated with normal melting point agarose. The slides were submersed in a freshly prepared cold (4°C) lysis solution (2.5 M NaCl, 100 mM EDTA-2Na, 10 mM Tris–HCl at pH 10-10.5, 1% Triton X-100 and 10% DMSO) for 2 hours. The slides were immersed in fresh electrophoresis buffer at 4°C for 30 min and then electrophoresed (25 V/300 Ma) for 25 min. After electrophoresis, the slides were stained with ethidium bromide, covered with a coverslip and analyzed using a Leica TCS SP5 confocal microscope (Leica, Germany). Comet Assay IV software was used to assess the DNA damage score.

Immunocytochemistry

PBMCs were incubated with dexamethasone (1 μM) or 1, 25(OH) 2 D3 (100 nM) for 30 minutes. PBMCs were immuno-stained for glucocorticoid receptor antibodies (1:500 dilution) (sc-1004, Santa Cruz Biotechnology). Tetramethylrhodamine isothio-cyanate (TRITC)–conjugated anti-rabbit secondary Abs or fluorescein isothiocyanate (FITC)-were used to probe the primary Abs. The nucleus was stained with DAPI reagent. The slides were analyzed with a Leica TCS SP5 confocal microscope (Leica, Germany).

Western blot

Cells were homogenized in radioimmunoprecipitation assay (RIPA) lysis buffer for the western blot analysis. Lysates (20 μg) were run on 10% SDS polyacrylamide gel at 100 V for 2 hours and transferred to a microporous polyvinylidene difluoride (PVDF) membrane at 100 mA for 2 hours. The membrane was blotted with goat polyclonal OGG-1 antibodies (1:1000)(CAT. # sc-12076), mouse polyclonal actin antibodies (1:1000)(CAT. # sc-8432), mouse polyclonal NFκB antibodies (1:1000) (CAT. # sc-8414), and phospho- NFκB rabbit polyclonal antibodies (Ser311 of p65, 1:1000) (CAT. # sc-166748) (Santa Cruz Biotechnology, Inc.) and processed via enhanced chemiluminescence (Pierce) [21].

Statistical analysis

The data are expressed as the mean ± standard error. The statistical analysis was performed using ANOVA (Tukey's post hoc) or Student's t-test and the level of significance was defined as $P<0.05$ between any 2 groups. The data were analyzed using SPSS 13.0 software.

Results

Description of asthma with severe asthma

The clinical characteristics of asthma with severe asthma exacerbation are presented in Table 1. The mean age and gender of the patients with severe asthma exacerbation and V-D-deficiency (vitamin D3 <30 ng/ml) or V-D-sufficiency (vitamin D3>30 ng/ml) were not significantly different from the mean age and gender of the normal controls. Severe asthma exacerbation showed increased peripheral white blood cell counts and neutrophils compared to those in the normal controls ($p = 0.001$). Severe asthma exacerbation with V-D-deficiency or V-D-sufficiency showed higher PCO_2 and lower PO_2; however, there was no difference in the PCO_2 and PO_2 between severe asthma exacerbation with V-D-deficiency and V-D-sufficiency (Table 1, $p = 0.067$). Severe asthma exacerbation with V-D-deficiency did not show a difference in the endotoxin level compared to that in severe asthma exacerbation with V-D-sufficiency (Table 1, $p = 0.056$).

V-D-deficiency enhances oxidative stress and DNA damage in severe asthma exacerbation

The effects of oxidative stress on asthma remain unclear. ROS level and DNA damage in PBMCs from the normal controls, severe asthma exacerbation and V-D-deficiency or V-D-sufficiency were directly measured.Using an ROS probe, we found that severe asthma exacerbation exhibited increased ROS in PBMC compared to that in the normal controls. V-D-deficiency showed increased ROS-positive cells and ROS density in severe asthma exacerbation compared to that in V-D-sufficiency (vitamin D> 30 ng/ml) (Figure 1A and B, $p = 0.0001$ and $0.00012, n = 16$). Additionally, DNA damage in PBMC was detected by comet assay. DNA damage in PBMC exhibited differential increases in severe asthma exacerbation. A total damage score for each slide in V-D-deficiency was significantly increased compared to the scores in V-D-sufficiency (Figure 1C, $p = 0.002, n = 16$). These results indicate that V-D-deficiency shown increased oxidative stress and DNA damage in severe asthma exacerbation.

V-D-deficiency showed lower FEV1%, SOD and increased TNF-α, NFκB in severe asthma exacerbation

To reflect the physiological relevance of Vitamin D deficiency, we evaluated FEV1%. We found that FEV1% was significantly decreased in severe asthma exacerbation compared to the normal controls (. V-D-deficiency patients (n = 16) showed lower FEV1% in severe asthma exacerbation compared to V-D-sufficiency patients (n = 16) (p = 0.015, Figure 2A). It was demonstrated that SOD is inactivated in bronchial brush material obtained from patients with mild asthma [22]. In this study, the serum SOD value in V-D-deficiency (n = 16) was significantly decreased compared to that in V-D-sufficiency ($p = 0.0018$, Figure 2B). The results indicate that V-D-deficiency aggravated the oxidative milieu changes in severe asthma exacerbation. TNF-α is a critical proinflammatory cytokine that might play an important role in severe refractory disease [23]. In our studies, serum TNF-α in V-D-deficiency in severe asthma exacerbation (n = 16) was significantly increased compared to that in V-D-sufficiency (n = 16) ($p = 0.028$, Figure 2C). Severe asthma exacerbation increased the expression and phosphorylation of NFκB in V-D-deficiency and V-D-sufficiency compared to that in the normal controls. V-D-deficiency increased the expression and phosphorylation of NFκB in severe asthma exacerbation compared to that in V-D-sufficiency (Figure 2D). Additionally, 8-Oxoguanine-DNA glycosylase (OGG-1) is a base excision DNA repair enzyme associated with oxidative stress damage [21]. In this study, V-D-deficiency increased the OGG1 expression in severe asthma exacerbation compared to that in V-D-sufficiency (Figure 2D). These results indicate that V-D-deficiency is associated with increased expres-

Table 1. Characteristics of severe asthma exacerbation.

	control	vitamin D>30ng/ml	vitamin D>30ng/ml
sample	16	16	16
Age(year)	46±4	45±15	50±10
Sexes	8F 8M	9F 7M	8F 8M
Leucocyte10*9	7.5±1.8	11.2±4	12.97±4.7
Neutrophils10*9	4.7±1.0	8. 9±4.5	10.6±4.4
Lymphocyte10*9	2.0±1.7	1.5±1.0	1.3±0.5
Eosinophils 10*9	0.25±0.04	0.20±0.09	0.19±0.13
PO2(mmHg)		57±10	53±22
PCO2(mmHg)		56±6	60±12
PH		7.4±0.03	7.32±0.06
Endotoxin(pg/ml)		19.15±4.95	21.91±7.06
FEV1%	92.56±9.14	42.5±3.98	32.25±4.02

*Statistically significant (P ≤ 0.05). F for female, and M for male.

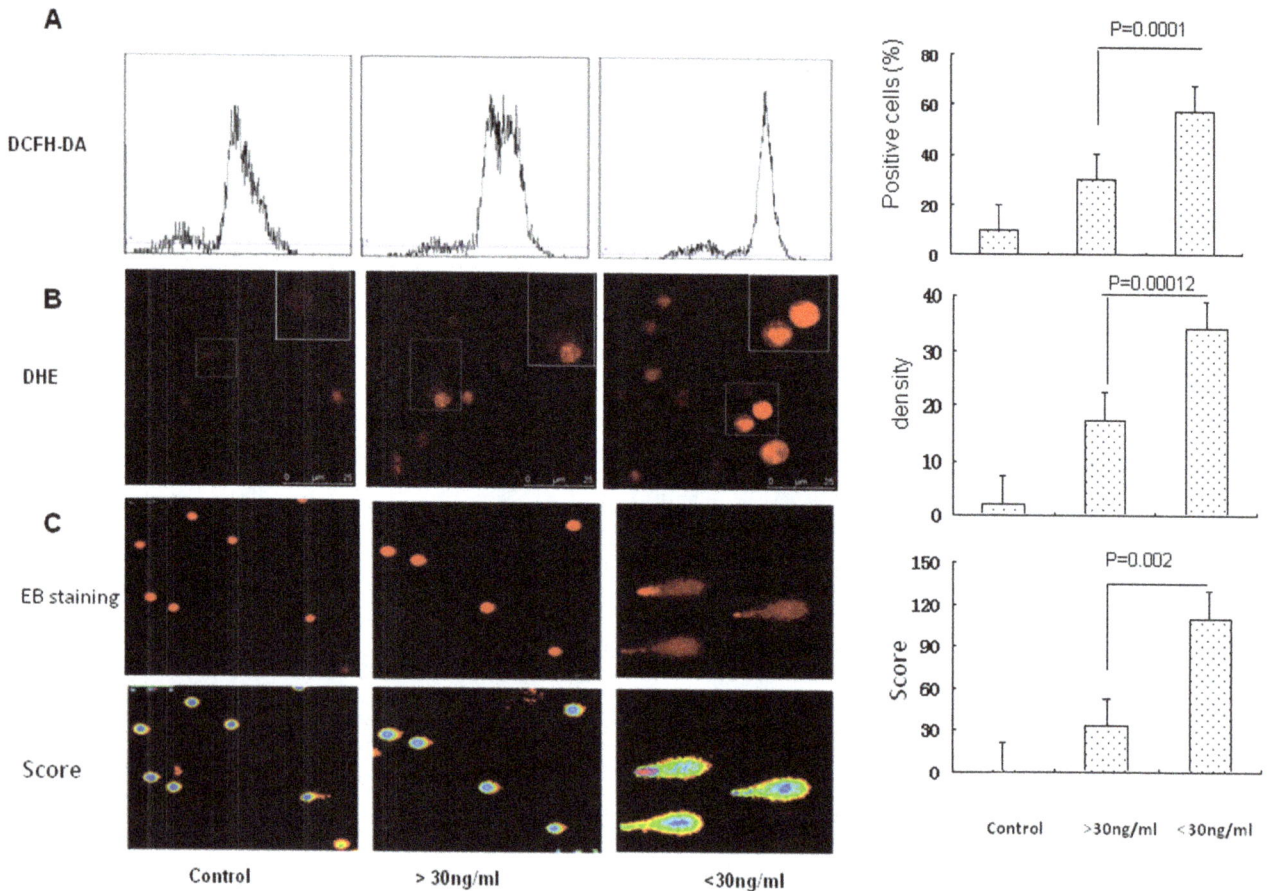

Figure 1. Oxidative stress and DNA damage in severe asthma exacerbation. A: The intracelluar ROS levels in PBMCs from the normal controls, severe asthma exacerbation and V-D-deficiency (vitamin D3 <30 ng/ml) or V-D-sufficiency (vitamin D3>30 ng/ml) were detected by flow cytometry using DCFH-DA, which is oxidized to DCF in the presence of ROS. The ROS level was represented by the percentage of ROS positive cells. B: The intracellular ROS levels in PBMCs from these asthmatic participants were detected by a confocal microscope using a DHE probe. The ROS level in PBMCs from these asthmatic participants was represented by the fluorescence intensity (X400). C: The DNA damage in PBMCs from these asthmatic participants was detected by comet assay using a confocal microscope(X400). The DNA damage score was analyzed with **Comet Assay IV** software.

sion levels of TNF-α, OGG1 and NFκB as well as NFκB phosphorylation.

V-D-deficiency decreased the corticosteroid response in severe asthma exacerbation

Oxidative stress contributes to the low response to glucocorticoids through the down-regulation of histone deacetylase (HDAC) activity [24]. In this study, the asthma patients with severe asthma exacerbation were treated with 80 mg/day of methylprednisolone for 7 days. The asthma patients with V-D-deficiency in V-D supplement (n = 8) were additionally injected with 7.5 mg vitamin of D3 at day 1 and 4. The FEV1%, ROS levels and DNA damage were detected after 7 days. The rates of FEV1 change in the V-D-deficiency patients treated with methylprednisolone (no V-D supplement,n = 8) were significantly lower than those in the V-D-sufficiency patients treated with methylprednisolone and vitamin D3 (n = 8) (p = 0.036, Figure 3A). These results demonstrated that V-D-deficiency decreased the corticosteroid response in severe asthma exacerbation. Vitamin D3 administration significantly increased the rates of FEV1 in the V-D-deficiency patients treated with methylprednisolone (V-D supplement, n = 8) (p = 0.0002,

Figure 3A). These results indicate that vitamin D3 improved the response to methylprednisolone in severe asthma exacerbation with V-D-deficiency. The ROS levels in the V-D-deficiency patients treated with methylprednisolone were significantly higher than those in the V-D-sufficiency patients treated with methylprednisolone (Figure 3B, p = 0.0001). The ROS levels were significantly decreased in the V-D-deficiency patients treated with methylprednisolone and vitamin D3 (V-D supplement, n = 8) compared to the ROS levels in the V-D-sufficiency patients treated with methylprednisolone (no V-D supplement,n = 8) (Figure 3B, P = 0.0003). The DNA damage scores in the V-D-deficiency patients treated with methylprednisolone were significantly increased, compared to the DNA damage scores of the V-D-sufficiency patients treated with methylprednisolone (Figure 3C, P = 0.0001). In the V-D-deficiency asthma patients treated with methylprednisolone, the DNA damage scores in the patients treated with vitamin D3 (V-D supplement, n = 8) were significantly decreased compared to the patients treated without vitamin D3 (no V-D supplement, n = 8) (Figure 3C, P = 0.0001). These data suggest that supplemental vitamin D3 decreased oxidative stress in severe asthma exacerbation with V-D deficiency

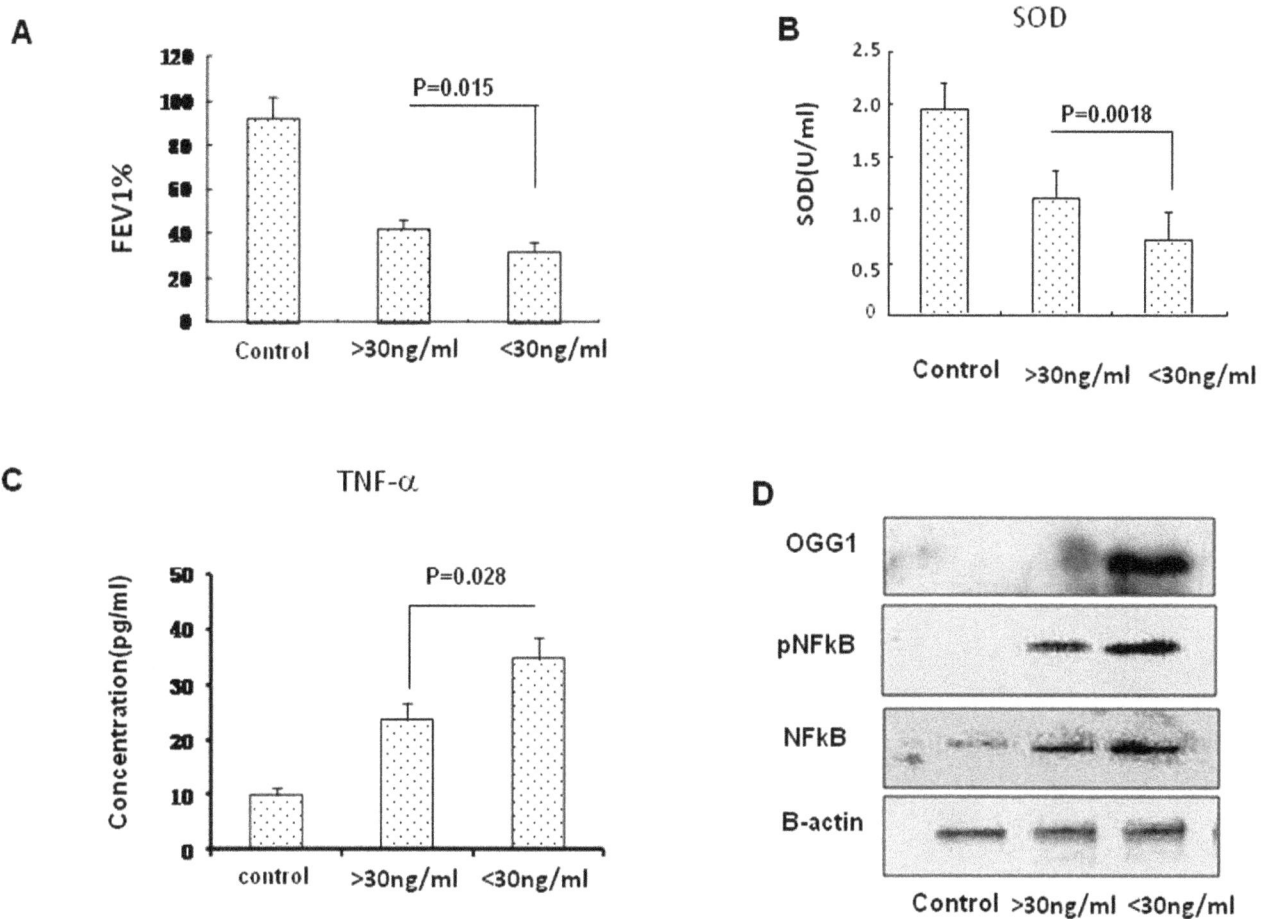

Figure 2. FEV1%, SOD activity, TNF-α, OGG1 and NFκB in severe asthma exacerbation. A: FEV1% in severe asthma exacerbation with V-D-deficiency and V-D-sufficiency. B: The serum SOD activity was measured using an SOD assay kit. C: Standard ELISA was performed to determine the levels of TNF-α in serum. D: OGG1 and NFκB in PBMC from severe asthma exacerbation with V-D-deficiency and V-D-sufficiency were analyzed by western blot. β-actin was used as the loading controls. The data are the means ± SEM.

Vitamin D3 inhibited LPS-induced oxidative stress and TNF-α and NFκB in airway epithelial cells

High endotoxin levels have been detected in bronchoalveolar lavage (BAL) fluid from subjects with corticosteroid-resistant (CR) asthma. LPS exposure contributes to CR asthma [8]. To assess the effect of vitamin D3 on LPS-induced oxidative stress and DNA damage, airway epithelial cells (16HBE) were stimulated with LPS for 24 hours, and vitamin D3 was added. Using a ROS probe, we found that LPS prime increased the ROS-positive cells compared to the control cells, and vitamin D3 decreased the ROS-positive cells, compared to the LPS-stimulated cells (Figure 4A). LPS caused oxidative stress. The DNA damage scores in the LPS-stimulated cells were significantly increased compared to that in the control cells. The vitamin D3 supply decreased the DNA damage scores compared to that in the LPS-stimulated cells (without vitamin D3) (Figure 4B). TNF-α was significantly increased in the LPS-stimulated cells compared to in the control cells. Vitamin D3 inhibited TNF-α in the LPS-stimulated cells (Figure 4C). The effect of vitamin D3 on LPS–induced NFκB remains unclear. Figure 4D shows that 10 μg/ml LPS significantly increased the expression and phosphorylation of NFκB, and vitamin D3 inhibited the LPS-induced expression and phosphorylation of NFκB (Figure 4D).

Vitamin D3 inhibited H_2O_2-induced oxidative stress and increased the nuclear translocation of the glucocorticoid receptors

Glucocorticoid receptor (GR) nuclear translocation play a critical role in glucocorticoid therapy [25]. However, 1, 25(OH) 2 D3 impacts GR nuclear translocation in asthma remains unclear. To assess the effect of vitamin D3 on GR nuclear translocation in H_2O_2-induced oxidative stress, airway epithelial cells (16HBE) were stimulated with H_2O_2 for 1 hours in the presence or absence of 1, 25(OH) 2D3. Treatment of 16HBE cells with 100nM μg H_2O_2 induced ROS production as compared to untreated 16HBE cells with 1, 25(OH) 2 D3. Pretreatment of 16HBE cells with 10nM and 100nM 1, 25(OH) 2 D3 for 1 hours caused a significant decrease in ROS in H_2O_2-stimulated 16HBE cells as compared to untreated 16HBE cells with 1, 25(OH) 2 D3 (Figure 5A). It have been confirmed that H2O2 inhibited the ligand-stimulated nuclear translocation of glucocorticoid receptor [26]. The effect of 1, 25(OH) 2 D3 on GR nuclear translocation in H_2O_2-stimulated cells has not been demonstrated. In our studies, H_2O_2 decreased GR nuclear translocation in 16HBE cells following dexamethasone stimulation, which induced GR nuclear translocation. 1, 25-hydroxyvitamin D3 pretreatment enhanced the dexamethasone induced-GR nuclear translocation in H_2O_2-stimulated cells (Figure 5B). To evaluate the clinical relevance of

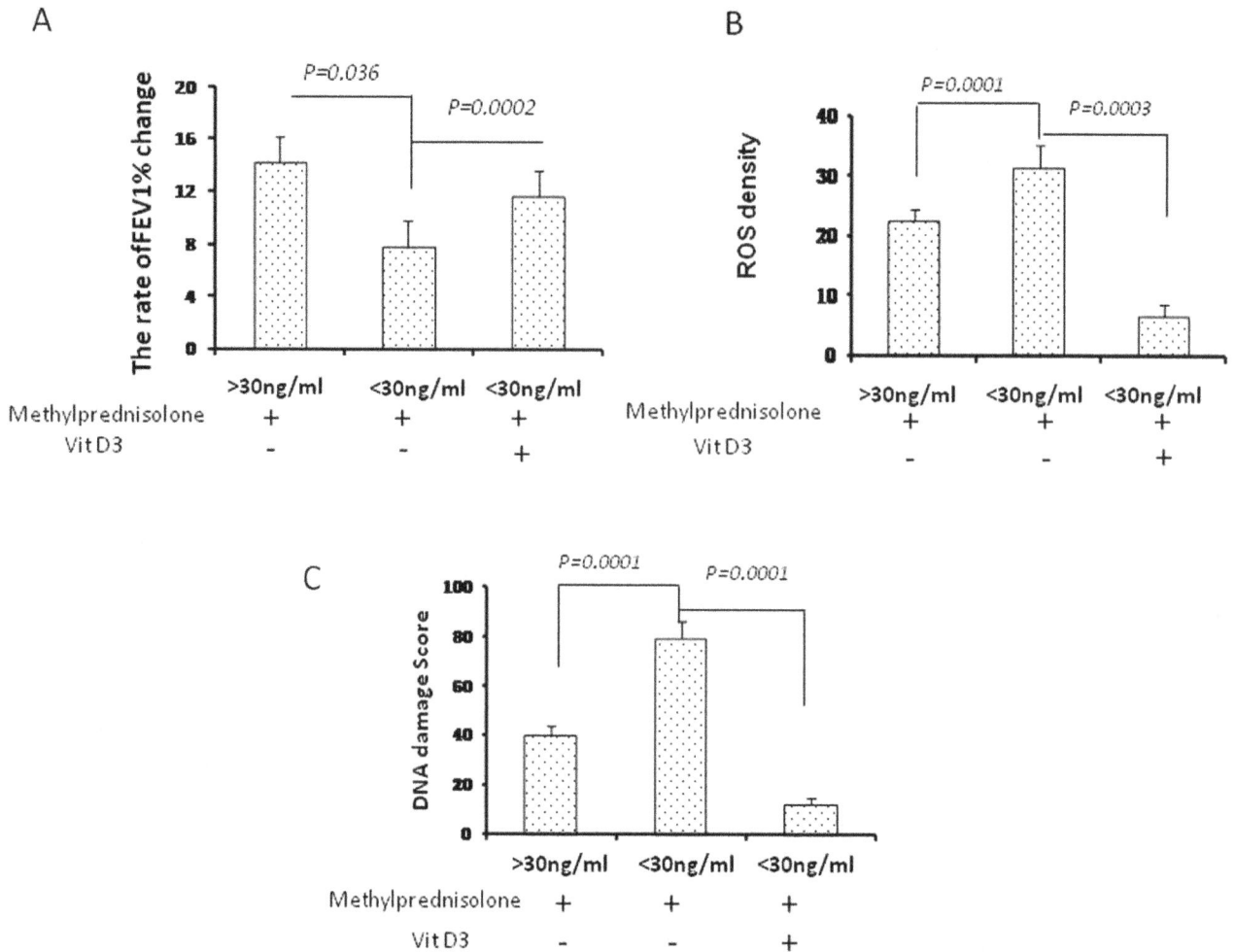

Figure 3. The change in FEV1%, ROS and DNA damage in severe asthma exacerbation treated with methylprednisolone and vitamin D3. A: The rates of the FEV1 change in severe asthma exacerbation treated with methylprednisolone and vitamin D3. B: The intracellular ROS in PBMCs from these asthmatic participants were detected by confocal microscopy using a DCFH-DA probe. The ROS levels were represented by the fluorescence intensity. The quantification of the ROS positive cell density in 10-random cell fields containing 500 cells(X400). C: The DNA damage in PBMCs from these asthmatic participants was detected by comet assay using confocal microscopy (X400). The DNA damage score was analyzed with **Comet Assay IV** software.

cellular studies, we measured GR nuclear translocation in monocytes from V-D deficiency and V-D-sufficiency severe asthma patients. Our studies found that V-D-sufficiency asthma patients showed normal GR nuclear translocation in monocytes following dexamethasone stimulation. The dexamethasone induced-GR nuclear translocation in monocytes in the V-D deficiency severe asthma patients was significantly decreased compared to that in the V-D-sufficiency asthma patients (Figure 5C). In the monocytes from the V-D-deficiency asthma patients, the 1, 25-hydroxyvitamin D3 pretreatment enhanced the dexamethasone induced-GR nuclear translocation (Figure 5C).

Discussion

Respiratory infections such as viruses, chlamydia and mycoplasma might cause wheezing and acute exacerbation of asthma; however, bacterial infection-induced acute exacerbation of asthma remains undefined [27,28]. Bacterial colonization of the lower airways has been reported to be typical in patients with chronic severe asthma. One study reports that 52% of chronic severe asthma cases showed positive sputum cultures, predominantly with *H influenzae*, *P aeruginosa*, *S aureus* and *S pneumoniae* strains [29]. Vitamin D deficiency predisposes to viral respiratory tract infections. A lack of vitamin D suppresses adaptive immunity and increases the risk and severity of asthma [30]. In this study, acute exacerbations of asthma with a radiological diagnosis of pneumonia were excluded from the study. The patients with acute exacerbation of asthma exhibited more pronounced blood neutrophils. V-D-deficiency in acute exacerbation of asthma showed significantly increased blood neutrophils. The results suggested that V-D-deficiency may be associated with the phenotype of neutrophilic inflammation in asthma exacerbation.

Oxidative stress has been recognized as contributing significantly to the inflammatory pathology of bronchial asthma. Dunstan et al., found that higher antioxidant levels were not associated with reduced allergen responsiveness in allergic adults [31]. The serum total antioxidant status was correlated with the severity criteria, and measurement of the total antioxidant status could be useful to evaluate asthma attacks [32]. Insufficient 25(OH) D levels increased oxidative/nitrosative stress, inflamma-

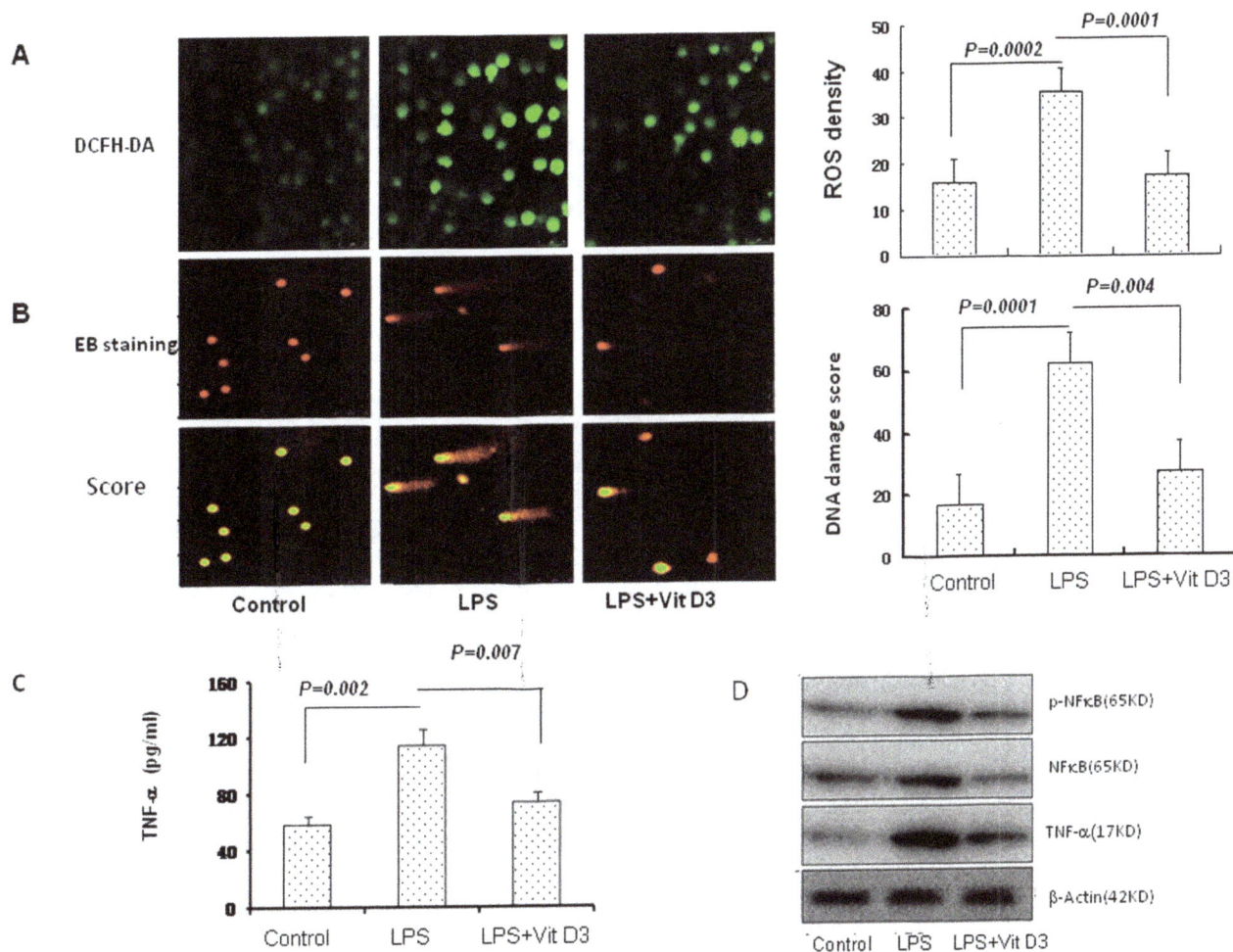

Figure 4. The effect of vitamin D3 on oxidative stress, DNA damage, TNF-α and NFκB in LPS-primed airway epithelial cells. The ROS and DNA damage in airway epithelial cells was measured in the presence or absence of vitamin D3 and treated with LPS for 24 hours. A: ROS was detected by confocal microscopy using a DCFH-DA probe. The ROS level was represented by fluorescence intensity (X400). B: The DNA damage was measured by comet assay. The DNA damage score was analyzed with **Comet Assay IV** software. **C**: Standard ELISA was performed to determine the levels of TNF-α. D: NFκB were analyzed by western blot. β-actin was used as the loading controls.

tion, and endothelial activation in severely obese children. Supplemental vitamin D3 decreased oxidative DNA damage in normal human colorectal mucosa [33,34]. The activity of SOD is as an intracellular antioxidant enzyme. SOD activity in the asthmatic patients was lower than that in the healthy controls [14]. The mechanism of oxidative stress in asthma remains unclear. In this study, the patients with severe asthma exacerbation showed increased ROS, DNA damage and OGG1 in the peripheral blood mononuclear cells. SOD in V-D-deficiency was significantly decreased compared to SOD in V-D-sufficiency in severe asthma exacerbation. The results indicated that V-D-deficiency aggravated the oxidative milieu changes in severe asthma exacerbation. V-D-deficiency increased oxidative stress and DNA damage in severe asthma exacerbation, and oxidative stress plays a key role in the pathophysiology of severe asthma exacerbation.

Oxidative stress is an important factor in corticosteroid insensitivity by the inhibition of HDAC-2 activity and expression. Antioxidants might be shown to be beneficial in restoring corticosteroid function [35]. The proposed extrarenal effects of 25-hydroxyvitamin D3 include increased antimicrobial peptide production, regulation of the inflammatory response, and airway remodeling [36]. Additionally, vitamin D deficiency is associated

with poorer lung function. Low vitamin D levels are associated with severe asthma exacerbation and decreased airway responsiveness in asthma [6,37]. In this study, a significant negative association was present between V-D-deficiency and corticosteroid response in severe asthma exacerbation, with severe asthma exacerbation with V-D-deficiency showing a decreased corticosteroid response. V-D-deficiency in acute exacerbation of asthma showed significantly a decreased FEV1%. FEV1% was significantly decreased in severe asthma exacerbation with V-D-deficiency compared to that in V-D-sufficiency. These observations indicated that the vitamin D status is related to a decreased FEV1% in severe asthma exacerbation. The FEV1 changes in severe asthma exacerbation with V-D-deficiency were significantly lower than those with V-D-sufficiency during methylprednisolone therapy. Supplemental vitamin D was beneficial for increased corticosteroid response and decreased oxidative stress. This study demonstrated an association between V-D-deficiency and corticosteroid response. The association between vitamin D and oxidative stress is supported by *in vivo* studies. Supplemental vitamin D significantly decreased oxidative stress and DNA damage in severe asthma exacerbation with V-D-deficiency.

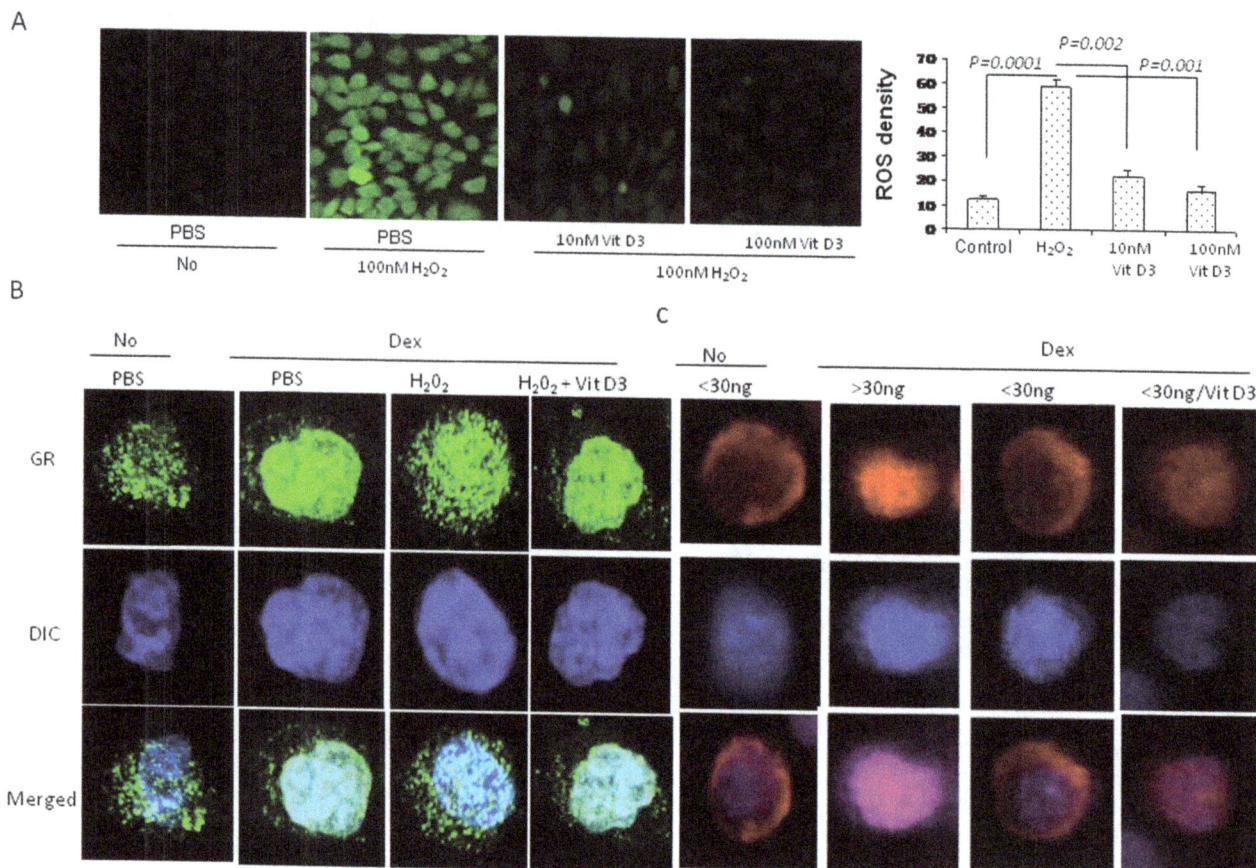

Figure 5. The effect of vitamin-D3 on oxidative stress and the nuclear translocation of the glucocorticoid receptor. A: The ROS in airway epithelial cells was detected by confocal microscopy using a DCFH-DA probe. The ROS level was represented by fluorescence intensity (X400).B: The nuclear translocation of GR was assessed by immunocytochemistry of the airway epithelial cells treated with Dex for 30 minutes. FITC-conjugated anti-rabbit secondary Abs (X400). C: The PBMC in severe asthma exacerbation with V-D-deficiency or V-D-sufficiency were incubated with or without vitamin D3 for 12 hours. The nuclear translocation of GR was assessed by immunocytochemistry of the PBMC treated with Dex for 30 minutes. TRITC–conjugated anti-rabbit secondary Abs (X400).

TNF-α plays an important role in severe refractory asthma [23]. Kox et al., reported that the plasma levels of vitamin D are not correlated with the LPS-induced TNF-α, IL-6 and IL-10 cytokine response in humans during experimental human endotoxemia [38]. However, Di Rosa et al., found that vitamin D facilitated the expression of inflammatory mediators such as IL-1β, IL-6 and TNF-α in human monocytes/macrophages [39]. Additionally, TNF-α mediated the vitamin D receptors. TNF-α-stimulation significantly decreased the expression and activity of vitamin D receptors in porcine coronary artery smooth muscle cells [40]. We found that severe asthma exacerbation with V-D-deficiency showed increased TNF-α, NFκB expression and NFκB phosphorylation compared to that with 25-hydroxyvitamin D-sufficiency.

A previous study confirmed that LPS-treated animals developed oxidative stress, and LPS-induced inflammatory responses were associated with oxidative stress. Some studies demonstrate that LPS-stimulated macrophages increased the production of TNF-α. The LPS-induced overexpression of inflammatory mediators in vascular smooth muscle cells was via the TLR4/MAPK/NFκB pathways [41,42]. A central event in the inflammatory response to LPS is the activation of transcription factor NFκB [43,44]. In our present study, TNF-α was significantly increased in the LPS-stimulated cells. Additionally, LPS induced NFκB expression and phosphorylation. In our studies, our results show that

LPS-stimulated airway epithelial cells caused increased ROS release and DNA damage. Supplemental vitamin D decreased the ROS release and DNA damage in LPS-stimulated airway epithelial cells. Vitamin D3 inhibited the LPS-induced expression of TNF-α, NFκB expression and NFκB phosphorylation. These results suggest that Vitamin D3 is a potential anti-inflammatory agent by attenuating the generation of TNF-α and blocking ROS generation and NFκB activation pathways in LPS-stimulated phagocytes.

Steroids could not contain the increased levels of T_H17 cytokines in steroid-resistant asthma; however, 1, 25(OH) 2D3 inhibited T_H17 cytokine production in all the patients [45] and demonstrated anti-inflammatory and corticosteroid-enhancing effects in the monocytes of asthma patients. The vitamin D3 pretreatment enhanced dexamethasone-induced GR binding and histone acetylation in monocytes from asthma [46]. Oxidative stress inhibited HDAC2 activity and expression through activation of phosphoinositide 3-kinase δ, which is a molecular mechanism of the steroid resistance in asthmatic patients [47]. In our present studies, H_2O_2 decreased GR nuclear translocation in 16HBE cells following dexamethasone stimulation. 1, 25-hydroxyvitamin D3 pretreatment enhanced the dexamethasone induced-GR nuclear translocation in H_2O_2-stimulated cells. V-D-deficiency asthma patients showed decreased nuclear translocation of glucocorticoid receptors in monocytes following dexamethasone stimulation. We used 1, 25-hydroxyvitamin D3 to pretreat monocytes from V-D-deficiency asthma patients and found that 1, 25-hydroxyvitamin D3 increased nuclear translocation of glucocorticoid receptors in monocytes following dexamethasone stimulation. Our studies represent a novel vitamin D mechanism in severe asthma exacerbation with V-D-deficiency.

This study of severe asthma exacerbation with V-D-deficiency showed oxidative stress and DNA damage in peripheral blood monocytes. V-D-deficiency increased the oxidative stress and DNA damage in exacerbation of severe asthma. Severe asthma exacerbation with V-D-deficiency increased TNF-α, NFκB expression and NFκB phosphorylation. Supplemental vitamin D increased the corticosteroid response and decreased oxidative stress. Supplemental vitamin D decreased ROS release and DNA damage in LPS-stimulated airway epithelial cells. Vitamin D3 down-regulates the expression of TNF-$\alpha$and NFκB as well as NFκB phosphorylation in LPS-stimulated airway epithelial cells, suggesting a possible mechanism for vitamin D3 therapy in severe asthma exacerbation. Our studies suggest that V-D-deficiency intensifies oxidative stress and DNA damage, suggesting a possible mechanism for corticosteroid resistance in severe asthma exacerbation.

Author Contributions

Conceived and designed the experiments: G. Li ZL NZ. Performed the experiments: NL G. Luo YC Xing Wang YZ Xiaoyun Wang. Analyzed the data: XY TX G. Luo G. Li. Wrote the paper: XY TX G. Luo G. Li.

References

1. Papiris S, Kotanidou A, Malagari K, Roussos C (2002) Clinical review: severe asthma. Crit Care 6: 30–44.
2. Williams LK, Peterson EL, Wells K, Ahmedani BK, Kumar R, et al. (2011) Quantifying the proportion of severe asthma exacerbations attributable to inhaled corticosteroid nonadherence. J Allergy Clin Immunol 128: 1185–1191.e1182.
3. Chung KF, Wenzel SE, Brozek JL, Bush A, Castro M, et al. (2014) International ERS/ATS guidelines on definition, evaluation and treatment of severe asthma. The European respiratory journal: official journal of the European Society for Clinical Respiratory Physiology 43: 343–373.
4. Bozzetto S, Carraro S, Giordano G, Boner A, Baraldi E (2012) Asthma, allergy and respiratory infections: the vitamin D hypothesis. Allergy 67: 10–17.
5. Berry DJ, Hesketh K, Power C, Hypponen E (2011) Vitamin D status has a linear association with seasonal infections and lung function in British adults. Br J Nutr 106: 1433–1440.
6. Brehm JM, Acosta-Perez E, Klei L, Roeder K, Barmada M, et al. (2012) Vitamin D insufficiency and severe asthma exacerbations in Puerto Rican children. Am J Respir Crit Care Med 186: 140–146.
7. Peden DB (2011) The role of oxidative stress and innate immunity in O(3) and endotoxin-induced human allergic airway disease. Immunol Rev 242: 91–105.
8. Goleva E, Hauk PJ, Hall CF, Liu AH, Riches DW, et al. (2008) Corticosteroid-resistant asthma is associated with classical antimicrobial activation of airway macrophages. J Allergy Clin Immunol 122: 550–559 e553.
9. Liu AH (2002) Endotoxin exposure in allergy and asthma: reconciling a paradox. J Allergy Clin Immunol 109: 379–392.
10. Goleva E, Jackson LP, Harris JK, Robertson CE, Sutherland ER, et al. (2013) The effects of airway microbiome on corticosteroid responsiveness in asthma. Am J Respir Crit Care Med 188: 1193–1201.
11. Kratzer E, Tian Y, Sarich N, Wu T, Meliton A, et al. (2012) Oxidative stress contributes to lung injury and barrier dysfunction via microtubule destabilization. Am J Respir Cell Mol Biol 47: 688–697.
12. Rosanna DP, Salvatore C (2012) Reactive oxygen species, inflammation, and lung diseases. Curr Pharm Des 18: 3889–3900.
13. Knaapen AM, Schins RP, Polat D, Becker A, Borm PJ (2002) Mechanisms of neutrophil-induced DNA damage in respiratory tract epithelial cells. Mol Cell Biochem 234–235: 143–151.
14. Ahmad A, Shameem M, Husain Q (2012) Relation of oxidant-antioxidant imbalance with disease progression in patients with asthma. Ann Thorac Med 7: 226–232.
15. Marotta F, Naito Y, Jain S, Lorenzetti A, Soresi V, et al. (2012) Is there a potential application of a fermented nutraceutical in acute respiratory illnesses? An in-vivo placebo-controlled, cross-over clinical study in different age groups of healthy subjects. J Biol Regul Homeost Agents 26: 285–294.
16. Hamden K, Carreau S, Jamoussi K, Miladi S, Lajmi S, et al. (2009) 1Alpha,25 dihydroxyvitamin D3: therapeutic and preventive effects against oxidative stress, hepatic, pancreatic and renal injury in alloxan-induced diabetes in rats. J Nutr Sci Vitaminol (Tokyo) 55: 215–222.
17. Peng X, Vaishnav A, Murillo G, Alimirah F, Torres KE, et al. (2010) Protection against cellular stress by 25-hydroxyvitamin D3 in breast epithelial cells. J Cell Biochem 110:1324–1333.
18. Bousquet J, Mantzouranis E, Cruz AA, Ait-Khaled N, Baena-Cagnani CE, et al. (2010) Uniform definition of asthma severity, control, and exacerbations: document presented for the World Health Organization Consultation on Severe Asthma. J Allergy Clin Immunol 126: 926–938.
19. Tse SM, Kelly HW, Litonjua AA, Van Natta ML, Weiss ST, et al. (2012) Corticosteroid use and bone mineral accretion in children with asthma: effect modification by vitamin D. J Allergy Clin Immunol 130: 53–60.e54.
20. Shermatov K, Zeyrek D, Yildirim F, Kilic M, Cebi N, et al. (2012) DNA damage in children exposed to secondhand cigarette smoke and its association with oxidative stress. Indian Pediatr 49: 958–962.
21. Li G, Yuan K, Yan C, Fox J, 3rd, Gaid M, et al. (2012) 8-Oxoguanine-DNA glycosylase 1 deficiency modifies allergic airway inflammation by regulating STAT6 and IL-4 in cells and in mice. Free Radic Biol Med 52: 392–401.
22. Janssen-Heininger Y, Ckless K, Reynaert N, van der Vliet A (2005) SOD inactivation in asthma: bad or no news? Am J Pathol 166: 649–652.
23. Brightling C, Berry M, Amrani Y (2008) Targeting TNF-alpha: a novel therapeutic approach for asthma. J Allergy Clin Immunol 121: 5-10; quiz 11–12.
24. Milara J, Navarro A, Almudever P, Lluch J, Morcillo EJ, et al. (2011) Oxidative stress-induced glucocorticoid resistance is prevented by dual PDE3/PDE4 inhibition in human alveolar macrophages. Clin Exp Allergy 41: 535–546.
25. Ito K, Yamamura S, Essilfie-Quaye S, Cosio B, Ito M, et al. (2006) Histone deacetylase 2-mediated deacetylation of the glucocorticoid receptor enables NF-kappaB suppression. J Exp Med 203: 7–13.
26. Asaba K, Iwasaki Y, Yoshida M, Asai M, Oiso Y, et al. (2004). Attenuation by reactive oxygen species of glucocorticoid suppression on proopiomelanocortin gene expression in pituitary corticotroph cells. Endocrinology 145: 39–42
27. Sevin CM, Peebles RS, Jr. (2010) Infections and asthma: new insights into old ideas. Clin Exp Allergy 40: 1142–1154.
28. Renz H, Herz U (2002) The bidirectional capacity of bacterial antigens to modulate allergy and asthma. Eur Respir J 19: 158–171.
29. Zhang Q, Illing R, Hui CK, Downey K, Carr D, et al. (2012) Bacteria in sputum of stable severe asthma and increased airway wall thickness. Respir Res 13: 35.
30. Hansdottir S, Monick MM (2011) Vitamin D effects on lung immunity and respiratory diseases. Vitam Horm 86: 217–237.
31. Dunstan JA, Breckler L, Hale J, Lehmann H, Franklin P, et al. (2006) Associations between antioxidant status, markers of oxidative stress and immune responses in allergic adults. Clin Exp Allergy 36: 993–1000.
32. Katsoulis K, Kontakiotis T, Leonardopoulos I, Kotsovili A, Legakis IN, et al. (2003) Serum total antioxidant status in severe exacerbation of asthma: correlation with the severity of the disease. J Asthma 40: 847–854.
33. Codoner-Franch P, Tavarez-Alonso S, Simo-Jorda R, Laporta-Martin P, Carratala-Calvo A, et al. (2012) Vitamin D status is linked to biomarkers of oxidative stress, inflammation, and endothelial activation in obese children. J Pediatr 161: 848–854.
34. Fedirko V, Bostick RM, Long Q, Flanders WD, McCullough ML, et al. (2010) Effects of supplemental vitamin D and calcium on oxidative DNA damage marker in normal colorectal mucosa: a randomized clinical trial. Cancer Epidemiol Biomarkers Prev 19: 280–291.
35. Chung KF, Marwick JA (2010) Molecular mechanisms of oxidative stress in airways and lungs with reference to asthma and chronic obstructive pulmonary disease. Ann N Y Acad Sci 1203: 85–91.
36. Finklea JD, Grossmann RE, Tangpricha V (2011) Vitamin D and chronic lung disease: a review of molecular mechanisms and clinical studies. Adv Nutr 2: 244–253.
37. Wu AC, Tantisira K, Li L, Fuhlbrigge AL, Weiss ST, et al. (2012) Effect of vitamin D and inhaled corticosteroid treatment on lung function in children. Am J Respir Crit Care Med 186: 508–513.
38. Kox M, van den Berg MJ, van der Hoeven JG, Wielders JP, van der Ven AJ, et al. (2013) Vitamin D status is not associated with inflammatory cytokine levels during experimental human endotoxaemia. Clin Exp Immunol 171: 231–236.
39. Di Rosa M, Malaguarnera G, De Gregorio C, Palumbo M, Nunnari G, et al. (2012) Immuno-modulatory effects of vitamin D3 in human monocyte and macrophages. Cell Immunol 280: 36–43.
40. Gupta GK, Agrawal T, Del Core MG, Hunter WJ 3rd, Agrawal DK (2012) Decreased expression of vitamin D receptors in neointimal lesions following coronary artery angioplasty in atherosclerotic swine. PLoS One 7: e42789.
41. He X, Shu J, Xu L, Lu C, Lu A (2012) Inhibitory effect of Astragalus polysaccharides on lipopolysaccharide-induced TNF-a and IL-1beta production in THP-1 cells. Molecules 17: 3155–3164.

42. Meng Z, Yan C, Deng Q, Gao DF, Niu XL (2013) Curcumin inhibits LPS-induced inflammation in rat vascular smooth muscle cells in vitro via ROS-relative TLR4-MAPK/NF-kappaB pathways. Acta Pharmacol Sin 34: 901–911.

43. Okamoto T, Gohil K, Finkelstein EI, Bove P, Akaike T, et al. (2004) Multiple contributing roles for NOS2 in LPS-induced acute airway inflammation in mice. Am J Physiol Lung Cell Mol Physiol 286: L198–209.

44. Huang CH, Yang ML, Tsai CH, Li YC, Lin YJ, et al. (2013) Ginkgo biloba leaves extract (EGb 761) attenuates lipopolysaccharide-induced acute lung injury via inhibition of oxidative stress and NF-kappaB-dependent matrix metalloproteinase-9 pathway. Phytomedicine 20: 303–309.

45. Nanzer AM, Chambers ES, Ryanna K, Richards DF, Black C, et al. (2013) Enhanced production of IL-17A in patients with severe asthma is inhibited by 1alpha,25-dihydroxyvitamin D3 in a glucocorticoid-independent fashion. J Allergy Clin Immunol 132: 297–304.e293.

46. Zhang Y, Leung DY, Goleva E (2014) Anti-inflammatory and corticosteroid-enhancing actions of vitamin D in monocytes of patients with steroid-resistant and those with steroid-sensitive asthma. J Allergy Clin Immunol 133: 1744–1752.e1.

47. To Y, Ito K, Kizawa Y, Failla M, Ito M, Kusama T, et al (2010). Targeting phosphoinositide-3-kinase-delta with theophylline reverses corticosteroid insensitivity in chronic obstructive pulmonary disease. Am J Respir Crit Care Med. 182(7):897–904.

6

Neem Leaf Glycoprotein Prophylaxis Transduces Immune Dependent Stop Signal for Tumor Angiogenic Switch within Tumor Microenvironment

Saptak Banerjee, Tithi Ghosh, Subhasis Barik, Arnab Das, Sarbari Ghosh, Avishek Bhuniya, Anamika Bose⁹, Rathindranath Baral*⁹

Department of Immunoregulation and Immunodiagnostics, Chittaranjan National Cancer Institute (CNCI), Kolkata, India

Abstract

We have reported that prophylactic as well as therapeutic administration of neem leaf glycoprotein (NLGP) induces significant restriction of solid tumor growth in mice. Here, we investigate whether the effect of such pretreatment (25µg/mice; weekly, 4 times) benefits regulation of tumor angiogenesis, an obligate factor for tumor progression. We show that NLGP pretreatment results in vascular normalization in melanoma and carcinoma bearing mice along with downregulation of CD31, VEGF and VEGFR2. NLGP pretreatment facilitates profound infiltration of CD8$^+$ T cells within tumor parenchyma, which subsequently regulates VEGF-VEGFR2 signaling in CD31$^+$ vascular endothelial cells to prevent aberrant neovascularization. Pericyte stabilization, VEGF dependent inhibition of VEC proliferation and subsequent vascular normalization are also experienced. Studies in immune compromised mice confirmed that these vascular and intratumoral changes in angiogenic profile are dependent upon active adoptive immunity particularly those mediated by CD8$^+$ T cells. Accumulated evidences suggest that NLGP regulated immunomodulation is active in tumor growth restriction and normalization of tumor angiogenesis as well, thereby, signifying its clinical translation.

Editor: Rupesh Chaturvedi, Jawaharlal Nehru University, India

Funding: The work was partially supported by Council of Scientific and Industrial Research, New Delhi (grant no. 09/030(0050)/2008-EMR-I to S. Banerjee, grant no. 09/030(0063)/2011-EMRI to S. Barik and grant SRA, Scientists' Pool Scheme No: 8463A to A. Bose). The funders had no role in study design, data collection and analysis, decision to publish, or preparation of the manuscript.

Competing Interests: The authors have declared that no competing interests exist.

* Email: baralrathin@hotmail.com

⁹ These authors contributed equally to this work.

Introduction

In 2000, Hanahan and Weinberg described angiogenesis as one of the most important hallmark criterion for cancer [1]. In spite of fundamental role of angiogenesis in fetal development and in many physiological conditions like wound healing [2,3] tumors exploit it to promote blood vessel growth and fuel a tumor's transition from benign to a malignant state [4,5]. Likewise, these malignant transformations need evasion from immune destruction, which has been included recently, in 2011, as another important hallmark of cancer growth [6]. Angiogenesis and immune evasion, these two apparently parallel cancer-intrinsic phenomenon actually possess bidirectional link and convergely promote malignant growth, metastasis and ultimately regulate therapeutic outcome [7]. In cancer, immune system can regulate angiogenesis with both pro- and anti-angiogenic activities [8,9]. Angiogenic molecules by differentially regulating immune system help in the development of sustained immunosuppressive mechanisms within tumor microenvironment (TME) [10,11]. This immunosuppressive mechanism may promote angiogenesis and tumor growth and inhibits infiltration and homing of activated immune cells within TME. Promoted angiogenesis then deregulates the proliferation and migration of vascular endothelial cells (VECs), thereby, causing neovascularization. These results in aberrant tumor vasculature associated with distorted and enlarged vessels, increased permeability, irregular blood flow and micro-hemorrhages [10,12,13]. Therefore, in recent years different works have shown that, for optimum immune-mediated tumor destruction, normalization of tumor vasculature is preferred over complete blockade of tumor angiogenesis [14].

Neem leaf glycoprotein (NLGP), a nontoxic immunomodulator reported previously have significant murine tumor growth restricting potential in prophylactic [15,16] as well as therapeutic [17,18] settings. NLGP facilitates anti-tumor activity by modulating both systemic and local immunity including: i) suppression of regulatory T cells [19], ii) activation of effector NK, NKT and T cells [20,21], iii) modulation of antigen presenting cells by maturing dendritic cells (DCs) towards DC1 phenotype [22,23] and macrophages [24], iv) regulation of cytokine-chemokine balance [25,26] and v) preventing anergy and exhaustion of effector T cells [17,18]. Recently in two consecutive studies, we have reported that therapeutic effectiveness of NLGP is associated with profound tumor infiltration of CD8$^+$ T cells [27] and normalization of tumor-immune-microenvironment [27,28].

Therefore, in the present study, we prophylactically applied NLGP in murine carcinoma and melanoma bearing mice to boost antitumor immune responses and subsequently analyzed the mode of NLGP counteraction on the tumor angiogenesis. We report that NLGP pretreatment associated immune-stimulation, particularly CD8$^+$ T cell activation, regulates the balance between pro- and anti-angiogenic molecules to induce vascular normalization without affecting normal physiological angiogenesis.

Results

NLGP prophylaxis prevents tumor angiogenesis and normalizes tumor vasculature

'Dormant' tumor requires both angiogenic switch and immune escape to proceed towards malignancy [7,9]. As prophylaxis with neem leaf preparation, precursor of NLGP, previously reported to be associated with significant immune-mediated tumor growth restriction [16,29], here, we intended to study how NLGP prophylaxis regulates pathological tumor angiogenesis. Consistent with our previous results prophylactic NLGP administration (4×) significantly restricts Ehrlich's carcinoma and B16 melanoma tumor growth (Figure 1a). Repeated investigations confirmed 4 immunizations with NLGP are required for optimum immune activation [15–18,27–29]. Angiogenic profiles were studied in mice after establishment of tumor (in between day 21 to 32) (Figure 1A.1 and A.2) and visual observations suggested a significant decrease in heavy, very thick, thick blood vessels, while thin blood vessels were retained substantially in NLGP pretreated carcinoma and melanoma tumor bearing mice group compared to PBS controls (Figure 1A.3). Additionally, histological analysis of tumor sections demonstrated less number of blood vessels with more regularized pattern in NLGP pretreated tumors than PBS mice. This regularized pattern of blood vessels is further evidenced by downregulation of CD31, a marker of VECs (Figure 1B). Correlating angiogenic profile with tumor volume revealed that normalized angiogenesis associated with NLGP prophylaxis represents restricted tumor growth, whereas, chaotic angiogenesis is correlated well with bigger tumor volume (Table 1; Figure 1C). Therefore, these data furnish evidences that NLGP can normalize tumor vasculature by decreasing only the thick and 'tortured' blood vessels while retaining the more compact thin blood vessels within tumor to maintain the optimum interstitial pressure and vaccine mediated immune benefits.

NLGP mediated vascular normalization is associated with down regulation of CD31, VEGF and VEGFR2

As VEGF-VEGFR2 signaling axis represents the key event in promoting tumor angiogenesis [30–32], expression of these molecules along with other pro-angiogenic molecules were next analyzed in NLGP pretreated carcinoma and melanoma bearing mice. Evidences obtained from RT-PCR (Figure 2A.1 and A.2)and Western Blot analyses demonstrated downregulation of VEGF, VEGFR2, CD31 in tumor from NLGP pretreated mice (Figure 2B.1 and B.2), in comparison to tumor obtained from PBS treated mice. Consistently, immunohistochemical analysis also revealed the significant decrease in expression level of VEGF and its receptor, VEGFR2, along with endothelial cell associated protein CD31 in harvested tumors with NLGP pre-therapy (Figure 2C.1). However, minimal decrease in VEGFR1 and NG2 level (Figure 2C.1 and C.2) was observed with similar treatment. Dual immunofluorescence staining of CD31 with NG2 (Figure 2C.3) indicated optimum and close pericyte coverage over VECs that may help in stabilization of blood vessels in NLGP treated mice group while, in PBS treated mice NG2$^+$ pericytes

were found detached from endothelial cells (Figure 2C.2), rendering the blood vessels thick, dilated and leaky. Therefore, obtained results clearly suggest that NLGP mediated alteration of pericytes' nature and/or that attachment along the vessel wall is intimately associated with observed vascular normalization within tumor.

NLGP mediated vascular normalization requires host's intact immune-system

Several recent studies have demonstrated that angiogenesis and suppressed cell-mediated immunity interdependently play central role in the pathogenesis of malignant disease facilitating tumor growth [33,34]. As NLGP prophylaxis reciprocally regulate tumor immune surveillance and angiogenesis to restrict murine tumor growth, next, we used two types of mice models (drug-induced immunosuppressive mice and immunocompromised athymic nude mice) to assess the immune involvement in NLGP mediated angiogenic modulation. As shown in (Figure 3A.1, A.2), mice were divided into three groups and two groups were injected with NLGP prophylactically, while one group was retained as control. Between these two NLGP pretreated mice groups, one group received immunosuppressant cyclosporine before EC tumor challenge as mentioned in 'Materials and Methods'. Analysis of their angiogenic profile revealed that NLGP pretreatment caused significant normalization of tumor vasculature than control group, as demonstrated in Figure 3A.1 However, in cyclosporine group, NLGP pretreatment failed to normalize angiogenesis, and so they showed prominent with prominent dilated and fragile blood vessels (Figure 3A.1, A.2-D.1, D.2). Observed results clearly indicated that NLGP modulates angiogenesis or vascular normalization by activating immune system.

Corroborately, in a separate set of experiments, tumor growth and associated angiogenesis were studied in three groups of NLGP-cyclosporin treated EC bearing mice. Two such groups of mice adoptively received non-adherent immune cells from either NLGP or PBS immunized normal mice (Figure 3A.3). Mice from all the 3 groups were sacrificed after tumor reached a considerable volume (1500 mm^3 to 2000 mm^3 approximately) and their angiogenic profiles were analyzed (Figure 3B.3–D.3). Enhanced angiogenesis related to the cyclosporine mediated immunosuppression in NLGP pretreated mice was observed to be almost normalized due to adoptive transfer of splenic immune cells from NLGP treated mice (Figure 3B.3–D.3). These findings might further conclude that NLGP mediated normalization of angiogenesis is immune dependent.

To further validate the influence of NLGP-conditioned immune system to restrain tumor angiogenesis, immune-compromised athymic nude mice were pretreated with NLGP before tumor (EC) inoculation. However, NLGP pretreated nude mice failed to normalize tumor angiogenesis (Figure 3A.4–D.4) and adoptive transfer of syngenic non-adherent immune cells or isolated T cells of NLGP immunized normal mice showed tumor growth restriction and vascular normalization or inhibition in angiogenesis in comparison to PBS treated or only NLGP treated group (data not shown).

Tumors harvested from mice with different compromised immune systems with either pretreatment with NLGP or adoptive transfer of immune cells were analyzed for the expression status of VEGF, VEGFR2 and CD31, as we earlier found that NLGP downregulates the elevated expression levels of these molecules during tumor growth. Immunosuppression, either by means of cyclosporine treatment or in nude mice, abrogated the NLGP mediated downregulation of VEGF, VEGFR2 and CD31

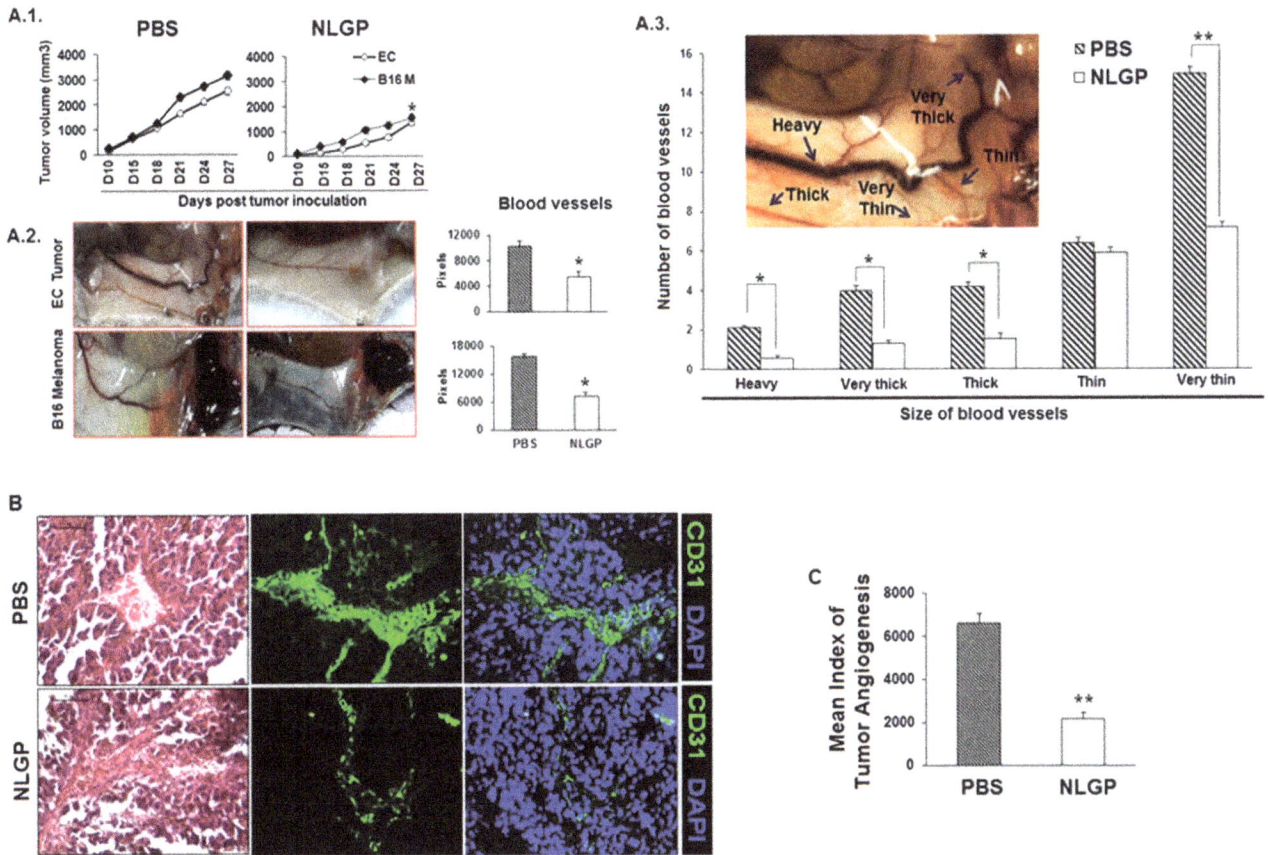

Figure 1. NLGP normalizes tumor vasculature. Swiss and C57BL/6 mice were pretreated with NLGP (25µg) once a week for four weeks in total followed by inoculation of EC (1×10^6 cells/mice) and B16 melanoma cells (2×10^5 cells/mice) subcutaneously. **A.1.** Tumor growth curve till day 27 is presented. *$p < 0.01$. **A.2.** Mice were sacrificed and their angiogenic profile was studied and presented in photographs and bar diagrams (Mean±SD of pixel values). *$p < 0.01$. **A.3.** Differentially dilated angiogenic vessels as shown in a representative figure (*inset*) were counted from NLGP and PBS treated mice and presented in bar diagram. *$p < 0.05$; **$p < 0.001$. **B.** Angiogenic blood vessels within tumors were studied by routine histology after H&E staining and CD31$^+$ VECs were studied by immunofluorescence staining. Representative figures in each case are presented. **C.** Mean index of tumor angiogenesis is presented in bar diagram. **$p < 0.001$.

Table 1. MITA* relating tumor volume and angiogenesis in NLGP pretreated mice.

PBS			NLGP		
Tumor Volume (in mm³)	Angiogenesis (in raw score)	Index for Tumor Angiogenesis	Tumor Volume (in mm³)	Angiogenesis (in raw score)	Index for Tumor Angiogenesis
220	+ (1)	220	126	+ (1)	126
600	++ (2)	1200	245	+ (1)	245
907	++ (2)	1814	665	++ (2)	1330
2025	++++ (4)	8100	1267	+++ (3)	3801
1152	+++ (3)	3456	445	+ (1)	445
3240	++++ (4)	12960	1568	++ (2)	3136
5292	++++ (4)	21168	1436	+++ (3)	4308
1352	+++ (3)	4056	1008	++ (2)	2016
Mean		**6622**			**1926**

*Mean index of tumor angiogenesis. Mean is presented in Figure 1C

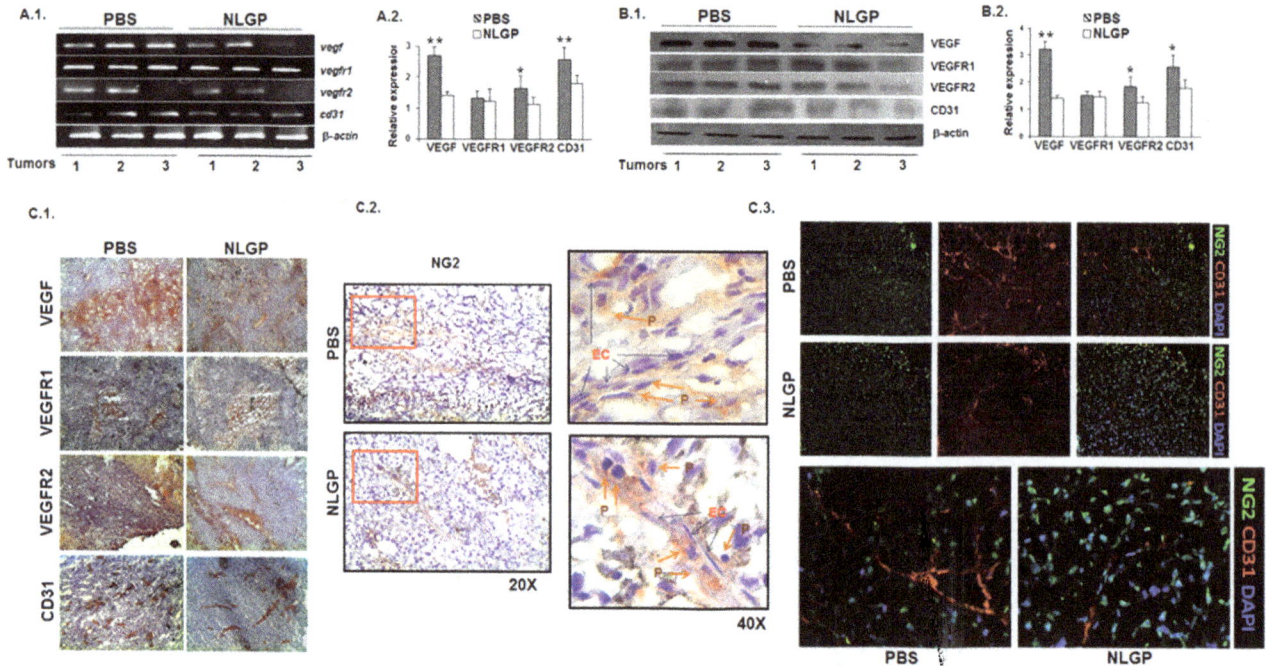

Figure 2. NLGP normalizes tumor microenvironment by downregulating expression of VEGF, VEGFR2 and CD31. B16 melanoma tumors (100 mm^3) harvested from either PBS or NLGP pretreated C57BL/6 mice representing tumor microenvironment were used for different analysis. **A.1.** Representative presentation of mRNA expression levels of *vegf, vegfr1, vegfr2, cd31* by RT-PCR analysis (n = 3). **A.2.** Densitometric analysis of three individual observations is presented with Mean ± SD. *p<0.05; **p<0.01. **B.1.** Another portion (100 mg) of tumors was lysed by freeze-thaw cycles in PBS used for Western Blotting to check the expression of various angiogenic proteins. Representative presentation of expression levels of different molecules as mentioned by Western blot analysis (n = 3) is shown. **B.2.** Densitometric analysis of three individual observations and Mean ± SD are presented. *p<0.05; **p<0.01. **C.1.** Immunohistochemistry with monoclonal antibodies, specific for VEGF, VEGFR1, VEGFR2 and CD31 and **C.2.** NG2 were detected on tumor sections. Arrows showed the pericyte coverage on endothelial cell lining on blood vessels. **D.** Fluorescence tagged monoclonal antibodies, specific for NG2$^+$ (green) and CD31$^+$ (Red) cells were used to study tumor vasculature. Nuclear staining was performed by DAPI.

(Figure 3E). Thus, NLGP may normalize angiogenesis by restricting availability of pro-angiogenic molecules.

CD8$^+$ T cells play vital role in NLGP mediated immune dependent vascular normalization

Since, above experiments clearly indicate that immune system has a regulatory role in NLGP driven normalization of tumor angiogenesis, next, we studied the histological sections from carcinoma and melanoma tumors of NLGP and PBS pretreated mice. Prominent infiltration of immune cells was noticed in tumors from NLGP pretreated mice (Figure 4A.1). Flow cytometric analysis of cells from PBMC of either PBS or NLGP treated tumor bearing mice revealed increased CD8$^+$ T cells in NLGP treated mice group (Figure 4A.2 and A.3). To validate the role of CD8$^+$ T cells (if any), such cells were depleted using specific antibody, as work plan is schematically presented in Figure 4B.1. CD8$^+$ T cell depletion was confirmed flow cytometrically (Figure 4B.2).

As we observed significant enhancement of CD8$^+$ T cells within tumors from NLGP pretreated mice, we wanted to decipher the contributing role of these effector cells in NLGP mediated normalization of angiogenesis by *in vivo* depletion of CD8$^+$ T cells as described in Materials and Methods and Fig. 4B.1. When mice were sacrificed on day 28 post B16F10 tumor inoculation, analysis of angiogenesis at that time point clearly suggested a predominant role for CD8$^+$ T cells in NLGP driven immune-mediated vascular normalization, since CD8$^+$ T cell depletion completely abolished anti-angiogenic potential of NLGP pretreatment (Figure 4C). NLGP mediated downregulation of VEGF,

VEGFR2 and CD31 was again upregulated in mice group with CD8$^+$ T cell depletion, as indicated by RT-PCR (Figure 4D.1, D.2) and immunohistochemical (Figure 4D.3) analysis.

NLGP mediated vascular normalization is not due to the T cell mediated apoptosis of CD31$^+$ cells rather due to unavailability of VEGF

Since CD8$^+$ T cells are found to be responsible for anti-angiogenic effect of NLGP-conditioned immune system (preferentially achieved by downregulation of VEGR2$^+$CD31$^+$ endothelial cells), initially we analyzed direct cytolytic effect of CD8$^+$ T cells on CD31$^+$ VECs. CD31$^+$ cells were flow sorted from solid B16F10 tumors (Figure S1) and exposed to CD8$^+$ T cells from NLGP pretreated tumor bearing mice. Co-incubation study suggested that CD8$^+$ T cells are unable to exert any direct cytolytic effect *in vitro* against tumor derived CD31$^+$ endothelial cells (Figure 5A). Furthermore, analysis of pro-apoptotic and apoptotic/necrotic VECs using Annexin V and PI respectively within tumor revealed that NLGP pretreatment has no effect on early apoptosis or late apoptosis/necrosis of CD31$^+$ cells (Figure 5B.1, B.2).

Analysing these two above mentioned results and considering the importance of VEGF as rate limiting factor for uncontrolled VEC proliferation and survival (necessary for neovascularization) next we assessed *in situ* VEGF concentration and its influence in NLGP mediated vascular normalization. Evidences obtained from ELISA clearly suggested that availability of VEGF is low in tumor

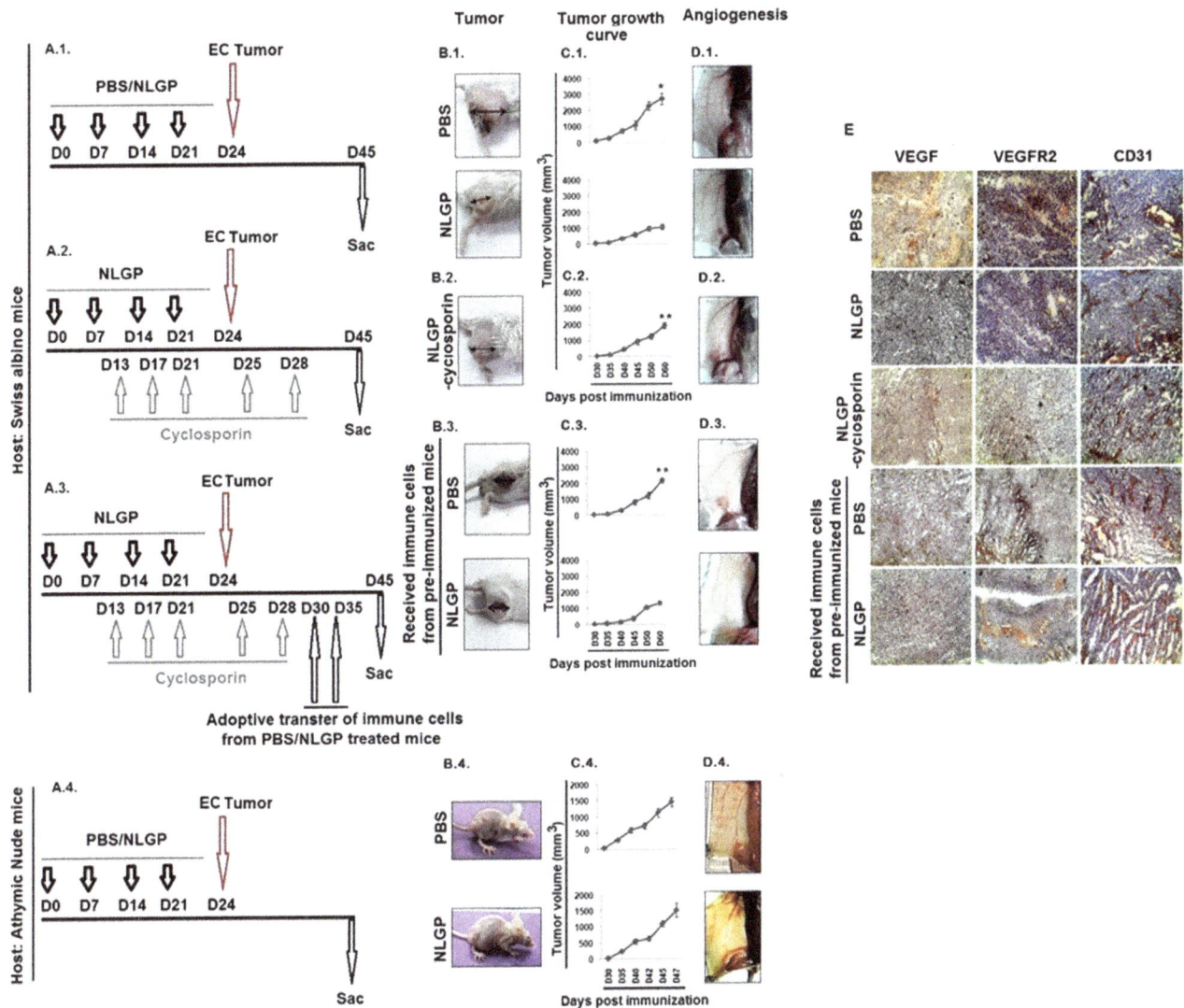

Figure 3. NLGP mediated normalization of angiogenesis is absent in immunocompromised mice. Schematic presentation of NLGP prophylaxis in **A.1.** normal mice, **A.2.** and **A.3.** cyclosporine treated/immunocompromised and **A.4.** athymic nude mice. **B.1.-B.4.** Representative photographs of murine tumors with **B.1.** PBS, NLGP, **B.2.** NLGP-Cyclosporin pretreatment, **B.3.** NLGP pretreatment with adoptive transfer of immune cells and **B.4.** NLGP and PBS pretreatment (athymic nude mice). **C.1.-C.4.** Tumor growth curve presenting Mean ± SD. *$p<0.001$, **$p<0.01$, in comparison to NLGP group with other above mentioned group and **D.1.-D.4.** Angiogenic profile of mice with **D.1.** PBS, NLGP, **D.2.** NLGP-Cyclosporin pretreatment, **D.3.** NLGP pretreatment with adoptive transfer of immune cells and **D.4.** NLGP and PBS pretreatment (athymic nude mice). **E.** Immunohistochemical detection of VEGF, VEGFR2 and CD31 in tumor sections as mentioned in **A.1–A.3.**

in situ from NLGP pretreated mice (Figure 5C), which might regulate CD31$^+$ endothelial cell proliferation. To further verify this possibility, CD31$^+$Ki67$^+$ proliferating cells were analyzed in B16F10 tumor from NLGP pretreated mice by flow cytometric (Figure 5D.1) and immunofluorescence analysis (Figure 5D.2). Consistently, *in vivo* BrdU labeling and analysis of CD31$^+$BrdU$^+$ proliferating cells within harvested cells from tumors indicated significant lowering of proliferating cells in tumor bearing mice pretreated with NLGP (Figure 5D.3). The obtained results clearly suggested that the presence of proliferating endothelial cells is significantly less in NLGP pretreated mice than control mice. Again, peripheral blood mononuclear cells (PBMC) from EC bearing PBS and NLGP treated mice were co-cultured with tumor (EC) cells and culture supernatant was analyzed for VEGF and IFNγ content. Analysis of such supernatants revealed low content of VEGF and high IFNγ (in NLGP-PBMC-EC cell-culture), in

comparison to those where PBS-PBMC was used (Figure 5E.1, E.2). Furthermore, flow-sorted CD31$^+$ cells were *in vitro* exposed to supernatants from NLGP-PBMC-EC cell co-culture and proliferation (monitored by Ki67 staining) of CD31$^+$ endothelial cells was monitored, where significantly less proliferation was noted due to supplementation of supernatant from NLGP-PBMC-EC cell co-culture (Figure 5E.3). Therefore, these results clearly pointed out the prominent role of VEGF downregulation caused after NLGP-instructed CD8$^+$ T cell infiltration in the reciprocal regulation of VEC proliferation and vascular normalization.

NLGP mediated vascular normalization has no adverse effect on normal wound healing process in mice

Given the potential safety concerns of systemic toxicity for strategies targeting tumor angiogenesis, we also intended to

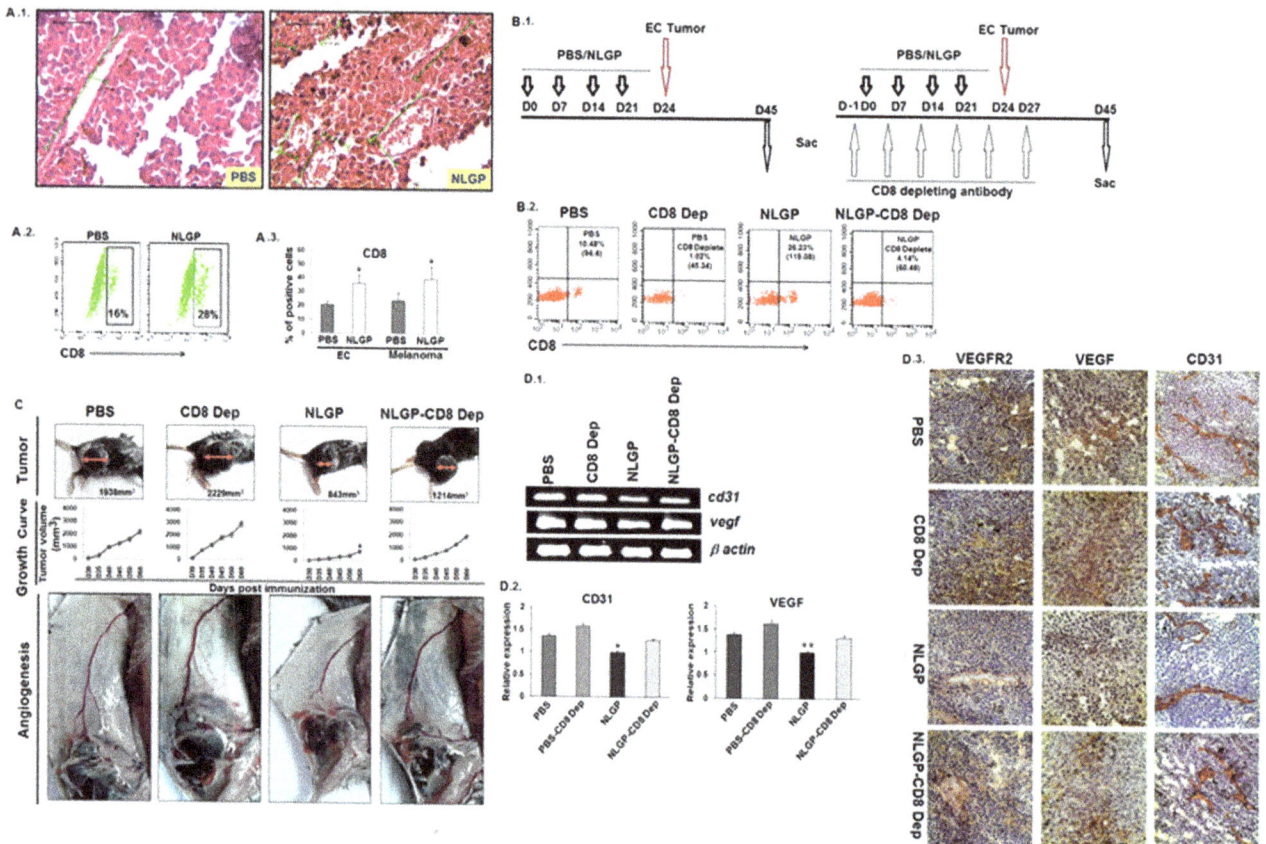

Figure 4. NLGP mediated normalization of tumor vasculature is dependent on CD8+ T cells. B16 melanoma tumors were harvested from both PBS and NLGP pretreated C57BL/6 mice. **A.1.** Immune infiltration within tumors from PBS and NLGP treated mice were assessed histologically (H&E). **A.2.** Status of CD8+ T cells in blood was assessed by flow cytometry. **A.3.** Bar diagram shows the status of CD8+ T cells within carcinoma and melanoma tumors. *$p<0.01$. **B.1.** Schematic presentation of control and CD8+ T cell depletion in either PBS or NLGP pretreated mice. **B.2.** Status of CD8+ T cells in all four mice groups (PBS, NLGP, PBS-CD8 dep and NLGP CD8 dep) were presented with representative figures. **C.** Representative picture of tumors, tumor growth curve and angiogenesis of PBS and NLGP pretreated mice with or without CD8+ T cell depletion. $p<0.001$. **D.1.** Total RNA was isolated from tumors of PBS, NLGP, PBS-CD8 depleted group (PBS-CD8 dep) and NLGP-CD8 depleted mice (NLGP-CD8-Dep) group (n = 3 in each case) to analyze genes, like, *cd31 and vegf* at transcriptional level by RT-PCR and **D.2.** densitometric analysis of band intensities from 3 individual observations (Mean ± SD) is presented. *$p<0.001$, **$p<0.01$. **D.3.** Immunohistochemical analysis of tumors obtained from PBS and NLGP pretreated mice with or without CD8 depletion were performed using monoclonal antibodies, specific for CD31, VEGF and VEGFR2.

evaluate the impact of NLGP on cutaneous wound healing process (model of physiological angiogenesis). Mice were treated with NLGP or PBS as described earlier and 4 mm² wounds were made in the skin of upper back. As shown in (Figure 6A) extent of wound closure in early days (between 4–7) was slightly higher in NLGP treated group, but in later stages (on day 9–14) healing was faster in PBS group and finally all wounds healed fully within a 2-week period. Furthermore, histological analysis revealed no observable differences in skin from both group of mice showing signature of wound healing (rapid epithelialization along with adipose layer were observed and hair follicles were formed) (Figure 6B). Immunofluorescence analysis on CD31+ and NG2+ cells on skin clearly showed no significant changes in wound healed skin from NLGP and PBS pretreated mice (Figure 6C). Therefore, our results clearly suggest that modulatory effect of NLGP on tumor angiogenesis does not hamper the normal physiological angiogenic process.

Discussion

We have reported significant restriction of murine sarcoma, carcinoma and melanoma growth due to administration of NLP/

NLGP in prophylactic [15,16,29] and therapeutic [17,18] settings. This tumor growth restriction is strictly dependent upon modulation of host-tumor immune interaction [20,25], since NLGP is unable to induce direct tumor cell apoptosis [19,35]. Apart from the already discussed immunomodulation by NLGP in cancer [18,20,22], angiogenic normalization property of this molecule is described here for the first time.

As results suggest, prophylactic administration of NLGP (with an interval of 7 days for 4 times) is inhibitory towards neovascularization initiated after tumor challenge and the antiangiogenic effect is indeed associated with the decrease in heavily dilated (thick)/fragile as well as very thin blood vessels. However, the thin and compact vessels were observed to be retained, probably to facilitate the trafficking of immune effector cells. Based on the available data, we reasoned that NLGP pretreatment causes significant reduction in proliferating Ki67+CD31+ VECs within tumor and thereby reduces the tumor micro vessel density (an indicator of tumor angiogenesis). Since proliferation of CD31+ cells corroborates neovascularization [36,37], such reduction plays a great role in angiogenic normalization. Unlike VECs, NLGP do not decrease the number of NG2+ pericytes, but effectively preserve their maturity and coverage of these cells on blood

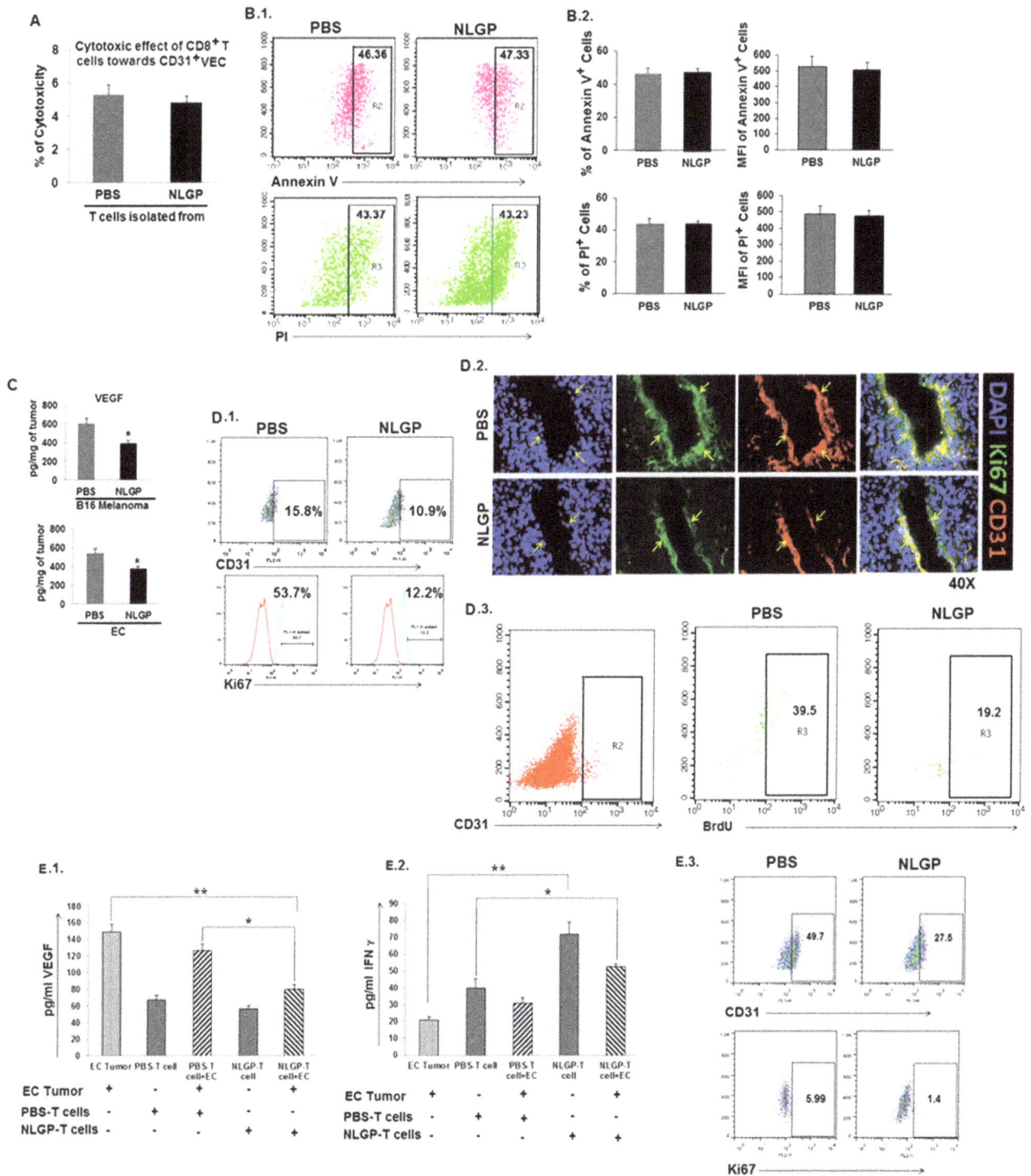

Figure 5. NLGP mediated vascular normalization is not due to CD8[+] T cell mediated apoptosis of CD31[+] cells. Mice were inoculated with B16 melanoma cells (2×10^5 cells/mice) to grow tumor. After reaching the tumor volume to a considerable size (1372 mm^3 approximately), tumor was harvested and CD31[+] VECs were isolated by flow sorting. CD8[+] T lymphocytes were isolated from NLGP or PBS pretreated ($4 \times$) mice by MACS purification and CD8[+] T cells were co-cultured with the CD31[+] VECs. **A.** Cytotoxicity was measured by LDH release assay. NLGP pretreated C57BL/6 mice were inoculated with B16 melanoma cells as mentioned earlier. **B.1.** As tumor reached a considerable volume (1372 mm^3 approximately), tumors were harvested, single cells prepared and stained with anti-CD31 antibody along with either Annexin V or Propidium Iodide (PI). Representative figures of Annexin-V and PI[+] cells from CD31 gated population. **B.2.** Bar diagram showing % positive cells and MFI. **C.** Cell lysates prepared from carcinoma and melanoma tumors of PBS and NLGP pretreated mice were used to quantitate the level of VEGF by ELISA. Cytokines were measured as pg/mg of tissue ± SE and Mean ± SD of 3 individual observations are presented in bar diagram. *$p<0.01$. **D.1.** Obtained cells as mentioned in **B.1**, were stained for CD31, along with Ki67. Gated CD31[+] population was assessed for Ki67 staining using Flowjo software and presented in histogram. **D.2.** Cryo-sections obtained from tumors of NLGP and PBS pretreated mice were stained with fluorescence labeled anti-CD31 (red) and anti-Ki67 (green) antibodies, along with DAPI (blue). Representative figures from 3 separate sets of experiments are presented. **D.3.**

PBS and NLGP pretreated tumor bearing mice were injected with BrdU within tumor and sacrificed after 48 hours. Single cells were prepared to check BrdU staining after gating the CD31 population, as shown in a representative figure. **E.1, E.2.** PBMC were isolated from both PBS and NLGP treated tumor bearing mice and cultured with EC cells (2×10^5 cells) for 24 hours and cell free supernatant were measured in pg/ml for VEGF (E.1) and IFNγ (E.2) by ELISA. Cytokines were quantitated as pg/ml $\pm$ SE. *$p<0.001$, **$p<0.01$. **E.3.** Flow sorted CD31$^+$ ECs isolated from tumor microenvironment were cultured with the above mentioned supernatants (NLGP-PBMC+EC vs PBS-PBMC+EC) for 48 hours and assessed for the EC proliferation flow cytometrically after Ki67 labeling.

vessels. Under NLGP influence, their tight association with VECs restore the vessel integrity and prevents leakiness. Therefore, by differentially regulating the two important stromal cell features, NLGP controls aberrant tumor vasculature. In context to host-antitumor benefits such results are encouraging as recent preclinical and clinical findings suggest that vascular normalization, rather than restriction of blood flow, is necessary to maintain the surge of effector immune cells and chemical regimens for cancer therapy [38].

Evidences are accumulated from present study suggesting the interference of NLGP in balancing tumor growth-supportive pro- and anti-angiogenic molecules. Several previous studies show that the VEGF family proteins, which signals through VEGFRs [39–41] are major factors involved in tumor-induced angiogenesis. Tumor and residing stromal cells secrete several growth factors particularly VEGF [42,43] to stimulate VEGFR$^+$ endothelial cell proliferation and in turn these cells provide the lining of newly formed blood vessels to supply nutrient to growing tumor [39]. Among all VEGFRs, VEGFR2 is mainly found on newly proliferating endothelial cells and targeting of VEGFR2 has been shown in some tumor models to reverse neo-vascularization [44].

Accordingly, NLGP selectively targets the VEGF-VEGFR2 signaling in proliferating endothelial cells to create a 'vascular normalization window' that might facilitate a decrease in interstitial pressure, enhanced tumor oxygenation and ultimately leads to a better therapeutic response [39,40] in terms of restricted tumor growth [27].

In view of our consistent observation on central involvement of immune system in NLGP-mediated eradication or prevention of murine tumor growth [17–20], the present study additionally evaluated the involvement of NLGP-instructed immune-modulation in controlling tumor-angiogenesis. Interestingly, we observed a significant abolition of NLGP mediated both anti-angiogenic and anti-tumor effect in cyclosporine [45,46] treated mice having prominent immunosuppression. However, adoptive transfer of immune cells from mice with NLGP therapy again restores both anti-angiogenic and tumor growth restricting effects of NLGP. Analysing these data, we speculated that NLGP-driven immune activation might be involved in anti-angiogenic process. To further validate our hypothesis, we used immunocompromised athymic nude mice and here also NLGP prophylaxis was unable to prevent neovascularization as well as tumor growth. Next, we directly

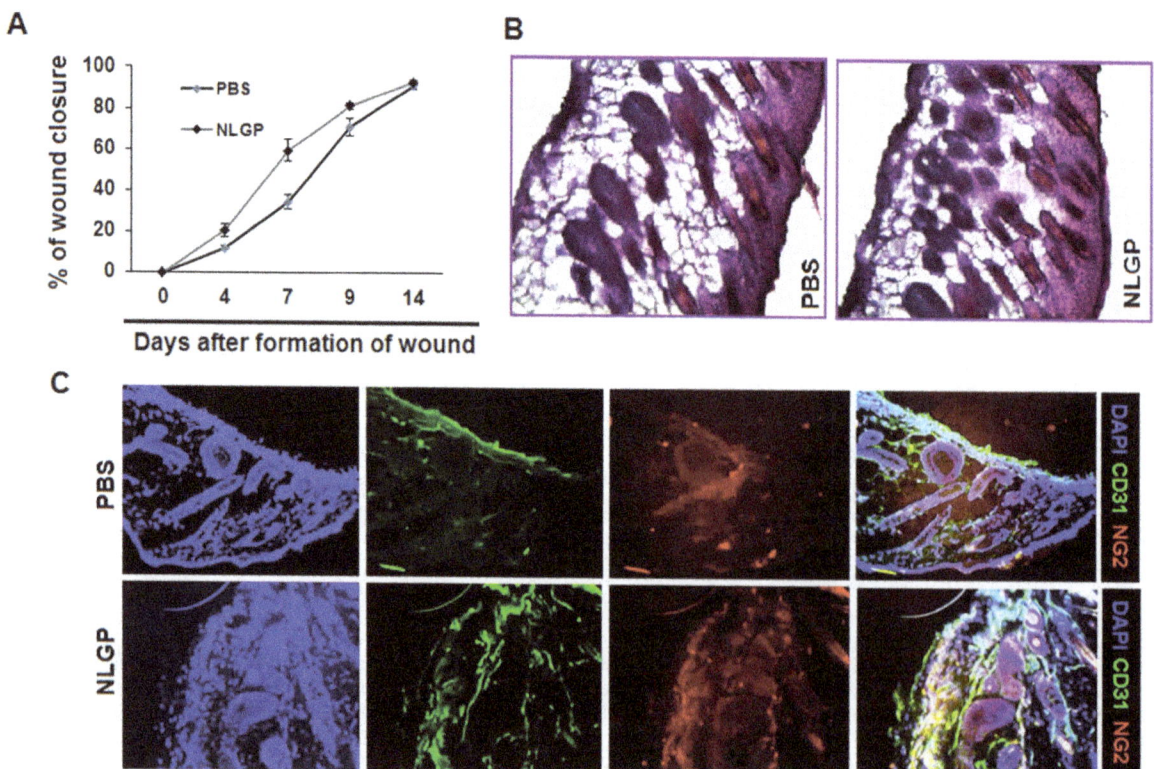

Figure 6. NLGP mediated vascular normalization has no adverse effect on normal wound healing process. Swiss mice were pretreated with NLGP (25µg) and PBS once in a week for four weeks and 4 mm^3 wound was made on the back of both groups of mice. **A.** Diameter of wounds was measured every two days and percentages of wound closure were calculated and data presented as Mean $\pm$ SD of 6 individual observations. **B.** Histological sections of wound beds were stained with H&E and assessed microscopically. Representative figures are presented. **C.** Cryo-sections of wound beds were stained with fluorescence labeled anti-CD31 (red) and anti-NG2 (green) antibodies along with DAPI.

focussed on the contribution of CD8[+] effector T cells, since NLGP selectively increases the trafficking of these effector cells into tumor parenchyma and therapeutic NLGP mediated tumor growth restriction is abrogated completely in CD8[+] T cell depleted mice [17,18]. However, infiltrating CD8[+] T cells often unable to show cytotoxic effect because, several tumor microenvironmental factors upregulate expression of inhibitory molecules like PD1 and CTLA4 on T cells to attenuate its effector functions and effector cytokine production [47]. In this context, modulatory effect of NLGP on TME is already reported [18,27,28]. More importantly, NLGP minimizes TME-induced anergy and exhaustion of CD8[+] T cells, as observed by downregulation of anergy related molecules DGKa, Grail, EGRs etc. [18] and exhaustion related molecules TIM3, LAG3, PD1 and CTLA4 [17,19] to preserve the optimum functional efficacy of infiltrated CD8[+] T cells. Likewise, in present study, NLGP administration followed by CD8[+] T cell depletion was unable to produce anti-angiogenic effect, as dilated tortuous (thick) blood vessels are seen in these groups of animals. Moreover, NLGP mediated reduction of proliferating CD31[+] endothelial cells or VEGF-VEGFR2 expression within tumor is abrogated in CD8[+] T cell depleted tumor bearing mice.

Considering this important contribution of CD8[+] T cells in NLGP mediated anti-angiogenesis, initially we assumed that CD8[+] T cells might be directly involved in killing of CD31[+] VECs. In several previous studies, it was demonstrated that VEGFR2-specific CTL can be directly involved in the killing of proliferating VECs [48]. Contrary to these reports in our system we do not observe any cytolytic activity of CD8[+] T cells isolated from NLGP treated mice towards flow sorted CD31[+] VECs. To solve this puzzle, we checked involvement of VEGF, for which sorted CD31[+] VECs were incubated with supernatants from co-culture of PBMC from NLGP/PBS EC bearing mice and EC cells. Interestingly, CD31[+] VECs proliferated less with NLGP-PBMC+EC cells culture supernatant (having comparatively high level of VEGF), which was again compensated with addition of recombinant VEGF. In vivo BrdU labeling study also suggests less number of CD31[+]BrdU[+] proliferating cells within tumors from NLGP pretreated mice, where VEGF content is significantly less. Therefore, finally, we concluded that unavailability of VEGF might be the predominant rate limiting factor of reduced VEC growth and vascular normalization. Considering the infiltration and essential role of CD8[+] T cells, we further assumed that, NLGP treatment may enhance DC migration to lymph node to prime CD8[+] T cells, which eventually infiltrates tumor parenchyma to kill tumor cells (that serves as one of the prime source for VEGF). It could also be possible that infiltrated CD8[+] T cells produce IFNγ and/or infiltrated DC produce IL-12 and either of these immunomodulatory cytokines possess anti-angiogenic effects by altering pro-angiogenic mediators [29,49]. Interestingly, our previous studies suggested the effectiveness of NLGP to influence CD8[+] T cells and DC to produce IFNγ and IL-12 respectively [20–22]. On the other-hand, in a separate in vitro study, we observed that NLGP can directly modulate B16 melanoma tumor cells by reducing HIF1α and VEGF in normoxic as well in hypoxic condition (unpublished observation).

In summary, our results suggest that NLGP prophylaxis educate whole immune system in such a way that after tumor challenge antigen presenting cells efficiently prime effector CD8[+] T cells, which in due course kill tumor cells to reduce tumor promoting growth factor burden within TME. These reduced availability of growth factor especially VEGF subsequently impede the growth of endothelial cells without affecting the vessel integrity to maintain the proper trafficking of immune effector cells within TME. More importantly this strategy does not affect the normal wound healing process, since immune-elimination is not obligate here. However, whether these infiltrated CD8[+] T cells affect other VEGF producing cells or any other parallel cascade operational in this NLGP-instructed immune system-mediated anti-angiogenic process needs further evaluation. Considering the limitation of anti-angiogenic immunotherapy [50,51] combination therapy integrating anti-angiogenic therapy along with immunotherapy or other conventional therapy was proposed by several groups [52,53]. In this context, NLGP treatment would be more promising in the field of cancer management because of its multidirectional fine tuning ability of tumor vasculature as well as of systemic/local immunity without any adverse physiological consequence.

Methods

Ethics statement on mice experiments

For maintenance and experimentation on mice, the relevant guidelines were followed and the Chittaranjan National Cancer Institute animal ethical committee approved the study.

Mice and tumors

Female C57BL/6 and Swiss mice (Age: 4–6 weeks; Body weight: 24–27 g) were obtained from the National Centre for Laboratory Animal Sciences (NCLAS), Hyderabad and Institutional Animal Care and Maintenance Department, Chittaranjan National Cancer Institute (CNCI), Kolkata, India respectively and maintained under standard laboratory conditions. Immuno-compromised athymic nude mice (4–6 weeks old) were purchased from NCLAS, Hyderabad and maintained in a specific pathogen free facility. Autoclaved dry pellet diet (Epic Laboratory Animal Feed, West Bengal Govt, Kalyani, India) and water were supplied ad libitum. Ehrlich Carcinoma (EC) was maintained by regular in vivo intraperitoneal passage in Swiss mice. B16F10 melanoma cell line was cultured in vitro in DMEM supplemented with 10% (v/v) FBS, 2 mM L-glutamine and penicillin-streptomycin (100μg/ml) at 37°C humidified conditions. To develop solid tumors in vivo, C57BL/6 and Swiss mice were inoculated subcutaneously (s.c.) in right hind leg quarters with B16F10 melanoma cells (2×10^5) and EC cells (1×10^6) respectively.

Antibodies and reagents

RPMI 1640, DMEM, and FBS were purchased from Invitrogen (NY, USA). Lymphocyte separation media (LSM) was procured from MP Biomedicals, Irvine, CA, USA and HiMedia, Mumbai, India. Fluorescence conjugated different anti-mouse antibodies (CD4, CD8, Ki67) and purified CD31 were procured from either BD-Pharmingen or Biolegends (both in, San Diego, CA, USA). Fluorescence- or peroxidase-labeled secondary antibodies were procured from e-Biosciences (San Diego, CA, USA). Purified anti-mouse Foxp3, VEGF, VEGFR1, VEGFR2, were procured from Santa Cruz Biotech (California, USA). IFNγ/IL-10 estimation kits (OptEIA, BD Biosciences, San Jose, CA, USA) 3,3′,5,5′-tetra-methylbenzidine (TMB) substrate solutions (for ELISA), CytoFix/CytoPerm kit (for intracellular staining), AnnexinV-Propidium iodide apoptosis detection kit were obtained from BD Pharmin-gen, San Dieago, CA, USA. LDH release assay kit for cytotoxicity and BrdU kit for proliferation were obtained from Roche Diagnostics, Mannheim, Germany. Western lightning chemilu-minescence and immunoperoxidase color detection kit were purchased from Pierce (Rockford, IL, USA) and Vector labora-tories Inc (Burlingame, CA, USA) respectively. Optimal cutting temperature (OCT) compound was purchased from Sakura Finetek, Torrance, CA, USA. RT-PCR primers were procured from MWG-Biotech AG (Bangalore, India). DAPI was purchased from Sigma, St. Louis, MO, USA.

Neem leaf glycoprotein

Mature neem *(Azadirachta indica)* leaves of identical size and color (indicative of similar age), taken from a standard source were shed-dried and pulverized. Leaf powder was soaked overnight in phosphate buffered saline (PBS), pH 7.4 and supernatant was collected by centrifugation at 1500 rpm, termed neem leaf preparation (NLP) [16,54]. NLP was then extensively dialyzed against PBS and concentrated by Centricon Membrane Filter (Millipore Corporation, Bedford, MA, USA) with 10 KDa molecular weight cut off. Active component of this preparation is a glycoprotein, as characterized earlier [55] and designated as Neem leaf glycoprotein (NLGP). Protein concentration of NLGP solution was measured by Lowry's method [56] using Folin's Phenol reagent. Purity of the NLGP was confirmed by HPLC [22] before use.

NLGP injection and tumor growth restriction assay

Two groups (n = 8, in each group) of either C57BL/6 or Swiss mice were immunized once weekly (25μg/100μl PBS/mice s.c.) for 4 weeks in total at left hind leg quarter with NLGP, keeping other group as PBS control. Immunized mice were inoculated with B16F10 and EC tumors respectively as mentioned above to develop solid tumors. Growth of solid tumor (in mm^3) was monitored biweekly by caliper measurement using the formula: $(width^2 \times length)/2$. Survival of mice was noted regularly, till tumor size reached to 25 mm in either direction.

Angiogenesis study with blood vessels

To study the role of NLGP on tumor angiogenesis, both groups of NLGP and PBS pre-treated tumor bearing mice were sacrificed and skin were removed carefully from peritoneal region without disturbing the angiogenic vessels adjacent to tumors. These blood vessels were counted macroscopically using convex lens depending on the thickness of the blood vessels and categorized as heavy, very thick, thick, thin and very thin. Area of blood vessels was calculated using Photoshop software (Adobe Systems Incorporated, San Jose, California, USA) and presented in Pixels. Extent of angiogenesis was categorized as 4 (++++), 3 (+++), 2 (++) and 1 (+). Tumor volume (in mm^3) and extent of angiogenesis (in raw score) was multiplied to obtain an index for tumor angiogenesis. Mean of score from all mice was presented as Mean Index for Tumor and Angiogenesis (MITA).

Angiogenesis in immunocompromised mice

To study the role of immune system in tumor angiogenesis, Swiss mice were divided into three groups (n = 3) and two groups received NLGP immunization as said before, keeping other group as PBS control. One of these NLGP treated mice group was immune suppressed by three consecutive peritoneal cyclosporine injections (15 mg/Kg) on day 13, 17 and 21. Mice of all groups were inoculated s.c. with EC (1×10^6 cells) on day 24. Again, cyclosporine was injected on day 25 and 28. Similar study was conducted on immune compromised athymic nude mice, where one group received NLGP with another PBS control group. Following completion of immunization all mice received EC (1×10^6 cells) s.c. and tumor growth and survivability were monitored biweekly. Pattern of angiogenesis was noted after sacrificing the mice.

To reconfirm the same, NLGP immunized Swiss mice were similarly divided in three groups (n = 3, in each group) and immunologically suppressed with consecutive peritoneal injection of cyclosporine as mentioned above. Then all three groups of mice were injected with 1×10^6 viable EC cells. Following establishment of tumor (64 mm^3 in average), first group was kept as control, second group received splenic immune cells (1×10^7) i.v. through tail vein from PBS treated mice and third group of mice received same number of immune cells from $4 \times$ NLGP (25μg/100μl/mice) immunized mice. When tumor reached a considerable volume (25 mm) in mice from PBS pretreated group, mice from both groups were sacrificed (on day 45) for comparative monitoring of angiogenesis, as described above. Identical experiment was performed in athymic nude mice with similar cell transfer from either PBS or NLGP injected mice.

Angiogenesis in CD8+ T cell depleted mice

Within several immune cells, to study the specific role of CD8+ T cells in the process of angiogenesis, C57BL/6 mice were divided in four groups (n = 4 in each group). Two groups of mice were immunized with NLGP as said before while other two groups of mice were injected with PBS. One NLGP and one PBS treated mice group were peritoneally injected with CD8 depleting antibody (100μg/50μl) on day -1, 6, 13, 20 and 27 as shown in Fig. 4BI. CD8+ T cell depletion status was monitored regularly by analyzing peripheral blood using flow cytometry. On day 24, B16F10 tumors (2×10^5 cells/mice) were inoculated s.c. to the left flank of hind leg. Tumor volumes were monitored biweekly and on reaching a considerable size (25 mm) in mice from PBS pretreated group, mice from both groups (PBS and NLGP) were sacrificed for comparative monitoring in angiogenesis, as described above.

Tumor infiltrated immune cells

After attaining considerable size, tumors of either type were harvested from sacrificed mice. Portions of tumors were separately preserved for histology, immunohistochemistry, immunofluorescence studies, western blot, flow cytometry and RT-PCR analysis.

A piece of tumor was cleaned with PBS and chopped into small pieces and treated with mixture of collagenase (2μg/ml) and hyaluronidase (2μg/ml) and passed through the nylon mesh to prepare single cell suspensions. Tumor infiltrating lymphocytes (TILs) were then separated from tumor cells by differential gradient centrifugation at 2000 rpm for 30 minutes to analyze their proportions.

Histology, immunohistochemistry and immunofluorescence studies

Tumors were fixed in 10% formalin for standard histological preparations and embedded in paraffin. Sections (4–5 μm) were prepared and stained with hematoxylin-eosin (H&E) according to standard protocol. Representative tumors were selected for immunohistochemical analysis. Fresh tumor tissues were also frozen for cryo-sectioning. Sections were immunostained for CD31, NG2, VEGF, VEGFR1 and VEGFR2 by the method described [27]. In some cases, tumor or skin sections were snap-frozen in OCT compound. Sections (5 μm) were prepared using cryostat (Leica, Germany), air-dried and fixed in ice-cold methanol for 20-30 min. The sections were blocked with 5% BSA solution and stained with different anti-mouse antibodies (CD31-PE, NG2-FITC, Ki67-FITC) by the method described earlier [27].

Western blot analysis

Tumor lysate or cellular lysate (50 μg) were separated on 6–20% SDS–polyacrylamide gel and transferred onto a PVDF membrane for Western Blotting. Incubation was performed for different primary antibodies, e.g., CD31, NG2, VEGF, VEGFR1 and VEGFR2, and the procedure followed the method as published [18].

RT-PCR analysis

Total RNA was isolated from solid tumors (from PBS and NLGP treated mice) using the TRIZOL Reagent (Ambion, Austin, Texas, USA). The cDNA synthesis was carried out using RevertAid First Strand cDNA Synthesis Kit (Fermentas, K1622) following the manufacturer's protocol and RT-PCR was carried out using gene-specific primers. The primer sequences of mouse CD31, VEGF, VEGFR1, VEGFR2, NG2 and β-Actin are described in the Table 2. PCR products were identified by image analysis software for gel documentation (Gel Doc XR+ system, BioRad) following electrophoresis on 1.5%–2% agarose gels and staining with ethidium bromide [18,27].

Flow cytometric staining

Single cell preparation from harvested tumors were labeled with $0.5\mu l$ (for 1×10^6 cells) FITC or PE conjugated antibodies, specific for mouse CD8, CD31, Ki67 markers, and surface or intracellular flow cytometry was performed by the method described [17].

Annexin V-PI staining for apoptosis

Harvested tumors from PBS and NLGP treated mice were minced to make single cell suspension as mentioned before. Freshly collected single cells were mixed with $1 \times$ binding buffer $(100 \ \mu l)$ and kept for 2 min at room temp. Then $5\mu l$ of each Annexin-V and PI were added and incubated for 15 mins and then finally analyzed by flow cytometry.

Flow sorting of CD31⁺ cells

Single cell suspension obtained from harvested tumors was washed with PBS (containing 1% FBS) and passed through cell strainer. This cell pellet was stained with primary anti-mouse-CD31 antibody (30 minutes) and further tagged with appropriate FITC labeled secondary antibody and CD31⁺ cells were purified by Flow sorting with BD FACS Aria, San Jose, CA.

Mechanistic studies on downregulation of CD31⁺ endothelial cells

CD8⁺ T cells were purified by MACS from the spleen of both PBS and NLGP treated tumor bearing mice by the method described [17,18]. Flow sorted CD31⁺ endothelial cells were co-cultured with CD8⁺ T cells in 1:10 dilution in serum free media and checked for cytotoxicity by LDH release assay. Cell-free supernatants were used to measure the level of released LDH using the formula: % Cytotoxicity = (Lysis from Effector-Target Mixture – Lysis from Effector only) – Spontaneous Lysis/ (Maximum Lysis – Spontaneous Lysis) $\times 100$.

In a separate experiment, splenic cells were purified from EC bearing PBS and NLGP treated mice and co-cultured with EC cells (10:1 ratio) for 24 hrs. Cell free culture supernatants were collected and assessed for VEGF and IFNγ content by ELISA. Purified CD31⁺ endothelial cells were also incubated with such culture supernatants for 48 hrs and their proliferation was assessed by Ki67 staining by the method described [15]. In a parallel experiment NLGP ($4\times$) pretreated mice were injected with anti-mouse BrdU antibody injected in tumor as per manufacturer's manual. After 48 hours of injection both groups of mice were sacrificed to harvest tumors and single cells were prepared as described before. Single cells were stained with anti-CD31 antibody and assessed flow cytometrically as per standard protocol.

Wound healing assay

Mice were pretreated with PBS and NLGP as described earlier. Mice were then anesthetized with peritoneal injection of 0.3 ml of 2-2-2-tribromoethanol (Avertin, Sigma, St. Louis, MO) and back portion was properly shaved to remove all fur and cleaned with 70% alcohol. Subsequently using dual puncher 4 mm² wound was created on both side of their back and kept in sterile environment. After every 3 days interval wound closure was measured henceforth by a vernier caliper and the wound healing was analyzed. Finally on day 15 mice of both groups were sacrificed and their skins were fixed and sectioned using cryostat. Routine histology and immunofluorescence study was performed in skins.

Statistical analysis

All results represent the average of separate *in vivo* and *in vitro* experiments. Number of experiments is mentioned in result section and legends to figures. In each experiment a value represents the mean of three individual observations and presented as mean $\pm$ standard deviation (SD). Statistical significance was established by Student's t-test using INSTAT 3 Software (GraphPad Software, Inc.), with differences between groups attaining a p value <0.05 considered as significant.

Table 2. Primer sequences of various cytokine genes studied.

Name	Primer sequences (5′–3′)	Product size
β-Actin-forward	CAACCGTGAAAAGATGACCC	228 bp.
β-Actin-reverse	ATGAGGTAGTCTGTCAGGTC	
VEGFR2-forward	ACAGACAGTGGGATGGTCC	271 bp
VEGFR2-reverse	AAACAGGAGGTGAGCGCAG	
VEGFR1-forward	CCAACTACCTCAAGAGCAAAC	315 bp
VEGFR1-reverse	CCAGGTCCCGATGAATGCAC	
CD31-forword	AGCCCACCAGAGACATGGAA	337 bp
CD31-reverse	CTGGCTCTGTTGGAGGCTGT	
VEGF-forward	GGACCCTGGCTTTACTGCTG	201 bp
VEGF-reverse	CACAGGACGGCTTGAAGATG	

Supporting Information

Figure S1 Purification of CD31⁺ cells by flow sorting.
Solid B16 melanoma tumors were harvested from PBS treated C57BL/6 mice and single cell preparation was made. Cells were labeled with anti-CD31 antibody and positive cells were sorted in flow cytometer (BD FACS Aria). A. FSC/SSC plot of single cell population under study. B. Unstained cell population in FL1 (CD31)/FSC plot. C. CD31⁺ cells in FL1 (CD31)/FSC plot. D. Purified CD31⁺ vascular endothelial cells after flow sorting. (TIF)

References

1. Hanahan D, Weinberg RA (2000) The hallmarks of cancer. Cell 7:57–70.
2. Breier G (2000) Angiogenesis in embryonic development- A review. Placenta 21:S11–15.
3. Tonnesen MG, Feng X, Clark RA (2000) Angiogenesis in wound healing. J Invest Dermatol Symp Proc 5:40–46.
4. Sihvo EI, Ruohtula T, Auvinen MI, Koivistoinen A, Harjula AL, et al. (2003) Simultaneous progression of oxidative stress and angiogenesis in malignant transformation of Barrett esophagus. J Thorac Cardiovasc Surg 126:1952–1957.
5. Khan M, Nayyar AS, Gayitri HC, Bafna UD, Siddique A (2012) Tumor angiogenesis: A potential marker of the ongoing process of malignant transformation in leukoplakia patients, removing the veil. Clin Cancer Invest J 1:127–134.
6. Sonnenschein C, Soto AM (2013) The aging of the 2000 and 2011 Hallmarks of Cancer reviews: A critique. J Biosci 38:651–663.
7. Hanahan D, Folkman J (1996) Patterns and emerging mechanisms of the angiogenic switch during tumorigenesis. Cell 86:353–364.
8. Zou W (2006) Regulatory T cells, tumour immunity and immunotherapy. Nat Rev Immunol 6: 295–307.
9. Ribatti D, Crivellato E (2009) Immune cells and angiogenesis. J Cell Mol Med 13:2822–2833.
10. Terme M, Colussi O, Marcheteau E, Tanchot C, Tartour E, et al. (2012) Modulation of Immunity. Antiangiogenic Molecules in Cancer. Clin Dev Immunol 2012:1–8.
11. Tartour E, Pere H, Maillere B, Terme M, Merillon N, et al. (2011) Angiogenesis and immunity: a bidirectional link potentially relevant for the monitoring of antiangiogenic therapy and the development of novel therapeutic combination with immunotherapy. Cancer Metastasis Rev 30:83–95.
12. Shiao SL, Ganesan AP, Rugo HS, Coussens LM (2011) Immune microenvironments in solid tumors: new targets for therapy. Genes Dev 25:2559–2572.
13. Munn LL (2003) Aberrant vascular architecture in tumors and its importance in drug-based therapies. Drug Discov Today 8:396–403.
14. Jain RK (2005) Normalization of tumor vasculature: an emerging concept in antiangiogenic therapy. Science 307:58–62.
15. Haque E, Mandal I, Pal S, Baral R (2006) Prophylactic dose of neem (Azadirachta indica) leaf preparation restricting murine tumor growth is nontoxic, hematostimulatory and immunostimulatory. Immunopharmacol Immunotoxicol 28:33–50.
16. Baral R, Chattopadhyay U (2004) Neem (Azadirachta indica) leaf mediated immune activation causes prophylactic growth inhibition of murine Ehrlich carcinoma and B16 melanoma. Int Immunopharmacol 4:355–366.
17. Mallick A, Barik S, Goswami KK, Banerjee S, Ghosh S, et al. (2013) Neem leaf glycoprotein activates CD8(+) T cells to promote therapeutic anti-tumor immunity inhibiting the growth of mouse sarcoma. PLoS One 8:e47434.
18. Barik S, Banerjee S, Mallick A, Goswami KK, Roy S, et al. (2013) Normalization of tumor microenvironment by neem leaf glycoprotein potentiates effector T cell functions and therapeutically intervenes in the growth of mouse sarcoma. PLoS One 8:e66501.
19. Chakraborty T, Bose A, Barik S, Goswami KK, Banerjee S, et al. (2011) Neem leaf glycoprotein inhibits CD4+CD25+Foxp3+ Tregs to restrict murine tumor growth. Immunotherapy 3:949–969.
20. Bose A, Chakraborty K, Sarkar K, Goswami S, Chakraborty T, et al. (2009) Neem leaf glycoprotein induces perforin-mediated tumor cell killing by T and NK cells through differential regulation of IFNgamma signaling. J Immunother 32:42–53.
21. Bose A, Baral R (2007) NK cellular cytotoxicity of tumor cells initiated by neem leaf preparation is associated with CD40-CD40L mediated endogenous production of IL-12. Human Immunol 68:823–831.
22. Goswami S, Bose A, Sarkar K, Roy S, Chakraborty T, et al. (2010) Neem leaf glycoprotein matures myeloid derived dendritic cells and optimizes anti-tumor T cell functions. Vaccine 28:1241–1252.
23. Roy S, Goswami S, Bose A, Chakraborty K, Pal S, et al. (2011) Neem leaf glycoprotein partially rectifies suppressed dendritic cell functions and associated

T cell efficacy in patients with stage IIIB cervical cancer. Clin Vaccine Immunol 18:571–579.
24. Goswami KK, Barik S, Sarkar M, Bhowmick A, Biswas J, et al. (2014) Targeting STAT3 phosphorylation by neem leaf glycoprotein prevents immune evasion exerted by supraglottic laryngeal tumor induced M2 macrophages. Mol Immunol 59:119–127.
25. Bose A, Chakraborty K, Sarkar K, Goswami S, Haque E, et al. (2009) Neem leaf glycoprotein directs T-bet-associated type 1 immune commitment. Hum Immunol 70:6–15.
26. Chakraborty K, Bose A, Chakraborty T, Sarkar K, Goswami S, et al. (2010) Restoration of dysregulated CC chemokine signaling for monocyte/macrophage chemotaxis in head and neck squamous cell carcinoma patients by neem leaf glycoprotein maximizes tumor cell cytotoxicity. Cell Mol Immunol 7:396–408.
27. Barik S, Bhuniya A, Banerjee S, Das A, Sarkar M, et al. (2013) Neem leaf glycoprotein is superior than Cisplatin and Sunitinib malate in restricting melanoma growth by normalization of tumor microenvironment. Int Immunopharmacol 17:42–49.
28. Barik S, Banerjee S, Sarkar M, Bhuniya A, Roy S, et al. (2013) Neem leaf glycoprotein optimizes effector and regulatory functions within tumor microenvironment to intervene therapeutically the growth of B16 melanoma in C57BL/6 mice. Trials in Vaccinology, e-pub on Dec 6, 2013.
29. Haque E, Baral R (2006) Neem (Azadirachta indica) leaf preparation induces prophylactic growth inhibition of murine Ehrlich carcinoma in Swiss and C57BL/6 by activation of NK cells and NK-T cells. Immunobiology 211:721–731.
30. Chatterjee S, Heukamp LC, Siobal M, Schöttle J, Wieczorek C, et al. (2013) Tumor VEGF:VEGFR2 autocrine feed-forward loop triggers angiogenesis in lung cancer. J Clin Invest 123:1732–1740.
31. Daniel WM, Vosseler S, Mirancea N, Hicklin DJ, Bohlen P, et al. Rapid Vessel Regression, Protease Inhibition, and Stromal Normalization upon Short-Term Vascular Endothelial Growth Factor Receptor 2 Inhibition in Skin Carcinoma Heterotransplants. Am J Pathol 167:1389–1403.
32. Vosseler S, Mirancea N, Bohlen P, Mueller MM, Fusenig NE (2005) Angiogenesis inhibition by vascular endothelial growth factor receptor-2 blockade reduces stromal matrix metalloproteinase expression, normalizes stromal tissue, and reverts epithelial tumor phenotype in surface heterotransplants. Cancer Res 65:1294–1305.
33. Facciabene A, Motz GT, Coukos G (2012) T-regulatory cells: key players in tumor immune escape and angiogenesis. Cancer Res 72: 2162–2171.
34. Kujawski M, Kortylewski M, Lee H, Herrmann A, Kay H, et al. (2008) Stat3 mediates myeloid cell–dependent tumor angiogenesis in mice. J Clin Invest 118:3367–3377.
35. Bose A, Haque E, Baral R (2007) Neem leaf preparation induces apoptosis of tumor cells by releasing cytotoxic cytokines from human peripheral blood mononuclear cells. Phytother Res 21: 914–920.
36. Wang D, Stockard CR, Harkins L, Lott P, Salih C, et al. (2008) Immunohistochemistry for the evaluation of angiogenesis in tumor xenografts. Biotech Histochem 83:179–189.
37. Kim H, Cho HJ, Kim SW, Liu B, Choi YJ, et al. (2010) CD31+ cells represent highly angiogenic and vasculogenic cells in bone marrow novel role of nonendothelial CD31+ cells in neovascularization and their therapeutic effects on ischemic vascular disease. Circ Res 107:602–614.
38. Goel S, Wong AH, Jain RK (2012) Vascular normalization as a therapeutic strategy for malignant and nonmalignant disease. Cold Spring Harb Perspect Med 2:a006486. doi: 10.1101/cshperspect.a006486.
39. Dudley AC (2012) Tumor endothelial cell. Cold Spring Harb Perspect Med 2:a006536.
40. Jain RK (2005) Normalization of tumor vasculature: an emerging concept in antiangiogenic therapy. Science 307:58–62.
41. Batchelor TT1, Sorensen AG, di Tomaso E, Zhang WT, Duda DG, et al. (2007) AZD2171, a pan-VEGF receptor tyrosine kinase inhibitor, normalizes tumor vasculature and alleviates edema in glioblastoma patients. Cancer Cell 11:83–95.

Acknowledgments

We acknowledge Director, CNCI, Kolkata, India, for providing necessary facilities. Thanks to Dr. Subrata Laskar, Burdwan University, India, for his help in characterization of NLGP. Thanks to Dr. Abhijit Rakshit for providing experimental animals. We also extend our thanks to Dr. P. S. Dasgupta for his help and suggestions in angiogenic study.

Author Contributions

Conceived and designed the experiments: A. Bose S. Banerjee RB. Performed the experiments: S. Banerjee S. Barik TG SG AD A. Bhuniya. Analyzed the data: S. Banerjee A. Bose TG S. Barik RB. Contributed reagents/materials/analysis tools: RB. Wrote the paper: A. Bose S. Banerjee RB.

42. Kaigler D, Krebsbach PH, Polverini PJ, Mooney DJ (2003) Role of vascular endothelial growth factor in bone marrow stromal cell modulation of endothelial cells. Tissue Engineering 9:95-103.

43. Guillem EB, Nyhus JK, Wolford CC, Friece CR, Sampsel JW (2002) Vascular endothelial Growth factor secretion by tumor-infiltrating macrophages essentially supports tumor angiogenesis and IgG immune complexes potentiate the process. Cancer Res 62:7042–7049.

44. Niethammer AG, Xiang R, Becker JC, Wodrich H, Pertl U, et al. (2002) A DNA vaccine against VEGF receptor 2 prevents effective angiogenesis and inhibits tumor growth. Nat Med 8: 1369–1375.

45. Rafiee P, Heidemann J, Ogawa H, Johnson NA, Fisher PJ, et al. (2004) Cyclosporin A differentially inhibits multiple steps in VEGF induced angiogenesis in human microvascular endothelial cells through altered intracellular signaling. Cell Commun Signal 2:3.

46. Hernández GL, Volpert OV, Iñiguez MA, Lorenzo E, Martínez-Martínez S, et al. (2001) Selective inhibition of vascular endothelial growth factor-mediated angiogenesis by cyclosporin A: roles of the nuclear factor of activated T cells and cyclooxygenase 2. J Exp Med 193:607–620.

47. Duraiswamy J, Kaluza KM, Freeman GJ, Coukos G (2013) Dual blockade of PD-1 and CTLA-4 combined with tumor vaccine effectively restores T-cell rejection function in tumors. Cancer Res 73: 3591–3603.

48. Zhou H, Luo Y, Mizutani M, Mizutani N, Reisfeld RA, et al. (2005) T cell-mediated suppression of angiogenesis results in tumor protective immunity. Blood 106:2026–2032.

49. Qin Z, Schwartzkopff J, Pradera F, Kammertoens T, Seliger B, et al. (2003) A Critical Requirement of Interferon γ-mediated Angiostasis for Tumor Rejection by CD8+ T Cells. Cancer Research 63:4095–4100.

50. Abdollahi A, Folkman J (2010) Evading tumor evasion: current concepts and perspectives of anti-angiogenic cancer therapy. Drug Resist Update 13:16–28.

51. Itasaka S, Komaki R, Herbst RS, Shibuya K, Shintani T, et al. (2007) Endostatin improves radioresponse and blocks tumor revascularization after radiation therapy for A431 xenografts in mice. Int J Radiat Oncol Biol Phys 7:870–878.

52. Cirone P, Bourgeois JM, Shen F, Chang PL (2004) Combined immunotherapy and antiangiogenic therapy of cancer with microencapsulated cells. Hum Gene Ther 15:945–959.

53. Shi S, Wang R, Chen Y, Song H, Chen L, et al. (2013) Combining Antiangiogenic Therapy with Adoptive Cell Immunotherapy Exerts Better Antitumor Effects in NonSmall Cell Lung Cancer Models. PLoS One 8: e65757.

54. Baral R, Mandal I, Chattopadhyay U (2005) Immunostimulatory neem leaf preparation acts as an adjuvant to enhance the efficacy of poorly immunogenic B16 melanoma surface antigen vaccine. Int Immunopharmacol 5:1343–1352.

55. Chakraborty K, Bose A, Pal S, Sarkar K, Goswami S, et al. (2008) Neem leaf glycoprotein restores the impaired chemotactic activity of peripheral blood mononuclear cells from head and neck squamous cell carcinoma patients by maintaining CXCR3/CXCL10 balance. Int Immunopharmacol 8:330–340.

56. Bailey JL (1967) Miscellaneous analytical methods. In: Bailey JL (ed) Techniques in Protein Chemistry, Elsevier Science, NY, USA.

7

Progranulin Facilitates Conversion and Function of Regulatory T Cells under Inflammatory Conditions

Fanhua Wei[1,2], Yuying Zhang[1], Weiming Zhao[2], Xiuping Yu[2], Chuan-ju Liu[1,3]*

1 Department of Orthopaedic Surgery, New York University Medical Center, New York, New York, United States of America, 2 Institute of Pathogenic Biology, Shandong University School of Medicine, Jinan, China, 3 Department of Cell Biology, New York University School of Medicine, New York, New York, United States of America

Abstract

The progranulin (PGRN) is known to protect regulatory T cells (Tregs) from a negative regulation by TNF-α, and its levels are elevated in various kinds of autoimmune diseases. Whether PGRN directly regulates the conversion of CD4+CD25-T cells into Foxp3-expressing regulatory T cells (iTreg), and whether PGRN affects the immunosuppressive function of Tregs, however, remain unknown. In this study we provide evidences demonstrating that PGRN is able to stimulate the conversion of CD4+CD25-T cells into iTreg in a dose-dependent manner *in vitro*. In addition, PGRN showed synergistic effects with TGF-β1 on the induction of iTreg. PGRN was required for the immunosuppressive function of Tregs, since PGRN-deficient Tregs have a significant decreased ability to suppress the proliferation of effector T cells (Teff). In addition, PGRN deficiency caused a marked reduction in Tregs number in the course of inflammatory arthritis, although no significant difference was observed in the numbers of Tregs between wild type and PGRN deficient mice during development. Furthermore, PGRN deficiency led to significant upregulation of the Wnt receptor gene Fzd2. Collectively, this study reveals that PGRN directly regulates the numbers and function of Tregs under inflammatory conditions, and provides new insight into the immune regulatory mechanism of PGRN in the pathogenesis of inflammatory and immune-related diseases.

Editor: Srinivas V. Kaveri, INSERMU1138, France

Funding: This work was supported partly by NIH research grants R01AR062207, R01AR061484, R56AI100901, and a Disease Targeted Research Grant from Rheumatology Research Foundation. The authors state that the funders had no role in study design, data collection and analysis, decision to publish, or preparation of the manuscript.

Competing Interests: The authors have declared that no competing interests exist.

* Email: chuanju.liu@nyumc.org

Introduction

CD4+CD25+Foxp3+ regulatory T cells (Tregs) play a critical role in maintenance of peripheral tolerance and prevention of chronic inflammation and autoimmune diseases [1], [2]. Tregs can be divided into two main types: naturally occurring regulatory T cells (nTreg) and adaptive/inducible regulatory T cells (iTreg). nTreg are generated in thymus and represent a stable subpopulation and suppress the proliferation of self reactive T cells in the secondary lymphoid tissues [3]. In contrast, iTreg are generated in peripheral lymphoid tissues, which have variable expression of Foxp3 and may lose regulatory properties after their generation. Recent studies have shown that iTreg can be differentiated from the conventional CD4+CD25- T cells in the presence of TGF-β [4]. Since iTreg play essential roles in self-tolerance and autoimmunity, an investigation of iTreg induction and function would be of great importance in their therapeutic potential [5–7]. A global sequencing revealed that Foxp3 and Wnt target genes are considerably overlapped, suggesting a crucial role of Wnt signaling in Treg function [8]. In addition, stable expression of β-catenin enhanced the survival of Treg cells and rendered pathogenic CD4+CD25- T cells anergic [9].

Progranulin (PGRN), also called granulin epithelin precursor (GEP), PC-cell-derived growth factor (PCDGF), proepithelin, and acrogranin, is a 593-amino-acid secreted growth factor [10], [11]. PGRN is known to play an important role in a variety of physiologic

and pathological processes, including wound healing, inflammation response, neurotrophic factor, and host defense [12]. PGRN can be induced in many cell types during inflammatory conditions, including immune cells and epithelial cells [13]. PGRN associates with some members in the TNF receptor superfamily, including TNFR1, TNFR2 and DR3 [12], [14–16], and possesses the ability to suppress inflammation in various kinds of conditions [12], [17–23]. The association between PGRN levels and systemic inflammation and autoimmunity has been reported [24–28], for instance, serum levels of PGRN were elevated in systemic lupus erythematosus and related with disease activity [25]. Auto-antibodies against PGRN have also been found in several autoimmune diseases, including rheumatoid arthritis, psoriatic arthritis, and inflammatory bowel disease, and such antibodies promoted a proinflammatory environment in a subgroup of patients [29–31]. Furthermore, PGRN was found to protect Tregs from a negative regulation by TNF-α [12], [30]. However, the direct regulation of PGRN on Tregs has not been reported yet. In this study, we present direct evidences that PGRN stimulates Tregs formation and is also required for its immunosuppressive activity.

Materials and Methods

Mice

All of the animal studies were performed and approved by the Institutional Animal Care and Use Committee of New York

University (IACUC protocol #130202-01). C57BL/6, Foxp3-RFP mice (C57BL/6 background) were obtained from Jackson Laboratories. The generation of PGRN-deficient mice has been described previously [32]. All efforts were made to minimize animal suffering through anaesthesia.

Flow cytometry

Spleen cells and lymphocytes from wild type and PGRN-deficient mice were stained using antibodies to mice CD4-FITC, CD25-PE and Foxp3-Alex Flour 647 (all from eBioscience, San Diego, CA, USA). Intracellular staining for Foxp3 (eBioscience, San Diego, CA, USA) were conducted according to the manufacturers' instructions. Data were acquired on a LSRII (BD) and analyzed with FlowJo (Tree star, Ashland OR). For CFSE labeling, cells were incubating with 5 mM CFSE (Invitrogen, Carlsbad, CA, USA) in PBS (containing 0.1% BSA) at 37°C for 10 min.

Cell purification

For isolation of CD4+CD25- T cells, 1×10^7 lymphocytes of spleens from 6- to 8-week-old mice were incubated with 10 μl antibody cocktail (Miltenyi Biotech, Bergisch Gladbach, Germany) and 10 μl anti-CD25 (biotin labeling), followed by incubation with 20 μl anti-biotin microbeads according to the manufactures instructions (Miltenyi Biotech, Bergisch Gladbach, Germany). The purity of the CD4+CD25- T cells was above 95%, as examined by FACS method.

For isolation of CD4+CD25+ T cells, lymphocytes of spleens from 6- to 8-week-old mice were depleted of cells that were labeled with Ab-to-mouse B220 and CD8 by magnetic cell sorting using Mitenyi reagents and a MACS apparatus. Then the lymphocytes were stained with CD4-APC and CD25-PE antibodies, washed 2 times with staining buffer and resuspended with sorting buffer. CD4+CD25+ T cells were sorted by FACS MoFlo cytometer. The purity of sorted fraction was 90–95%.

PGRN immunization

The recombinant PGRN protein was prepared according to our previous publication [33]. One week-old Foxp3-RFP reporter mice were divided into two groups (n = 3). Two group mice were treated with 100 μg PGRN or PBS (serving as a control) by intraperitoneal injection every two days. After 1 week, the lymphocytes of spleen, peripheral lymph nodes (PLN), mesenteric lymph nodes (MLN), and Peyer's patches (PP) were collected for analysis by FACS.

In vitro naïve CD4+CD25- T cells conversion assay

Naïve CD+CD25- T cells were purified from lymphocytes of spleens from Foxp3-GFP mice (6- to 8-week-old) using Mitenyi reagents and a MACS apparatus according to the manufactures instructions. Naïve cells were stimulated with plate-bound anti-CD3 (10 μg/ml, BD, San Diego, CA, USA) and soluble anti-CD28 (1 μg/ml, BD, San Diego, CA, USA) for 3–4 days in the presence of IL-2 (20 U/ml, R&D, Minneapolis, MN, USA). Human TGF-β (0 ng/ml, 0.01 ng/ml) and recombinant PGRN protein (0 μg/ml, 0.2 μg/ml, 1 μg/ml) were added as indicated. The induction of Foxp3+ T cells in the CD4+ fraction was detected by flow cytometry based on the levels of GFP.

In vitro suppression assay

CD4+CD25- T cells were magnetic sorted from spleen lymphocytes of Thy1.1 mice (C57BL/6 background) using isolation kit from Miltenyi, and labeled with 5 mM CFSE as

responder cells (Teff). 1×10^6 spleen cells from TCRα-/-β-/- mice (C57BL/6 background) were lysed with red blood cell lysis buffer for 3 min, washed with pre-cooling PBS and treated with 1 μg mitomycin for 20 min, then resuspended with RPMI 1640 medium as antigen-presenting cells (APC). CD4+CD25+ T cells were FACS sorted from spleen lymphocytes of wild type and PGRN-deficient mice as suppressor cells.

For the analysis of suppression function, we performed assays in 96-well plate. Each well contained 0.5×10^5 responder cells, 1×10^5 mitomycin-treated APC cells and anti-CD3 at a concentration of 5 μg/ml. Suppressor cells were added at suppressor and responder cells rations of 1:2, 1:1, 2:1, 4:1 and 8:1. Responder cells proliferation with wild type CD4+CD25+ T cells or PGRN-deficient CD4+CD25+ T cells were analyzed by FACS method assessing CFSE dilution after 3 days.

BrdU incorporation assay

Wild type (n = 3) and PGRN-deficient mice (n = 3) were injected intraperitoneally with BrdU labeling reagent (BrdU, Sigma-Aldrich, St Louis, MO, USA) at a dose of 10 ml/kg body weight and sacrificed 2 hours later. Lymphocytes from spleen and lymph nodes were prepared. Then we performed cell surface staining with CD4-PerCP-cy5.5 and CD25-APC and permeabilized for intracellular staining of BrdU using the BrdU flow kit (BD, San Diego, CA, USA) according to the manufactures instructions.

Real-time PCR

CD4+CD25+T cells were purified from the splenocytes of both wild type and PGRN-deficient mice by FACS sorting. Total RNA was extracted from CD4+CD25+T cells using RNeasy mini kit (Qiagen, Valencia, CA, USA). 1 μg RNA samples were reverse-transcribed by use of ImProm-II^{TM} Reverse Transcription System (Promega, Madison, WI, USA). The primer pairs and expected length are in Table 1. Relative mRNA expression was measured as the fold increase in expression by 2-ΔΔct method and data was normalized to mRNA levels of GAPDH.

Induction of CIA

Chicken type II collagen (Chondrex, LLC, Seattle, WA) was emulsified with an equal volume of complete Freund's adjuvant (CFA) (Chondrex, LLC, Seattle, WA). Wild type mice (n = 6) and PGRN-deficient mice (n = 6) were intradermally immunized with 100 μl of the emulsion at the base of the tail. After 3 weeks, draining lymph nodes were extracted and CD4+CD25+Foxp3+ cells were analyzed by FACS.

Statistical Analysis

Data was represented as mean ± SEM. Differences between the groups were analyzed with unpaired, 2-tailed t tests. P values less than 0.05 were considered as significant. All experiments were repeated two to three times with similar results.

Results

PGRN deficiency does not alter the numbers of CD4+CD25+Foxp3+ Treg cells in vivo

To determine the role of PGRN in the development of naturally CD4+CD25+Foxp3+ cells, we used flow cytometry to analyze the numbers of CD4+CD25+Foxp3+ cells in lymphocytes of thymus, spleen, and lymph nodes from one-, three-, and six-week-old wild type and PGRN-deficient mice. As shown in Fig. 1A, one-week-old wild type and PGRN-deficient mice have comparable proportions of CD4+ and CD8+ T cells in thymus ($p > 0.05$),

Table 1. Primer sequences.

Gene name	Primer sequence (5′-3′)	Product length (bp)
Wnt 1	Forward- ATTTTGCGCTGTGACCTCTT	
	Reverse- AGCAACCTCCTTTCCCACTT	177
Wnt 2	Forward- GGTCAGCTCTTCATGGTGGT	
	Reverse- GGAACTGGTGTTGGCACTCT	176
Wnt 3a	Forward- TCGGAGATGGTGGTAGAGAAA	
	Reverse- CGCAGAAGTTGGGTGAGG	130
Wnt 4	Forward- AAGAGGAGACGTGCGAGA AA	
	Reverse- CACCACCTTCCCAAAGACAG	191
Wnt 5a	Forward- CAAATAGGCAGCCGAGAGAC	
	Reverse- TGCAACCACAGGTAGACAGC	109
Wnt 5b	Forward- TCTCCGCCTCACAAAAGTCT	
	Reverse- CACAGACACTCTCAAGCCCA	242
Wnt 7a	Forward- GACAAATACAACGAGGCCGT	
	Reverse- GGCTGTCTTATTGCAGGCTC	207
Wnt 8b	Forward- CCAGAGTTCCGGGAGGTAG	
	Reverse- GAGATGGAGCGGAAGGTGT	131
Wnt 11	Forward- TGCTTGACCTGGAGAGAGGT	
	Reverse- AGCCCGTAGCTGAGGTTGT	193
Wisp 2	Forward- GTTTTGTGCCGCTGTGATG	
	Reverse- CTGAGGAGGGCTGGATTG	175
Fzd 1	Forward- TGCCCAGTGTCTTTCTCCTT	
	Reverse- TCTCTTTAGCCTCTCCCAACC	192
Fzd 2	Forward- ATCTGGAAACCTCCCAATCC	
	Reverse- CGTTTTGTTGCCCATTCTCT	184
Fzd 4	Forward- TGACAACTTTCACGCCGCTC	
	Reverse-ACAAGCCAGCATCGTAGCCACAC	397
Fzd 6	Forward- AGCCACCACACTCAGCTTTT	
	Reverse- CTACACTCTCCCTGCCCAAC	180
Fzd 7	Forward- AGAGACAAAGCGGGAAACAA	
	Reverse- TGTGCCTGAATGGGTATGAA	177
Fzd 8	Forward- TCCGTTCAGTCATCAAGCAG	
	Reverse- ATAGAAAAGGCAGGCGACAA	131
Fzd 9	Forward- GAAGCTGGAGAAGCTGATGG	
	Reverse- AAGTCCATGTTGAGGCGTTC	108
Fzd 10	Forward- GCTGCCCACATAACACACAC	
	Reverse- TCCTCACCCTCACTTGGTTC	179
β-catenin	Forward- TGAAGGCGTGGCAACATAC	
	Reverse- ATCAGGCAGCCCATCAACT	322
TCF 1	Forward- TCAAGAGGTGGGGGATTAGA	
	Reverse- GCAGGAGAAGCATTTGTAGG	185
TCF 3	Forward- ACCCCTTCCTGATGATTCC	
	Reverse- CGACCTTGTGTCCTTGACT	143
Wisp 1	Forward- CCCCTACAAGTCCAAGACCA	
	Reverse- TTTACCCTGAGCCACACACC	195
Axin 2	Forward- AACCTATGCCCGTTTCCTCT	
	Reverse- CCACACATTTCTCCCTCTCC	177
GAPDH	Forward-ACGTCGGTGGTAACGGATTTG	
	Reverse-TGTAGACCATGTAGTTGAGGTCA	123

and no significant difference in the percentage of CD4+CD25+ Foxp3+ cells in thymus were found ($p>0.05$) (Fig. 1B). Equivalent numbers of CD4+CD25+Foxp3+ cells were found in the spleen and lymph nodes in three- and six-week-old PGRN-deficient mice, compared with wild type mice ($p>0.05$) (Fig. 1C–F). Thus, the results suggest that the absence of PGRN may not affect the generation of naturally CD4+CD25+Foxp3+ cells during development.

In a separate experiment, one-week-old Foxp3-RFP mice were treated with 100 µg PGRN every two days for 1 week, and the percentage of CD4+RFP+ cells in lymphoid tissues were analyzed by FACS. The results revealed that the numbers of CD4+RFP+ cells in spleen (15.1±0.8% RFP+ cells in PBS group versus 14.0±0.4% in PGRN group), peripheral lymph nodes (16.1±0.2% RFP+ cells in PBS group versus 16.0±0.1% in PGRN group), mesenteric lymph nodes (15.1±1.0%RFP+ cells in PBS group versus 15.9±1.6% in PGRN group), and Peyer's patches (15.3%±2.0 RFP+ cells in PBS group versus 12.3±1.8% in PGRN group) in these two groups was not significantly changed ($p>0.05$) (Fig. 2). In brief, these findings demonstrate that PGRN treatment does not change the proportions and numbers of CD4+ CD25+Foxp3+ cells under physiological conditions.

PGRN promotes the CD4+CD25- T cells conversion into Foxp3-expressing iTreg

Since iTreg cells are essential in immune tolerance and in the prevention of chronic inflammation [34], growth factors which can boost TGF-β-mediated the conversion of CD4+CD25- T cells into iTreg will be of great importance in inflammatory conditions. TGF-β was reported to induce Foxp3-expressing iTreg [35]. We sought to determine whether PGRN regulates the conversion of CD4+CD25- T cells into iTreg. In a loss-of-function study, we first

stimulated naïve wild type and PGRN-deficient CD4+CD25- T cells with plate-bound CD3 antibody and soluble CD28 antibody in the presence of IL-2 and cultured for 3-4 days with or without TGF-β. In the absence of TGF-β, PGRN-deficient CD4+CD25- T cells have comparable capacity to convert into iTreg cells (0.10±0.02% Foxp3+ cells in KO versus 0.12±0.01% in WT, $p>$ 0.05) (Fig. 3A). In addition, no difference were found in wild type and PGRN-deficient CD4+CD25- T cells conversion into iTreg cells in the presence of TGF-β at dose of 1 ng/ml (49.8±3.3% Foxp3+ cells in KO versus 48.3±1.0% in WT, $p>0.05$) and 10 ng/ml (84±1.4% Foxp3+ cells in KO versus 84.3±3.5% in WT, $p>0.05$) (Fig. 3B-C). Thus, the findings suggest endogenous PGRN may not be required for CD4+CD25- T cells conversion into iTreg.

We further performed the gain-of-function experiment, we treated CD4+GFP- T cells with different concentrations of PGRN and examined the change of GFP expression in CD4+ T cells. As shown in Fig. 4, PGRN significantly promoted the conversion of CD4+GFP- T cells into CD4+GFP+ T cells at a dose-dependent manner in the presence of 0.1 ng/ml TGF-β (2.74±0.70% GFP+ cells with no PGRN versus 4.33±0.98% GFP+ cells with 200 ng/ ml PGRN versus 12.3±2.85% GFP+ cells with 1 µg/ml PGRN, p <0.05) (Fig. 4D–F). Furthermore, in the absence of TGF-β, 1 µg/ ml of PGRN significantly induced the expression of GFP in 5.67±1.65% of the cells, when compared with 0.16±0.07% GFP+ cells without PGRN ($p<0.01$) (Fig. 4A and C). And low concentrations of PGRN also significantly induced GFP expression in CD4+ cells, when compared with no PGRN conditions (0.63±0.23% GFP+ cells versus 0.16±0.07% GFP+ cells, $p<$ 0.05) (Fig. 4B). Taken together, these results indicate that recombinant PGRN promotes and synergistically enhances TGF-β-mediated induction of inducible regulatory T cells *in vitro*.

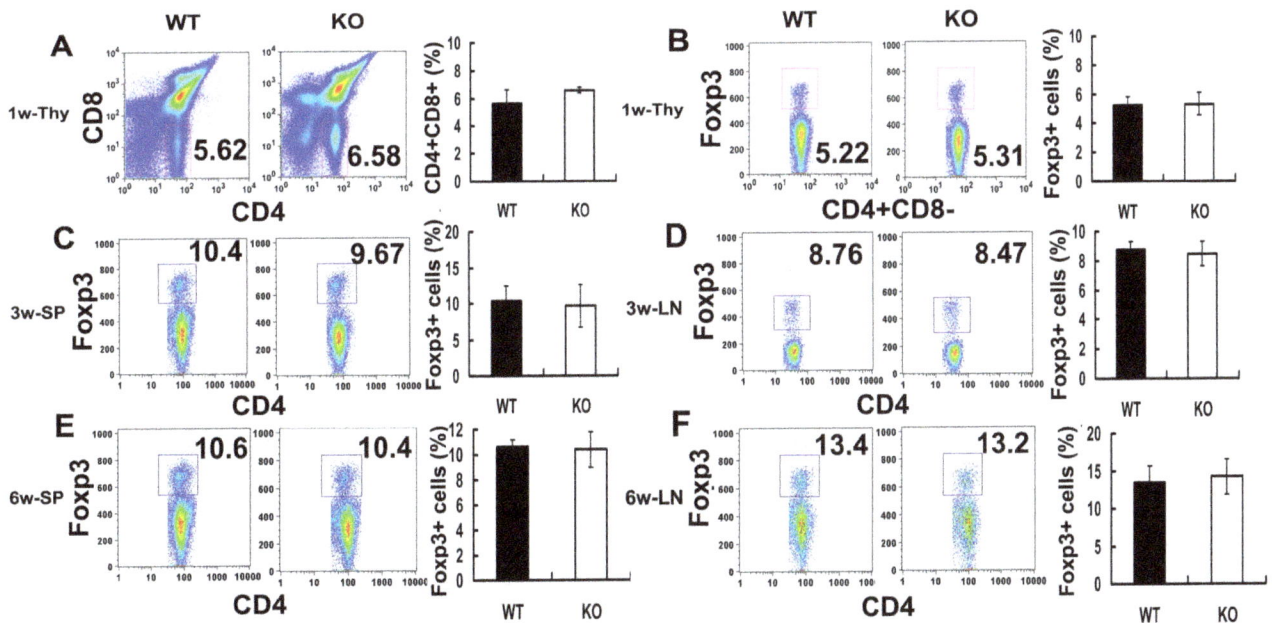

Figure 1. PGRN deficiency does not alter the generation of CD4+CD25+Foxp3+ T cells in vivo. Flow cytometric evaluation of CD4+CD25+ Foxp3+ T cells in one-, three-, and six-week-old wild type (WT) and PGRN-deficient mice. (A) The percentage of CD4+ and CD8+ T cells in thymus from one-week-old C57BL/6 mice and PGRN-deficient mice. (B) The percentage of CD4+CD25+Foxp3+ cells in thymus from one-week-old C57BL/6 mice and PGRN-deficient mice. (C) The proportion of CD4+CD25+Foxp3+ cells in spleen from three-week-old C57BL/6 mice and PGRN-deficient mice. (D) CD4+CD25+Foxp3+ cells in lymph nodes from three-week-old C57BL/6 mice and PGRN-deficient mice. (E) The proportion of CD4+CD25+Foxp3+ cells in spleen from six-week-old C57BL/6 mice and PGRN-deficient mice. (F) CD4+CD25+Foxp3+ cells in lymph nodes from six-week-old C57BL/6 mice and PGRN-deficient mice. All data was representative of three mice per group and indicated as mean ± SEM.

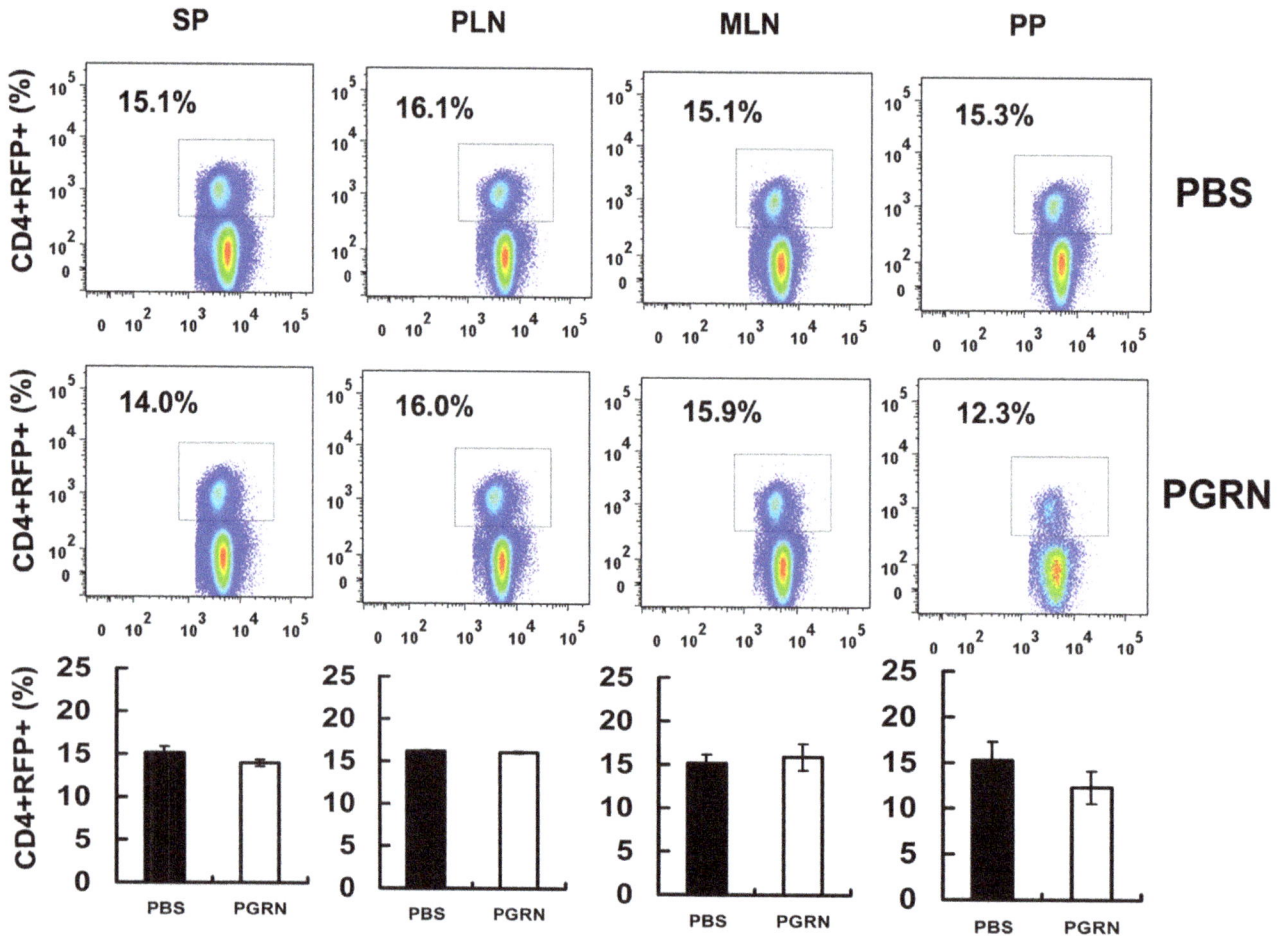

Figure 2. PGRN treatment does not change the proportions of CD4+CD25+Foxp3+ cells in normal conditions. One week-old Foxp3-RFP reporter mice were divided into two groups, three mice per group. PGRN group mice were treated with 100 μg PGRN every two days for 1 week, and PBS group mice were injected with the same volume of PBS as a control. The lymphocytes of spleen, peripheral lymph nodes (PLN), mesenteric lymph nodes (MLN), and Peyer's patches (PP) were isolated and analyzed by FACS. All data are representative of three independent experiments.

PGRN deficiency decreases the immunosuppressive function of CD4+CD25+ T cells

The proportion of normal CD4+CD25+ Tregs constitutes 5–10% of peripheral CD4+ T cells in mice and 1–2% in humans, and can potently suppress the proliferation of active CD4+CD25- and CD8+ T cells [36], [37]. To evaluate the role of PGRN signaling in regulation of CD4+CD25+ Tregs function, we performed in vitro CFSE-based proliferation suppression assay. 5×10^5 CFSE-labeling Teff cells were stimulated for 72 hours with CD3 antibody (5 μg/ml) in the presence of 1×10^5 APC cells and varying ratios of FACS purified WT or PGRN-deficient CD4+CD25+ Tregs, and CFSE dilution was evaluated by FACS. The CFSE proliferation in negative control and positive control group was $1.93 \pm 0.1\%$ and $94.2 \pm 3.2\%$, respectively (Fig. 5A and B). Our results demonstrate that wild type and PGRN-deficient CD4+CD25+ Tregs significantly suppress the CFSE proliferation when Teff co-cultured with Tregs at rations of 1:2, 1:1, 2:1 and 4:1, compared with positive control group ($p<0.05$) (Fig. 5B–F). PGRN-deficient Tregs significantly decreased suppressive capacity when Teff co-cultured with Tregs at ratios of 1:2 ($66.3 \pm 3.2\%$ CFSE dilution in KO versus $52.5 \pm 3.0\%$ CFSE dilution in WT, $p<0.01$, Fig. 5C) and 1:1 ($79.6 \pm 3.78\%$ CFSE dilution in KO versus $65.4 \pm 3.6\%$ CFSE dilution in WT, $p<0.01$, Fig. 5D),

compared with wild type Tregs. Suppressor cells were added at suppressor and responder cells rations of 2:1, PGRN-deficient Tregs showed a slightly lower suppressive capacity than wild type Tregs ($80.8 \pm 2.18\%$ CFSE dilution in KO versus $75.5 \pm 1.5\%$ CFSE dilution in WT, $p<0.05$, Fig. 5E). However, no significant difference were found between wild type and PGRN-deficient Tregs at ratios of 4:1 ($86.3 \pm 1.4\%$ CFSE proliferation in KO versus $83.8 \pm 1.7\%$ CFSE proliferation in WT, $p>0.05$, Fig. 5F) and 8:1 ($89.3 \pm 0.1\%$ CFSE dilution in KO versus $87.6 \pm 2.0\%$ CFSE dilution in WT, $p>0.05$, Fig. 5G). Collectively, PGRN is required for the immunosuppressive function of Tregs *in vitro*.

PGRN deficiency does not affect the proliferation of CD4+CD25+ Treg in vivo

5-Bromo-2-deoxyuridine (BrdU) is a pyrimidine analogue of thymidine, selectively incorporated into replicating DNA, effectively tagging dividing cells. To determine whether PGRN deficiency alters the proliferation of Tregs *in vivo*, we set a BrdU incorporation assay. We injected BrdU labeling reagent (BrdU, Sigma-Aldrich) at a dose of 10 ml/kg body weight into wild type and PGRN-deficient mice, three mice per group. Mice were sacrificed 2 hours after injection and intracellular staining of BrdU in lymphocytes of spleen (SP) and lymph nodes (LN) were stained

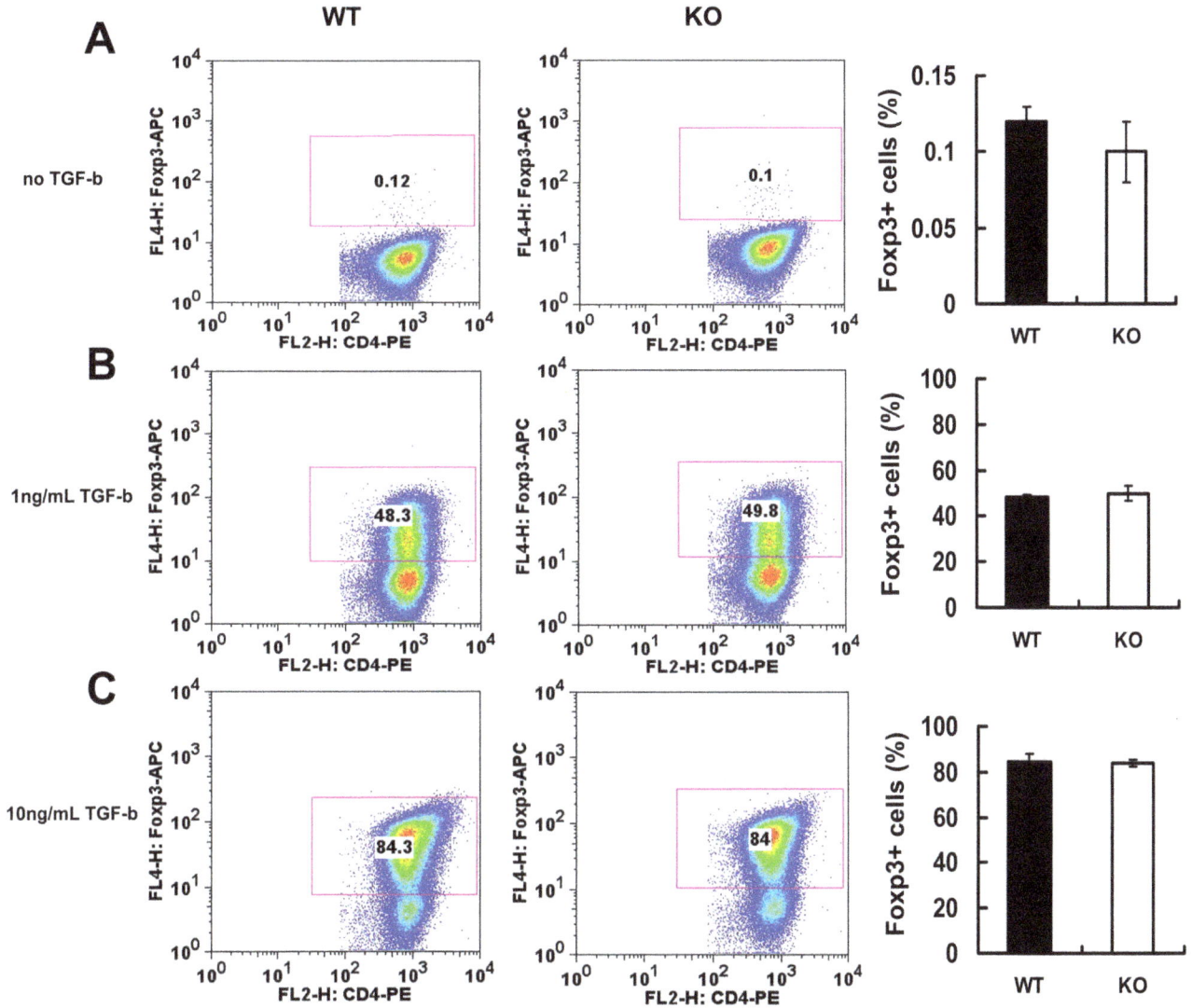

Figure 3. PGRN deficiency does not affect the conversion of naïve CD4+CD25- T cells into iTreg mediated by TGF-β. Naïve CD4+ CD25- T cells isolated from both wildtype (WT) and PGRN-deficient mice were stimulated with plate-bound CD3 Ab and solute CD28 Ab and cultured the cells for 3-4 days in the presence or absence of TGF-β, and the expression of GFP was measured by FACS. (A) The GFP levels in CD4+ T cells in the absence of TGF-β. (B) The GFP levels in CD4+ T cells in the presence of 1 ng/ml TGF-β. (C) The GFP levels in CD4+ T cells in the presence of 10 ng/ml TGF-β. All data were repeated three times with similar results.

with BrdU flow kit (BD Bioscience) and analyzed by FACS. We did not observe any significant changes in the number of CD4+ CD25+BrdU+ cells from splenocytes between wild-type and PGRN-deficient mice ($6.58 \pm 1.42\%$ BrdU+ cells in KO versus $5.68 \pm 0.11\%$ BrdU+ cells in WT, $p>0.05$) (Fig. 6A–B). In addition, $6.54 \pm 1.46\%$ of the cells in lymphocytes of lymph nodes are BrdU positive from PGRN-deficient mice, and comparable to $6.58 \pm 0.77\%$ BrdU+ cells seen in wild type mice ($p>0.05$) (Fig. 6C and D). These findings suggest that wild type and PGRN-deficient CD4+CD25+ Treg cells have a comparable proliferation and division capacity *in vivo*.

PGRN deficiency leads to fewer Treg cells in collagen-induced arthritis (CIA)

To determine whether the PGRN deficiency alters the number of Tregs in inflammatory conditions, we established a collagen-induced arthritis (CIA) model. Wild type and PGRN-deficient mice, six mice per group, were intradermally injected with 100 μl of the emulsion at the base of the tail. Two group mice were sacrificed 21 days after immunization and intracellular staining of Foxp3 in lymphocytes of draining lymph nodes (LN) was stained and analyzed by FACS. The results demonstrate that PGRN-deficient CD4+CD25- T cells have an impaired ability to generate iTreg in arthritis conditions (Fig. 7A–B). Arthritic PGRN-deficient mice shown a significant changes in the number of CD4+CD25+Foxp3+ cells from draining lymph nodes ($11.8 \pm 0.2\%$ CD4+CD25+Foxp3+ cells in arthritic KO mice versus $20.4 \pm 2.7\%$ CD4+CD25+Foxp3+ cells in arthritic WT mice, $p<0.01$, Fig. 7A–B). These findings suggest that PGRN deficiency leads to fewer CD4+CD25+ Foxp3+ Treg cells in collagen-induced arthritis conditions.

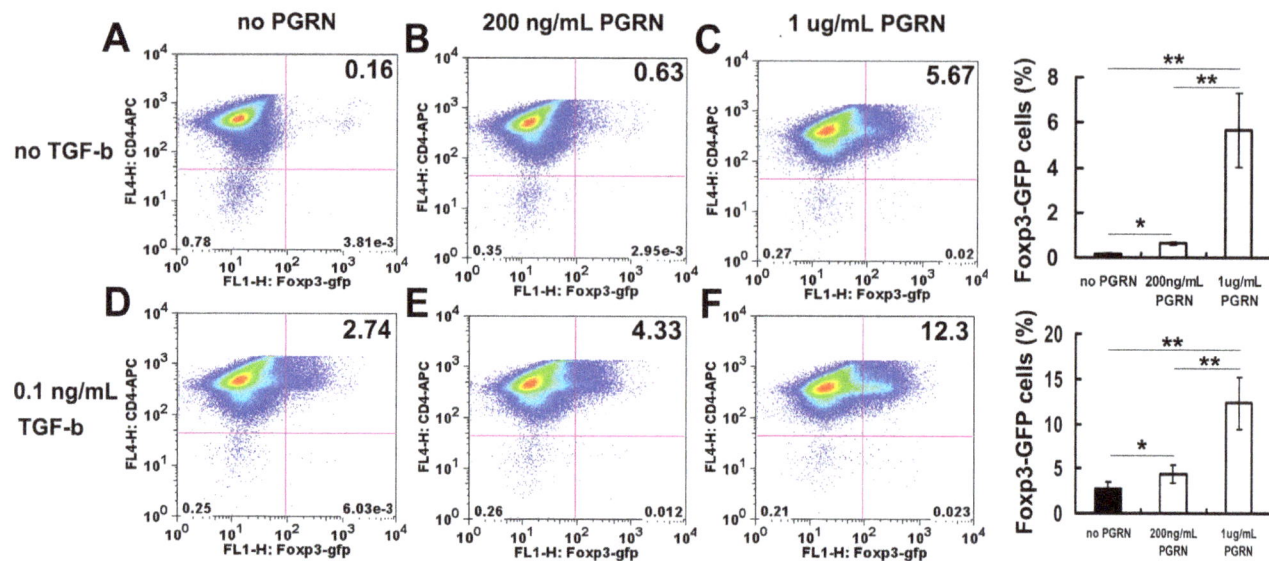

Figure 4. Recombinant PGRN promotes the induction of inducible regulatory T cells in vitro. Naïve CD4+GFP- cells in lymphocytes of spleen from Foxp3-GFP reporter mice were purified by using Mitenyi reagents and a MACS apparatus. The purity of cells was evaluated by FACS method. CD4+GFP- cells conversion assay was performed as described in Methods, and GFP expression in TGF-β-unstimulated CD4+GFP- cells was taken as a control. After 3-4 days, cells were washed and GFP expression was analyzed by FACS. Data represent three independent experiments are shown. (A) No TGF-β and no PGRN. (B) No TGF-β plus 200 ng/ml of PGRN. (C) No TGF-β plus 1 μg/ml of PGRN. (D) 0.1 ng/ml of TGF-β and no PGRN. (E) 0.1 ng/ml of TGF-βplus 200 ng/ml of PGRN. (F) 0.1 ng/ml of TGF-β plus 1 μg/ml of PGRN. Data represent as a means ±SE of a representative experiment. *$p < 0.05$; **$p < 0.01$.

PGRN deficiency upregulates the expression of Fzd2 in CD4+CD25+ T cells

Wnt signaling proteins can be divided into two subgroups according to the downstream molecules, the canonical pathway which stabilized β-catenin and activated target genes through the regulation of TCF/Lef transcription factors, and the noncanonical pathway did not dependent on the regulation of β-catenin and activated protein kinase C and G proteins, etc [38]. It was reported that Wnt signaling regulated PGRN-mediated fronto-temporal dementia (FTD) and PGRN and Wnt reciprocally regulated each other [38], [39]. Moreover, Wnt signaling was also reported to stabilize the survival of CD4+CD25+ Treg cells and to enhance their suppressive capacity [9], [40]. To further study the molecular events underlying PGRN-mediated regulation of CD4+CD25+ T cells, we purified CD4+CD25+ T cells from splenocytes of wild type and PGRN-deficient mice by FACS sorting and examined the gene expression of Wnt signaling components through real-time PCR. Our results did not found significantly change of Wnt1, Wnt2, Wnt3a, Wnt4, Wnt5a, Wnt5b, Wnt7a, Wnt8b, Wnt11, Wisp2, Fzd1, Fzd4, Fzd6, Fzd7, Fzd8, Fzd9, Fzd10, β-catenin, TCF1, TCF3, wisp1 and axin2 gene expression ($p > 0.05$) (Fig. 8). Interestingly, the mRNA level of Fzd2 gene in PGRN-deficient CD4+CD25+ T cells was significantly upregulated, when compared with its expression in wild type CD4+CD25+ T cells ($p < 0.01$) (Fig. 8). Collectively, this set of experiments indicated that PGRN deficiency upregulates the expression of Fzd2 gene in CD4+CD25+ T cells.

Discussion

Inducible CD4+CD25+Foxp3+ regulatory T cells (iTreg) develop outside of the thymus and play an essential role in controlling of chronic inflammation and autoimmunity [34]. Therefore, investigation of the growth factors which can convert naïve conventional T cells into iTreg may provide a new strategy for manipulating chronic inflammation and autoimmune diseases. In this study, we examine the role of PGRN in the conversion of CD4+CD25- T cells into Foxp3-expressing iTreg and immuno-suppressive function of CD4+CD25+ Tregs. Our findings demonstrate that PGRN significantly promotes the conversion of naïve CD4+CD25- T cells into iTreg mediated by lower concentration of TGF-β in a dose-dependent manner (Fig. 4D–F). PGRN alone also effectively induce the generation of iTreg, although less efficiently than the conversion capacity induced by TGF-β (Fig. 4A–C). The findings that PGRN alone or combined with TGF-β stimulates the production of iTreg may provide new insights into the conversion of naïve CD4+CD25- T cells into iTreg.

PGRN deficiency does not alter the numbers and percentage of CD4+CD25+Foxp3+ T cells in thymus, spleen, and lymph nodes in different ages of mice (Fig. 1). In addition, mice in PGRN-treated group have a comparable number of CD4+CD25+Fxop3+ T cells in spleen, peripheral lymph nodes, mesenteric lymph nodes, and Peyer's patches, when compared with the PBS group (Fig. 2). However, PGRN deficiency leads to a marked reduction of Treg number in collagen-induced inflammatory arthritis (Fig. 7). These results suggest that PGRN is important for the Tregs formation under inflammatory conditions, and does not influence the development of Tregs under normal immune homeostasis. A deficiency or defective function of Tregs is common in autoimmune diseases such as rheumatoid arthritis [41]. Furthermore, therapeutic agents that target Tregs can benefit rheumatoid arthritis. For instance, intravenous immunoglobulin (IVIg) also induces the expansion of Tregs and enhances their suppressive function and exerts beneficial effect in autoimmune diseases [42–46]. In addition, our previous report also supports this concept [12]. In CIA model, PGRN inhibits Th1 (IFNγ) cytokines production in Teff cells, decreases the levels of IL-6 expression in serum, prevents TNFα-induced downregulation of

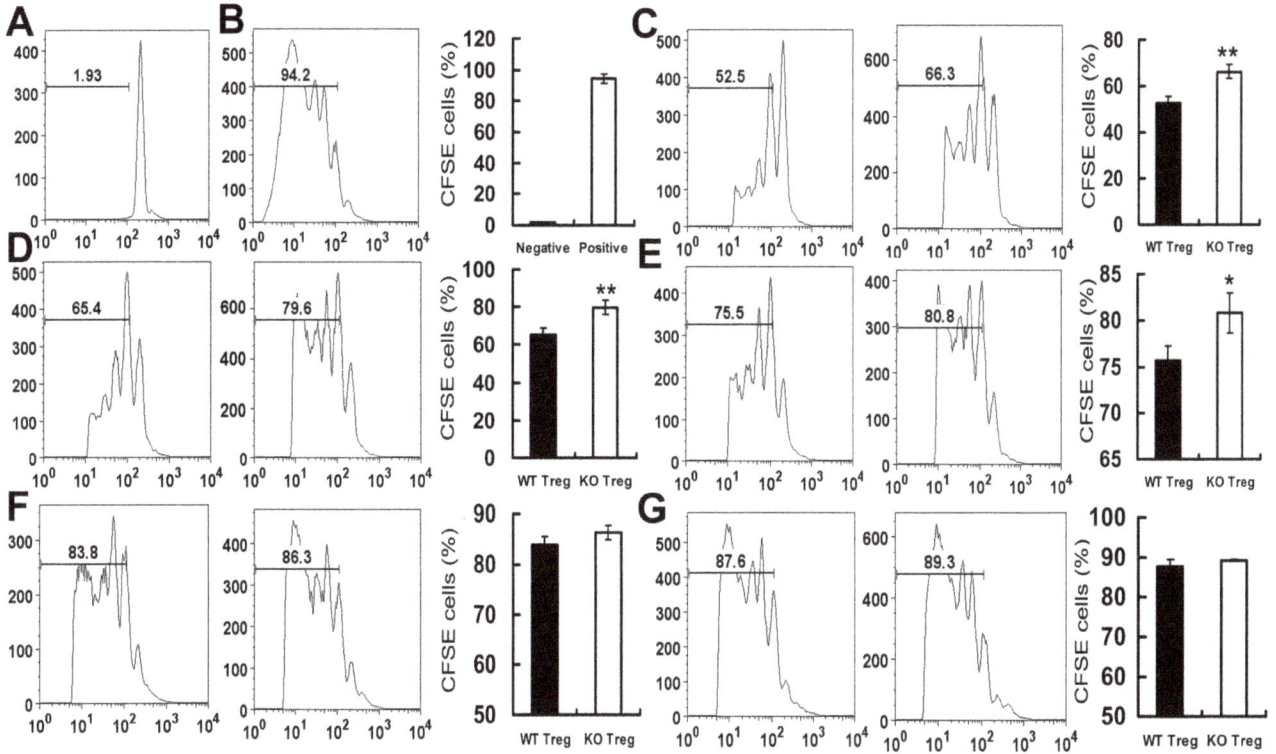

Figure 5. PGRN-deficient CD4+CD25+ Treg decreased the suppressive capacity to Teff proliferation. Freshly isolated, CFSE-labeled CD4+ CD25- T cells from Thy1.1 mice were used as Teff and co-cultured with Tregs at ratios of 1:2, 1:1, 2:1, 4:1 and 8:1. CFSE-based Teff proliferation suppression assay in vitro in which 5×10^5 CFSE-labeled Teff cells were stimulated with CD3 antibody in the presence of mitomycin-treated APC cells and different ratios of FACS sorted wild type or PGRN-deficient Tregs. The CFSE proliferation was evaluated by FACS. All data are representative of three separate experiments. (A) Negative control. (B) Positive control. (C) The CFSE dilution when Teff co-cultured with Tregs at ratios of 1:2. (D) The CFSE dilution when Teff co-cultured with Tregs at ratios of 1:1. (E) The CFSE dilution when Teff co-cultured with Tregs at ratios of 2:1. (F) The CFSE dilution when Teff co-cultured with Tregs at ratios of 4:1. (G) The CFSE dilution when Teff co-cultured with Tregs at ratios of 8:1. Data represent as a means $\pm$SE of a representative experiment. *$p < 0.05$; **$p < 0.01$.

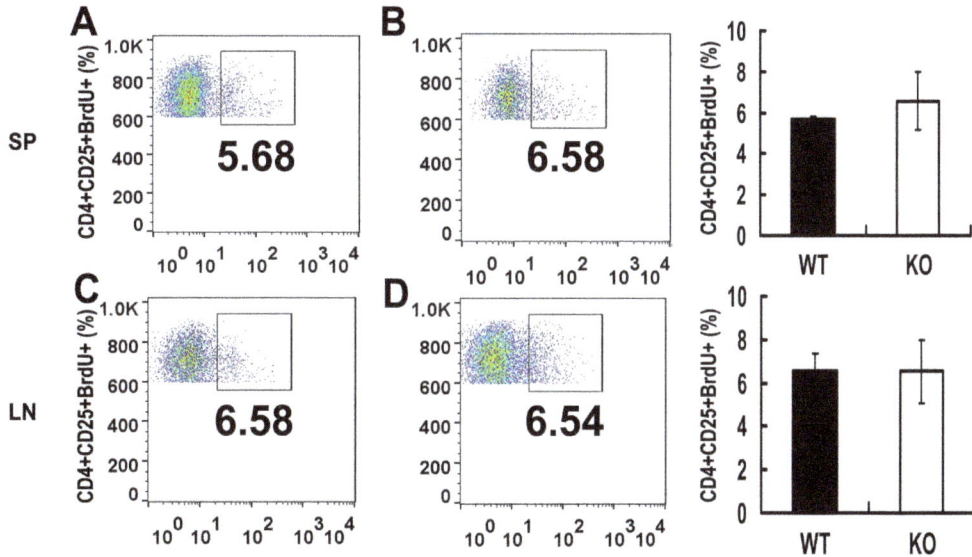

Figure 6. In vivo proliferation of CD4+CD25+ T cells from spleen and lymph nodes analyzed by BrdU corporation. Wild type and PGRN-deficient mice were injected intraperitoneally with BrdU labeling reagents, and the degrees of BrdU incorporation by CD4+CD25+ T cells from lymphocytes of spleen and lymph nodes were determined by FACS. (A) The BrdU incorporation of wild type CD4+CD25+ T cells from splenocytes. (B) The BrdU incorporation of PGRN-deficient CD4+CD25+ T cells from splenocytes. (C) The percentage of wild type CD4+CD25+ T cells from lymphocytes of lymph nodes that incorporated BrdU. (D) The percentage of PGRN-deficient CD4+CD25+ T cells from lymphocytes of lymph nodes that incorporated BrdU. All data was representative of three mice per group and indicated as mean $\pm$SEM.

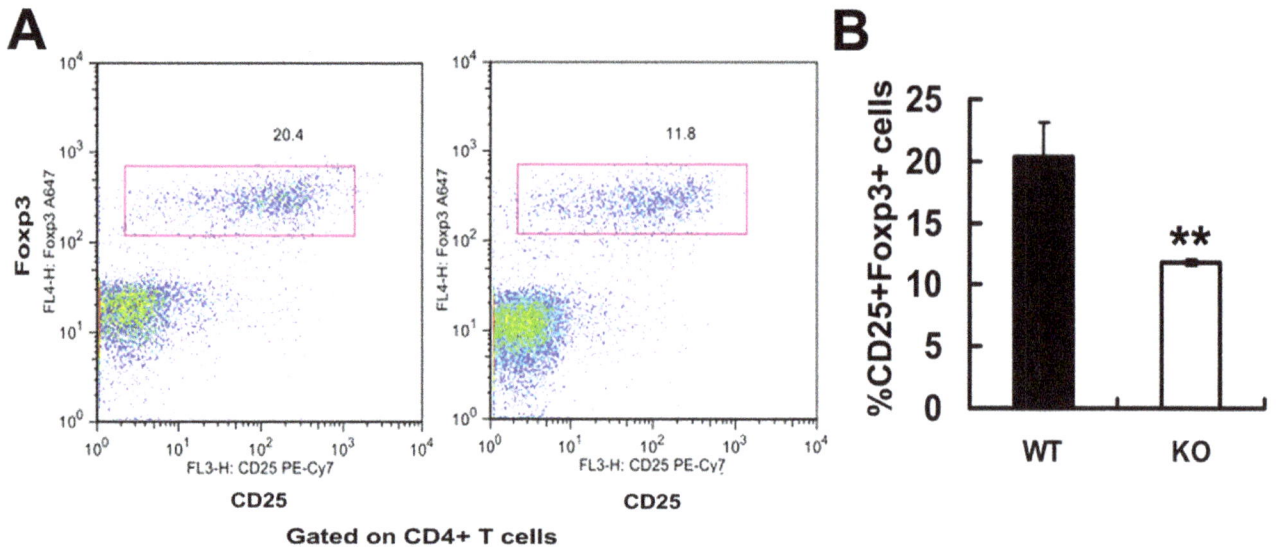

Figure 7. Fewer CD4+CD25+Foxp3+ Treg cells seen in PGRN-deficient CIA model. Wild type (n = 6) and PGRN-deficient mice (n = 6) were intradermally immunized with 100 μl of chicken type II collagen emulsified with an equal volume of complete Freund's adjuvant (CFA). 21 days post immunization, draining lymph nodes were extracted and CD4+CD25+Foxp3+ T cells were analyzed by FACS. Data represent as a means ±SE of a representative experiment. **$p < 0.01$.

Tregs suppressive function and inhibits inflammatory arthritis in mice [12].

CD4+CD25+ Tregs potently suppress the proliferation of active CD4+CD25- cells [36], [37]. In vitro Teff proliferation suppression assay demonstrated that PGRN deficiency led to significant reduction in the suppressive function of Tregs (Fig. 5C–E), indicating an important immunosuppressive role of PGRN in Tregs. PGRN insufficiency resulted from the mutations in the *GRN* gene was reported to cause reduced survival signaling and accelerated cell death in neurons [47–49]. PGRN deficiency does not affect the proliferation of Teff cells (data not show). Therefore, we further investigated the correlation between Tregs function and cell survival in PGRN-deficient mice using BrdU incorporation assay. Interestingly, we did not observe significant difference in CD4+CD25+BrdU+ numbers between wild type and PGRN-deficient mice (Fig. 6A–D), suggesting PGRN-deficiency may not impair Tregs survival and proliferation under normal immune homeostasis *in vivo*.

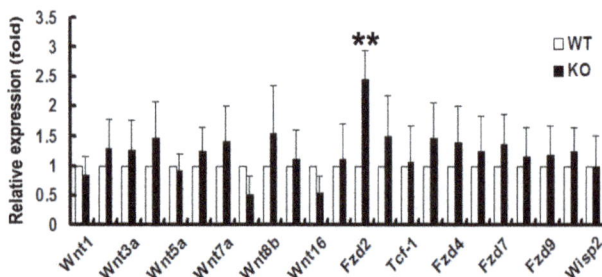

Figure 8. Wnt signaling components expression in wild type and PGRN-deficient CD4+CD25+ T cells measured by real-time PCR. All values are shown as a relative ratio to GAPDH measured by 2-ΔΔct method. Data represent as a means ±SE of a representative experiment. *$p < 0.05$; **$p < 0.01$.

It is known that Wnt signaling plays an important role in regulating CD4+CD25+ Tregs. For instance, β-catenin and Wnt3a both regulate Tregs function [8], [9], [40]. Fzd2 receptor was reported to be involved in the Wnt3a-dependent activation of β-catenin pathway and also required for Wnt5a-mediated β-catenin-independent pathway [50]. In our study, we found the level of Fzd2 was upregulated in PGRN-deficient Treg cells (Fig. 8). The finding is consistent with a recent report that Fzd2 is upregulated in PGRN-knockout mice using weighted gene coexpression network analysis (WGCNA) [39]. It is postulated that regulation of Fzd2 by PGRN may also contribute to the PGRN-mediated regulation of Tregs.

PGRN associates with some members in the TNF receptor superfamily, including TNFR1, TNFR2 and DR3 [12], [14–16], and possesses the ability to suppress inflammation in various kinds of conditions [12], [17–23]. Auto-antibodies against PGRN have been found in several autoimmune diseases, including rheumatoid arthritis, psoriatic arthritis, and inflammatory bowel disease, and such antibodies promoted a proinflammatory environment in a subgroup of patients [29–31]. In accordance with the finding that PGRN binds to TNFR, we found that PGRN protected Tregs from a negative regulation by TNF-α [12]. This finding has been also independently confirmed by other laboratories [30]. Chen and colleagues agreed that PGRN played an protective role in Tregs, but through enhancing TNF-α-induced Tregs proliferation [51]. The effect of TNF-α on the regulation of Tregs purified from mice and humans appears to be highly controversial. The data from Chen lab suggest that TNF-α promotes murine Tregs activity *in vitro* [51], whereas in humans, TNF-α inhibits the suppressive function of Tregs through negative regulation of Foxp3 expression [30], [52–55]. Although the effect of TNF-α on Tregs function remains controversy, the beneficial and therapeutic effects of Tregs in autoimmune diseases have been well-accepted by the scientific community [56], [57]. In addition, TNF-α inhibitors have been accepted as the most effective anti-inflammatory therapeutics.

In summary, this study provides evidences demonstrating that PGRN directly regulates the induction of iTreg and function of

Tregs *in vitro*, in addition to its antagonizing TNF-α-mediated negative regulation of Tregs. More importantly, PGRN deficiency leads to a significant reduction in Tregs in the course of inflammatory arthritis *in vivo*. Additionally, selective and significant upregulation of Fzd2 gene expression in PGRN deficient Tregs may contribute to the PGRN regulation of Tregs. These findings not only provide new insights into the role and regulation of PGRN in Tregs, but also present PGRN and/or its derivatives as therapeutic targets for treating chronic inflammatory and autoimmune diseases.

References

1. Takahashi T, Sakaguchi S (2003) Naturally arising CD25+CD4+ regulatory T cells in maintaining immunologic self-tolerance and preventing autoimmune disease. Current molecular medicine 3: 693–706.
2. Takahashi T, Sakaguchi S (2003) The role of regulatory T cells in controlling immunologic self-tolerance. International review of cytology 225: 1–32.
3. Ouyang W, Beckett O, Ma Q, Li MO (2010) Transforming growth factor-beta signaling curbs thymic negative selection promoting regulatory T cell development. Immunity 32: 642–653.
4. Xu L, Kitani A, Strober W (2010) Molecular mechanisms regulating TGF-beta-induced Foxp3 expression. Mucosal immunology 3: 230–238.
5. Dons EM, Raimondi G, Cooper DK, Thomson AW (2012) Induced regulatory T cells: mechanisms of conversion and suppressive potential. Human immunology 73: 328–334.
6. Schmitt EG, Williams CB (2013) Generation and function of induced regulatory T cells. Frontiers in immunology 4: 152.
7. Zhou X, Kong N, Zou H, Brand D, Li X, et al. (2011) Therapeutic potential of TGF-beta-induced CD4(+) Foxp3(+) regulatory T cells in autoimmune diseases. Autoimmunity 44: 43–50.
8. van Loosdregt J, Fleskens V, Tiemessen MM, Mokry M, van Boxtel R, et al. (2013) Canonical Wnt signaling negatively modulates regulatory T cell function. Immunity 39: 298–310.
9. Ding Y, Shen S, Lino AC, Curotto de Lafaille MA, Lafaille JJ, et al. (2008) Beta-catenin stabilization extends regulatory T cell survival and induces anergy in nonregulatory T cells. Nature medicine 14: 162–169.
10. Anakwe OO, Gerton GL (1990) Acrosome biogenesis begins during meiosis: evidence from the synthesis and distribution of an acrosomal glycoprotein, acrogranin, during guinea pig spermatogenesis. Biology of reproduction 42: 317–328.
11. Ong CH, Bateman A (2003) Progranulin (granulin-epithelin precursor, PC-cell derived growth factor, acrogranin) in proliferation and tumorigenesis. Histology and histopathology 18: 1275–1288.
12. Tang W, Lu Y, Tian QY, Zhang Y, Guo FJ, et al. (2011) The growth factor progranulin binds to TNF receptors and is therapeutic against inflammatory arthritis in mice. Science 332: 478–484.
13. Jian J, Konopka J, Liu C (2013) Insights into the role of progranulin in immunity, infection, and inflammation. Journal of leukocyte biology 93: 199–208.
14. Jian J, Zhao S, Tian Q, Gonzalez-Gugel E, Mundra JJ, et al. (2013) Progranulin directly binds to the CRD2 and CRD3 of TNFR extracellular domains. FEBS letters 587: 3428–3436.
15. Tian Q, Zhao Y, Mundra JJ, Gonzalez-Gugel E, Jian J, et al. (2014) Three TNFR-binding domains of PGRN act independently in inhibition of TNF-alpha binding and activity. Frontiers in bioscience (Landmark edition) 19: 1176–1185.
16. Li M, Liu Y, Xia F, Wu Z, Deng L, et al. (2014) Progranulin is required for proper ER stress response and inhibits ER stress-mediated apoptosis through TNFR2. Cellular signalling 26: 1539–1548.
17. Zhu J, Nathan C, Jin W, Sim D, Ashcroft GS, et al. (2002) Conversion of proepithelin to epithelins: roles of SLPI and elastase in host defense and wound repair. Cell 111: 867–878.
18. Kessenbrock K, Frohlich L, Sixt M, Lammermann T, Pfister H, et al. (2008) Proteinase 3 and neutrophil elastase enhance inflammation in mice by inactivating antiinflammatory progranulin. The Journal of clinical investigation 118: 2438–2447.
19. Egashira Y, Suzuki Y, Azuma Y, Takagi T, Mishiro K, et al. (2013) The growth factor progranulin attenuates neuronal injury induced by cerebral ischemia–reperfusion through the suppression of neutrophil recruitment. Journal of neuroinflammation 10: 105.
20. Kawase R, Ohama T, Matsuyama A, Matsuwaki T, Okada T, et al. (2013) Deletion of progranulin exacerbates atherosclerosis in ApoE knockout mice. Cardiovascular research 100: 125–133.
21. Vezina A, Vaillancourt-Jean E, Albarao S, Annabi B (2014) Mesenchymal stromal cell ciliogenesis is abrogated in response to tumor necrosis factor-alpha and requires NF-kappaB signaling. Cancer letters 345: 100–105.
22. Zhao YP, Tian QY, Liu CJ (2013) Progranulin deficiency exaggerates, whereas progranulin-derived Atsttrin attenuates, severity of dermatitis in mice. FEBS letters 587: 1805–1810.
23. Guo Z, Li Q, Han Y, Liang Y, Xu Z, et al. (2012) Prevention of LPS-induced acute lung injury in mice by progranulin. Mediators of inflammation: 540794.
24. Qiu F, Song L, Ding F, Liu H, Shu Q, et al. (2013) Expression level of the growth factor progranulin is related with development of systemic lupus erythematosus. Diagnostic pathology 8: 88.
25. Tanaka A, Tsukamoto H, Mitoma H, Kiyohara C, Ueda N, et al. (2012) Serum progranulin levels are elevated in patients with systemic lupus erythematosus, reflecting disease activity. Arthritis research & therapy 14: R244.
26. Yamamoto Y, Takemura M, Serrero G, Hayashi J, Yue B, et al. (2014) Increased Serum GP88 (Progranulin) Concentrations in Rheumatoid Arthritis. Inflammation.
27. Miller ZA, Rankin KP, Graff-Radford NR, Takada LT, Sturm VE, et al. (2013) TDP-43 frontotemporal lobar degeneration and autoimmune disease. Journal of neurology, neurosurgery, and psychiatry 84: 956–962.
28. De Riz M, Galimberti D, Fenoglio C, Piccio LM, Scalabrini D, et al. (2010) Cerebrospinal fluid progranulin levels in patients with different multiple sclerosis subtypes. Neuroscience letters 469: 234–236.
29. Thurner L, Preuss KD, Fadle N, Regitz E, Klemm P, et al. (2013) Progranulin antibodies in autoimmune diseases. Journal of autoimmunity 42: 29–38.
30. Thurner L, Stoger E, Fadle N, Klemm P, Regitz E, et al. (2014) Proinflammatory Progranulin Antibodies in Inflammatory Bowel Diseases. Digestive diseases and sciences.
31. Thurner L, Zaks M, Preuss KD, Fadle N, Regitz E, et al. (2013) Progranulin antibodies entertain a proinflammatory environment in a subgroup of patients with psoriatic arthritis. Arthritis research & therapy 15: R211.
32. Yin F, Banerjee R, Thomas B, Zhou P, Qian L, et al. (2010) Exaggerated inflammation, impaired host defense, and neuropathology in progranulin-deficient mice. The Journal of experimental medicine 207: 117–128.
33. Feng J, Guo F, Jiang B, Zhang Y, Frenkel S, et al. (2010) Granulin epithelin precursor: a bone morphogenic protein 2-inducible growth factor that activates Erk1/2 signaling and JunB transcription factor in chondrogenesis. FASEB Journal 24: 1879–1892.
34. Curotto de Lafaille MA, Lafaille JJ (2009) Natural and adaptive foxp3+ regulatory T cells: more of the same or a division of labor? Immunity 30: 626–635.
35. Fantini MC, Becker C, Monteleone G, Pallone F, Galle PR, et al. (2004) Cutting edge: TGF-beta induces a regulatory phenotype in CD4+CD25- T cells through Foxp3 induction and down-regulation of Smad7. J Immunol 172: 5149–5153.
36. Shevach EM (2002) CD4+ CD25+ suppressor T cells: more questions than answers. Nature reviews 2: 389–400.
37. Yamano Y, Takenouchi N, Li HC, Tomaru U, Yao K, et al. (2005) Virus-induced dysfunction of CD4+CD25+ T cells in patients with HTLV-I-associated neuroimmunological disease. The Journal of clinical investigation 115: 1361–1368.
38. Wexler EM, Rosen E, Lu D, Osborn GE, Martin E, et al. (2011) Genome-wide analysis of a Wnt1-regulated transcriptional network implicates neurodegenerative pathways. Science signaling 4: ra65.
39. Rosen EY, Wexler EM, Versano R, Coppola G, Gao F, et al. (2011) Functional genomic analyses identify pathways dysregulated by progranulin deficiency, implicating Wnt signaling. Neuron 71: 1030–1042.
40. Bluestone JA, Hebrok M (2008) Safer, longer-lasting regulatory T cells with beta-catenin. Nature medicine 14: 118–119.
41. Maddur MS, Othy S, Hegde P, Vani J, Lacroix-Desmazes S, et al. (2010) Immunomodulation by intravenous immunoglobulin: role of regulatory T cells. Journal of clinical immunology Suppl 1: S4–8.
42. Kessel A, Ammuri H, Peri R, Pavlotzky ER, Blank M, et al. (2007) Intravenous immunoglobulin therapy affects T regulatory cells by increasing their suppressive function. Journal of immunology 179: 5571–5575.
43. Ephrem A, Chamat S, Miquel C, Fisson S, Mouthon L, et al. (2008) Expansion of CD4+CD25+ regulatory T cells by intravenous immunoglobulin: a critical factor in controlling experimental autoimmune encephalomyelitis. Blood 111: 715–722.
44. Bayry J, Mouthon L, Kaveri SV (2012) Intravenous immunoglobulin expands regulatory T cells in autoimmune rheumatic diseases. The journal of rheumatology 39: 450–451.
45. Trinath J, Hegde P, Sharma M, Maddur MS, Rabin M, et al. (2013) Intravenous immunoglobulin expands regulatory T cells via induction of

Acknowledgments

We thank Dr. Juan Lafaille for providing TCRα-/-β-/- (C57BL/6 background), Thy1.1 (C57BL/6 background), and Foxp3-GFP (C57BL/6 background) mice.

Author Contributions

Conceived and designed the experiments: CJL FHW. Performed the experiments: YYZ FHW. Analyzed the data: WMZ XPY CJL. Contributed reagents/materials/analysis tools: YYZ. Wrote the paper: YYZ CJL.

cycooxygenase-2-dependent prostaglandin E2 in human dendritic cells. Blood 122: 1419–1427.

46. Bayry J, Sibéril S, Triebel F, Tough DF, Kaveri SV (2007) Rescuing CD4+ CD25+ regulatory T-cell functions in rheumatoid arthritis by cytokine-targeted monoclonal antibody therapy. Drug discovery today 12: 548–552.

47. He Z, Ismail A, Kriazhev L, Sadvakassova G, Bateman A (2002) Progranulin (PC-cell-derived growth factor/acrogranin) regulates invasion and cell survival. Cancer research 62: 5590–5596.

48. Van Damme P, Van Hoecke A, Lambrechts D, Vanacker P, Bogaert E, et al. (2008) Progranulin functions as a neurotrophic factor to regulate neurite outgrowth and enhance neuronal survival. The Journal of cell biology 181: 37–41.

49. Xu J, Xilouri M, Bruban J, Shioi J, Shao Z, et al. (2011) Extracellular progranulin protects cortical neurons from toxic insults by activating survival signaling. Neurobiology of aging 32: 2326 e2325–2316.

50. Sato A, Yamamoto H, Sakane H, Koyama H, Kikuchi A (2010) Wnt5a regulates distinct signalling pathways by binding to Frizzled2. The EMBO journal 29: 41–54.

51. Hu Y, Xiao H, Shi T, Oppenheim JJ, Chen X (2014) Progranulin promotes tumour necrosis factor-induced proliferation of suppressive mouse CD4(+) Foxp3(+) regulatory T cells. Immunology 142: 193–201.

52. Ehrenstein MR, Evans JG, Singh A, Moore S, Warnes G, et al. (2004) Compromised function of regulatory T cells in rheumatoid arthritis and reversal by anti-TNFalpha therapy. The Journal of experimental medicine 200: 277–285.

53. Valencia X, Stephens G, Goldbach-Mansky R, Wilson M, Shevach EM, et al. (2006) TNF downmodulates the function of human CD4+CD25hi T-regulatory cells. Blood 108: 253–261.

54. Zanin-Zhorov A, Ding Y, Kumari S, Attur M, Hippen KL, et al. (2010) Protein kinase C-theta mediates negative feedback on regulatory T cell function. Science (New York, NY 328: 372–376.

55. Nie H, Zheng Y, Li R, Guo TB, He D, et al. (2013) Phosphorylation of FOXP3 controls regulatory T cell function and is inhibited by TNF-alpha in rheumatoid arthritis. Nature medicine 19: 322–328.

56. Miyara M, Ito Y, Sakaguchi S (2014) T-cell therapies for autoimmune rheumatic diseases. Nat Rev Rheumatol.

57. Lan Q, Fan H, Quesniaux V, Ryffel B, Liu Z, et al. (2012) Induced Foxp3(+) regulatory T cells: a potential new weapon to treat autoimmune and inflammatory diseases? Journal of molecular cell biology 4: 22–28.

8

Persistent and Compartmentalised Disruption of Dendritic Cell Subpopulations in the Lung following Influenza A Virus Infection

Deborah H. Strickland[1,9], Vanessa Fear[1], Seth Shenton[1,2], Mathew E. Wikstrom[1], Graeme Zosky[1,3], Alexander N. Larcombe[1], Patrick G. Holt[1,4], Cassandra Berry[2], Christophe von Garnier[1,5,9], Philip A. Stumbles[1,2*,9]

1 Telethon Institute for Child Health Research and Centre for Child Health Research, University of Western Australia, Perth, W.A., Australia, 2 School of Veterinary and Life Sciences, Murdoch University, Perth, W.A., Australia, 3 School of Medicine, University of Tasmania, Hobart, Tasmania, Australia, 4 Queensland Children's Medical Research Institute, University of Queensland, Brisbane, Qld., Australia, 5 Pulmonary Medicine, Bern University Hospital and Department of Clinical Research, Berne University, Berne, Switzerland

Abstract

Immunological homeostasis in the respiratory tract is thought to require balanced interactions between networks of dendritic cell (DC) subsets in lung microenvironments in order to regulate tolerance or immunity to inhaled antigens and pathogens. Influenza A virus (IAV) poses a serious threat of long-term disruption to this balance through its potent pro-inflammatory activities. In this study, we have used a BALB/c mouse model of A/PR8/34 H1N1 Influenza Type A Virus infection to examine the effects of IAV on respiratory tissue DC subsets during the recovery phase following clearance of the virus. In adult mice, we found differences in the kinetics and activation states of DC residing in the airway mucosa (AMDC) compared to those in the parenchymal lung (PLDC) compartments. A significant depletion in the percentage of AMDC was observed at day 4 post-infection that was associated with a change in steady-state CD11b$^+$ and CD11b$^-$ AMDC subset frequencies and significantly elevated CD40 and CD80 expression and that returned to baseline by day 14 post-infection. In contrast, percentages and total numbers of PLDC were significantly elevated at day 14 and remained so until day 21 post-infection. Accompanying this was a change in CD11b$^+$ and CD11b$^-$ PLDC subset frequencies and significant increase in CD40 and CD80 expression at these time points. Furthermore, mice infected with IAV at 4 weeks of age showed a significant increase in total numbers of PLDC, and increased CD40 expression on both AMDC and PLDC, when analysed as adults 35 days later. These data suggest that the rate of recovery of DC populations following IAV infection differs in the mucosal and parenchymal compartments of the lung and that DC populations can remain disrupted and activated for a prolonged period following viral clearance, into adulthood if infection occurred early in life.

Editor: Ulrich A. Maus, Hannover School of Medicine, Germany

Funding: This work was supported by the National Health and Medical Research Council of Australia (APP ID 211912, 437200; www.nhmrc.gov.au). The funders had no role in study design, data collection and analysis, decision to publish, or preparation of the manuscript.

* Email: p.stumbles@murdoch.edu.au

9 These authors contributed equally to this work.

Introduction

Continuous exposure of the respiratory tract to environmental antigens poses a major challenge to the maintenance of local immunological homeostasis at this site. Inhaled foreign proteins and pathogens must be efficiently screened by the immune system for their potential "danger" to the host and either ignored in the case of harmless proteins (ignorance or tolerance), or translated into signals for induction of innate and adaptive immunity in the case of pathogens such as respiratory viruses. There is a close association between respiratory viral infections, bronchiolitis, wheezing and development of allergic asthma, particularly a subset of susceptible infants and children [1]. Human Rhinovirus (HRV), Respiratory Syncytial Virus (RSV) and Influenza A Virus (IAV) have high burdens of hospitalisation in children younger than 5 years, and particularly in those under 2 years of age [2,3]. Airways inflammation resulting from viral infections in infancy have been linked to wheezing in pre-school years, with associations for IAV, RSV and to a lesser extent other respiratory viral infections being documented [4-6]. Although the development of allergic asthma involves a complex series of interactions between genes and environment, there is data associating respiratory viral infections and atopy to the development of asthma, particularly in children with atopic sensitisation by the age of 2 years [3]. While the underlying pathogenesis of virally induced allergic asthma remains unclear, experimental evidence suggests that viral infections disrupt tolerance to aeroallergens across mucosal barriers together with enhanced pro-allergic immune responses [7,8].

Under normal circumstances, immunological homeostasis within the respiratory tract is maintained via the surveillance activities of local dendritic cell (DC) populations. These are distributed within respiratory tissues as integrated networks, playing a crucial role in sampling of inhaled antigens including viruses and allergens and in the initiation of subsequent tolerance and/or adaptive T cell-mediated immune responses in draining lymph nodes (DLN) [9]. Earlier observations from our group in a rat model were the first to demonstrate the rapid expansion of airway mucosal DC (AMDC) during acute viral (parainfluenza) infection, and the apparent persistence of this response beyond viral clearance [10]. This was subsequently confirmed in a mouse RSV model with respect to whole lung DC and similar observations have been reported in humans for nasal mucosal DC populations in children post RSV and HRV infections [11,12]. Given the key role that these frontline DC populations in local immune surveillance for all classes of environmental antigens, their long-term disruption following viral infection has significant implications in regards to maintenance of general immunological homeostasis within the respiratory tract. With this in mind we have sought to confirm and extend these earlier observational studies, aiming to more comprehensively identify which DC subsets are susceptible to the effects of virus, and in which precise tissue microenvironments within the respiratory tree; moreover we have extended the studies to encompass immunologically immature weanling animals, similar to the age range described above for maximal susceptibility to severe virus associated airways inflammation in humans.

Early studies in rodent models demonstrated the capacity of respiratory tract DC to direct the outcome of $CD4^+$ T cell responses to inhaled allergens and a number of subsequent studies have confirmed the essential requirement for DC migration to DLN for induction of $CD4^+$ T cell mediated allergic airways inflammation and asthmatic syndromes [13,14]. Furthermore, our previous work in rodents identified a subdivision of function based on anatomical location, with AMDC being functionally distinct from their counterparts in parenchymal lung tissue, most likely due to micro-environmental differences between these anatomical locations [15,16]. Consistent with airway mucosal surfaces being the first site of exposure to inhaled allergens and viruses, AMDC show high levels of endocytic activity and rapid turn-over and drainage to airway DLN, defining their proposed role as "gatekeepers" for the initiation of adaptive immunity to inhaled allergens and pathogens [15,17-19].

A number of DC subsets have been described in rodents and humans with differing capacities to influence naïve and memory $CD4^+$ and $CD8^+$ T cell responses [20]. In the mouse, major populations of classical (also termed "myeloid" or "conventional") DC (cDC) and plasmacytoid DC (pDC) have been identified, as well as a number of cDC subsets with distinct phenotypic and transcriptional profiles [21]. In the mouse respiratory tract, two dominant cDC subsets based on the reciprocal expression of CD11b and the alpha (E) integrin CD103 have been described, whereby $CD11b^{lo}$ ($CD103^+$) DC express tight junction proteins, reside within the airway epithelium and increase in numbers during allergic airways inflammation, while the $CD11b^{hi}$ ($CD103^-$) subset readily produces a number of chemokines that regulate $CD4^+$ T cell activity [16,22,23]. During IAV infection, both DC subsets have been shown to be infected and be capable of presenting viral antigens to T cells, however the $CD11b^{lo}$ subset appears to be the predominant subset for migration to DLN and for either direct or cross-presentation of viral antigens to $CD8^+$ T

cells although, other subsets in tissue and DLN are likely to be involved [24–27]. In addition to cDC, other non-myeloid lineages such as plasmacytoid DC (pDC) in lungs, as well as resident lymphoid-origin DC in DLN, may also play important roles in initiating T cell immunity to IAV [27–29].

In this study we have characterised the impact of IAV infection on the frequency and activation of cDC in anatomical compartments of the respiratory tract of BALB/c mice following IAV infection. IAV infection was shown to have a differential impact on DC numbers and activation status in airway mucosal and parenchymal lung tissues, which represent two anatomically and immunologically distinct compartments of the respiratory tract. Furthermore, IAV infection of juvenile mice induced long-term alterations on the frequency and activation states of parenchymal lung DC subsets that persisted into adulthood.

Results

Clinical features of the BALB/c mouse model of influenza A virus (IAV) infection

An adult BALB/c mouse model of IAV infection was established, using intranasal (i.n.) delivery of an optimised dose of the mouse-adapted A/PR/8/34 (H1N1) type A influenza virus (IAV). Using this protocol, mice developed peak clinical symptoms on d9 to d10 post-infection (p.i.) as evidenced by body weight loss (Fig. 1A) and clinical score (Fig. 1B), with mice recovering to pre-infection clinical score and weight by d14 and d21 p.i. respectively. Lung tissue viral titres were elevated at d3 p.i. and completely resolved by d14 p.i. (Fig. 1C). Lung mechanics were also altered at d4 p.i., with IAV infected mice showing increased airway resistance at functional residual capacity (FRC) ($p<0.001$), which was maintained throughout inflation up to 20 cmH_2O transrespiratory pressure ($p<0.001$) (Fig. 1D, left panel). Similarly, IAV infected mice had increased tissue damping (0 cm H_2O, $p<0.01$) (Fig. 1D, middle panel) and tissue elastance (0 cm H_2O, $p = 0.002$; 20 cm H_2O, $p <0.001$) (Fig. 1D, right panel), although at high pressures there was no difference in tissue damping between influenza infected mice and controls.

Total cell counts in bronchoalveolar lavage fluids (BALF) from IAV infected mice showed a significant increase at d4 p.i. ($p < 0.01$), and peak increase at d7 p.i. ($p<0.01$), when compared to control mice, declining by d14 p.i. but still remaining significantly elevated above control levels at d21 p.i. ($p<0.05$). (Fig. 2A) Differential cell counts of BALF showed significantly elevated macrophage numbers at d4 p.i. ($p<0.01$) that mirrored the kinetics of total cell counts (Fig. 2B). An early neutrophil response was observed, with a peak at d4 p.i. ($p <0.0001$) that declined but remained significantly elevated above control levels at d14 p.i. ($p <0.05$), and at d21 p.i. ($p<0.05$) (Fig. 2C). Total lymphocyte counts were also significantly elevated by d4 p.i. ($p<0.0001$) with a peak at d7 p.i. ($p<0.0001$), declining but remaining significantly elevated above control levels at d14 and d21 p.i. ($p<0.0001$). (Fig. 2D). Calculation of the percentage of each cell type in BALF showed a significant decrease in the percentage of macrophages from d4 to d21 p.i. (Fig. 2E), and significant increases in the percentages of neutrophils (Fig. 2F) and lymphocytes (Fig. 2G) over the same time period.

Cytokine levels in BALF showed significantly elevated IFNα (Fig. 3A) and KC (Fig. 3B) levels at d4 p.i. ($p<0.05$) that declined to control levels by d14 for IFNα, whereas KC remained elevated until d21 p.i. ($p<0.05$). G-CSF showed a biphasic response, being significantly elevated at d4 and d7 p.i. ($p<0.0001$), returning to baseline levels at d14 p.i. and significantly increasing again at d21 p.i. ($p<0.0001$) (Fig. 3C). IL-12 p40 (but not IL-12p70, data not

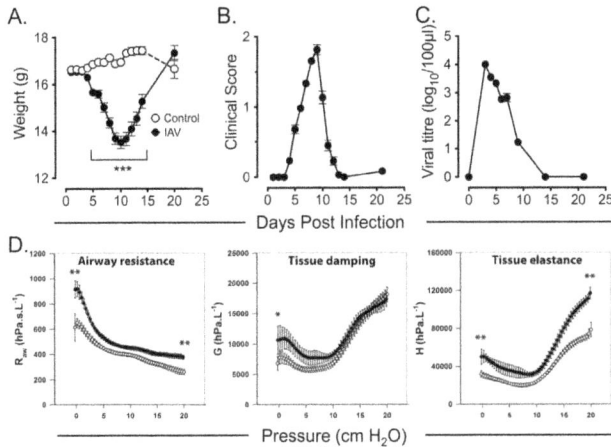

Figure 1. Clinical features of the adult BALB/c mouse model of A/PR8/34 H1N1 influenza A virus (IAV) infection. Eight week-old female BALB/c mice were inoculated i.n. with 1×10^2 TCID$_{50}$ A/PR/8/34 influenza A virus (IAV) in PBS and assessed at the indicated time points over the following 21 days for (A) body weight (B) clinical score and (C) lung tissue viral titres. Data are mean +/− SEM of groups of 20 to 60 mice per time point for weight measurements and clinical score, and 5 mice per time point for lung viral titres. Control mice received equivalent volumes of virus-free DMEM i.n. at day 0. (D) Measurement of airway resistance, tissue damping and tissue elastance at transrespiratory pressure during slow inflation manoeuvres up to 20cm H$_2$O in influenza infected mice (closed circles) and controls (open circles) at day 4 post infection. Influenza infected mice had impairments in Raw, G and H. Asterisks indicate statistical significance of IAV infected as compared to control mice as described in Materials and Methods. Data are means +/− SEM of 4 mice per group. * = $p<0.05$; ** = $p<0.01$; *** = $p< 0.001$.

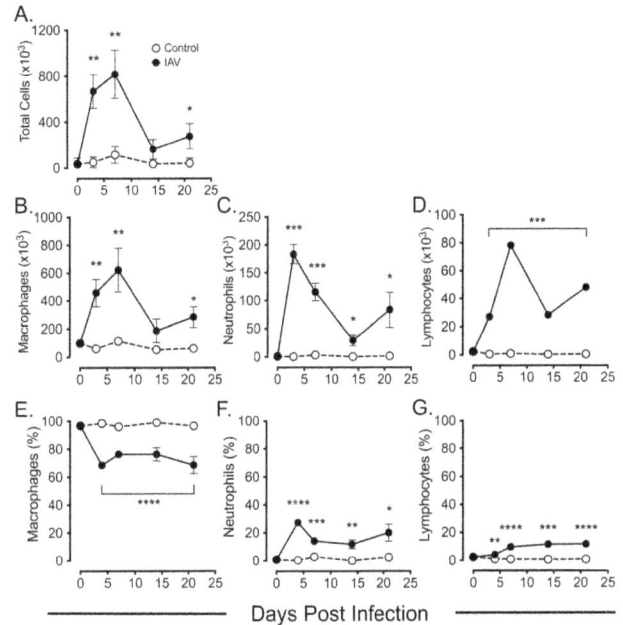

Figure 2. Bronchoalveolar lavage fluid (BALF) differential cell counts following IAV infection. Groups of 8 week old BALB/c mice were infected with IAV i.n. and BALF harvested on day 0 (pre-infection) and at the indicated time post-infection and assessed for total numbers of (A) total cells, (B) macrophages, (C) neutrophils and (D) lymphocytes and for percentages of cells by differential Leishman's staining for (E) macrophages, (F) neutrophils and (G) lymphocytes as described in Materials and Methods. Control mice received equivalent volumes of virus-free DMEM i.n. at day 0. Results are mean +/− SEM for 5 mice at each time point. * = $p<0.05$; ** = $p<0.01$; *** = $p<0.001$; **** = $p< 0.0001$.

shown) was significantly elevated at d4 and d7 p.i. ($p<0.0001$), declining but remaining significantly elevated at d21 p.i. ($p<0.05$) (Fig. 3D). Both IL-10 (Fig. 3E) and IFNγ (Fig. 3F) were significantly elevated ($p<0.05$) at d7 p.i., returning to control levels by d14 p.i.

Kinetics of airway mucosal and lung parenchymal DC subsets following acute IAV infection

Our previous mouse studies have identified functionally distinct populations of DC in the airway mucosa (AMDC) and parenchymal lung (PLDC), with AMDC displaying more rapid turnover rates (<12 h) compared to PLDC (>7 days) and more rapid activation in response to aeroallergen challenge [15,16]. Given that acute IAV infection is characterised by early infection and replication of the virus in epithelial cells of the airway mucosa, we initially examined the population dynamics of AMDC compared to their more peripheral PLDC counterparts following IAV infection. AMDC and PLDC were identified by flow cytometry using co-staining of tracheal and parenchymal lung tissue respectively for CD11c and MHC class II (I-A/E) as previously described [15], allowing gating of CD11c$^+$ I-A/E^{hi} AMDC and PLDC following IAV infection (Figs. 4A and 4D). This combination of markers also allowed identification of CD11c$^+$ I-A/E^{low} parenchymal lung macrophages (PLMac) [15], which were also tracked over the same time course post-IAV infection (Fig. 4G). In addition, as expression of I-A/E may possibly have modulated after IAV infection, we confirmed that these phenotypes remained stable by substituting the mouse DC marker CD205 for I-A/E (Fig. S1). A time course analysis of tracheal tissue showed a significant depletion of AMDC as a percentage of total cells ($p<$

0.01) (Fig. 4A and 4B), but not total cell numbers (Fig. 4C), at day 4 p.i. with the percentages of AMDC returning to baseline levels by d7-14 p.i. In contrast, percentages (Fig. 4D and 4E) and total numbers (Fig. 4F) of PLDC in peripheral lung tissue remained unchanged from controls at d4 p.i., but were then significantly increased above control levels from d14 p.i ($p <0.05$). Over the same time-course, a decrease in percentages (Fig. 4G and 4H) and total numbers (Fig. 4I) of PLMac was observed from d4 p.i., with a significant decrease in the percentage of PLMac at d4 and d14 p.i. ($p<0.01$), returning to near-baseline levels at d21 p.i.

In addition to anatomical location, we and others have shown that the myeloid marker CD11b functionally divides mouse lung DC, with CD11b^{hi} and CD11b^{lo} DC subsets showing different rates of capture and trafficking of inhaled antigens in the steady-state and during allergic inflammatory airways disease [15,16,30]. Furthermore, the CD11b^{lo} DC subset has been shown to be important for clearance of IAV and to have distinct functional properties in terms of T cell recruitment and activation [22,23]. In the current study, analysis of CD11b expression on respiratory tract DC populations following IAV infection showed a compartmentalised change. In the airway mucosa, IAV infection induced a significant decrease in the percentage of CD11b^{lo} AMDC (Fig. 5A), and corresponding increase in the percentage of CD11b^{hi} AMDC (Fig. 5B) at d4 and d7 p.i., returning to control levels for each subset at d14 p.i. Similarly, IAV infection also induced a decrease in the percentage of CD11b^{lo} PLDC (Fig. 5C), and increase in the percentage of CD11b^{hi} PLDC at d7 p.i. (Fig. 5D). However, in contrast to AMDC, changes in CD11b

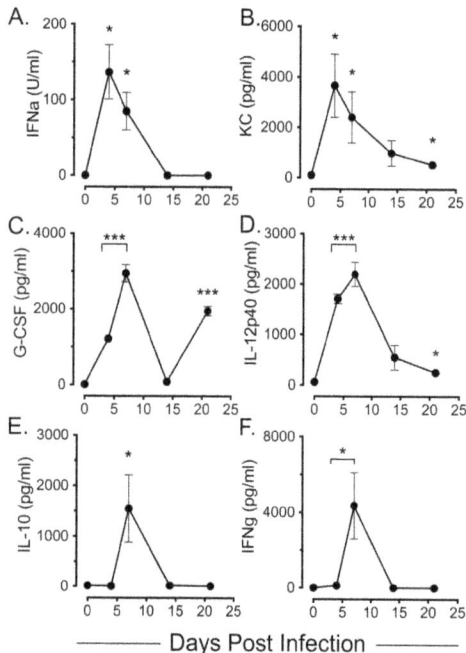

Figure 3. BALF cytokine analysis following IAV infection. Mice were infected with IAV i.n. and BALF fluids harvested at the indicated time points and assessed for *(A)* IFNα by bioassay as described in Materials and Methods, and by multiplex immunoassay assay for *(B)* KC, *(C)* G-CSF *(D)* IL-12 p40, *(E)* IL-10 and *(F)* IFNγ. Results shown are means +/− SEM of duplicate samples for 3 mice at each time point. Statistical significances were calculated for infected mice relative to control (d0) mice. * = *p*<0.05; *** = *p*<0.001.

expression on PLDC persisted, remaining significantly changed from control PLDC until d21 p.i. (Fig. 5C and 5D).

In summary, IAV infection induced a transient derangement of AMDC percentages and CD11b expression that generally resolved by d14 p.i., whereas these alterations persisted in PLDC. Therefore, restoration of homeostasis of DC populations following IAV infection is rapidly regulated at the mucosal surfaces of the conducting airways, but remains disrupted in the lung parenchymal compartment.

Expression of co-stimulatory markers on respiratory tract DC following acute IAV infection

We next examined the expression of the co-stimulatory markers CD40, CD80 and CD86 on AMDC and PLDC following IAV infection as indicators of cellular activation status. We have previously shown that CD40 is an early activation marker of AMDC, being upregulated in the early stages of allergic airways disease [16]. For AMDC, the percentages of cells expressing CD40 (Fig. 6A) and CD80 (Fig. 6B) were significantly increased at d4 p.i. when compared to control AMDC (Fig. S2), generally returning to control levels by d14 p.i. Although baseline expression levels of CD86 were constitutively high on AMDC, expression of this marker was also significantly upregulated at d4 p.i., returning to control levels by d7- d14 p.i. (Fig. 6C). For PLDC, CD40 (Fig. 6D) and CD80 (Fig. 6E) were upregulated at d4 p.i. (Fig. S2) and, in contrast to AMDC, remained elevated until d21 p.i. Again, as for AMDC, CD86 expression was constitutively high on PLDC and was further upregulated from d4 to d14 p.i., returning to normal levels by d21 p.i. (Fig. 6F). Expression of these co-stimulatory

markers was equally distributed amongst the CD11b[lo] and CD11b[hi] AMDC and PLDC subsets (data not shown).

In summary, AMDC showed a rapid and transient increase in co-stimulatory molecules following IAV infection that returned to baseline levels by d14 p.i., whereas PLDC showed a persistent increase in these molecules on both the CD11b[lo] and CD11b[hi] subsets. Therefore, control of DC activation following IAV infection is rapidly regulated in the airway mucosa, but remains dysregulated in the lung parenchymal compartment.

Frequency and activation status of respiratory tract APC populations following early-life IAV infection

We next addressed the question of the long-term impact of IAV on respiratory tract APC populations after early-life virus infection. To investigate this, post-weaning (28 day-old) BALB/c mice were infected with a weight-adjusted dose of IAV as described in the Materials and Methods, and tracheal and lung tissue isolated 35 days later (i.e. as 8 week-old adults) to examine AMDC and PLDC cell frequencies and their activation status. Early-life IAV infection resulted in a clinical syndrome that was very similar to that shown for adult mice (see Fig. 1B), with clinical scores peaking and declining at similar time-points p.i. (data not shown). Analysis of tracheal tissue of mice infected at 28 days of age and analysed as adults showed no significant difference in percentages or total numbers of AMDC compared to control mice (Fig. 7A and 7B), however significant increases were observed in the percentage of cells expressing CD40 (*p*<0.01) and CD86 (*p*< 0.01) (Fig. 7C). In contrast, analysis of peripheral lung tissue showed significantly elevated percentages (*p*<0.01, data not shown) and total numbers (*p*<0.05) of PLDC compared to control mice (Fig. 7D and 7E), and significantly up-regulated percentages of cells expressing CD40 and CD80 (*p*<0.01) (Fig. 7F). Analysis of PLMac showed a significant increase in the percentage of cells (*p*< 0.05, data not shown), but no significant increases in the percentages or total numbers of cells (Fig. 7G and 7H), and significant increases in the proportions of cells expressing CD40 and CD80 (Fig. 7I). Furthermore, a small but significant decrease in the intensity of MHC Class II expression was observed on PLDC (p<0.01), and a significant increase on PLMac (p<0.001) (Fig. S3).

In summary, early life IAV infection induced increases in PLDC numbers and increased expression of co-stimulatory molecules on AMDC, PLDC and PLMac that persisted into adulthood. These data indicate that restoration of respiratory APC homeostasis is persistently disrupted if IAV infection occurs in early life.

Discussion

This study examined the acute and long-term effects of A/PR8/ 34 H1N1 IAV infection on the depletion, reconstitution kinetics and activation state of DC populations in mucosal and parenchymal lung compartments. Uniquely, these were examined both in adult and juvenile mice for airway mucosal and parenchymal lung tissue sites, representing the two major anatomical compartments of the respiratory tract. We have argued previously that these sites differ in their induction and effector immunoregulatory functions in the mouse RT [15,16]. In this study, we have explored the hypothesis that these sites will respond differentially to IAV infection, and that the impact of IAV on immunological homeostasis in the RT will vary as a function of the age of infection.

An adult BALB/c mouse model of IAV infection was established utilising a sub-lethal dose of A/PR8/34, in which clinical signs peaking at days 8 to 9 p.i., with viral titres and lung

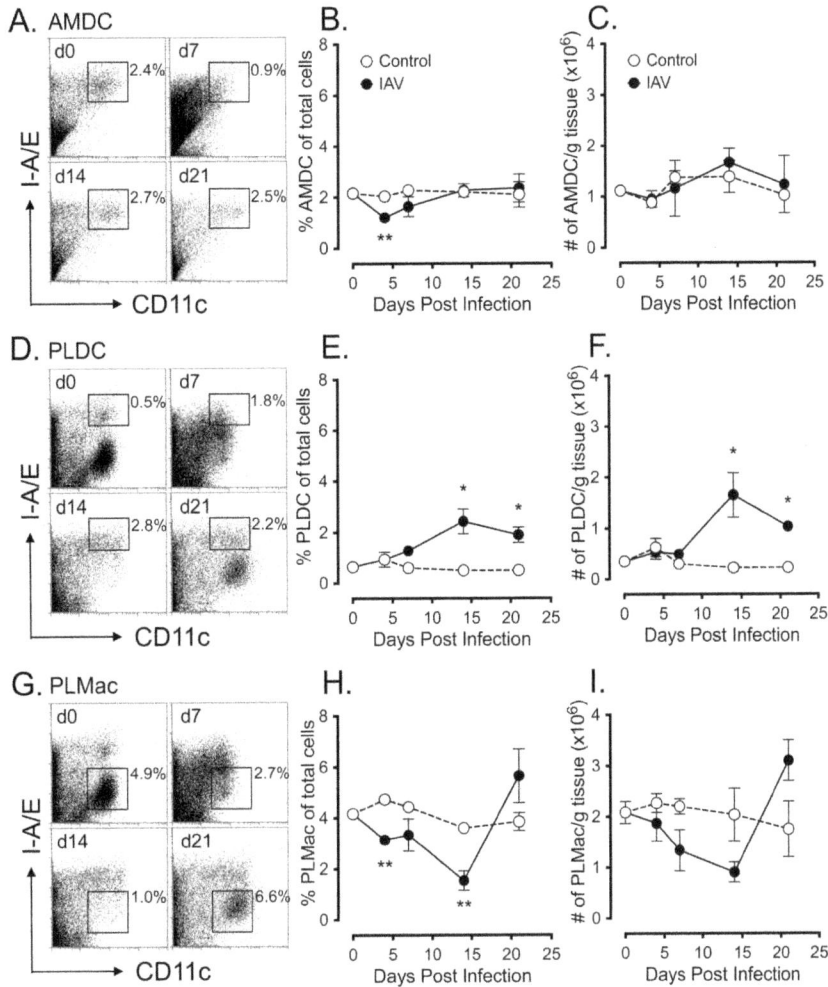

Figure 4. Kinetics of airway mucosal and parenchymal lung DC changes following IAV infection. *(A)* Representative FACS profiles showing gating for AMDC at the indicated time points p.i. *(B and C)* AMDC percentage frequencies *(B)* and total numbers *(C)* following IAV infection for control (open circles) and IAV infected mice (closed circles). *(D)* Representative FACS profiles showing gating for PLDC at the indicated time points p.i. *(E and F)* PLDC percentage frequencies *(E)* and total numbers *(F)* following IAV infection for control (open circles) and IAV infected mice (closed circles). *(G)* Representative FACS profiles showing gating for PLMac at the indicated time points p.i. *(H and I)* PLMac percentage frequencies *(H)* and total numbers *(I)* following IAV infection for control (open circles) and IAV infected mice (closed circles). Data are means +/− SEM for 3 independent infection experiments using pools of tissue from 3 to 4 mice for each experiment. * = $p < 0.05$; ** = $p < 0.01$.

histopathology reverting to background levels by day 14 p.i. Influenza infection resulted in significant and physiologically important deficits in lung mechanics of the conducting airways, peripheral airways and lung parenchyma that were maintained at high lung volume. Mice showed altered lung physiological responses at the peak of IAV infection, which was associated with the maximum of the neutrophil influx into alveolar space. These data are consistent with previous studies using the A/Mem/1/71(H3N1) strain of influenza virus in BALB/c mice, which showed heightened AHR at day 4 p.i. which had normalised by day 20 p.i. [31]. The acute phase of viral infection was also characterised by peak influxes of lymphocytes and neutrophils into BAL fluid as well as IFNα, the neutrophil chemoattractant KC (CXCL1) and IL-12 p70, which declined by day 14 p.i. The neutrophil response in particular was of interest, as these cells had not return to baseline levels by day 14 when virus had been cleared, and began to increase again by day 14. Interestingly, this second wave of neutrophil influx occurred without a concurrent increase in KC or detectable viral titres in lung tissue, suggesting a secondary

recruitment response independent of these factors was taking place. The reason for this is unclear, as we saw no indirect evidence of secondary bacterial infection in the mice, further supported by a lack of Type 1 IFN responses in BAL fluids after day 9 p.i., however this would need to be confirmed by bacteriology. However, the bi-phasic neutrophil response did correlate with a bi-phasic G-CSF response in BALF. This growth factor is a potent regulator of haemopoesis, and mediates neutrophil activation and survival [32]. It is possible that failure to correctly regulate G-CSF in the resolution phase of disease may lead to persistent neutrophil recruitment and activation and incomplete resolution of the inflammatory response. Recently, Narasaraju *et al.* showed a role for macrophages in limiting neutrophil influxes into lavage fluids following PR8 infection [33]. These late and persistent increases in inflammatory cells in BAL suggest that inflammation may never be fully resolved after IAV infection in BALB/c mice, which is consistent with what has been previously proposed and which may in part explain post-infective

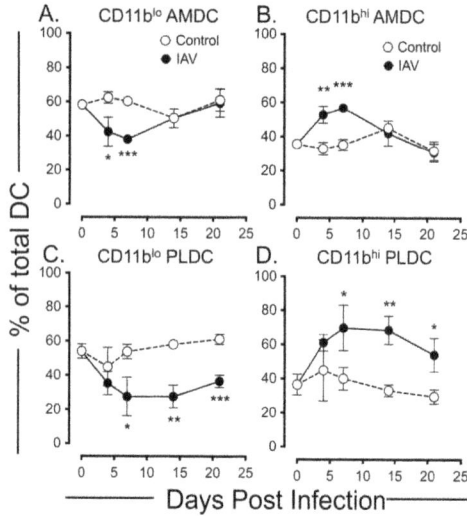

Figure 5. Time course of changes in the expression of CD11b on respiratory DC subsets in anatomical compartments of the respiratory tract following IAV infection. *(A and B)* Percentage frequency of CD11b^{lo} AMDC *(A)* and CD11b^{hi} AMDC *(B)* amongst total AMDC (gated as per Fig. 4A) in IAV infected (closed circles) and control mice (open circles). *(C and D)* Percentage frequency of CD11b^{lo} PLDC *(A)* and CD11b^{hi} PLDC *(B)* amongst total PLDC (gated as per Fig. 4D) in IAV infected (closed circles) and control mice (open circles). Data are means +/− SEM for 3 independent infection experiments using pools of tissue from 3 to 4 mice for each experiment. * = $p<0.05$; ** = $p<0.01$; *** = $p<0.001$.

bronchial hyperreactivity that may persist in humans for weeks or months after influenza infection [34,35].

A key objective of the current study was to examine the kinetics of changes in numbers and activation status of DC, in different anatomical compartments of the mouse respiratory tract after influenza infection. This was based on our previous mouse studies showing that AMDC displayed more rapid turnover rates and were activated early in response to aeroallergen challenge compared to their PLDC counterparts [15,16]. We reasoned that the responses of DC in these two compartments would differ given that AMDC are in intimate contact with airway epithelial cells, which represent the first site of influenza infection and replication, whereas PLDC reside within the alveolar septal walls that represent a distinct microenvironment that may be influenced by inflammatory responses later in the course of infection [36]. Dendritic cells play an important role in the initiation of anti-viral T cell responses, rapidly migrating to draining lymph nodes during early infection and being critical for the activation of both CD4$^+$ and CD8$^+$ viral-specific T cell responses that are essential for viral clearance and resolution of inflammation [27,36,37]. The findings of this study are in accordance with this, as we found that AMDC were being activated to express costimulatory markers early after infection, that correlated with induction of high levels of IAV-specific CD8$^+$ T cell proliferation and IFNγ production in draining lymph nodes at day 4 p.i. (Wikstrom, Stumbles, unpublished observations). Interestingly, associated with this was a significant decrease in the numbers of AMDC at day 4 p.i. but recovery by day 14 p.i., suggesting either cell death, or enhanced migration of AMDC to draining lymph nodes after IAV infection, consistent with the previous findings of others for pulmonary viral infections [37]. Previously we have shown that mouse AMDC and PLDC can be subdivided based on expression of the myeloid

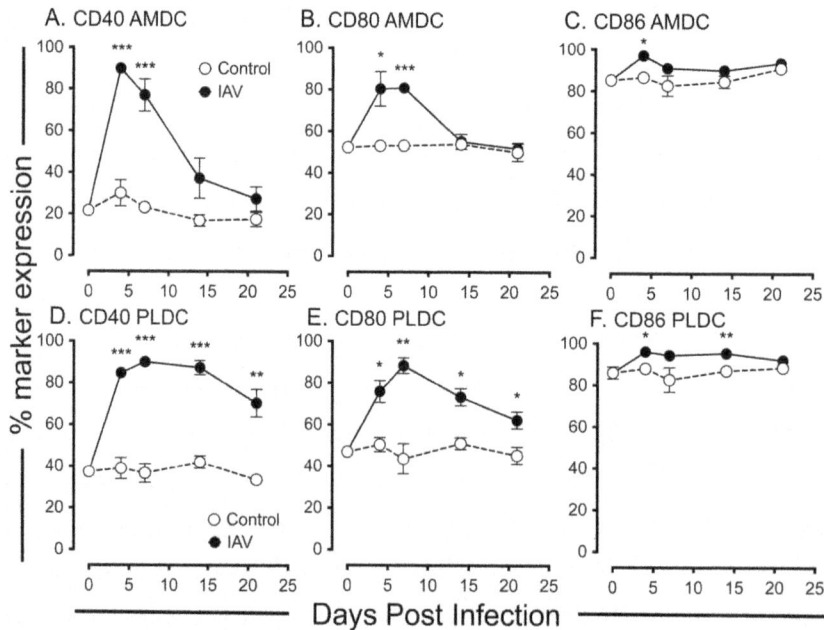

Figure 6. Expression of the co-stimulatory molecules CD40, CD80 and CD86 on respiratory DC subsets in anatomical compartments of the respiratory tract following IAV infection. *(A–C)* Time-course of expression of CD40 *(A)*, CD80 *(B)* and CD86 *(C)* on AMDC expressed as a percentage of cells expressing each marker of the total AMDC population (gated as per Fig. 4A). *(D–F)* Time-course of expression of CD40 *(D)*, CD80 *(E)* and CD86 *(F)* on PLDC expressed as a percentage of cells expressing each marker of the total PLDC population (gated as per Fig. 4D). Data are means +/− SEM for 3 independent infection experiments using pools of tissue from 3 to 4 mice for each experiment. The percentage expression of each marker was calculated based on histogram gates set using matching isotype control antibodies for each marker (Fig. S2) * = $p<0.05$; ** = $p<0.01$; *** = $p<0.001$.

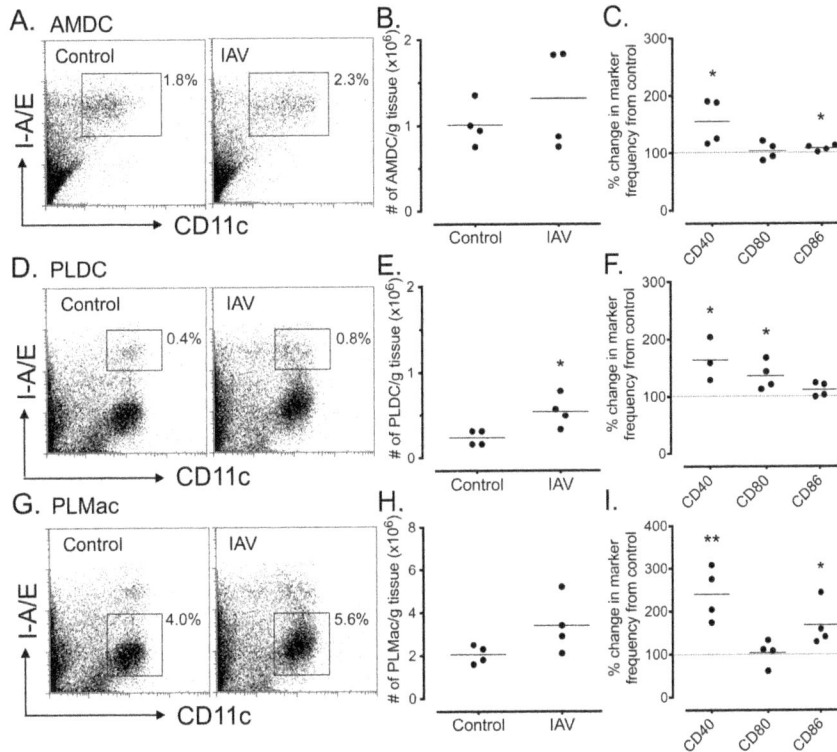

Figure 7. Long-term changes in total cell numbers of, and co-stimulatory molecule expression by, of respiratory APC populations following IAV infection in early life. Juvenile (28 day old) BALB/c mice were infected i.n. with a weight-adjusted dose of IAV as described in Materials and Methods, then respiratory tissues harvested 35 days later as 8 week-old adults. (A) Representative FACS profiles showing gating for AMDC in tracheal tissue of control (left) and IAV infected mice (right). (B and C) Total AMDC numbers (B) and percentage changes in co-stimulatory marker expression (C), expressed a percentage change from control mice. (D) Representative FACS profiles showing gating for PLDC in parenchymal lung tissue of control (left) and IAV infected mice (right). (E and F) Total PLDC numbers (E) and percentage changes in co-stimulatory marker expression (F), expressed a percentage change from control mice. (G) Representative FACS profiles showing gating for PLMac in parenchymal lung tissue of control (left) and IAV infected mice (right). (H and I) Total PLMac numbers (H) and percentage changes in co-stimulatory marker expression (I), expressed a percentage change from control mice. Data are shown for 4 independent infection experiments, using pools of tissue from 4 to 5 mice for each experiment. * = $p < 0.05$; ** = $p < 0.01$.

marker CD11b into CD11b^{hi} and CD11b^{lo} subsets that show different rates of capture of inhaled antigens *in vivo* [16,30]. Others have shown that the CD11b^{lo} subset, that co-expresses the surface marker CD103, is important in capturing viral antigens and migrating to draining lymph nodes for the activation of CD4$^+$ and CD8$^+$ T cells. This capacity also resides within the CD11b^{hi} subset, although to a lesser extent [26]. Furthermore, CD11b^{lo} and CD11b^{hi} DC in the mouse RT have been shown to express differing arrays of chemokines and have been proposed to play differing roles in lung homeostasis, with the CD11b^{lo} (CD103$^+$) subset expressing tight junction proteins and may play a major regulatory role in allergen-induced lung inflammation [22,23]. The findings in this study that the relative proportions of CD11b^{hi} PLDC remain persistently elevated amongst the PLDC population after viral clearance. The reason for this disrupted balance in CD11b-expressing subsets was not determined in the current study, but may relate to altered recruitment kinetics or local maturation of CD11b^{hi} and CD11b^{lo} subsets. In this regard, Lin et al., described a population of inflammatory CCR2$^+$ monocyte-derived DC recruited during acute IAV infection, that have a similar phenotype to the PLDC observed in our study (CD11c+ MHC Class II$^+$ CD11b^{hi}) [38]. Thus, these cells may be contributing to the enhanced proportions of CD11b$^+$ PLDC that persist following IAV infection in our study. Disruptions to the balance of CD11b-expressing PLDC subsets, along with persistent

elevation of co-stimulatory molecule expression on these cells, may have important implications for immune homeostasis at this site given that maintaining a balance in these subsets of DC is likely to be important for the correct regulation of T cell immunity to inhaled allergens. In this regard, it is of interest to note that IAV infection has been associated with enhanced IgE production and CD4$^+$ T cell sensitisation to inhaled allergens, an effect linked to altered function of respiratory dendritic cells [7,39–41]. Furthermore, IAV has been shown to disrupt the induction of T and B cell tolerance to inhaled antigens that normally occurs following exposure to inert proteins in immunologically naïve mice [8]. It is interesting to speculate that these observations may be linked to the findings in the current study of persistently increased proportions of activated CD11b^{hi} PLDC following IAV infection, that may act to promote aberrant local CD4$^+$ T cell activation to inhaled allergens in lung tissue.

Finally, we examined the impact of IAV infection in juvenile mice at the age of 28 days old, representing the post-weaning age of human infants. Juvenile mice infected with a weight-adjusted, adult-equivalent dosage of IAV developed a clinical disease of similar severity to adults, with peak clinical signs and resolution of symptoms occurring at the same time points. When these mice were examined at day 35 p.i., an age at which is mice are considered to have reached adult maturity, we observed persistent and significant increases in the numbers and activation status of parenchymal lung DC and Mac populations, but not in their airway mucosal counterparts. This was particularly evident for the PLMac populations, which displayed marked increases in MHC Class II, CD40 and CD86 expression above control mice, and for PLDC that displayed increased numbers and persistent CD40 and CD80 upregulation. Activation of PLMac was also observed in the adult model prior during the course of IAV infection, most likely as a result of TLR7 binding by viral components and NLR (NOD-like receptor) inflammasome activation [42]. Whether persistent PLMac and PLDC activation in juvenile and adult mice is a result of sustained TLR or NLR signalling, or some other sustained inflammatory response is unclear. However, this could have important down-stream consequences for immune homeostasis at in the lung, given that interactions between macrophages and DC are important for dampening DC function and T cell reactivity in parenchymal lung tissue and that long-lived APC expressing elevated levels of MHC Class II could act as depots for allergen persistence and reactivation of allergen-specific T cells [43,44].

In conclusion, in this study we have demonstrated that A/PR8/34 H1N1 IAV infection of BALB/c mice has differential effects on DC populations in differing anatomical locations of the respiratory tract, with persistent derangement in the numbers and activation states of DC in the parenchymal lung compartment as compared to the airway mucosa. Furthermore, these disruptions persisted for several weeks after clearance of the virus in adult mice, and persisted into adulthood in mice that were infected with IAV in early life. These data indicate that IAV has a severe and long-term impact on the balance and activation state of respiratory DC and other APC subsets, potentially disrupting the fine balance of immunological homeostatic mechanisms required for the prevention of respiratory inflammatory diseases to inert antigens.

Materials and Methods

Mice and Viral Inoculations

Ethics statement. All animal experiments were conducted in strict accordance with the recommendations of the National Health and Medical Research Council of Australia, Guidelines to Promote the Wellbeing of Animals used for Scientific Research. All procedures were approved by the Telethon Institute for Child Health Research Animal Experimentation Ethics Committee (permit numbers: 139 and 256) and Murdoch University Animal Ethics Committee (permit number: N2569/13). Intranasal (i.n.) viral inoculations were performed under light inhaled Isofluorane anaesthesia. Mice were sacrificed by i.p. injection of 100μl of Phenobarbitone Sodium performed under inhaled Isofluorane anaesthesia, with all efforts made to minimise animal suffering.

Specific pathogen free female BALB/c mice were obtained from the Animal Resources Centre (Perth, W.A., Australia) and used at either 28 days (juvenile) or 8 weeks (adult) of age. The mouse-adapted influenza H1N1 A/PR/8/34 virus was from the American Type Tissue Culture Collection and prepared in allantoic fluid of 9-day old embryonated hens eggs. Stock virus was sub-passaged through Mardin-Darby canine kidney (MDCK) cells in Dulbecco's modified Eagle's medium (DMEM; Gibco, Sydney, Australia), harvested as tissue culture supernatant and viral titres determined by cytopathic effects on MDCK cells and expressed as the mean $\log_{10}$ tissue culture infective dose that kills 50% of the cells ($TCID_{50}$) over a 5-day incubation period. Adult mice were inoculated intranasally (i.n.) under light inhalation anaesthesia with 0.5×10^2 $TCID_{50}$ PR8 diluted in 50μl DMEM [45]. Juvenile mice were obtained post-weaning and inoculated i.n. using a weight-for-age adjusted volume of 0.5×10^2 $TCID_{50}$ PR8/50μl adjusted to 2.5μl per gram body weight. Mock-infected

control mice received matched volumes of virus-free DMEM tissue culture medium by i.n. inoculation.

Animal Monitoring and Clinical Assessments

Mice were weighed daily during the acute period of infection (d0 to d14) and then every second day until day 21. Clinical disease scores were also assessed according ot the following criteria: 0-healthy; 1-barely ruffled fur; 2-ruffled fur, active; 3-ruffled fur, inactive; 4-ruffled fur, inactive, hunched. Mice were euthanized at indicated time points and lung tissue harvested for assessment of viral titres. Lung-tissue viral titres were determined by the $TCID_{50}$ assay described above, using 20% dilutions of clarified lung tissue homogenates. Results are expressed as $\log_{10}$ $TCID_{50}/100$μl of lung tissue homogenate. Broncho-alveolar lavage fluid (BALF) was harvested by slowly infusing and withdrawing 1 ml of PBS containing 20mg/ml bovine serum albumin (CSL, Victoria, Australia) and 35 mg/ml lidocaine (Sigma, St Louis, USA) from the lungs three times, and the cells pelleted and prepared for total cell counts and differential cell counts as previously described [46]. Briefly, the percentage of each cell type as identified by Leishman's stain (macrophage, neutrophil, lymphocyte) was calculated as a proportion of 300 counted cells, and this figure used to derive total numbers of each subset based on the total BALF cell count. The BALF supernatants were stored at -80°C for cytokine analysis. All cytokines were measured in undiluted BALF using a Bio-Plex Pro Mouse Cytokine Grp 1 Panel 23-Plex assay and Bio-Plex MAGPIX plate reader (BIO-RAD, USA) apart from acid stable Type I IFN (IFNα), which was measured by bioassay using encephalomyocarditis virus-induced cytopathic effect (CPE) of L929 monolayers as previously described [47].

Lung Function Testing

Lung mechanics were measured as described previously [48]. Briefly, mice (4 per experimental group) were anaesthetised by i.p. injection of a solution containing 40 mg.mL^{-1} ketamine and 2 mg.mL^{-1} xylazine at a dose of 0.1 mL.10 g^{-1} body weight. Mice were surgically tracheotomised and connected to a mechanical ventilator (tidal volume, 8 mL.kg-1; frequency, 450 breaths.min-1, PEEP, 2 cmH$_2$O). Following standardisation of lung volume history the ventilator was paused and a pseudorandom oscillatory signal (4-38 Hz) was delivered to the tracheal cannula by a loudspeaker via a wavetube of known impedance. A positive pressure was then applied via the wavetube in order to slowly (15–20s) inflate the lung up to 20 cmH$_2$O transrespiratory pressure. The oscillatory signal was applied throughout this manoeuvre in order to track changes in lung mechanics from functional residual capacity (FRC) to total lung capacity (TLC). A respiratory system impedance spectrum was then generated for each 0.5 s data epoch of the inflation manoeuvre. Data from each of these spectra was then fit to a 4 parameter mathematical model with constant phase tissue impedance which allowed us to partition lung mechanics into parameters representing airway resistance (Raw, resistance of the conducting airways), tissue damping (G, resistance of the small peripheral airways were airflow occurs by diffusion) and tissue elastance (H, stiffness of the lung parenchyma) [49].

Isolation and Preparation of Respiratory Tract Tissues

Lungs were perfused to isolate tracheal (airway mucosal) and parenchymal lung tissue and prepare single cell suspensions as previously described [50]. In brief, trachea or lungs were collected from pools of five mice and single-cell suspensions prepared by type IV collagenase digestion (1.5 mg/ml; Worthington Biochemical, Lakewood, NJ) with type I DNAse (0.1 mg/ml; Sigma

Aldrich). DLN (upper paratracheal and parathymic) were pooled separately from the same groups of mice, finely chopped with a scalpel, and digested with type IV collagenase and type I DNAse. All digestions and washes were performed in glucose sodium potassium buffer (11 mM D-glucose, 5.5 mM KCl, 137 mM NaCl, 25 mM Na_2HPO_4, 5.5 mM $NaH_2PO_4.2H_2O$) with debris and RBCs removed as previously described [51].

Analysis of Cell Surface Markers by Flow Cytometry

After preparation of single-cell suspensions, FcR were routinely blocked using 2.4G2 (BD Biosciences) for 10 min on ice to prevent non-specific binding of phenotyping antibodies subsequently added. Airway, lung and draining lymph node DC populations were identified in tracheal digests using combinations of fluorochrome labelled mAbs (all from BD Biosciences, NSW, Australia except where indicated) to mouse CD11c (clone N418), I-A/I-E (clone 2G9), CD205 (DEC205; Serotec, Oxford, UK), CD11b (clone M1/70), CD40 (clone 3/23), CD80 (clone 16-10A1) and CD86 (clone GL1). All labelling was performed in glucose sodium potassium buffer containing 0.2% BSA for 30 min on ice. All Abs were used as direct conjugates to FITC, Phycoerythrin (PE), PE-Cy7, allophycocyanin (APC), APC-Cy7, or biotin as required. Where appropriate, biotinylated antibodies were detected with Streptavidin conjugated PE-Cy5 (BD Biosciences). Appropriately matched and conjugated IgG isotype controls (BD Biosciences) were used in all experiments, and cytometer compensation settings were adjusted using single-stained controls for each experiment. Samples were collected using a FACSCalibur or LSRII flow cytometer (BD Biosciences) and analyzed using FlowJo software (TreeStar, Ca, USA).

Determination of Total Cell Counts

Total counts for AMDC, PLDC and PLMac were determined on the basis of tissue weight and total cell yield for each tissue (trachea and peripheral lung), and then calculated on the basis of the total percentage of each DC type as determined by FACS. Values are expresses as number of cells/g tissue according to the formula: (% frequency x total cells/g tissue)/100.

Statistical Analysis

Two-tailed, unpaired Student's t tests assuming equal variance were employed to calculate significances (GraphPad Prism, CA, USA), with p-values <0.05 considered statistically significant. Statistical significance is indicated as follows: $* = p<0.05$; $** = p<0.01$; $*** = p<0.001$; $**** = p<0.0001$.

References

1. Gern JE (2008) Viral respiratory infection and the link to asthma. Pediatr Infect Dis J 27: S97–103.
2. Iwane MK, Edwards KM, Szilagyi PG, Walker FJ, Griffin MR, et al. (2004) Population-based surveillance for hospitalizations associated with respiratory syncytial virus, influenza virus, and parainfluenza viruses among young children. Pediatrics 113: 1758–1764.
3. Kusel MM, de Klerk NH, Kebadze T, Vohma V, Holt PG, et al. (2007) Early-life respiratory viral infections, atopic sensitization, and risk of subsequent development of persistent asthma. J Allergy Clin Immunol 119: 1105–1110.
4. Lemanske RF Jr, Jackson DJ, Gangnon RE, Evans MD, Li Z, et al. (2005) Rhinovirus illnesses during infancy predict subsequent childhood wheezing. J Allergy Clin Immunol 116: 571–577.
5. Sigurs N, Gustafsson PM, Bjarnason R, Lundberg F, Schmidt S, et al. (2005) Severe respiratory syncytial virus bronchiolitis in infancy and asthma and allergy at age 13. Am J Respir Crit Care Med 171: 137–141.
6. Stein RT, Sherrill D, Morgan WJ, Holberg CJ, Halonen M, et al. (1999) Respiratory syncytial virus in early life and risk of wheeze and allergy by age 13 years. Lancet 354: 541–545.

Supporting Information

Figure S1　CD205 and CD11c staining of respiratory tissues. Tracheal (A) and parenchymal lung tissue (B and C) cells were prepared as per Methods, labelled for CD11c and CD205 and analysed by flow cytometry at the indicated time points after IAV infection. Representative dot plots of 3 experiments for each time point are shown, with AMDC (A), PLDC (B) and PLMac (C) gated as indicated.
(TIF)

Figure S2　Expression levels of co-stimulatory markers on AMDC and PLDC at d4 post-IAV infection. Adult BALB/c mice were infected with IAV and 4 days later (representing a time point of peak expression of each marker) tracheal and lung tissue were prepared for flow cytometry analysis for each marker on AMDC (A) and PLDC (B). Representative histograms (of 3 experiments) are shown for control and IAV infected mice, showing isotype controls (grey shaded) and specific marker (solid black) expression.
(TIF)

Figure S3　Changes in MHC Class II (I-A/E) expression on respiratory APC of adult mice following IAV infection at 4 weeks of age. Mice were infected with IAV at 4 weeks of age and respiratory tissue harvested 35 days later. The mean fluorescence intensity (MFI) of I-A/E expression on AMDC (A), PLDC (B) and PLMac (C) was then determined for IAV infected mice (black line) and control mice (grey shade), and expressed as a percentage change in MFI of IAV infected mice as compared to control mice (D). Histograms are representative of 4 independent experiments using pooled tissue from 5 mice in each, gated on DC populations as shown in Fig. S1. Panel D shows cumulative data of 4 independent experiments using pools of tissue from 5 mice in each experiment.
(TIF)

Acknowledgments

We thank Miranda Smith, Elizabeth Bozanich, Jenny Thomas, Siew Ping Lau and Sylvia Napoli for their excellent technical assistance during this study.

Author Contributions

Conceived and designed the experiments: PAS DHS CvG VF PGH GZ ANL. Performed the experiments: VF SS MEW GZ ANL CB. Analyzed the data: PAS DHS CvG MEW GZ VF SS CB. Contributed reagents/materials/analysis tools: PAS DHS CB GZ ANL. Wrote the paper: PAS DHS CvG VF MEW GZ.

7. Al-Garawi AA, Fattouh R, Walker TD, Jamula EB, Botelho F, et al. (2009) Acute, but not resolved, influenza A infection enhances susceptibility to house dust mite-induced allergic disease. J Immunol 182: 3095–3104.
8. Tsitoura DC, Kim S, Dabbagh K, Berry G, Lewis DB, et al. (2000) Respiratory infection with influenza A virus interferes with the induction of tolerance to aeroallergens. J Immunol 165: 3484–3491.
9. Holt P, Strickland D, Wikström M, Jahnsen F (2008) Regulation of immunological homeostasis in the respiratory tract. Nature reviews Immunology 8: 142–194.
10. McWilliam AS, Marsh AM, Holt PG (1997) Inflammatory infiltration of the upper airway epithelium during Sendai virus infection: involvement of epithelial dendritic cells. J Virol 71: 226–236.
11. Beyer M, Bartz H, Horner K, Doths S, Koerner-Rettberg C, et al. (2004) Sustained increases in numbers of pulmonary dendritic cells after respiratory syncytial virus infection. J Allergy Clin Immunol 113: 127–133.
12. Gill MA, Palucka AK, Barton T, Ghaffar F, Jafri H, et al. (2005) Mobilization of plasmacytoid and myeloid dendritic cells to mucosal sites in children with respiratory syncytial virus and other viral respiratory infections. J Infect Dis 191: 1105–1115.

13. Stumbles PA, Thomas JA, Pimm CL, Lee PT, Venaille TJ, et al. (1998) Resting respiratory tract dendritic cells preferentially stimulate T helper cell type 2 (Th2) responses and require obligatory cytokine signals for induction of Th1 immunity. J Exp Med 188: 2019–2031.

14. Lambrecht B, Hammad H (2010) The role of dendritic and epithelial cells as master regulators of allergic airway inflammation. Lancet 376: 835–878.

15. von Garnier C, Filgueira L, Wikström M, Smith M, Thomas JA, et al. (2005) Anatomical location determines the distribution and function of dendritic cells and other APCs in the respiratory tract. J Immunol 175: 1609–1618.

16. von Garnier C, Wikstrom ME, Zosky G, Turner DJ, Sly PD, et al. (2007) Allergic airways disease develops after an increase in allergen capture and processing in the airway mucosa. J Immunol 179: 5748–5759.

17. McWilliam AS, Napoli S, Marsh AM, Pemper FL, Nelson DJ, et al. (1996) Dendritic cells are recruited into the airway epithelium during the inflammatory response to a broad spectrum of stimuli. J Exp Med 184: 2429–2432.

18. Stumbles PA, Strickland DH, Pimm CL, Proksch SF, Marsh AM, et al. (2001) Regulation of dendritic cell recruitment into resting and inflamed airway epithelium: use of alternative chemokine receptors as a function of inducing stimulus. J Immunol 167: 228–234.

19. Wikstrom M, Stumbles P (2007) Mouse respiratory tract dendritic cell subsets and the immunological fate of inhaled antigens. Immunology and cell biology 85: 182–190.

20. Heath W, Carbone F (2009) Dendritic cell subsets in primary and secondary T cell responses at body surfaces. Nature immunology 10: 1237–1281.

21. Miller J, Brown B, Shay T, Gautier E, Jojic V, et al. (2012) Deciphering the transcriptional network of the dendritic cell lineage. Nature immunology 13: 888–899.

22. Beaty SR, Rose CE Jr, Sung SS (2007) Diverse and potent chemokine production by lung CD11b^{high} dendritic cells in homeostasis and in allergic lung inflammation. J Immunol 178: 1882–1895.

23. Sung SS, Fu SM, Rose CE Jr, Gaskin F, Ju ST, et al. (2006) A major lung CD103 (alphaE)-beta7 integrin-positive epithelial dendritic cell population expressing Langerin and tight junction proteins. J Immunol 176: 2161–2172.

24. Moltedo B, Li W, Yount J, Moran T (2011) Unique type I interferon responses determine the functional fate of migratory lung dendritic cells during influenza virus infection. PLoS pathogens 7(11): e1002345.

25. Ho AW, Prabhu N, Betts RJ, Ge MQ, Dai X, et al. (2011) Lung CD103$^+$ dendritic cells efficiently transport influenza virus to the lymph node and load viral antigen onto MHC class I for presentation to CD8 T cells. J Immunol 187: 6011–6021.

26. Kim TS, Braciale TJ (2009) Respiratory dendritic cell subsets differ in their capacity to support the induction of virus-specific cytotoxic CD8$^+$ T cell responses. PLoS One 4: e4204.

27. GeurtsvanKessel CH, Willart MA, van Rijt LS, Muskens F, Kool M, et al. (2008) Clearance of influenza virus from the lung depends on migratory langerin$^+$ CD11b$^-$ but not plasmacytoid dendritic cells. J Exp Med 205: 1621–1634.

28. Ingulli E, Funatake C, Jacovetty EL, Zanetti M (2009) Cutting edge: antigen presentation to CD8 T cells after influenza A virus infection. J Immunol 182: 29–33.

29. Belz G, Smith C, Kleinert L, Reading P, Brooks A, et al. (2004) Distinct migrating and nonmigrating dendritic cell populations are involved in MHC class I-restricted antigen presentation after lung infection with virus. Proceedings of the National Academy of Sciences of the United States of America 101: 8670–8675.

30. Fear VS, Burchell JT, Lai SP, Wikstrom ME, Blank F, et al. (2011) Restricted aeroallergen access to airway mucosal dendritic cells in vivo limits allergen-specific CD4$^+$ T cell proliferation during the induction of inhalation tolerance. J Immunol 187: 4561–4570.

31. Bozanich EM, Gualano RC, Zosky GR, Larcombe AN, Turner DJ, et al. (2008) Acute Influenza A infection induces bronchial hyper-responsiveness in mice. Respir Physiol Neurobiol 162: 190–196.

32. Eyles JL, Roberts AW, Metcalf D, Wicks IP (2006) Granulocyte colony-stimulating factor and neutrophils–forgotten mediators of inflammatory disease. Nat Clin Pract Rheumatol 2: 500–510.

33. Narasaraju T, Yang E, Samy RP, Ng HH, Poh WP, et al. (2011) Excessive neutrophils and neutrophil extracellular traps contribute to acute lung injury of influenza pneumonitis. Am J Pathol 179: 199–210.

34. Snelgrove R, Goulding J, Didierlaurent A, Lyonga D, Vekaria S, et al. (2008) A critical function for CD200 in lung immune homeostasis and the severity of influenza infection. Nature immunology 9: 1074–1083.

35. Sterk P (1993) Virus-induced airway hyperresponsiveness in man. The European respiratory journal 6: 894–902.

36. Yoo J-K, Kim T, Hufford M, Braciale T (2013) Viral infection of the lung: Host response and sequelae. The Journal of allergy and clinical immunology 132: 1263–1276.

37. Legge KL, Braciale TJ (2003) Accelerated migration of respiratory dendritic cells to the regional lymph nodes is limited to the early phase of pulmonary infection. Immunity 18: 265–277.

38. Lin KL, Suzuki Y, Nakano H, Ramsburg E, Gunn MD (2008) CCR2$^+$ monocyte-derived dendritic cells and exudate macrophages produce influenza-induced pulmonary immune pathology and mortality. J Immunol 180: 2562–2572.

39. Brimnes MK, Bonifaz L, Steinman RM, Moran TM (2003) Influenza Virus-induced Dendritic Cell Maturation Is Associated with the Induction of Strong T Cell Immunity to a Coadministered, Normally Nonimmunogenic Protein. J Exp Med 198: 133–144.

40. Dahl M, Dabbagh K, Liggitt D, Kim S, Lewis D (2004) Viral-induced T helper type 1 responses enhance allergic disease by effects on lung dendritic cells. Nature immunology 5: 337–343.

41. Suzuki S, Suzuki Y, Yamamoto N, Matsumoto Y, Shirai A, et al. (1998) Influenza A virus infection increases IgE production and airway responsiveness in aerosolized antigen-exposed mice. The Journal of allergy and clinical immunology 102: 732–740.

42. Ichinohe T, Lee HK, Ogura Y, Flavell R, Iwasaki A (2009) Inflammasome recognition of influenza virus is essential for adaptive immune responses. J Exp Med 206: 79–87.

43. Bilyk N, Holt PG (1993) Inhibition of the immunosuppressive activity of resident pulmonary alveolar macrophages by granulocyte/macrophage colony-stimulating factor. J Exp Med 177: 1773–1777.

44. Julia V, Hessel E, Malherbe L, Glaichenhaus N, O'Garra A, et al. (2002) A restricted subset of dendritic cells captures airborne antigens and remains able to activate specific T cells long after antigen exposure. Immunity 16: 271–283.

45. Southam DS, Dolovich M, O'Byrne PM, Inman MD (2002) Distribution of intranasal instillations in mice: effects of volume, time, body position, and anesthesia. Am J Physiol Lung Cell Mol Physiol 282: L833–839.

46. Zosky GR, von Garnier C, Stumbles PA, Holt PG, Sly PD, et al. (2004) The pattern of methacholine responsiveness in mice is dependent on antigen challenge dose. Respir Res 5: 15.

47. Cull V, Bartlett E, James C (2002) Type I interferon gene therapy protects against cytomegalovirus-induced myocarditis. Immunology 106: 428–437.

48. Hantos Z, Collins RA, Turner DJ, Janosi TZ, Sly PD (2003) Tracking of airway and tissue mechanics during TLC maneuvers in mice. J Appl Physiol 95: 1695–1705.

49. Hantos Z, Daroczy B, Suki B, Nagy S, Fredberg JJ (1992) Input impedance and peripheral inhomogeneity of dog lungs. J Appl Physiol 72: 168–178.

50. Stumbles P, Strickland D, Wikstrom M, Thomas J, von Garnier C, et al. (2010) Identification and isolation of rodent respiratory tract dendritic cells. Methods in molecular biology.pp. 249–312.

51. Wikstrom ME, Batanero E, Smith M, Thomas JA, von Garnier C, et al. (2006) Influence of mucosal adjuvants on antigen passage and CD4$^+$ T cell activation during the primary response to airborne allergen. J Immunol 177: 913–924.

9

NIAM-Deficient Mice Are Predisposed to the Development of Proliferative Lesions including B-Cell Lymphomas

Sara M. Reed[1,2], **Jussara Hagen**[1], **Viviane P. Muniz**[1,3], **Timothy R. Rosean**[4], **Nick Borcherding**[5], **Sebastian Sciegienka**[1], **J. Adam Goeken**[5], **Paul W. Naumann**[5], **Weizhou Zhang**[4,5], **Van S. Tompkins**[5], **Siegfried Janz**[4,5], **David K. Meyerholz**[5], **Dawn E. Quelle**[1,2,3,5]*

1 Department of Pharmacology, University of Iowa, Iowa City, Iowa, United States of America, 2 Medical Scientist Training Program, University of Iowa, Iowa City, Iowa, United States of America, 3 Molecular and Cellular Biology Program, University of Iowa, Iowa City, Iowa, United States of America, 4 Interdisciplinary Program in Immunology, University of Iowa, Iowa City, Iowa, United States of America, 5 Department of Pathology, University of Iowa, Iowa City, Iowa, United States of America

Abstract

Nuclear Interactor of ARF and Mdm2 (NIAM, gene designation *Tbrg1*) is a largely unstudied inhibitor of cell proliferation that helps maintain chromosomal stability. It is a novel activator of the ARF-Mdm2-Tip60-p53 tumor suppressor pathway as well as other undefined pathways important for genome maintenance. To examine its predicted role as a tumor suppressor, we generated *NIAM* mutant (*NIAM$^{m/m}$*) mice homozygous for a β-galactosidase expressing gene-trap cassette in the endogenous gene. The mutant mice expressed significantly lower levels of NIAM protein in tissues compared to wild-type animals. Fifty percent of aged *NIAM* deficient mice (14 to 21 months) developed proliferative lesions, including a uterine hemangioma, pulmonary papillary adenoma, and a Harderian gland adenoma. No age-matched wild-type or *NIAM$^{+/m}$* heterozygous animals developed lesions. In the spleen, *NIAM$^{m/m}$* mice had prominent white pulp expansion which correlated with enhanced increased reactive lymphoid hyperplasia and evidence of systemic inflammation. Notably, 17% of *NIAM* mutant mice had splenic white pulp features indicating early B-cell lymphoma. This correlated with selective expansion of marginal zone B cells in the spleens of younger, tumor-free *NIAM*-deficient mice. Unexpectedly, basal p53 expression and activity was largely unaffected by NIAM loss in isolated splenic B cells. In sum, *NIAM* down-regulation *in vivo* results in a significant predisposition to developing benign tumors or early stage cancers. These mice represent an outstanding platform for dissecting NIAM's role in tumorigenesis and various anti-cancer pathways, including p53 signaling.

Editor: Sumitra Deb, Virginia Commonwealth University, United States of America

Funding: This work was supported by the NIH through a pre-doctoral fellowship 5F30CA165736 (S.M.R.), pre-doctoral training grant 5T32AI007485 (T.R.R.), NCI Core Grant P30CA086862 in support of the University of Iowa Holden Comprehensive Cancer Center, and R01CA151354 (S.J.), as well as an Oberley Award through the Holden Comprehensive Cancer Center (S.J. and D.E.Q). The funders had no role in study design, data collection and analysis, decision to publish or preparation of the manuscript.

Competing Interests: The authors have declared that no competing interests exist.

* Email: dawn-quelle@uiowa.edu

Introduction

The p53 tumor suppressor forms the core of an extensive signaling network that protects cells against genomic instability and neoplastic transformation in response to genotoxic insults [1–3]. Once activated, p53 transactivates or represses a wide array of genes that cause cell cycle arrest, promote DNA repair, restrict metabolism or kill irreparably damaged cells, among other anti-cancer activities [4]. Loss of p53 function occurs in the vast majority of human cancers, if not all, due to *TP53* gene mutation or alteration of its many regulators and targets [2,5]. Mouse models that lack p53 or express naturally occurring p53 mutants are highly tumor prone and develop the broad range of malignancies found in humans with impaired p53 signaling [6–8]. Understanding how p53 activity is controlled, and the importance of its regulators in tumor biology, has been a top priority in cancer research for more than two decades [1–3,9].

NIAM (Nuclear Interactor of ARF and Mdm2, also called *Tbrg1*) is a new p53 regulator and anti-proliferative factor whose role in cancer is not yet defined [10–13]. Mechanistically, it engages the p53 pathway at multiple levels. First, NIAM promotes the relocalization of ARF (Alternative Reading Frame protein), a major activator of p53 [14], from nucleoli into the nucleoplasm where it is more effective at activating p53 [10,15,16]. Second, NIAM binds to Mdm2, the primary antagonist of p53 [17], and reduces the formation of p53-Mdm2 complexes [10,12]. As such, NIAM impairs Mdm2-mediated polyubiquitylation and proteasomal degradation of p53, thereby stabilizing and activating p53 signaling [12]. Third, NIAM is a chromatin-bound protein that associates with the histone acetyltransferase, Tip60 (Tat-interacting protein of 60 kDa) [12], which is essential for p53-dependent cell cycle arrest and death [18–20]. Tip60 knockdown studies demonstrated that it contributes to NIAM-mediated p53

Table 1. Reduced *NIAM* mRNA levels in cancer tissues.

Tumor Type	No. of Studies*	References
Brain	9	[63–67]
B-cell Lymphoma	7	[33–37]
Lung	2	[68]
Breast	10	[69–71]
Prostate	2	[72]

*Microarray analyses identified through ONCOMINE showing a statistically significant decrease in *NIAM* mRNA in tumors. (p<0.05).

activation, revealing that NIAM induces p53 activity through multiple mechanisms involving Tip60 association as well as Mdm2 inhibition [12]. Notably, like p53 and Tip60, NIAM is normally kept at low expression levels in cells by Mdm2-dependent ubiquitylation [10].

The interplay of NIAM with p53 and its established partners (ARF, Mdm2 and Tip60), all of which are frequently disrupted in human cancers [3,14,17,21,22], suggests NIAM may have tumor suppressive activity. That idea is supported by *in silico* evidence from microarray databases suggesting significant down-regulation of NIAM mRNA levels in many advanced human cancers [23,24]. Interestingly, NIAM can act independently of ARF-Mdm2-p53 signaling. It can inhibit proliferation in cells lacking ARF, Mdm2 and/or p53, and its depletion in *ARF/Mdm2/p53*-null mouse embryo fibroblasts results in chromosomal instability [10]. These findings imply that NIAM plays an important role in other anti-cancer pathways outside of the ARF-Mdm2-p53 tumor suppressor pathway.

Here, we describe the generation and initial characterization of the first *NIAM* mutant mouse model. These animals have hypomorphic *NIAM* alleles that result in greatly impaired expression of NIAM protein in tissues, similar to what may occur in human malignancies in which its mRNA expression is down-regulated. Spontaneous tumor formation was assessed and NIAM down-regulation found to increase tumor susceptibility in aged animals. B-cell lymphoma was among the tumors identified and this correlated with a marked expansion of splenic marginal zone B cells in young, tumor-free *NIAM*-deficient mice. Interestingly, p53 inactivation in B cells promotes splenic marginal zone B cell expansion and B-cell lymphoma [25,26], implicating impaired p53 function in the *NIAM* knockout phenotype. At least under non-stressed conditions, however, splenic B cells from young *NIAM*-deficient mice showed no significant effect on basal p53 activity. We suggest that the *NIAM* mutant mice described in this study represent a unique model of B-cell lymphoma that should help resolve NIAM's biological role in p53 signaling and other cancer pathways.

Results

Decreased NIAM mRNA expression in human tumors

It is well established that ARF-Mdm2-Tip60-p53 signaling plays a dominant role in carcinogenesis [1–3,17,21,27]. Since NIAM has important roles in regulating this pathway, we probed various online databases for the most recent information on *NIAM* alterations in human cancers. A previous analysis of the ONCOMINE microarray database in 2007 suggested that *NIAM* mRNA expression is down-regulated in multiple advanced human cancers [10]. The addition of large amounts of microarray results to ONCOMINE since that time only strengthens that conclusion,

once again suggesting significant reduction of *NIAM* mRNA levels in many cancers including lung, breast, brain, prostate, and B-cell lymphoma (**Table 1**). Recent RNA sequencing data from The Cancer Genome Atlas (TCGA) project is now available for certain cancers and verifies that there is a marked decrease in *NIAM* (gene name *Tbrg1*) mRNA levels in human lung, liver, bladder, and breast cancers as compared to paired, normal tissues (**Fig. 1**). These data demonstrate that *NIAM* expression is reduced in many different types of human malignancies, consistent with the prediction that it plays an important role in inhibiting tumorigenesis.

Generation of NIAM-deficient mice

A *NIAM* gene targeting construct was inserted between exon 1 (which contains the ATG start site) and exon 2 in C57BL/6N embryonic stem cells by the Knockout Mouse Project (KOMP) (**Fig. 2A**). The cassette contains a poly (A) adenylation site, a neomycin resistance gene (Neo), and β-galactosidase trap for tracking normal *NIAM* expression patterns in tissues. It also contains FRT sites for removal of neomycin and β-galactosidase cassettes by flippase, which would restore normal gene function of *NIAM*. Two intronic LoxP sites enable conditional deletion of exon 2 using Cre-expressing mice should the cassette not lead to sufficient loss of the *NIAM* gene. This construct is predicted to interfere with splicing or, at minimum, generate a severely

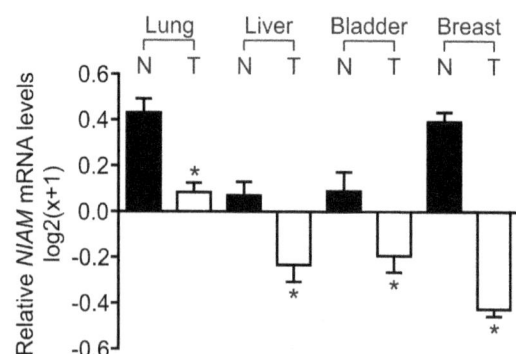

Figure 1. *NIAM* **mRNA expression is downregulated in multiple human cancers.** *NIAM* mRNA levels are significantly reduced in primary tumor (T) samples relative to normal (N) tissue, according to RNA-seq data obtained from the TCGA project database. The number of samples analyzed for each tissue was as follows: lung (N = 58, T = 488), liver (N = 50, T = 147), bladder (N = 19, T = 211), and breast (N = 108, T = 992). Error bars represent a 95% CI as calculated using the standard error, and an unpaired Welch's T-test was used to calculate statistical significance (*, p<0.0001).

truncated chimeric protein containing only 48 N-terminal residues of NIAM.

We obtained chimeric mice expressing the mutant (m) *NIAM* allele from KOMP and generated NIAM heterozygous (+/m) mice by crossing them to C57BL/6N breeders. After obtaining germline transmission, we interbred heterozygous mice to obtain homozygous offspring (m/m) (**Fig. 2B**). Heterozygous mouse matings (n = 31) produced litter sizes between 1 to 9 pups (avg = 5.58). The genotype (+/+, +/m, m/m) was determined for 173 mice and the expected Mendelian ratios of 1:2:1 were not met (p = 0.0035, using the χ^2-test) (**Fig. 2C**). The number of heterozygous $NIAM^{+/m}$ and homozygous $NIAM^{m/m}$ mice was higher than expected, possibly suggesting that *NIAM* loss may provide a selective advantage during embryogenesis. The $NIAM^{m/m}$ mice also successfully mated and produced offspring demonstrating no crucial effects of NIAM on fertility and viability.

To determine if the gene-trap cassette effectively interfered with *NIAM* expression, mouse tissues from each genotype were obtained and assessed for levels of NIAM protein. NIAM expression was greatly diminished although some level of expression remained in all $NIAM^{m/m}$ mouse tissues examined, demonstrating that these animals have hypomorphic *NIAM* alleles (**Fig. 3**). Effective down-regulation of NIAM expression was observed in the bladder, lung, pancreas and spleen of homozygous m/m mice. By comparison, protein extracts from the brain (**Fig 3**) and testes (not shown) of the $NIAM^{m/m}$ mice showed decreased yet substantial remaining expression of NIAM as compared to wild-type mice. Interestingly, many bands for NIAM protein were detected in some tissues, such as brain, consistent with database predictions for the existence of numerous alternative transcripts of *NIAM*. Tissues were also examined for expression of p53, Mdm2 and p21. NIAM would be predicted to reduce their levels; however, we did not expect to detect significant changes in their expression since p53 signaling is generally kept off in normal tissues under non-stressed conditions. Indeed, basal expression of all three factors was low, and in some cases undetectable, in whole tissue lysates with no consistent differences observed between $NIAM^{m/m}$ and wild-type mice (data not shown). Immunohistochemical analyses of tissues to identify cell-specific changes in naïve versus stressed mice exposed to p53 activating stimuli (e.g., irradiation) should more effectively reveal effects of NIAM down-regulation on the p53 pathway *in vivo*. Overall, a significant decrease in NIAM expression was observed in $NIAM^{+/m}$ and $NIAM^{m/m}$ mice relative to wild-type controls, indicating these

animals are a useful model for examining the biological effects of reduced NIAM expression *in vivo*.

Loss of NIAM *in vivo* promotes spontaneous tumor formation

$NIAM^{m/m}$ mice grow to adulthood and normal size, are fertile, and are externally indistinguishable from wild-type mice. Moreover, full pathological examination of young *NIAM* mutant animals at approximately 8 weeks of age showed no apparent tissue abnormalities, suggesting that tissue development is unaffected by *NIAM* deficiency. However, NIAM carries out a variety of anti-cancer activities in cultured cells [10,12] and our database analyses (**Table 1** and **Fig. 1**) indicate its expression is down-regulated in many human cancers, suggesting it may normally prevent tumor development. Thus, we assessed aged mice of all three *NIAM* genotypes for spontaneous tumorigenesis. As shown in **Table 2**, 50% of $NIAM^{m/m}$ mice developed a neoplastic lesion whereas no wild-type and heterozygous mice of similar age showed obvious signs of tumorigenesis (p = 0.0025, Fisher's exact test). The $NIAM^{m/m}$ mice developed different types of benign tumors including a uterine hemangioma (**Fig. 4A**), an early lung papillary adenoma (**Fig. 4B**), and a Harderian gland adenoma (**Fig. 4C**). In addition, a focus of cellular alteration (FCA) was seen in the liver of one $NIAM^{m/m}$ mouse (**Fig. 4D**), a precancerous lesion seen in other mouse models [28]. These histopathological findings suggest that NIAM normally suppresses neoplasia.

Inflammation and early B-cell lymphoma develop in $NIAM^{m/m}$ mice

A prominent finding within the cohort was the pathological changes in the spleens of older *NIAM* mutant mice, which were significantly increased in size compared to wild-type and heterozygous mouse spleens (p <0.05) (**Fig. 5A**). Hematoxylin and Eosin (H&E) staining showed that NIAM deficiency led to a significant expansion of the splenic white pulp compared to control age matched cohorts (**Fig. 5B, C**). These white pulp changes in $NIAM^{m/m}$ mice were often due to reactive hyperplasia. This, along with perivascular lymphoid aggregates in various visceral organ, was consistent with systemic inflammation in mice [29]. In addition, one $NIAM^{m/m}$ mouse had severe diffuse eosinophilic crystalline pneumonia (ECP) whereas only one control had minor localized ECP disease (**Fig. 5D**). ECP may be seen in certain strains of mice including those with immunodeficiency and Th2 prone inflammatory environments [30,31]. Altogether, these data suggest that NIAM mutant mice have a

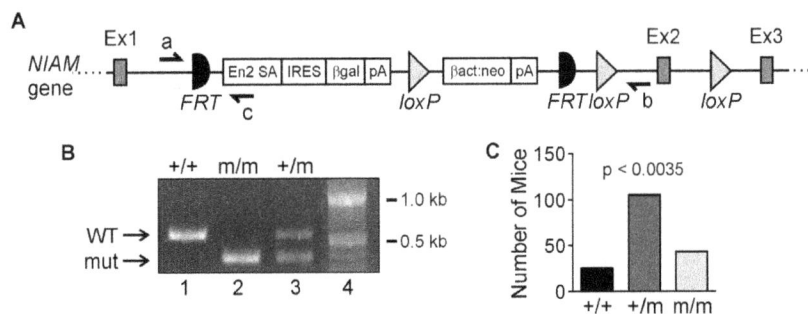

Figure 2. Generating and verifying *NIAM* gene disruption in mice. A. The targeted *NIAM* gene locus for the conditional-ready mouse knockout model. Cre-recombinase LoxP sites and Flippase targeted FRT sites are shown, as are locations for the PCR primers to detect the endogenous *NIAM* allele (a+b) or the mutant allele (a+c). Ex, exon. **B.** PCR amplification of the mutant (mut) allele results in a 380 bp product whereas the 548 bp product reflects the wild-type (WT) *NIAM* allele. DNA standards are shown in lane 4. **C.** Number of mice with each genotype (+/+, +/m, m/m) from heterozygous mouse crossings. Chi-square analysis shows a statistically significant difference from the Mendelian distribution of 1:2:1.

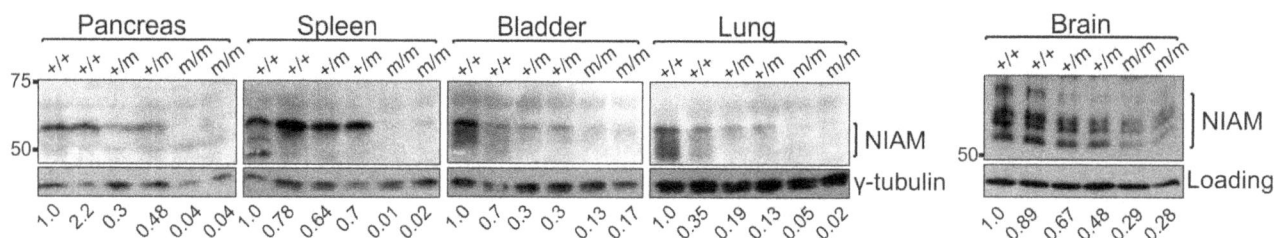

Figure 3. NIAM protein expression in tissues of *NIAM* mutant mice. NIAM protein levels were assessed in mouse tissues from two mice of each genotype (+/+, +/m, m/m). Equivalent amounts of protein lysates from spleen, bladder, lung, brain, and pancreas were analyzed by immunoblotting with antibodies to NIAM and γ-tubulin. The relative expression of NIAM in each sample, as compared to the first wild-type (+/+) sample in each tissue set, is denoted below the lanes. Relative NIAM levels were determined by Image J analysis of band intensities followed by normalization of those values to quantified intensities of the loading control (γ-tubulin or the non-specific band in brain lysates) in each sample.

proinflammatory phenotype. Additionally, two of the twelve (17%) $NIAM^{m/m}$ mice developed early B-cell lymphoma. Their spleens had multifocal loss of the white pulp architecture (e.g. small lymphocytes, germinal centers and tingible body macrophages) with replacement by highly mitotic centrocytic and centroblastic cells (**Fig. 5E**) [32]. When considered with the development of various benign neoplasms in other $NIAM^{m/m}$ animals, these results indicate that NIAM expression is required to prevent spontaneous tumorigenesis.

Marginal zone B cells are increased in $NIAM^{m/m}$ mice

Since aged $NIAM^{m/m}$ mice have enlarged spleens and some develop B-cell lymphoma, we evaluated B cell development in younger, tumor-free mice (6 months of age, 3 of each *NIAM* genotype) to identify potential pre-malignant changes that could give rise to B-cell tumors. Analysis of B cell development in the bone marrow of $NIAM^{m/m}$ mice revealed no alterations compared to wild-type control animals (**Fig. S1**). Specifically, there were no significant differences in the frequency of pro/pre (B220+IgM-, p = 0.4783), immature (B220+IgM+, p = 0.7693) or mature (B220^{hi}IgM+, p = 0.8048) B cells. Analysis of B cells from the spleen likewise showed no difference in the frequency of transitional (CD21^{lo}/CD23-) or follicular (CD21+/CD23+) B cells (**Fig. 6A, B**; p values of 0.5068 and 0.9325, respectively). In contrast, splenic marginal zone B cells (CD21^{hi}/CD23-) were significantly increased in frequency (p = 0.0281) and number (p = 0.0144) in $NIAM^{m/m}$ mice compared to wild-type controls (**Fig. 6**). These results uncover a specific sensitivity of splenic marginal zone B cells to NIAM loss, which may suggest that NIAM normally restricts their proliferation.

Selective expansion of splenic marginal zone B cells also occurs in mice with conditional inactivation of p53 in B cells and it is associated with their development of B-cell lymphomas [25,26]. Since NIAM is a positive regulator of p53 expression and

transcriptional activation [12], and some NIAM mice developed B-cell lymphoma, we wondered if the B cell phenotype in $NIAM^{m/m}$ mice could be associated with reduced p53 signaling. Therefore, we examined p53 status in LPS-stimulated splenic B cells isolated from five wild-type $NIAM^{+/+}$ and five mutant $NIAM^{m/m}$ mice. Western analyses showed complete NIAM loss in $NIAM^{m/m}$ cells compared to wild-type B cells (**Fig. 7**). We expected NIAM loss would reduce p53 levels and activity, but surprisingly it had no effect on basal expression of p53 or its targets, Mdm2 and p21, in the B cells of most $NIAM^{m/m}$ mice (4 of 5) relative to NIAM-positive B cells (**Fig. 7**, set A). These results were seen in B cells isolated from both 8 week and 6 month old mice, suggesting the marginal zone B cell expansion in 6 month old *NIAM* mutant mice is likely independent of p53. Notably, one *NIAM* mutant mouse had decreased B cell expression of p53 although this did not correlate with reduced expression of Mdm2 or p21, at least under these stress-free conditions (**Fig. 7**, set B). These analyses show that NIAM is not required for basal p53 activity in splenic B cells but may, depending on the context, predispose to p53 down-regulation. Additional studies examining p53 stimulation and checkpoint activation following DNA damage or other genotoxic insults in *NIAM*-deficient B cells are warranted.

Discussion

This study is the first investigation of NIAM function *in vivo* using newly generated *NIAM*-deficient mice. A tumor suppressor role for NIAM was anticipated given its ability to activate p53 and other currently undefined anti-cancer pathways involved in growth inhibition and genome maintenance [10,12]. Consistent with that prediction, reduced NIAM expression in mice yielded a tumor phenotype characterized by the development of both benign and cancerous lesions, including early B-cell lymphoma. No neoplasms developed in similarly aged heterozygote or wild-type controls, strongly suggesting that tumor formation was due to

Table 2. Neoplastic lesions in *NIAM*-deficient mice.

Genotype	Avg. Age at Necropsy (weeks)	# of mice with Neoplasms*	Types of neoplasms
$NIAM^{+/+}$	68.2	0/8	-
$NIAM^{+/m}$	68.5	0/8	-
$NIAM^{m/m}$	66	6/12	Early B-cell lymphoma (2) Uterine hemangioma (1) Preputial gland cyst (1) Harderian gland adenoma (1) Lung adenoma (1)

*, p<0.0025 by Fisher's Exact Test between control ($NIAM^{+/+}$ and $NIAM^{+/m}$) mice and $NIAM^{m/m}$ mice.

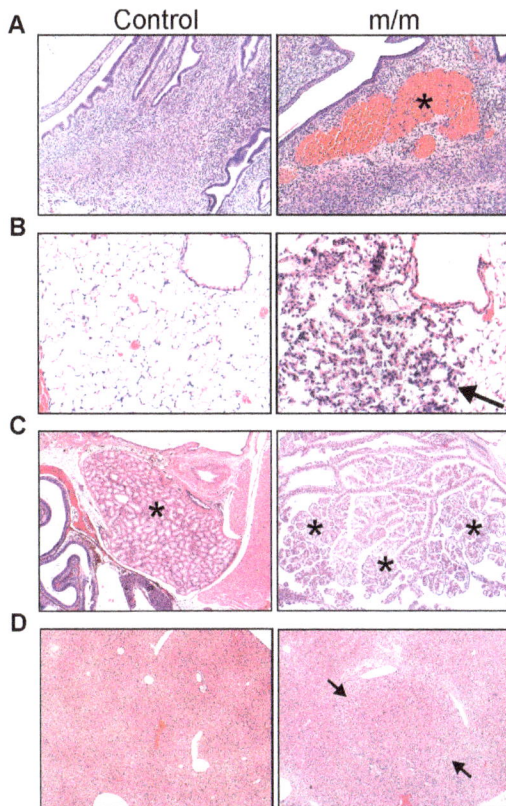

Figure 4. NIAM^{m/m} mice are predisposed to proliferative lesions. Histopathologic analyses of multiple mouse tissues. **A**. A hemangioma (asterisk, right panel) found in the uterus of a NIAM^{m/m} mouse compared to normal uterine tissue (left panel). (H&E, 100x) **B**. Pulmonary papillary adenoma in a homozygous NIAM^{m/m} mouse (arrow, right panel). A depiction of normal lung tissue from a control mouse is shown (left panel). (H&E, 20x) **C**. Harderian gland adenoma of a NIAM^{m/m} mouse (asterisks, right panel). A representative image of a normal Harderian gland (asterisk) from a control mouse is depicted (left panel). (H&E, 40x) **D**. A representative image of a normal liver from a control mouse (left panel) versus a focus of cellular alteration (arrows) in a NIAM^{m/m} mouse (right panel). (H&E, 40x) Controls represent tissues from similarly aged wild-type (panels B and C) and NIAM^{+/m} heterozygous (panels A and D) mice, which were found to be indistinguishable in our analyses.

NIAM loss. It is noteworthy that systemic inflammation was seen in multiple mice as that often precedes tumorigenesis. Although mice from each genotype (+/+, +/m, m/m) in our cohort showed signs of heightened inflammation, only the NIAM^{m/m} animals develop lesions. Thus, it is possible that reduced NIAM expression may accelerate or exacerbate the tumor promoting effects of a chronic inflammatory response.

The development of B-cell lymphoma in NIAM^{m/m} mice is consistent with several observations. First, microarray analyses suggest that NIAM mRNA levels are significantly reduced in human B-cell lymphomas [33–37]. Second, NIAM's functional partners, ARF, Mdm2, and p53 each play a critical role in that disease. ARF and p53 are commonly inactivated whereas Mdm2 is overexpressed in a majority of B-cell lymphomas in patients [38–40], and genetically engineered mice that mimic those alterations effectively model the disease [41–43]. Finally, NIAM is a growth inhibitor whose activation of p53 in cultured cells results in induction of p21 (CDKN1A/Waf1/Cip1) [10,12], a key transcriptional target of p53 [44,45]. Others previously showed that a

significant fraction (14%) of tumors that develop in p21 knockout mice are B-cell lymphomas [46], which is similar in incidence (17%) to the B-cell lymphomas arising in NIAM^{m/m} mice.

Our data show that NIAM contributes to tumor suppression but to a lesser extent than p53 or ARF. Half of NIAM^{m/m} mice developed benign and early cancerous lesions at an average age of 16.5 months (66 weeks). By comparison, mice lacking p53 in all tissues develop a range of malignancies (mainly T-cell lymphomas and sarcomas) with full penetrance at approximately 5 months of age [6,7]. Less pronounced in vivo effects are observed for disruption of p53 regulators and targets relative to loss of p53 itself [2]. For example, animals lacking ARF, a major positive regulator of p53, develop tumors at a slower rate (~10 months average age) than p53-null mice [47,48]. Among p53 targets, loss of PUMA causes no increased susceptibility to tumorigenesis [49] while deletion of p21 yields a moderate tumor phenotype [46]. Specifically, p21-null animals develop tumors at an average age of 16 months and with reduced incidence (27% in females, 55% in males) compared to mice lacking p53. Thus, a milder tumor phenotype for NIAM^{m/m} mice is not surprising since it represents just one of many p53 regulators [1,3].

We currently know very little about the normal physiological or pathological signals that control NIAM expression and where its function is required. The expression of β-galactosidase in these mutant mice will provide an excellent surrogate for tracking normal patterns of NIAM expression during development, in particular tissue and cell types, and in response to different stimuli. The interplay between NIAM, p53, and ARF, as well as NIAM's regulation of p21 expression, may be instructive. For instance, loss of each factor (p53, ARF, or p21) is associated with impaired stem cell maintenance and renewal for a variety of cellular lineages, including hematopoietic and neuronal cells, suggesting a possible contribution by NIAM to those processes and cell types [50–52]. Similarly, one of the most significant cellular stresses that stimulate p53 activity is DNA damage [1]. We recently found that treatment of MCF10A mammary epithelial cells causes NIAM protein upregulation (**Fig. S2**), implying a role for NIAM in the DNA damage response. The importance of NIAM to p53 activation and maintenance of DNA integrity in different tissues in response to DNA damage or other diverse stimuli may now be evaluated in an in vivo context.

A link between NIAM and p53 in B cell development and lymphoma was strongly suggested by findings that mice lacking those genes each display splenic marginal zone B cell expansion and B-cell lymphoma ([25,26] and this study). Yet NIAM loss had minimal effects on basal p53 expression and activity in B cells from young animals, with just one of five NIAM^{m/m} mice displaying lower p53 levels. That unexpected result suggests the splenic marginal zone B cell enrichment in young NIAM^{m/m} mice is independent of p53. However, it remains to be determined if p53 function in response to DNA damage or other cellular stresses is diminished in NIAM^{m/m} cells and contributes to tumor development in older animals. Indeed, it is conceivable that lower basal p53 expression in splenic B cells observed in some NIAM^{m/m} mice impairs stress-induced p53 signaling and checkpoint activation, ultimately fostering B-cell lymphomagenesis in aging mice. Future studies will assess that possibility.

Crosses between NIAM mutant mice with other genetic models of cancer will be instrumental in determining NIAM's contribution to p53 signaling as well as other cancer pathways. In that regard, in vivo studies should help resolve the biological relevance of NIAM's association with the ARF tumor suppressor [10–12]. Initial studies showed NIAM is capable of mobilizing ARF into the nucleoplasm [10], where ARF is known to more effectively bind

Mdm2 and activate p53 [15,16], yet NIAM and ARF can nonetheless act independent of each other to transiently activate p53 [10,12]. It is possible that NIAM's inhibition of Mdm2 and association with Tip60 may help sustain ARF-p53 signaling and promote senescence in cells following DNA damage or oncogene activation. If so, this would represent an important anti-cancer function since p53-mediated cellular senescence (induced by ARF or other mechanisms) is thought to play a pivotal role in tumor suppression [53–56].

Earlier work on NIAM and much of this Discussion has revolved around the idea that NIAM would prevent tumorigenesis, at least in part, through its effects on p53. However, it is likely that NIAM has significant anti-cancer functions *in vivo* that are independent of p53. One reason is that NIAM can inhibit proliferation and promote chromosomal stability independent of ARF, Mdm2, and p53, indicating it acts in other important pathways relevant to maintaining genomic stability [10]. Moreover, in this study basal p53 expression in splenic B cells was unchanged by NIAM loss in most animals. One factor besides p53 that could contribute to the tumor phenotype in $NIAM^{m/m}$ mice is transforming growth factor beta 1 (TGF-β1). NIAM was originally identified as a TGF-β1 responsive gene [13] and we previously found it is induced in TGF-β1-arrested cells [10]. TGF-β1 is a potent inhibitor of proliferation in many cell types (epithelial, endothelial, hematopoietic, etc), but alterations of its signaling components in neoplastic cells ultimately causes it to drive proliferation and cancer progression [57,58]. If NIAM is an effector of TGF-β signaling, its down-regulation in $NIAM^{m/m}$ mice may diminish the anti-proliferative activities of the pathway and consequently enhance its tumor-promoting effects.

Another factor of interest is the nuclear transcription factor, NF-kappa B. NF-κB was originally identified in B cells, contributes to marginal zone B cell formation, and is often constitutively activated in numerous inflammatory conditions and human cancers, including B cell lymphomas [59,60]. NF-κB is activated by a multitude of stimuli and cross-talks with many essential molecules (e.g., p53 and STAT3) and complex signaling pathways (including TGF-β) that control inflammation, cell survival and cell proliferation, among other key biological processes. The enrichment of marginal zone B cells as well as progressive expansion of splenic white pulp and development of B-cell lymphomas in NIAM mutant mice supports the prediction that NF-κB signaling may be hyper-activated when NIAM is down-regulated.

Overall, our data show that NIAM deficiency is associated with a proinflammatory phenotype and facilitates spontaneous tumorigenesis. Based on the literature, we speculate that the marginal

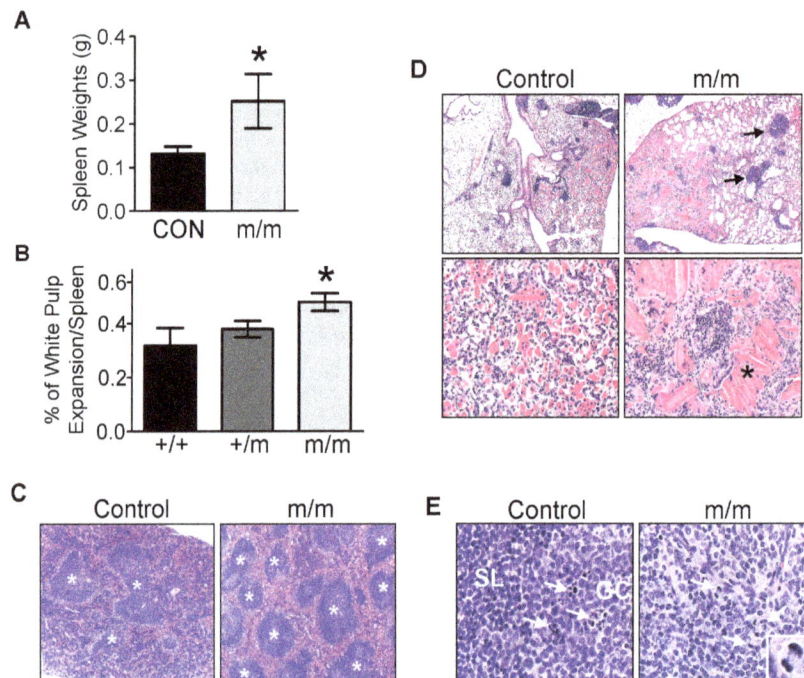

Figure 5. Loss of NIAM promotes reactive lymphoid hyperplasia and B-cell lymphoma in the spleen. A. Weights of spleens from +/+ and +/m mice (CON, n = 15) compared to $NIAM^{m/m}$ mice (m/m, n = 12). Note: one WT (+/+) mouse with an incidental case of severe chronic pyometra was excluded from the analysis. Statistical significance was shown by a Mann-Whitney test (*, p<0.05) **B**. The percentage of splenic white pulp per total splenic area was calculated for each genotype. $NIAM^{m/m}$ mice (n = 8) are statistically different from both wild-type (+/+, n = 5) and heterozygous (+/m, n = 6) mice as calculated by an unpaired two-tailed T-test. (*, p<0.05) Note: one WT (+/+) and one mutant (m/m) mouse were excluded from the analysis because extensive extramedullary hematopoiesis prevented accurate visualization of the white pulp **C**. Representative images of spleens from control wild-type (+/+) and homozygous m/m mice (H&E, 40x). Splenic white pulp (asterisks) was increased in $NIAM^{m/m}$ mice. Note: these samples show a range of variation in the extent of red pulp extramedullary hematopoiesis that was seen for both groups. **D**. Eosinophilic crystalline pneumonia in the lungs of control $NIAM^{+/m}$ heterozygous and $NIAM^{m/m}$ mice. Loss of NIAM resulted in more severe disease with extensive pulmonary lymphoid inflammation (arrows) and large extracellular crystals (asterisks) in the affected $NIAM^{m/m}$ mouse. (H&E, 40 × top and 100 × bottom panels) **E**. White pulp from control $NIAM^{+/m}$ heterozygous and $NIAM^{m/m}$ homozygous mice (H&E, 600x). A spleen from a heterozygous mouse with chronic ulcerative dermatitis and reactive hyperplasia of white pulp characterized by a germinal center (GC) and tingible body macrophages full of cellular debris (arrows) on a background of small lymphocytes (SL) (left panel). In two homozygous m/m mice, typical white pulp architecture was multifocally depleted and effaced by centroblasts and centrocytes with multiple mitotic figures (inset and arrows) (right panel). Note that $NIAM^{+/m}$ heterozygous and $NIAM^{+/+}$ wild-type mice appeared identical in our analyses and were therefore used interchangeably as controls.

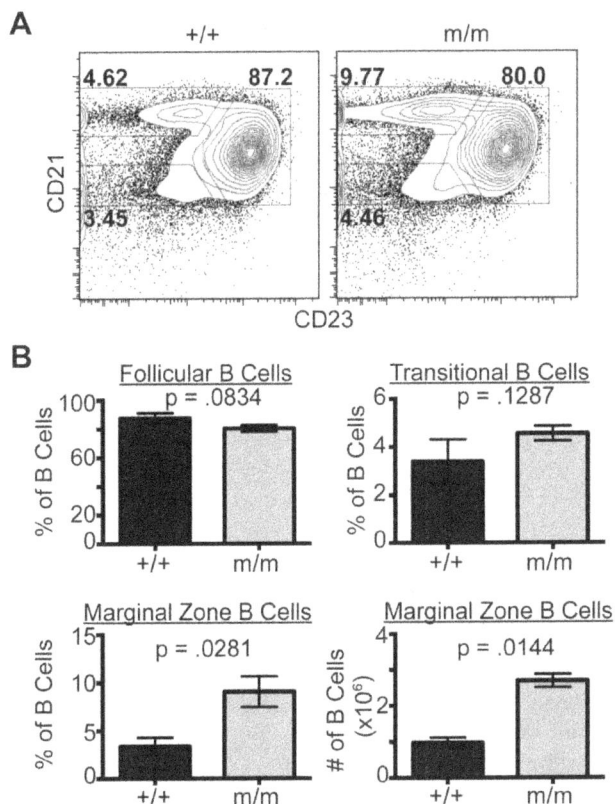

Figure 6. Marginal zone B cells are increased in NIAM^{m/m} mice. Flow cytometric analyses of splenic B cell development. Splenic B cells were isolated from young, 6 month old tumor-free wild-type (+/+) and NIAM mutant (m/m) mice (three of each genotype). **A.** Representative flow cytometry plots of NIAM wild-type versus m/m IgM positive splenocytes. Transitional (CD21^{lo}/CD23-), follicular (CD21+/CD23+) and marginal zone (CD21^{hi}/CD23-) B cells are identified. **B.** Average frequency of follicular (top left), transitional (top right), and marginal zone (bottom left) B cells from mice of the indicated genotypes. Average marginal zone B cell numbers are also shown (bottom right). All p values were calculated using unpaired, two-tailed Student's T tests.

zone B cell expansion in NIAM mutant mice is intimately related to their development of systemic inflammation [61] and B cell lymphomagenesis [25,26]. We also predict that NIAM, as a regulator of ARF-Mdm2-Tip60-p53 signaling and other undefined pathways affecting maintenance of chromosomal stability, normally cooperates with multiple anti-cancer pathways to suppress tumor development. The NIAM^{m/m} mice described here are an outstanding model to explore those concepts.

Materials and Methods

Animal Husbandry and Ethics Statement

Mice were housed in the University of Iowa Animal Care barrier facility. Mice were kept in rooms with a 12 hour light-dark cycle and free access to water and food. All mouse experiments were conducted according to protocols approved by the University of Iowa Institutional Animal Care and Use Committee (protocol#1204079). All efforts were made to minimize suffering. Mice were euthanized using carbon dioxide inhalation.

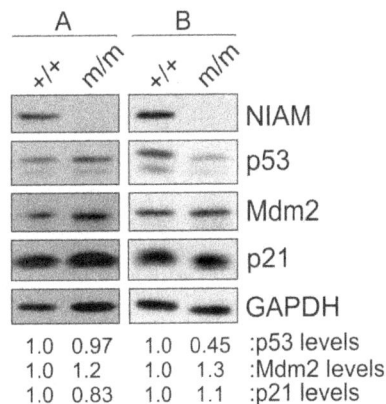

Figure 7. NIAM is not required for basal p53 activity in splenic B cells. Splenic B cells from young, tumor-free wild-type NIAM^{+/+} or NIAM^{m/m} homozygous mutant mice were isolated and expression of endogenous NIAM, p53, Mdm2 and p21 proteins was assessed by western blotting. Relative levels of p53, Mdm2 and p21 (normalized to GAPDH loading and compared to the untreated, wild-type control sample) were determined following quantification of bands using Image J. Representative results from 4 of 5 pairs of mice (both 8 week and 6 months of age) are shown in Set A, while Set B shows data for one pair of 6 month old mice. Set A and B samples were analyzed on separate gels, and lanes within each set were spliced together from the same autoradiogram for image clarity.

Generation of NIAM Mutant Mice

The Knockout Mouse Project (KOMP) generated male chimeras by injecting embryonic stem cells containing a NIAM (TBRG1) allele with a β-galactosidase cassette and LoxP sites around Exon2 into C57BL/6 blastocysts (www.komp.org, Project ID: CSD41510). Chimeric mice were then bred with C57BL/6N females to obtain germline transmission of the mutant TBRG1 allele. To confirm mouse genotypes, the REDExtract-N-Amp Tissue PCR Kit (Sigma Aldrich, XNAT-100RXN) was used to isolate DNA from mouse tails and to perform PCR. PCR genotyping primers were: Primer a: 5'- GGTCAAAGCTG-TAAGCATAGAGAGTC -3'; Primer b: 5'- CTTGAGG-CTCCTTTCTGGTG -3'; Primer c: 5'- CCAACTGACCT-TGGGCAAGAACAT -3'. PCR reactions consisted of 2 μL DNA added to 5 μl RedExtract PCR Master Mix (Sigma Aldrich), 0.8 μl of each primer and 0.6 μL PCR grade water to a total reaction volume of 10 μL. PCR was performed as follows: 95°C for 5 min, 35 cycles of 95°C for 1 min, annealing of primers at 54°C for 1 min, and extension at 72°C for 1.5 min on a PCR Sprint thermal cycler (Thermo Scientific Hybaid).

Database Analyses

The Cancer Genome Atlas Pan-Cancer analysis project's individual RNAseq datasets were downloaded from the UCSC Cancer Genome Browser (https://genome-cancer.ucsc.edu/). The UCSC Cancer Browser Team utilized level 3 TCGA RNAseq datasets (available at https://tcga-data.nci.nih.gov/tcga/), log2(x+1) transformed, and renormalized to the expression of all available TCGA cancer cohorts. PanCan normalized, log2(x+1) expression for available paired normal and primary tumor samples were compared for each TCGA cancer cohort utilizing an unpaired Welch's T-test.

Protein Analyses in Mouse Tissues

Mouse tissues were isolated, flash frozen in liquid nitrogen, and crushed into a powder by mortar and pestle. Tissues were lysed with RIPA buffer (50 mM Tris, pH 8.0, 150 mM NaCl, 1% Triton X-100, 0.1% SDS, 0.5% Sodium deoxycholate) supplemented with 1 mM NaF, protease inhibitor cocktail (Sigma, P8340), phosphatase inhibitor cocktail (Sigma, P0044), and 30 μM phenylmethylsulfonyl fluoride for 1 hour on ice. After brief sonication (2×5s pulses), protein lysates were centrifuged at 14,000 rpm for 15 min at 4°C. The concentration of protein for each tissue was assessed by BCA assay (Pierce, Rockford, IL). Equivalent amounts of total cellular protein was loaded and separated by SDS-PAGE, transferred to polyvinylidene difluoride (PVDF) membranes (Millipore), and analyzed by immunoblotting. Proteins were detected on membranes by ECL (Amersham Biosciences) with antibodies against NIAM (rabbit polyclonal antibody at 1.5 μg/ml [10] and mouse monoclonal antibody [clone 11E12] at 1:5 dilution [62]) and γ-tubulin (Sigma, T6557, mouse monoclonal antibody, 1:10,000).

Primary B Cell Analyses

Bone marrow and spleens were harvested from wild-type and NIAM mutant mice (three 6 month old littermate males per genotype) and minced between frosted glass slides to liberate cells. ACK lysis (Lonza, Radnor, PA) was used to lyse red blood cells. For flow cytometric analyses of B cells, one million lymphocytes were washed and resuspended in staining buffer that consisted of balanced salt solution, 5% bovine calf serum and 0.1% sodium azide. Non-specific binding of antibody was blocked using 10 μl rat serum (Jackson Immunoresearch, West Grove, PA) and 10 μg 2.4G2 (BioXCell, West Lebanon, NH). Cells were then incubated on wet ice in the dark with antibodies to B220-PE-Cy7 (6B2, eBioscience, San Diego, CA), CD23-PE (B3B4, eBioscience), CD21-APC (7G6, BD Biosciences, San Jose, CA), and IgM-FITC (RMM-1, Biolegend, San Diego, CA). Samples were run on a BD FACSCANTO II instrument (Becton Dickinson, San Jose, CA) and data were analyzed using FlowJo (Tree Star, Ashland, OR).

For analyses of p53, B cells were isolated from spleens of 6 month and 8 week old wild-type and NIAM mutant mice using B220 micro beads (Miltenyi Biotec, San Diego, CA) according to manufacturer's specifications. Cells were plated at 5×10^5 c/ml in B-cell media (RPMI, 10% fetal calf serum, 2 mM Glutamine, 1 mM Sodium Pyruvate, 0.055 mM β-mercaptoethanol and 100 units/ml of penicillin with 100 μg/ml streptomycin) supplemented with LPS (Sigma) at 20 μg/ml to maintain viability. After overnight incubation at 37°C, 5% CO_2, cells were harvested and lysed directly in 1× SDS-PAGE sample buffer. Samples (1×10^6 cell equivalents) were subjected to SDS-PAGE and protein expression examined by western blotting as described above using antibodies to p53 (Santa Cruz, Sc-6243 [FL-393] rabbit polyclonal, 1:200), Mdm2 (2A10 mouse monoclonal, 1:10), p21 (Calbiochem, PC55 [Ab-5], rabbit polyclonal, 2 μg/ml), and GAPDH (Abcam, Ab8245, mouse monoclonal, 1:20,000).

Mouse Necropsy and Histopathological Analyses

Individual organs were harvested from mice euthanized by CO_2 asphyxiation. A total of 28 mice (8 $NIAM^{+/+}$, 8 $NIAM^{+/m}$ and 12 $NIAM^{m/m}$) between the ages of 14 to 21 months were subjected to pathological examination. Organs assessed by macroscopic and histopathological analyses included pancreas, liver, spleen, gastrointestinal tract, reproductive tract for males and females, kidney, urinary bladder, lung, heart, head sections (e.g., eyes, nasal cavity, etc), and sagittal section of the brain (cerebellum, cerebrum and brain stem). Organ weights (e.g., spleen and liver) were collected and then tissues were formalin fixed and paraffin embedded. Tissue sections (~4 μm) were made from paraffin blocks and stained with hematoxylin and eosin (H&E). Mouse tissues were analyzed and reviewed for abnormal findings by a pathologist. Quantification of the white pulp of individual mouse spleens stained with H&E was measured by Image J software. The splenic white pulp was evaluated as a percentage of the total splenic area in tissue sections.

Supporting Information

Figure S1 Early B cell development is not altered in NIAM-deficient mice. Flow cytometric analysis of early B cell development. **A**. Representative flow cytometry plots of bone marrow lymphocytes from *NIAM* wild-type (+/+) or mutant (m/m) mice. Early (B220+/IgM-), immature (B220+/IgM+) and mature (B220high/IgM+) B cells are identified. **B**. Average frequency of immature (left), mature (middle) and early (right) B cells in *NIAM* +/+ versus m/m mice. No significant differences were observed. For these studies, bone marrow was isolated and analyzed from six mice total (the same analyzed in Figure 6), three of each genotype.
(TIF)

Figure S2 Sustained DNA damage induces NIAM expression. Western analyses show that endogenous NIAM protein is induced by DNA damage caused by exposure to doxorubicin (Dxn, 66 ng/mL) for the indicated times (hrs) in human MCF10A mammary epithelial cells. GAPDH levels serve as control for equivalent loading.
(TIF)

Acknowledgments

The authors thank Jennifer Stivers for technical assistance and personnel in the animal care facility for their mouse expertise and guidance. We also thank Drs. Adam Dupuy and Fred Quelle for helpful discussions.

Author Contributions

Conceived and designed the experiments: SMR TRR VST DKM DEQ. Performed the experiments: SMR JH VPM TRR NB SS JAG PN VST DKM DEQ. Analyzed the data: SMR DEQ WZ NB DKM JAG PN TRR VST SJ. Contributed reagents/materials/analysis tools: WZ SJ DKM DEQ. Wrote the paper: SMR TRR DKM DEQ.

References

1. Vousden KH, Prives C (2009) Blinded by the Light: The Growing Complexity of p53. Cell 137: 413–431.
2. Vogelstein B, Lane D, Levine AJ (2000) Surfing the p53 network. Nature 408: 307–310.
3. Levine AJ, Oren M (2009) The first 30 years of p53: growing ever more complex. Nature Reviews Cancer 9: 749–758.
4. Riley T, Sontag E, Chen P, Levine A (2008) Transcriptional control of human p53-regulated genes. Nat Rev Mol Cell Biol 9: 402–412.
5. Muller PAJ, Vousden KH (2013) p53 mutations in cancer. Nat Cell Biol 15: 2–8.
6. Donehower LA, Harvey M, Slagle BL, McArthur MJ, Montgomery CA Jr, et al. (1992) Mice deficient for p53 are developmentally normal but susceptible to spontaneous tumours. Nature 356: 215–221.

7. Jacks T, Remington L, Williams BO, Schmitt EM, Halachmi S, et al. (1994) Tumor spectrum analysis in p53-mutant mice. Current Biology 4: 1–7.
8. Garcia PB, Attardi LD (2014) Illuminating p53 function in cancer with genetically engineered mouse models. Seminars in Cell & Developmental Biology.
9. Lane DP (1992) p53, guardian of the genome. Nature 358: 15–16.
10. Tompkins VS, Hagen J, Frazier AA, Lushnikova T, Fitzgerald MP, et al. (2007) A Novel Nuclear Interactor of ARF and MDM2 (NIAM) That Maintains Chromosomal Stability. Journal of Biological Chemistry 282: 1322–1333.
11. Tompkins V, Hagen J, Zediak VP, Quelle DE (2006) Identification of novel ARF binding proteins by two-hybrid screening. Cell Cycle 5: 641–646.

12. Reed SM, Hagen J, Tompkins V, Thies K, Quelle FW, et al. (2014) Nuclear Interactor of ARF and Mdm2 regulates multiple pathways to activate p53. Cell Cycle 13: 1288–1298.

13. Babalola GO, Schultz RM (1995) modulation of gene-expression in the preimplantation mouse embryo by TGF-alpha and TGF-beta. Molecular Reproduction and Development 41: 133–139.

14. Sherr CJ (2006) Divorcing ARF and p53: an unsettled case. Nature Reviews Cancer 6: 663–673.

15. Llanos S, Clark PA, Rowe J, Peters G (2001) Stabilisation of p53 by p14ARF without relocalization of Mdm2 to the nucleolus. Nature Cell Biology 3: 445–452.

16. Korgaonkar C, Hagen J, Tompkins V, Frazier AA, Allamargot C, et al. (2005) Nucleophosmin (B23) Targets ARF to Nucleoli and Inhibits Its Function. Molecular and Cellular Biology 25: 1258–1271.

17. Momand J, Wu HH, Dasgupta G (2000) MDM2 - master regulator of the p53 tumor suppressor protein. Gene 242: 15–29.

18. Legube G, Linares LK, Tyteca S, Caron C, Scheffner M, et al. (2004) Role of the Histone Acetyl Transferase Tip60 in the p53 Pathway. Journal of Biological Chemistry 279: 44825–44833.

19. Sykes SM, Mellert HS, Holbert MA, Li K, Marmorstein R, et al. (2006) Acetylation of the p53 DNA-Binding Domain Regulates Apoptosis Induction. Molecular Cell 24: 841–851.

20. Tang Y, Luo J, Zhang W, Gu W (2006) Tip60-dependent acetylation of p53 modulates the decision between cell-cycle arrest and apoptosis. Molecular Cell 24: 827–839.

21. Sapountzi V, Logan IR, Robson CN (2006) Cellular functions of TIP60. International Journal of Biochemistry & Cell Biology 38: 1496–1509.

22. Senturk E, Manfredi JJ (2012) Mdm2 and Tumorigenesis: Evolving Theories and Unsolved Mysteries. Genes & Cancer 3: 192–198.

23. Rhodes DR, Yu JJ, Shanker K, Deshpande N, Varambally R, et al. (2004) ONCOMINE: A cancer microarray database and integrated data-mining platform. Neoplasia 6: 1–6.

24. Rhodes DR, Kalyana-Sundaram S, Mahavisno V, Varambally R, Yu J, et al. (2007) Oncomine 3.0: Genes, pathways, and networks in a collection of 18,000 cancer gene expression profiles. Neoplasia 9: 166–180.

25. Gostissa M, Bianco JM, Malkin DJ, Kutok JL, Rodig SJ, et al. (2013) Conditional inactivation of p53 in mature B cells promotes generation of nongerminal center-derived B-cell lymphomas. Proceedings of the National Academy of Sciences of the United States of America 110: 2934–2939.

26. Chiang YJ, Difilippantonio MJ, Tessarollo L, Morse HC, Hodes RJ (2012) Exon 1 Disruption Alters Tissue-Specific Expression of Mouse p53 and Results in Selective Development of B Cell Lymphomas. Plos One 7: e49305.

27. Lowe SW, Sherr CJ (2003) Tumor suppression by Ink4a-Arf: progress and puzzles. Current Opinion in Genetics & Development 13: 77–83.

28. Carter JH, Carter HW, Deddens JA, Hurst BM, George MH, et al. (2003) A 2-year dose-response study of lesion sequences during hepatocellular carcinogen-esis in the male B6C3F(1) mouse given the drinking water chemical dichloroacetic acid. Environmental Health Perspectives 111: 53–64.

29. Percy DH, Barthold SW (2007) Pathology of laboratory rodents and rabbits 2nd Edition: 90.

30. Liu Q, Cheng LI, Yi L, Zhu N, Wood A, et al. (2009) p47(phox) Deficiency Induces Macrophage Dysfunction Resulting in Progressive Crystalline Macro-phage Pneumonia. American Journal of Pathology 174: 153–163.

31. Hoenerhoff MJ, Starost MF, Ward JM (2006) Eosinophilic crystalline pneumonia as a major cause of death in 129S4/SvJae mice. Veterinary Pathology 43: 682–688.

32. Ward JM, Rehg JE, Morse HC III (2012) Differentiation of Rodent Immune and Hematopoietic System Reactive Lesions from Neoplasias. Toxicologic Pathology 40: 425–434.

33. Alizadeh AA, Eisen MB, Davis RE, Ma C, Lossos IS, et al. (2000) Distinct types of diffuse large B-cell lymphoma identified by gene expression profiling. Nature 403: 503–511.

34. Rosenwald A, Wright G, Chan WC, Connors JM, Campo E, et al. (2002) The use of molecular profiling to predict survival after chemotherapy for diffuse large-B-cell lymphoma. New England Journal of Medicine 346: 1937–1947.

35. Brune V, Tiacci E, Pfeil I, Doering C, Eckerle S, et al. (2008) Origin and pathogenesis of nodular lymphocyte-predominant Hodgkin lymphoma as revealed by global gene expression analysis. Journal of Experimental Medicine 205: 2251–2268.

36. Eckerle S, Brune V, Doering C, Tiacci E, Bohle V, et al. (2009) Gene expression profiling of isolated tumour cells from anaplastic large cell lymphomas: insights into its cellular origin, pathogenesis and relation to Hodgkin lymphoma. Leukemia 23: 2129–2138.

37. Storz MN, van de Rijn M, Kim YH, Mraz-Gernhard S, Hoppe RT, et al. (2003) Gene expression profiles of cutaneous B cell lymphoma. Journal of Investigative Dermatology 120: 865–870.

38. Ghobrial IM, McCormick DJ, Kaufmann SH, Leontovich AA, Loegering DA, et al. (2005) Proteomic analysis of mantle-cell lyrnphoma by protein microarray. Blood 105: 3722–3730.

39. Watanabe T, Ichikawa A, Saito H, Hotta T (1996) Overexpression of the MDM2 oncogene in leukemia and lymphoma. Leukemia & Lymphoma 21: 391–397.

40. Wilda M, Bruch J, Harder L, Rawer D, Reiter A, et al. (2004) Inactivation of the ARF-MDM-2-p53 pathway in sporadic Burkitt's lymphoma in children. Leukemia 18: 584–588.

41. Eischen CM, Weber JD, Roussel MF, Sherr CJ, Cleveland JL (1999) Disruption of the ARF-Mdm2-p53 tumor suppressor pathway in Myc- induced lympho-magenesis. Genes & Development 13: 2658–2669.

42. Alt JR, Greiner TC, Cleveland JL, Eischen CM (2003) Mdm2 haplo-insufficiency profoundly inhibits Myc-induced lymphomagenesis. EMBO Journal 22: 1442–1450.

43. Wang P, Greiner TC, Lushnikova T, Eischen CM (2006) Decreased Mdm2 expression inhibits tumor development induced by loss of ARF. Oncogene 25: 3708–3718.

44. el-Deiry WS, Tokino T, Velculescu VE, Levy DB, Parsons R, et al. (1993) WAF1, a potential mediator of p53 tumor suppression. Cell 75: 817–825.

45. el-Deiry WS, Harper JW, O'Connor PM, Velculescu VE, Canman CE, et al. (1994) WAF1/CIP1 is induced in p53-mediated G1 arrest and apoptosis. Cancer Research 54: 1169–1174.

46. Martin-Caballero J, Flores JM, Garcia-Palencia P, Serrano M (2001) Tumor Susceptibility of p21Waf1/Cip1-deficient Mice. Cancer Research 61: 6234–6238.

47. Kamijo T, Zindy F, Roussel MF, Quelle DE, Downing JR, et al. (1997) Tumor suppression at the mouse INK4a locus mediated by the alternative reading frame product p19(ARF). Cell 91: 649–659.

48. Kamijo T, Bodner S, van de Kamp E, Randle DH, Sherr CJ (1999) Tumor spectrum in ARF-deficient mice. Cancer Research 59: 2217–2222.

49. Jeffers JR, Parganas E, Lee Y, Yang CY, Wang JL, et al. (2003) Puma is an essential mediator of p53-dependent and -independent apoptotic pathways. Cancer Cell 4: 321–328.

50. Kippin TE, Martens DJ, van der Kooy D (2005) P21 loss compromises the relative quiescence of forebrain stem cell proliferation leading to exhaustion of their proliferation capacity. Genes & Development 19: 756–767.

51. Cheng T, Rodrigues N, Shen HM, Yang YG, Dombkowski D, et al. (2000) Hematopoietic stem cell quiescence maintained by p21(cip1/waf1). Science 287: 1804–1808.

52. Yu H, Yuan YZ, Shen HM, Cheng T (2006) Hematopoietic stem cell exhaustion impacted by p18(INK4C) and p21(Cip1/Waf1) in opposite manners. Blood 107: 1200–1206.

53. Jiang D, Attardi LD (2013) Engaging the p53 metabolic brake drives senescence. Cell Res 23: 739–740.

54. Christophorou MA, Ringshausen I, Finch AJ, Swigart LB, Evan GI (2006) The pathological response to DNA damage does not contribute to p53-mediated tumour suppression. Nature 443: 214–217.

55. Ventura A, Kirsch DG, McLaughlin ME, Tuveson DA, Grimm J, et al. (2007) Restoration of p53 function leads to tumour regression in vivo. Nature 445: 661–665.

56. Xue W, Zender L, Miething C, Dickins RA, Hernando E, et al. (2007) Senescence and tumour clearance is triggered by p53 restoration in murine liver carcinomas. Nature 445: 656–660.

57. Massague J, Blain SW, Lo RS (2000) TGF beta signaling in growth control, cancer, and heritable disorders. Cell 103: 295–309.

58. Derynck R, Akhurst RJ, Balmain A (2001) TGF-beta signaling in tumor suppression and cancer progression. Nature Genetics 29: 117–129.

59. Hoesel B, Schmid JA (2013) The complexity of NF-kappa B signaling in inflammation and cancer. Molecular Cancer 12: 86.

60. Gerondakis S, Siebenlist U (2010) Roles of the NF-kappa B Pathway in Lymphocyte Development and Function. Cold Spring Harbor Perspectives in Biology 2: a000182.

61. Cerutti A, Cols M, Puga I (2013) Marginal zone B cells: virtues of innate-like antibody-producing lymphocytes. Nature Reviews Immunology 13: 118–132.

62. Hagen J, Tompkins V, Dudakovic A, Weydert JA, Quelle DE (2008) Generation and characterization of monoclonal antibodies to NIAM: A nuclear interactor of ARF and Mdm2. Hybridoma 27: 159–166.

63. Bredel M, Bredel C, Juric D, Harsh GR, Vogel H, et al. (2005) Functional network analysis reveals extended gliomagenesis pathway maps and three novel MYC-interacting genes in human gliomas. Cancer Research 65: 8679–8689.

64. Sun LX, Hui AM, Su Q, Vortmeyer A, Kotliarov Y, et al. (2006) Neuronal and glioma-derived stem cell factor induces angiogenesis within the brain. Cancer Cell 9: 287–300.

65. Liang Y, Diehn M, Watson N, Bollen AW, Aldape KD, et al. (2005) Gene expression profiling reveals molecularly and clinically distinct subtypes of glioblastoma multiforme. Proceedings of the National Academy of Sciences of the United States of America 102: 5814–5819.

66. French PJ, Swagemakers SMA, Nagel JHA, Kouwenhoven MCM, Brouwer E, et al. (2005) Gene expression profiles associated with treatment response in oligodendrogliomas. Cancer Research 65: 11335–11344.

67. Murat A, Migliavacca E, Gorlia T, Lambiv WL, Shay T, et al. (2008) Stem cell-related "Self-Renewal" signature and high epidermal growth factor receptor expression associated with resistance to concomitant chemoradiotherapy in glioblastoma. Journal of Clinical Oncology 26: 3015–3024.

68. Hou J, Aerts J, den Hamer B, van Ijcken W, den Bakker M, et al. (2010) Gene Expression-Based Classification of Non-Small Cell Lung Carcinomas and Survival Prediction. Plos One 5: e10312.

69. Zhao HJ, Langerod A, Ji Y, Nowels KW, Nesland JM, et al. (2004) Different gene expression patterns in invasive lobular and ductal carcinomas of the breast. Molecular Biology of the Cell 15: 2523–2536.

70. Blum JL, Kohles J, McKenna E, Scotto N, Hu S, et al. (2011) Association of age and overall survival in capecitabine-treated patients with metastatic breast cancer in clinical trials. Breast Cancer Research and Treatment 125: 431–439.

71. Richardson AL, Wang ZGC, De Nicolo A, Lu X, Brown M, et al. (2006) X chromosomal abnormalities in basal-like human breast cancer. Cancer Cell 9: 121–132.

72. Tomlins SA, Mehra R, Rhodes DR, Cao X, Wang L, et al. (2007) Integrative molecular concept modeling of prostate cancer progression. Nature Genetics 39: 41–51.

10

Erythrocytic Mobilization Enhanced by the Granulocyte Colony-Stimulating Factor Is Associated with Reduced Anthrax-Lethal-Toxin-Induced Mortality in Mice

Hsin-Hou Chang[1,2], Ya-Wen Chiang[1], Ting-Kai Lin[1], Guan-Ling Lin[2], You-Yen Lin[2], Jyh-Hwa Kau[3], Hsin-Hsien Huang[4], Hui-Ling Hsu[4], Jen-Hung Wang[5], Der-Shan Sun[1,2]*

1 Department of Molecular Biology and Human Genetics, Tzu-Chi University, Hualien, Taiwan, **2** Institute of Medical Sciences, Tzu-Chi University, Hualien, Taiwan, **3** Department of Microbiology and Immunology, National Defense Medical Center, Taipei, Taiwan, **4** Institute of Preventive Medicine, National Defense Medical Center, Taipei, Taiwan, **5** Department of Medical Research, Tzu Chi General Hospital, Hualien, Taiwan

Abstract

Anthrax lethal toxin (LT), one of the primary virulence factors of *Bacillus anthracis*, causes anthrax-like symptoms and death in animals. Experiments have indicated that levels of erythrocytopenia and hypoxic stress are associated with disease severity after administering LT. In this study, the granulocyte colony-stimulating factor (G-CSF) was used as a therapeutic agent to ameliorate anthrax-LT- and spore-induced mortality in C57BL/6J mice. We demonstrated that G-CSF promoted the mobilization of mature erythrocytes to peripheral blood, resulting in a significantly faster recovery from erythrocytopenia. In addition, combined treatment using G-CSF and erythropoietin tended to ameliorate *B. anthracis*-spore-elicited mortality in mice. Although specific treatments against LT-mediated pathogenesis remain elusive, these results may be useful in developing feasible strategies to treat anthrax.

Editor: Nupur Gangopadhyay, University of Pittsburgh, United States of America

Funding: This work was supported by grants of National Science Council http://web1.nsc.gov.tw/mp.aspx (NSC 96-2311-B-320-005-MY3 and NSC 99-2311-B-320-003-MY3) and Tzu-Chi University http://www.tcu.edu.tw/ (610400130). The funders had no role in study design, data collection and analysis, decision to publish, or preparation of the manuscript.

Competing Interests: The authors have declared that no competing interests exist.

* Email: dssun@mail.tcu.edu.tw

Introduction

Infection with *Bacillus anthracis*, a gram-positive spore-forming bacterium, can lead to life-threatening anthrax [1]. Anthrax lethal toxin (LT) is comprised of a protective antigen (PA, 83 kDa) and lethal factor (LF, 90 kDa) [2–4], and is one of the primary virulence factors of *B. anthracis*. LF is a specific metalloprotease for mitogen-activated protein kinase (MAPK) kinases (MKKs/MEKs) [5], and can thus disrupt MAPK signaling cascades including p38 MAPK, p42/44 extracellular signal-regulated kinase (ERK), and c-Jun N-terminal kinase (JNK) [6,7]. All of these 3 MAPK pathways are critical in maintaining fundamental cellular homeostasis, including cell proliferation, differentiation, and apoptosis [8]. LF can be delivered into cells by PA, a cell-receptor binding component [3,9]. Although experimental LT treatments may not reproduce the full pathogenesis of anthrax, LT studies in cell or animal models have revealed certain pathogenic progressions. Various cell types, which include macrophages [10,11], dendritic cells [12], lymphocytes [13,14], erythrocytes [15], and megakaryocytes [16], cardiomyocytes [17], and smooth muscle [17], are sensitive to LT treatment. LT has been shown to suppress the differentiation and maturation of the progenitors of macrophages, megakaryocytes, and erythrocytes [15,16,18]. In addition, blood cell count analyses have indicated that LT treatment significantly reduced levels of circulating red blood cells (RBCs) and platelets in mice [15,16], suggesting multiple targets of

LT in hematopoietic lineage cells. Deficiencies of platelets and RBCs may lead to hemorrhage and lethal hypoxic damage [19,20]. Because high levels of LT accumulate in the body when anthrax enters the bacteremia stage, death is typically inevitable even after aggressive antibiotic treatments. This suggests that a specific treatment to overcome the toxic effect is crucial in controlling the disease [21]. Unfortunately, an effective therapeutic approach against LT remains elusive.

Cytokine treatments, particularly hematopoietic growth factors, have been used in various clinical settings to rescue pathological defects [22]. Our previous demonstration was the first to indicate that thrombopoietin (TPO), a megakaryopoiesis-enhancing cytokine [23], can ameliorate LT-induced thrombopoiesis suppression, thrombocytopenia, and likely reduce the mortality in mice [16]. Our data also revealed that erythropoietin (EPO), a potent erythropoiesis-stimulating cytokine [24], ameliorated LT-induced erythropoiesis suppression (particularly those precursors in early erythropoiesis stages), erythrocytopenia, and reduced mortality rates from 100% to 50% after lethal-dose LT challenges in experimental mice [15]. Bone marrow is the primary stem niche supporting erythropoiesis, displaying technically-divided 4-differentiation stages of erythroblasts based on the expression levels of surface markers CD71 and TER-119 [25]. The transferrin receptor (CD71) is first expressed on early erythroblasts, such as erythroid burst-forming units (BFU-Es) and erythroid colony-forming units (CFU-Es) cells. Erythrocytic CD71 is downregulated by more mature erythroblasts [26]. By contrast, TER-119 is primarily expressed on relatively mature erythroblasts, reticulocytes, and mature erythrocytes [27]. Accordingly, 4 cell populations (CD71^{high}TER-119^{med}, CD71^{high}TER-119^{high}, CD71^{med}-TER-119^{high}, and CD71^{low}TER-119^{high}) can be defined, which are morphologically equivalent to proerythroblasts (flow cytometry-gated region 1; R1), basophilic erythroblasts (R2), late basophilic and polychromatophilic erythroblasts (R3), and orthochromatophilic erythroblasts (R4), from the early to late stages of erythroid differentiation, respectively [25]. Following these approaches, we are thus able to characterize the mechanism to use hematopoietic cytokines/growth factors as ameliorative agents to rescue anthrax LT-induced mortality [15,16].

The granulocyte colony-stimulating factor (G-CSF) has been found to regulate granulopoiesis [28], and is a multifunctional cytokine. For example, it has been found to stimulate cell proliferation, differentiation, enhance hematopoiesis, mobilize hematopoietic stem cells, and induce anti-apoptotic and anti-inflammatory effects [29–31]. Both G-CSF and EPO are U.S. FDA-approved drugs. Although the mechanism remains unclear, combined treatments using G-CSF and EPO were shown to ameliorate aplastic anemia in patients with myelodysplastic syndrome [32–36]. Given that EPO treatments are beneficial for LT-challenged mice [15], we hypothesized that combining G-CSF and EPO may be useful in treating anthrax. Consequently, we used mouse models to discuss the combined treatments of G-CSF and EPO on reduced anthrax LT and spore-induced mortality. In addition, we also discussed the differential erythropoietic regulation in response to G-CSF and EPO treatments.

Materials and Methods

Ethics Statement

Our research approaches involving experimental mice were approved by the Institutional Animal Care and Use Committee of Tzu Chi University (Approval ID: 98104) and the National Defense Medical Center (Approval ID: AN-100-04).

Toxins and spores

B. anthracis-derived LT was purified according to previously described procedures [49]. LT was delivered in a 1:5 ratio of LF and PA [16]. Spores derived from the *B. anthracis*-nonencapsulated mutant strain (pXO1$^+$, pXO2$^-$) were purchased from the American Type Culture Collection (Manassas, VA, USA) (ATCC 14186).

Erythroid colony-forming cell assay

The erythroid colony-forming cell assay was conducted according to the manufacturer's instructions (MethoCult M3334, StemCell Technologies). For the *in vitro* erythroid colony-forming cell assay, bone marrow cells were collected from the femurs and tibiae of C57BL/6J mice. C57BL/6J mice (males, 8–10 wk of age) were obtained from the National Laboratory Animal Center (Taipei, Taiwan) and kept in a specific pathogen-free (SPF) environment in the experimental animal center of Tzu Chi University. For the *ex vivo* erythroid colony-forming cell assay, C57BL/6J mice were retro-orbitally injected with 55 μg/kg/d of recombinant human G-CSF (Filgrastim, Kirin, Tokyo, Japan) in 250 μl saline, once daily for 5 d, initiated 5 d before the challenges of a lethal dose of LT (1.5 mg/kg in 250 μl saline, retro-orbitally injected). Treatments using saline, G-CSF, and LT alone were used as comparison controls. Bone marrow cells were collected at 69 h after LT treatment and flushed with Roswell Park Memorial Institute medium (RPMI)-1640 containing 20% anticoagulant acid

citrate dextrose formula A (ACD-A: 38 mM citric acid, 75 mM trisodium citrate, 139 mM D-glucose, 12.5 mM EDTA [15]). After depleting RBCs by adding a hypotonic buffer (153 mM NH$_4$Cl and 17 mM Tris-HCl) at room temperature for 10 min, 100 μl of remaining cells (9×10^5/ml) were resuspended in Iscove's Modified Dulbecco's Medium (IMDM) (StemCell Technologies) and mixed with 1 ml of semisolid methylcellulose-based medium containing 3 units of EPO. Finally, each 1.1 ml of methylcellulose-cell suspension was mixed with or without a dose of G-CSF (20 ng/ml or 764 ng/ml) and duplicate seeded in 35-mm dishes. A G-CSF dose of 20 ng/ml was used in the colony-forming cell assay for hematopoietic cells [50]. Because the volume of mice blood is 70–80 ml/kg [51], a dose of 764 ng/ml approximated the dose used to ameliorate LT-induced mortality in the experiments. Two doses of G-CSF (20 ng/ml and 764 ng/ml) were added to the medium supplement of the erythroid colony-forming cell assay. The cultures were incubated at 37°C for 14 d. Dynamic changes in colony number were measured on Days 3, 7, and 14 after initiating the colony assay. The erythroid colonies were separated into 3 groups by size: small (8–50 cells), medium (more than 50, but less than 200 cells), and large (more than 200 cells).

Analysis of erythropoiesis in bone marrow

Bone marrow cells were purified and blocked with 5% bovine serum albumin in RPMI medium at 37°C for 1 h and incubated in 500 μl RPMI-1640 medium with 1 μl of fluorescein (FITC)-conjugated rat anti-mouse CD71 antibody (BioLegend) and 3 μl of R-Phycoerythrin (R-PE)-conjugated rat anti-mouse TER-119 antibody (BD Immunocytometry System) at 37°C for 1 h. After washing with phosphate-buffered saline (PBS), the cells were measured and analyzed using a FACSCalibur flow cytometer and the CellQuest^{TM} Pro program (Becton-Dickinson).

Flow cytometry analysis of peripheral blood cells of G-CSF-treated EGFP mice

EGFP mice [C57BL/6J-Tg (Pgk1-EGFP) 03Narl, males, 10–12 wk of age] were obtained from the National Laboratory Animal Center (Taipei, Taiwan) and maintained in the aforementioned SPF environments. EGFP mice were retro-orbitally injected with G-CSF (55 μg/kg/d in 250 μl saline) once daily for 4 d. To detect the erythrocytes' specific surface markers, 50 μl of retro-orbital blood samples were obtained 22, 44, 66, and 94 h after the initial G-CSF injection, and subsequently mixed with 450 μl of anticoagulant ACD-A (1:9). Cells were incubated in 300 μl of RPMI-1640 medium with 3 μl of the R-Phycoerythrin (R-PE)-conjugated rat anti-mouse TER-119 antibody (BD Immunocytometry System) at 37°C for 1 h. After washing with PBS, the cells were analyzed using a FACSCalibur flow cytometer and the CellQuest^{TM} Pro program.

G-CSF treatment to reduce LT-induced mortality

C57BL/6J mice (males, 8–10 wk of age) were retro-orbitally injected with 55 μg/kg/d of recombinant human G-CSF in 250 μl saline, once daily for 5 d, initiated 5 d before or 1 d after the challenges of a lethal dose of LT (1.5 mg/kg in 250 μl saline, retro-orbitally injected). Treatments using saline, G-CSF, and LT alone were used as comparison controls. Because no suitable potential predictor of death/survival exists for LT-challenged mice, we used death as an endpoint for the survival experiment. The survival time and mortality of mice were recorded after the LT challenges. LT treatment in mice did not induce obvious discomfort and body weight loss, except for reducing activities. The experimental mice were continually monitored up to 250 h

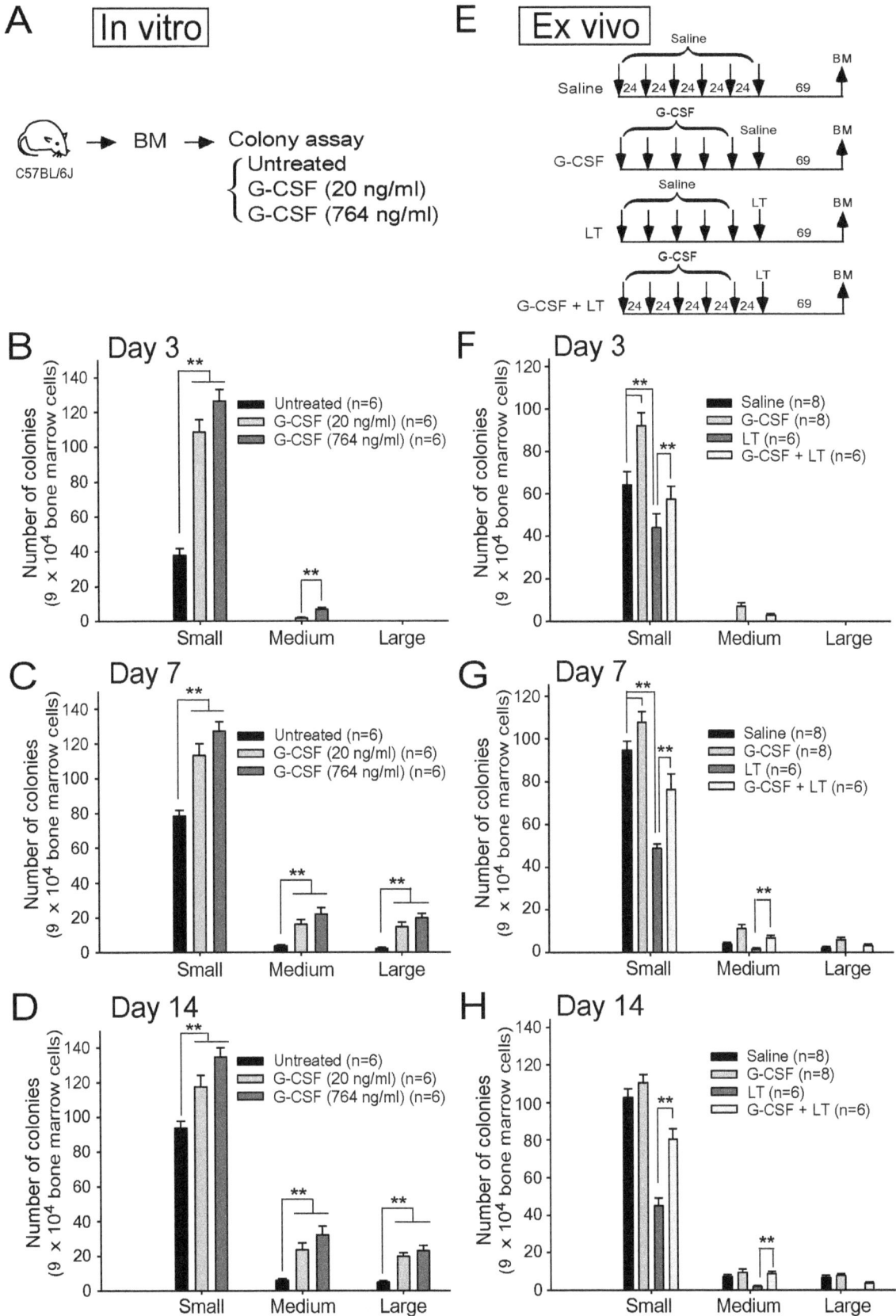

Figure 1. Erythroid colony-forming cell assays to measure the effect of G-CSF on erythropoiesis. The experimental outlines of *in vitro* (A) and *ex vivo* (E) analyses are shown. An *in vitro* assay was performed using murine bone marrow (BM) cells that were incubated with [20 ng/ml (n = 6) or 764 ng/ml (n = 6)], or without G-CSF (n = 6). The colonies were quantified on Days 3 (B), 7 (C), and 14 (D). Untreated bone marrow cells were used

as a control. Colony numbers of bone marrow cells from mice, which were treated with G-CSF (n=8), LT (n=6), or G-CSF and LT (n=6), were measured on Days 3 (F), 7 (G), and 14 (H) following the *ex vivo* colony assay. Bone marrow cells from saline treated mice (n=8) served as controls. **P<0.01 was compared between the indicated groups. Data are shown as mean ± standard deviation (SD) and represent results from 2 independent experiments. The mouse drawing used in this and all following figures was originally published in *Blood*. Huang, H. S., Sun, D. S., Lien, T. S. and Chang, H. H. Dendritic cells modulate platelet activity in IVIg-mediated amelioration of ITP in mice. *Blood*. 2010; 116: 5002–5009. © the American Society of Hematology.

for every 4–6 h. All surviving mice were monitored each day for 2 subsequent mo. For hematopoietic parameters, 50 µl of retro-orbital blood samples were collected at 22, 44, and 66 h after LT challenges and analyzed by an automated hematology analyzer (KX-21, Sysmex Corporation).

Combined treatments with G-CSF and EPO to reduce anthrax-spore-induced mortality

C57BL/6J mice were retro-orbitally injected with G-CSF (55 µg/kg/d in 250 µl saline) daily for 5 consecutive d or injected with a combination of recombinant human EPO (rhEPO, Neorecormon, Roche, Mannheim, Germany) (2 IU/g, in 250 µl saline) twice at 24 and 48 h after injecting spores (1×10^7 in 1 ml saline, intraperitoneal injection). The survival times and mortality of mice were recorded. Because no suitable potential predictor of death/survival exists for spore-challenged mice, we used death as an endpoint for the survival experiment. Spore treatment in mice did not induce obvious discomfort and body weight loss, except for reducing activities. The experimental mice were continually

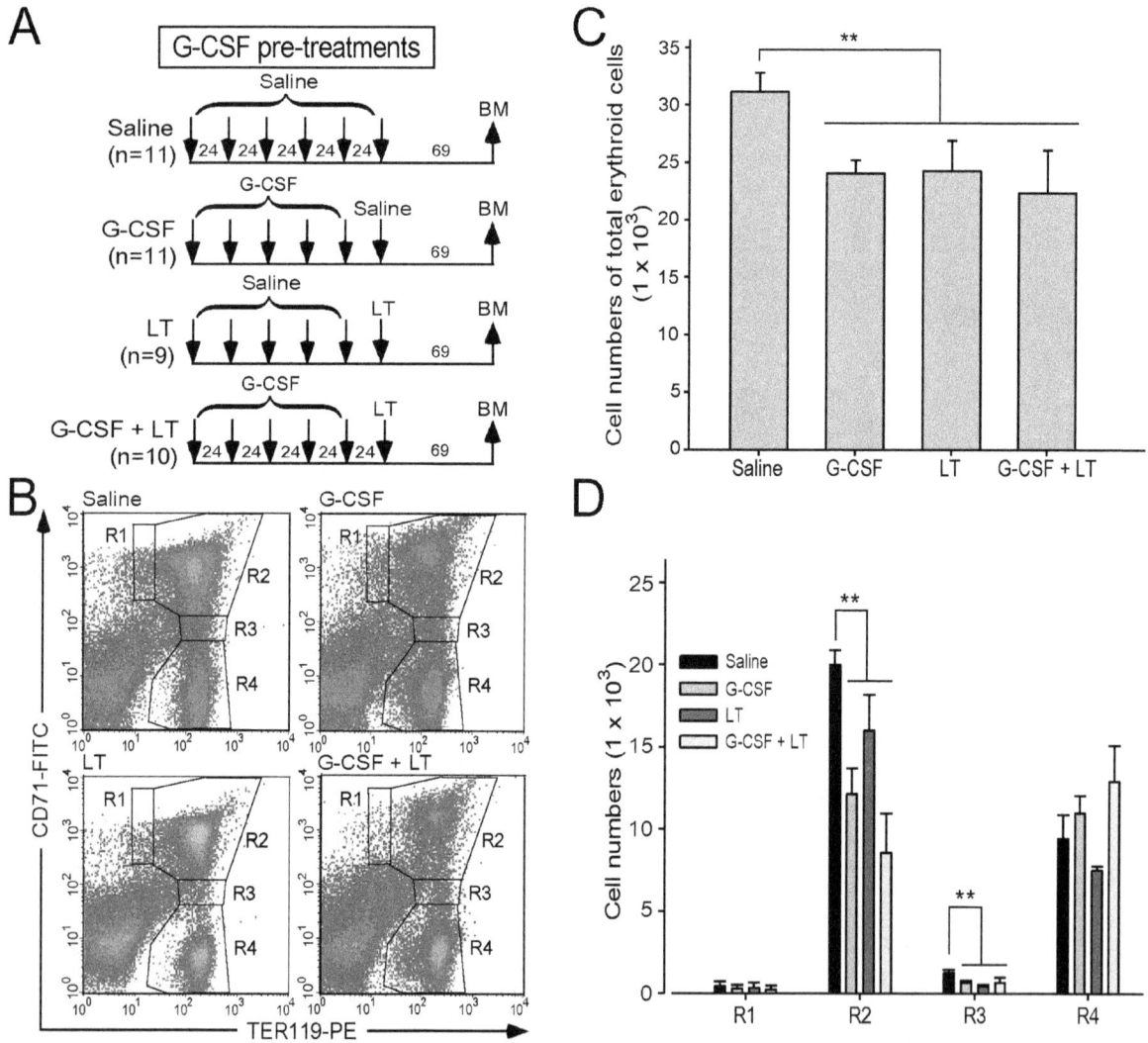

Figure 2. Regulation of G-CSF on bone marrow erythroblast populations. The experimental outlines are illustrated (A). Mice were treated with saline (n=11), G-CSF (n=11), LT (n=9), or G-CSF plus LT (n=10). Flow cytometry analysis analyzed erythroblast populations of BM cells at 69 h after LT challenges. The erythroblast cells were gated as R1 (CD71^{high}, TER-119^{med}), R2 (CD71^{high}, TER-119^{high}), R3 (CD71^{med}, TER-119^{high}), and R4 (CD71^{low}, TER-119^{high}) in all groups (B) as described [25]. The cell numbers of all erythroblast cells (sum of R1 to R4) (C) and individual erythroblast (R1, R2, R3, and R4) (D) in each group were quantified. **P<0.01 was compared between indicated groups. Data are showed as mean ± SD and represent the results from 2 independent experiments.

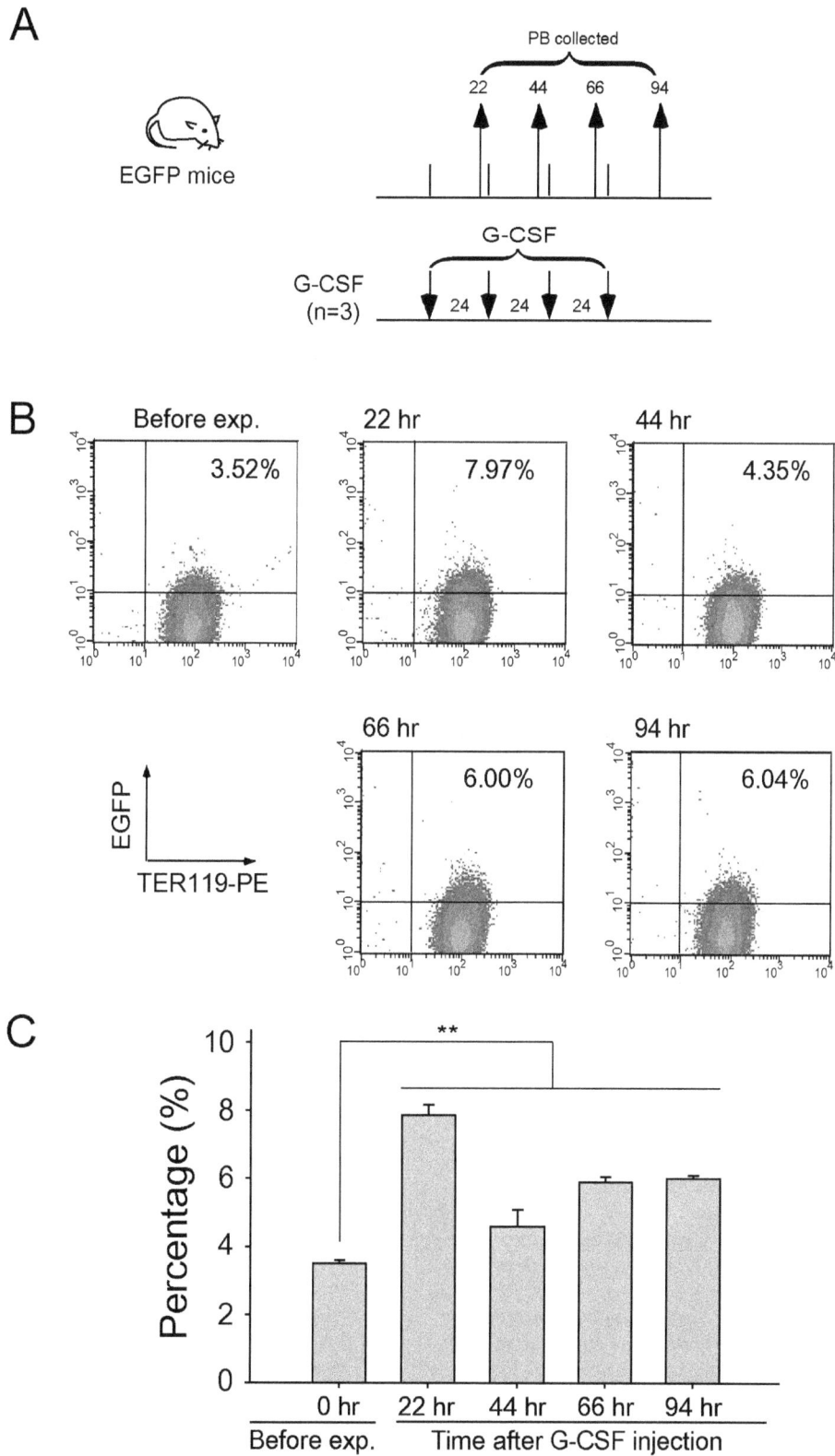

Figure 3. Mobilization of newly synthesized erythrocytes into peripheral blood by G-CSF. The experimental outline is illustrated (A). The EGFP mice were injected with G-CSF (n = 3). The percentage of EGFP[+]/TER119[+] cells in peripheral blood (PB) was analyzed by flow cytometry (B) and quantified (C) at 22, 44, 66, and 94 h after G-CSF injection. PB collected from mice before G-CSF injection served as the negative control. **$P < 0.01$ was compared to the negative control. Data are shown as mean ± SD.

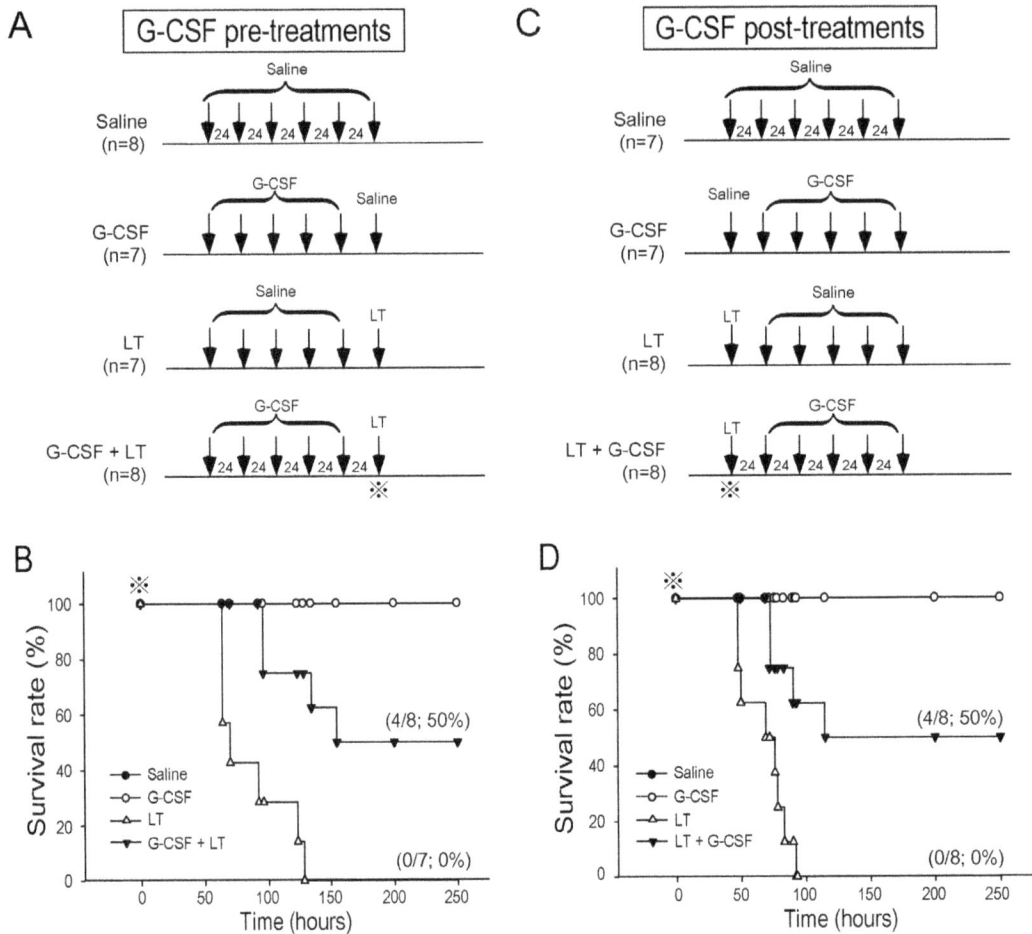

Figure 4. G-CSF treatments ameliorated LT-elicited mortality in mice. The experimental timetable (A), (C), and the survival rates of mice pre-treated (B) and post-treated (D) with G-CSF, LT, or G-CSF and LT are indicated. Saline treated mice served as negative controls. The symbol (※) in (A) to (D) indicates the onset time point for recording survival rates.

monitored up to 15 d for every 4–6 h. All surviving mice were monitored each day for 2 subsequent mo.

Statistics

All results are presented as the mean ± SD (standard deviation) for each group. Data significance was examined by one-way ANOVA followed by the post-hoc Bonferroni-corrected t-test. Univariate Kaplan-Meier analysis was used to compare the difference in survival rate between groups with various treatments. P-values were calculated and log-rank tests were performed to determine statistical significance. A probability of type 1 error $\alpha = 0.05$ was recognized as the threshold of statistical significance. Statistical analysis was conducted using the statistical software SPSS, version 17.0 (SPSS Inc., Chicago, IL, USA).

Results

G-CSF treatment promoted erythrocytic differentiation and proliferation *in vitro* and *ex vivo*

To elucidate the role of G-CSF on erythrocytic differentiation and proliferation, an *in vitro* erythroid colony-forming cell assay was performed to quantify BFU-Es and CFU-Es. Control groups without using filgrastim G-CSF supplements formed only medium-sized colonies by Day 7 (Figure 1C). By contrast, G-CSF treatments accelerated the formation of medium-sized colonies, which appeared earlier by Day 3 (Figure 1B). Following G-CSF treatment, the numbers of colonies in all colony sizes were greater than those in the untreated control groups (Figure 1B–1D). Based on the traditional concept that G-CSF primarily regulates granulopoiesis [28], those colonies to be affected by G-CSF treatment may not be exclusively erythroid-origin cells. Consequently, 3, 3′-diaminobenzidine tetrahydrochloride (DAB) [37] was used to identify erythroid colonies, and the pseudoperoxidase activity of erythroid cells was stained on Day 14. Compared with the untreated groups, the number of DAB+ colonies was greater in G-CSF-treated groups (Figure S1). This data indicated that G-CSF treatment enhances the proliferation and differentiation of erythrocytes *in vitro*. Further experiments were performed to investigate the effect of G-CSF and LT treatments *ex vivo* (Figure 1E). The number of erythroid colonies sharply decreased with LT treatment on Days 3, 7 and 14 (Figure 1F–1H). Medium-sized colonies first appeared on Day 3 in G-CSF treated groups (Figure 1F), compared with saline and LT-treated groups, whereas medium-sized colonies only appeared on Day 7 (Figure 1G). In addition, G-CSF treatments ameliorated LT-induced suppression on erythropoiesis in the *ex vivo* erythroid colony-forming cell assay (Figure 1F–1H). These results indicated that G-CSF promoted erythrocytic proliferation and differentiation *in vitro* and *ex vivo*

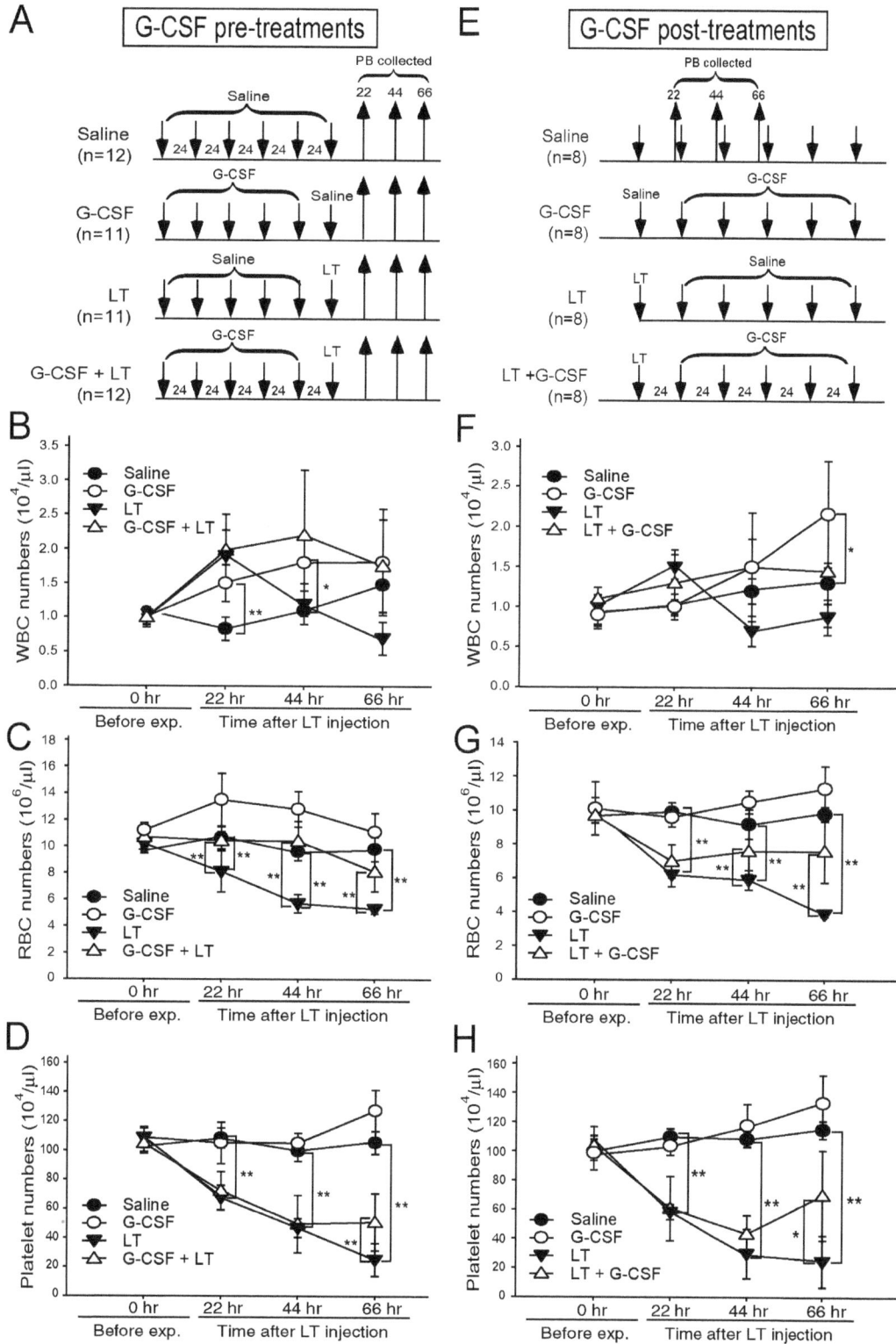

Figure 5. Amelioration of LT-induced erythrocytopenic response by G-CSF. The experimental outlines are indicated (A), (E). Mice were treated with saline (n = 12), G-CSF (n = 11), LT (n = 11), and G-CSF plus LT (n = 12) before (A) or saline (n = 8), G-CSF (n = 8), LT (n = 8), and LT plus G-CSF (n = 8) after (E) the LT challenges; their WBC, RBC, and platelet counts were subsequently analyzed at 22, 44, and 66 h after the LT challenges. Saline-treated mice were used as negative controls. *$P < 0.05$, **$P < 0.01$ were compared between the indicated groups. Data are shown as mean ± SD and represent the results from 2 independent experiments.

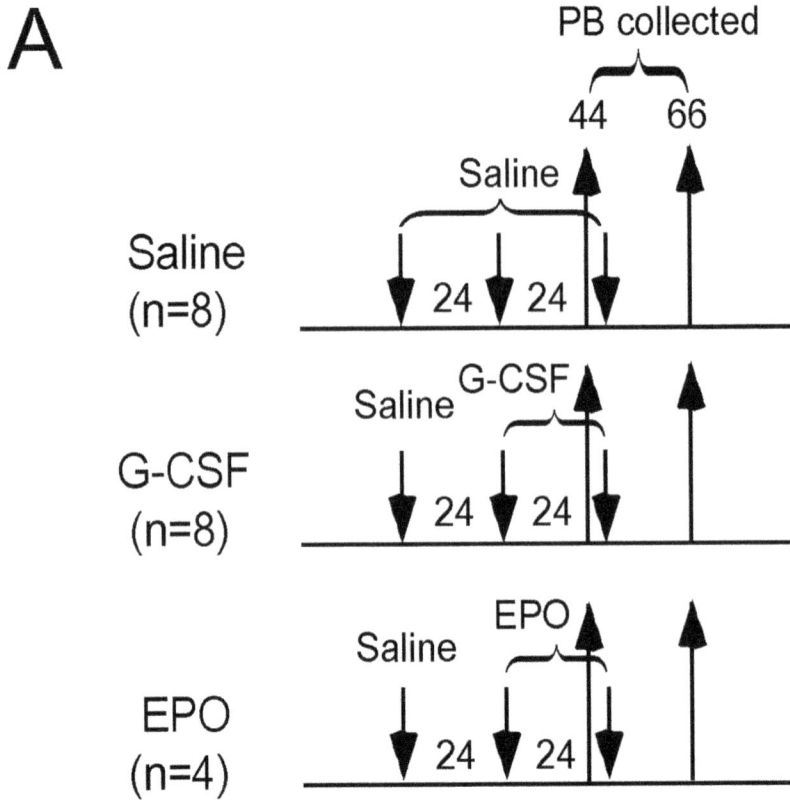

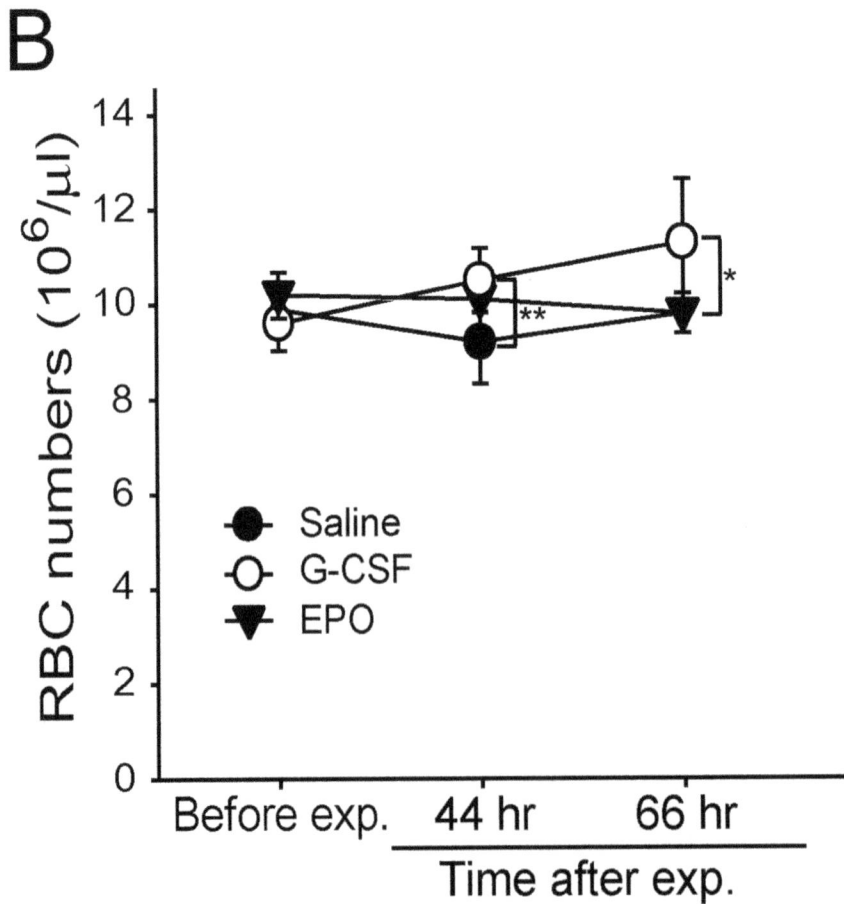

Figure 6. Fast mobilization of erythrocytes into peripheral blood by G-CSF versus EPO treatments. Experimental outline for measuring the PB-RBC counts of mice treated with G-CSF (n = 8) or EPO (n = 4) for 2 consecutive d (A). The PB RBC counts were measured before the experiments and at 44 and 66 h after the first saline injection (B). Data are shown as mean ± SD and represent the results from 2 independent experiments. Saline treated groups (n = 8) were used as the negative control. *P<0.05, **P<0.01 were compared to the negative control.

and ameliorated LT-induced erythropoiesis suppression in the *ex vivo* erythroid colony-forming cell assay.

G-CSF treatment promoted mobilization of newly synthesized RBC to peripheral blood

After the promising analyses *in vitro* and *ex vivo*, this study investigated the erythropoietic progression *in vivo*. Our previous report revealed that LT suppressed erythropoiesis in bone marrow [15]. Following similar approaches [15,25], we used surface expression of CD71 and TER-119 to verify the maturation status of various bone marrow erythroblasts under the G-CSF treatments with or without anthrax LT challenges. Although we found that G-CSF treatment rescued LT-induced erythrocytopenia (please see the following section), G-CSF pre-treatments could not overcome LT-mediated suppression on the cell numbers of both total erythroblast and individual subpopulations of erythroblast (R1 to R4 populations) (Figure 2C and 2D). This prompted us to verify whether G-CSF could mobilize mature erythrocytes into peripheral blood; we employed C57BL/6J mice with the whole-body-expressing enhanced-green-fluorescence-protein (EGFP) transgene. Prior to G-CSF analyses, we found that only a small fraction of EGFP⁺ RBCs was detectable in the peripheral blood of normal control groups (Figure 3, 3.5% cells, before exp. groups). This is likely because mature erythrocytes do not have a nucleus, and that newly differentiated RBCs, rather than aged RBCs, express detectable EGFP. We employed an acute hemorrhage model, in which 35% of total blood was removed, to provoke the natural induction of erythropoiesis to investigate whether newly synthesized erythrocytes contain additional fluorescence. Our data revealed that EGFP⁺/TER-119⁺ erythrocytes increased consistently by Days 2, 4, and 6 after acute anemia (Figure S2). This suggested that EGFP⁺/TER-119⁺ cells are newly synthesized erythrocytes. Using the same strategy, analyses revealed that G-CSF treatment can mobilize newly synthesized erythrocytes to peripheral blood in mice (Figure 3, beginning at 22 h after G-CSF injections).

G-CSF treatment reduced LT-mediated mortality, erythrocytopenia, and thrombocytopenia

To investigate the ameliorative effect of G-CSF on LT, C57BL/6J mice were treated with G-CSF according to the manufacturer's instructions (once daily for 5 d). Treatments of G-CSF were initiated 5 d before (Figure 4A) or 1 d after (Figure 4C) the challenges of a lethal dose of LT (Figure 4C). LT initiated mortality within 48 to 129 h (Figure 4B and 4D, LT groups). Administration of 5 doses of G-CSF before (Figure 4A) and after (Figure 4C) the LT challenges significantly improved survival rates (Figure 4B and 4D) (P<0.01). Treatments using saline, G-CSF, and LT alone served as the controls (Figure 4B and 4D). The peripheral white blood cell (WBC) counts of the G-CSF-treated groups increased approximately 2-fold at 22 and 44 h (Figure 5A and 5B), as well as at 66 h (Figure 5E and 5F) following the implementation of differing G-CSF regimens; this is in consistent with a previous G-CSF report [38]. Notably, both G-CSF treatments significantly ameliorated LT-induced erythrocytopenia (Figure 5C, G-CSF + LT vs. LT; Figure 5G, LT + G-CSF vs. LT). Compared with RBC counts, the ameliorative effect of G-CSF on LT-induced thrombocytopenia was somewhat later and was observed at

approximately 66 h after LT treatment (Figure 5D and 5H). These results indicated that G-CSF positively regulated both RBC and platelet counts.

G-CSF treatment induced erythrocytes to mobilize into peripheral blood faster than EPO

Our previous study showed that EPO up-regulated RBC counts in peripheral blood [15]. To compare the EPO and G-CSF treatments in their efficiency at increasing RBC counts, mice were injected with 2 doses of either G-CSF or EPO. The circulating RBC counts were measured (Figure 6). Our data revealed that G-CSF induced a faster increase of RBC counts, within 20 h of the first G-CSF administration, than the EPO treatment, in which no increased RBC counts were observed (Figure 6B, G-CSF vs. EPO). These results suggested that G-CSF induced a faster mobilization of erythrocytes into peripheral blood than that of EPO.

Combined G-CSF and EPO had an ameliorative effect on anthrax-spore-induced mortality in C57BL/6J mice

Our previous report suggested that EPO ameliorates LT-mediated erythrocytopenia by enhancing erythropoiesis [15]. Because G-CSF increases the erythrocyte supply through a diverse mechanism by enhancing the mobilization of erythrocytes into peripheral blood, these results prompted us to investigate whether combined treatments using G-CSF and EPO may be more effective than respective single treatments alone. The analysis indicated that EPO treatment did not exert a protective effect on anthrax-spore-challenged mice (Figure 7B, Spore + EPO vs. Spore only). This is consistent with another line of evidence; the survival rates of anthrax LT-challenged mice increased only 25% following EPO post-treatment (Figure S3, LT + EPO vs. LT, P = 0.101). By contrast, G-CSF treatments with or without EPO effectively increased the survival rate of anthrax spore-challenged mice from 18.75% to 37.5% (Figure 7, Spore + G-CSF vs. Spore only). Post-treatments combining G-CSF and EPO prolonged the survival period of anthrax-spore-challenged mice (Figure 7, Spore + G-CSF + EPO vs. Spore + G-CSF). Statistical analysis revealed that the P value is marginally significant (Figure 7, P = 0.094, Spore + G-CSF + EPO vs. Spore; P = 0.088, Spore + G-CSF + EPO vs. Spore + EPO). These results suggested that combined treatment using G-CSF and EPO tended to ameliorate anthrax-spore-induced mortality in mice.

Discussion

This study demonstrated that G-CSF, a stimulating factor for granulopoiesis, enhanced erythrocytic mobilization, by which it enhanced RBC counts in peripheral blood. This likely therefore rescued anthrax LT-induced anemia and mortality in mice.

Our *in vitro* (Figure 1A–1D) and *ex vivo* (Figure 1E–1H) evidence suggested that G-CSF may promote erythropoiesis. The *in vivo* analyses revealed that G-CSF ameliorated LT-induced erythrocytopenia in peripheral blood (Figure 5C and 5G), but did not increase erythroblast cell numbers in bone marrow (Figure 2). Therefore, the effects of G-CSF on erythropoiesis *in vivo* require clarification. One study demonstrated that G-CSF had a negative effect on bone marrow erythropoiesis in mice [39].

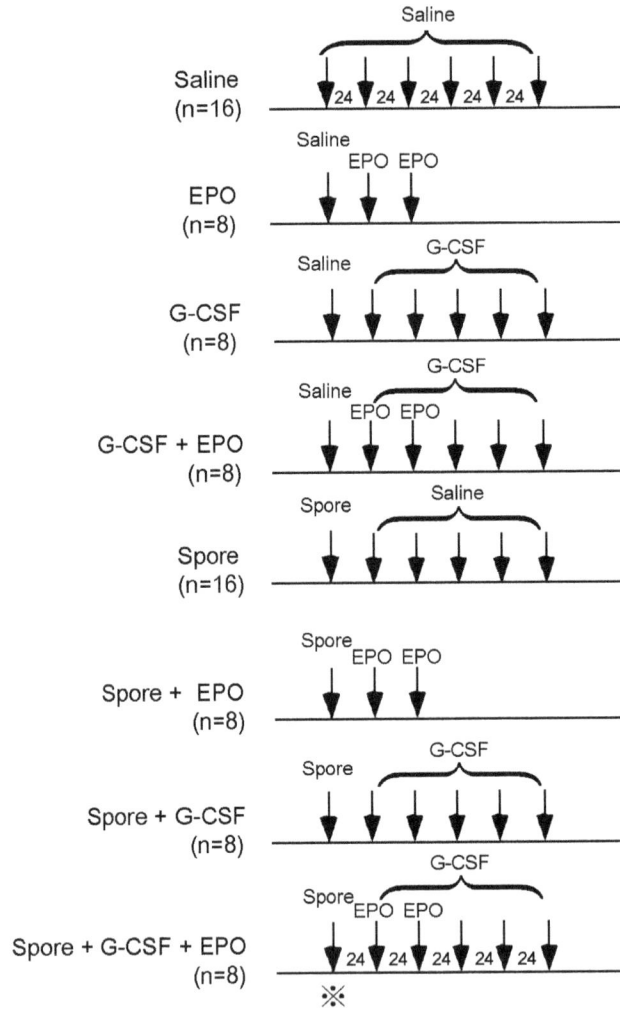

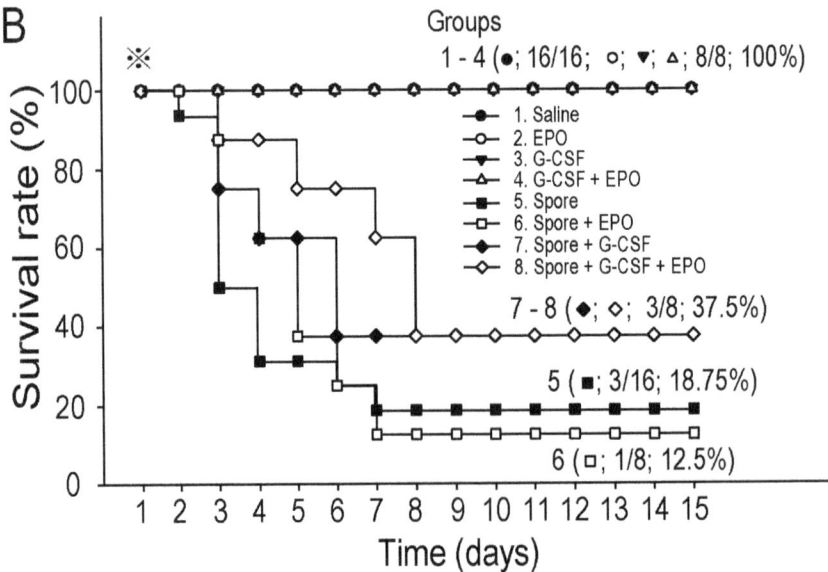

Figure 7. Post-treatments of G-CSF and EPO tended to ameliorate anthrax spore elicited-lethality in mice. Experimental outlines (A) and the survival rates of mice treated with G-CSF (n = 8), EPO (n = 8), and G-CSF combined with EPO (n = 8) after anthrax spore injection (B). Saline (n = 16), EPO (n = 8), G-CSF (n = 8), G-CSF and EPO (n = 8), and anthrax spore (n = 16) injected groups were used for comparisons. The symbol (※) in (A) and (B) indicates the onset time point for recording survival rates. Data represent the results from 2 independent experiments.

However, another study demonstrated that G-CSF treatments in humans increased immature reticulocytes in peripheral blood [40]. Clinical observations also found that the reticulocyte fraction, an assessment of immature erythroid cells in peripheral blood, was an early surrogate marker for the rise of CD34$^+$ hematopoietic stem cells during G-CSF mobilization [41]. This evidence suggests that G-CSF is involved in regulating erythroid precursor cells in humans.

G-CSF induced fast mobilization of RBCs to peripheral blood within 20 h of the first G-CSF administration, compared with the EPO treatment (Figure 6). This data is consistent with the EGFP mice experiment, regarding the time in which G-CSF treatment increased the percentage of newly synthesized erythrocytes in peripheral blood (Figure 3). Thus, a single post-treatment dose of G-CSF was sufficient to save approximately 40% of mice within 24 h (Figure 4D, 100% and 60% survival rates in LT + G-CSF and LT, 48 h groups, respectively). The advantage of fast mobilization of RBCs of G-CSF can also be confirmed by the higher survival rate of G-CSF compared with EPO in LT-induced (Figure 4D vs. Figure S3B) and LT-spore-induced (Figure 7B) mortality in mice.

G-CSF is a multi-function cytokine that stimulates the proliferation and differentiation of myeloid precursors and modulates mature cells [29]. G-CSF is also used to prevent or shorten neutropenia in chemotherapy-induced or primary congenital neutropenia [42], and mobilize hematopoietic stem cells to peripheral blood for transplantation [43]. Probably because of the anti-apoptotic and anti-inflammatory effects, G-CSF has also been used to treat nonhematopoietic targets including cerebral ischemia [44], spinal cord ischemia [45], infarct heart [46], and end stage liver disease [47]. Consequently, the effects of G-CSF on other cell types (e.g., macrophage, lymphocyte, endothelial, dendritic cells, cardiomyocytes, and smooth muscle) may not be completely excluded from the rescue mechanism of G-CSF. Although the mechanism is unclear, combination therapy using G-CSF and EPO has been used to treat myelodysplastic anemia in clinical settings [32–36,48]. This suggests that the medical community has empirically recognized the RBC-enhancing effect of the combination treatment using G-CSF and EPO. One critical aspect of G-CSF is the rapid induction of peripheral RBCs, a property superior to EPO, which may be applied to anthrax or other diseases with urgent RBC and oxygen demands. Further detailed and well-designed clinical studies are required to explore the therapeutic potential of combination treatment using G-CSF and EPO.

In this study, we demonstrated that G-CSF mobilized erythrocytes into peripheral blood. In addition, combined treatments of G-CSF and EPO tended to ameliorate anthrax spore-induced mortality. An optimized rescue protocol may provide new perspectives and assist the development of a feasible therapeutic strategy against anthrax.

Supporting Information

Figure S1   G-CSF treatments enhanced bone marrow erythroid colony numbers. An *in vitro* erythroid colony-forming cell assay was performed using murine bone marrow (BM) cells incubated with [20 ng/ml (n = 6) or 764 ng/ml (n = 6)] or without G-CSF (n = 6). The erythroid colonies were confirmed by 3, 3′-diaminobenzidine tetrahydrochloride (DAB) staining (A) and quantified on Day 14 (B). Untreated BM cells were used as the control. **P<0.01 was compared to the untreated groups. Scale bar: 500 μm. Data are shown as mean ± SD.
(TIF)

Figure S2   Mobilization of newly synthesized erythrocytes (EGFP$^+$/TER-119$^+$) into peripheral blood by acute anemia in EGFP transgenic mice. Experimental timetable used in acute anima assay (A). During acute anima (after aspirating 35% of total blood), the population of EGFP$^+$/TER-119$^+$ cells in peripheral blood (PB) of EGFP mice was gated as R1 and quantified. The total cell number was defined as 100%. The percentage of R1 was analyzed by flow cytometry (B) on Day 2, 4, and 6 after the removal of 35% of total blood. PB samples from mice before acute anemia were used as negative controls. Data were collected from 2 representative EGFP mice.
(TIF)

Figure S3   Post-treatments of EPO increased the survival rates of LT-challenged mice. Experimental timetable (A). The survival rates of mice challenged with EPO (n = 4), LT (n = 4), or LT plus EPO (n = 4) are shown (B). Saline-treated mice were used as controls (n = 4). C57BL/6J mice were retro-orbitally injected with recombinant human EPO (rhEPO, Neorecormon, Roche, Mannheim, Germany) (2 IU/g, in 250 μl saline) twice every 24 h after the challenges of a lethal dose of LT (1.5 mg/kg in 250 μl saline, retro-orbitally injected). The symbol (※) in (A) and (B) indicates the onset time point for recording the survival rates of mice.
(TIF)

Methods S1   Supplemental experimental procedures.
(DOC)

Acknowledgments

We wish to thank Professor Yu MS for providing 3, 3′-diaminobenzidine tetrahydrochloride (DAB) tablets. We also wish to thank Professor Wang MH and his team, the Experimental Animal Center of Tzu-Chi University for animal care.

Author Contributions

Conceived and designed the experiments: HHC DSS. Performed the experiments: YWC TKL GLL YYL JHK HHH HLH. Analyzed the data: HHC JHW DSS. Contributed reagents/materials/analysis tools: JHK HHH HLH JHW. Wrote the paper: HHC DSS.

References

1. Mock M, Fouet A (2001) Anthrax. Annu Rev Microbiol 55: 647–671.
2. Brossier F, Mock M (2001) Toxins of Bacillus anthracis. Toxicon 39: 1747–1755.
3. Collier RJ, Young JA (2003) Anthrax toxin. Annu Rev Cell Dev Biol 19: 45–70.
4. Mourez M (2004) Anthrax toxins. Rev Physiol Biochem Pharmacol 152: 135–164.
5. Bardwell AJ, Abdollahi M, Bardwell L (2004) Anthrax lethal factor-cleavage products of MAPK (mitogen-activated protein kinase) kinases exhibit reduced binding to their cognate MAPKs. Biochem J 378: 569–577.
6. Hagemann C, Blank JL (2001) The ups and downs of MEK kinase interactions. Cell Signal 13: 863–875.
7. Wada T, Penninger JM (2004) Mitogen-activated protein kinases in apoptosis regulation. Oncogene 23: 2838–2849.
8. Raman M, Chen W, Cobb MH (2007) Differential regulation and properties of MAPKs. Oncogene 26: 3100–3112.
9. Moayeri M, Leppla SH (2004) The roles of anthrax toxin in pathogenesis. Curr Opin Microbiol 7: 19–24.
10. Kau JH, Sun DS, Huang HS, Lien TS, Huang HH, et al. (2010) Sublethal doses of anthrax lethal toxin on the suppression of macrophage phagocytosis. PLoS One 5: e14289.
11. Muehlbauer SM, Evering TH, Bonuccelli G, Squires RC, Ashton AW, et al. (2007) Anthrax lethal toxin kills macrophages in a strain-specific manner by apoptosis or caspase-1-mediated necrosis. Cell Cycle 6: 758–766.
12. Alileche A, Serfass ER, Muehlbauer SM, Porcelli SA, Brojatsch J (2005) Anthrax lethal toxin-mediated killing of human and murine dendritic cells impairs the adaptive immune response. PLoS Pathog 1: e19.

13. Comer JE, Chopra AK, Peterson JW, Konig R (2005) Direct inhibition of T-lymphocyte activation by anthrax toxins in vivo. Infect Immun 73: 8275–8281.

14. Fang H, Xu L, Chen TY, Cyr JM, Frucht DM (2006) Anthrax lethal toxin has direct and potent inhibitory effects on B cell proliferation and immunoglobulin production. J Immunol 176: 6155–6161.

15. Chang HH, Wang TP, Chen PK, Lin YY, Liao CH, et al. (2013) Erythropoiesis suppression is associated with anthrax lethal toxin-mediated pathogenic progression. PLoS One 8: e71718.

16. Chen PK, Chang HH, Lin GL, Wang TP, Lai YL, et al. (2013) Suppressive effects of anthrax lethal toxin on megakaryopoiesis. PLoS One 8: e59512.

17. Liu S, Zhang Y, Moayeri M, Liu J, Crown D, et al. (2013) Key tissue targets responsible for anthrax-toxin-induced lethality. Nature 501: 63–68.

18. Kassam A, Der SD, Mogridge J (2005) Differentiation of human monocytic cell lines confers susceptibility to Bacillus anthracis lethal toxin. Cell Microbiol 7: 281–292.

19. Kau JH, Sun DS, Tsai WJ, Shyu HF, Huang HH, et al. (2005) Antiplatelet activities of anthrax lethal toxin are associated with suppressed p42/44 and p38 mitogen-activated protein kinase pathways in the platelets. J Infect Dis 192: 1465–1474.

20. Moayeri M, Haines D, Young HA, Leppla SH (2003) Bacillus anthracis lethal toxin induces TNF-alpha-independent hypoxia-mediated toxicity in mice. J Clin Invest 112: 670–682.

21. Rainey GJ, Young JA (2004) Antitoxins: novel strategies to target agents of bioterrorism. Nat Rev Microbiol 2: 721–726.

22. Wadhwa M, Thorpe R (2008) Haematopoietic growth factors and their therapeutic use. Thromb Haemost 99: 863–873.

23. Debili N, Wendling F, Katz A, Guichard J, Breton-Gorius J, et al. (1995) The Mpl-ligand or thrombopoietin or megakaryocyte growth and differentiative factor has both direct proliferative and differentiative activities on human megakaryocyte progenitors. Blood 86: 2516–2525.

24. Fisher JW (2003) Erythropoietin: physiology and pharmacology update. Exp Biol Med (Maywood) 228: 1–14.

25. Socolovsky M, Nam H, Fleming MD, Haase VH, Brugnara C, et al. (2001) Ineffective erythropoiesis in Stat5a(−/−)5b(−/−) mice due to decreased survival of early erythroblasts. Blood 98: 3261–3273.

26. Trowbridge IS, Lesley J, Schulte R (1982) Murine cell surface transferrin receptor: studies with an anti-receptor monoclonal antibody. J Cell Physiol 112: 403–410.

27. Kina T, Ikuta K, Takayama E, Wada K, Majumdar AS, et al. (2000) The monoclonal antibody TER-119 recognizes a molecule associated with glycophorin A and specifically marks the late stages of murine erythroid lineage. Br J Haematol 109: 280–287.

28. Hubel K, Dale DC, Liles WC (2002) Therapeutic use of cytokines to modulate phagocyte function for the treatment of infectious diseases: current status of granulocyte colony-stimulating factor, granulocyte-macrophage colony-stimulating factor, macrophage colony-stimulating factor, and interferon-gamma. J Infect Dis 185: 1490–1501.

29. Morstyn G, Burgess AW (1988) Hemopoietic growth factors: a review. Cancer Res 48: 5624–5637.

30. Metcalf D (2008) Hematopoietic cytokines. Blood 111: 485–491.

31. Xiao BG, Lu CZ, Link H (2007) Cell biology and clinical promise of G-CSF: immunomodulation and neuroprotection. J Cell Mol Med 11: 1272–1290.

32. Bessho M, Hirashima K, Asano S, Ikeda Y, Ogawa N, et al. (1997) Treatment of the anemia of aplastic anemia patients with recombinant human erythropoietin in combination with granulocyte colony-stimulating factor: a multicenter randomized controlled study. Multicenter Study Group. Eur J Haematol 58: 265–272.

33. Greenberg PL, Sun Z, Miller KB, Bennett JM, Tallman MS, et al. (2009) Treatment of myelodysplastic syndrome patients with erythropoietin with or without granulocyte colony-stimulating factor: results of a prospective randomized phase 3 trial by the Eastern Cooperative Oncology Group (E1996). Blood 114: 2393–2400.

34. Hellstrom-Lindberg E, Gulbrandsen N, Lindberg G, Ahlgren T, Dahl IM, et al. (2003) A validated decision model for treating the anaemia of myelodysplastic syndromes with erythropoietin + granulocyte colony-stimulating factor: significant effects on quality of life. Br J Haematol 120: 1037–1046.

35. Hellstrom-Lindberg E, Negrin R, Stein R, Krantz S, Lindberg G, et al. (1997) Erythroid response to treatment with G-CSF plus erythropoietin for the anaemia of patients with myelodysplastic syndromes: proposal for a predictive model. Br J Haematol 99: 344–351.

36. Negrin RS, Stein R, Doherty K, Cornwell J, Vardiman J, et al. (1996) Maintenance treatment of the anemia of myelodysplastic syndromes with recombinant human granulocyte colony-stimulating factor and erythropoietin: evidence for in vivo synergy. Blood 87: 4076–4081.

37. Ogawa M, Parmley RT, Bank HL, Spicer SS (1976) Human marrow erythropoiesis in culture. I. Characterization of methylcellulose colony assay. Blood 48: 407–417.

38. Kikuta T, Shimazaki C, Ashihara E, Sudo Y, Hirai H, et al. (2000) Mobilization of hematopoietic primitive and committed progenitor cells into blood in mice by anti-vascular adhesion molecule-1 antibody alone or in combination with granulocyte colony-stimulating factor. Exp Hematol 28: 311–317.

39. Nijhof W, De Haan G, Dontje B, Loeffler M (1994) Effects of G-CSF on erythropoiesis. Ann N Y Acad Sci 718: 312–324; discussion 324–315.

40. Park K, Im T, Sasaki A, Yamane T, Nakao Y, et al. (1991) Positive effect of granulocyte-colony stimulating factor on erythropoiesis in humans. Osaka City Med J 37: 123–132.

41. Remacha AF, Martino R, Sureda A, Sarda MP, Sola C, et al. (1996) Changes in reticulocyte fractions during peripheral stem cell harvesting: role in monitoring stem cell collection. Bone Marrow Transplant 17: 163–168.

42. Page AV, Liles WC (2011) Colony-stimulating factors in the prevention and management of infectious diseases. Infect Dis Clin North Am 25: 803–817.

43. Rankin SM (2012) Chemokines and adult bone marrow stem cells. Immunol Lett 145: 47–54.

44. Abe K, Yamashita T, Takizawa S, Kuroda S, Kinouchi H, et al. (2012) Stem cell therapy for cerebral ischemia: from basic science to clinical applications. J Cereb Blood Flow Metab 32: 1317–1331.

45. Chen WF, Jean YH, Sung CS, Wu GJ, Huang SY, et al. (2008) Intrathecally injected granulocyte colony-stimulating factor produced neuroprotective effects in spinal cord ischemia: the mitogen-activated protein kinase and Akt pathways. Neuroscience 153: 31–43.

46. Baldo MP, Davel AP, Damas-Souza DM, Nicoletti-Carvalho JE, Bordin S, et al. (2011) The antiapoptotic effect of granulocyte colony-stimulating factor reduces infarct size and prevents heart failure development in rats. Cell Physiol Biochem 28: 33–40.

47. Gaia S, Smedile A, Omede P, Olivero A, Sanavio F, et al. (2006) Feasibility and safety of G-CSF administration to induce bone marrow-derived cells mobilization in patients with end stage liver disease. J Hepatol 45: 13–19.

48. Jadersten M, Montgomery SM, Dybedal I, Porwit-MacDonald A, Hellstrom-Lindberg E (2005) Long-term outcome of treatment of anemia in MDS with erythropoietin and G-CSF. Blood 106: 803–811.

49. Kau JH, Lin CG, Huang HH, Hsu HL, Chen KC, et al. (2002) Calyculin A sensitive protein phosphatase is required for Bacillus anthracis lethal toxin induced cytotoxicity. Curr Microbiol 44: 106–111.

50. Sarma NJ, Takeda A, Yaseen NR (2010) Colony forming cell (CFC) assay for human hematopoietic cells. J Vis Exp.

51. Harkness JE, Wagner JE (1995) Clinical procedures: Biology and Medicine of Rabbits and Rodents 93.

11

Specific Activation of Dendritic Cells Enhances Clearance of *Bacillus anthracis* following Infection

Iain J. T. Thompson[1], Elizabeth R. Mann[2], Margaret G. Stokes[1], Nicholas R. English[2], Stella C. Knight[2], Diane Williamson[1]*

1 Biomedical Sciences Department, Defence Science and Technology Laboratory, Porton Down, Salisbury, Wiltshire, SP4 0JQ, United Kingdom, **2** Antigen Presentation Research Group, Imperial College London, Northwick Park and St. Mark's Campus, Watford Road, Harrow, HA1 3UJ, United Kingdom

Abstract

Dendritic cells are potent activators of the immune system and have a key role in linking innate and adaptive immune responses. In the current study we have used *ex vivo* pulsed bone marrow dendritic cells (BMDC) in a novel adoptive transfer strategy to protect against challenge with *Bacillus anthracis*, in a murine model. Pre-pulsing murine BMDC with either recombinant Protective Antigen (PA) or CpG significantly upregulated expression of the activation markers CD40, CD80, CD86 and MHC-II. Passive transfusion of mice with pulsed BMDC, concurrently with active immunisation with rPA in alum, significantly enhanced (p<0.001) PA-specific splenocyte responses seven days post-immunisation. Parallel studies using *ex vivo* DCs expanded from human peripheral blood and activated under the same conditions as the murine DC, demonstrated that human DCs had a PA dose-related significant increase in the markers CD40, CD80 and CCR7 and that the increases in CD40 and CD80 were maintained when the other activating components, CpG and HK *B. anthracis* were added to the rPA in culture. Mice vaccinated on a single occasion intra-muscularly with rPA and alum and concurrently transfused intra-dermally with pulsed BMDC, demonstrated 100% survival following lethal *B. anthracis* challenge and had significantly enhanced (p< 0.05) bacterial clearance within 2 days, compared with mice vaccinated with rPA and alum alone.

Editor: Bernhard Kaltenboeck, Auburn University, United States of America

Funding: This work was supported by the United States Army Research Office and the Defense Advanced Research Projects Agency (DARPA). The funders had no role in study design, data collection and analysis, decision to publish, or preparation of the manuscript.

Competing Interests: The authors have declared that no competing interests exist.

* Email: dewilliamson@dstl.gov.uk

Introduction

Dendritic cells (DCs) are potent activators of the adaptive immune system [1] and are critical for host defence against pathogens. Naïve DCs perform a surveillance function, constantly sampling their environment, taking up antigen by phagocytosis and with increased efficiency by receptor-mediated endocytosis [2]. Upon maturation, DCs alter their phenotype and home to lymph nodes where they initiate and polarise an adaptive immune response by presentation of peptides on MHC-II molecules to CD4$^+$ T cells or by cross-priming on MHC-I molecules to CD8$^+$ T cells [3]. Their ability to induce antigen-specific T cell and antibody responses and their ability to be easily cultured *in vitro* has enabled DCs to be trialled as cellular vaccines, both for infectious diseases and in cancer, resulting in either tumour or infectious disease regression or eradication [4]. However, the passive transfusion of activated DC raises logistic and practical difficulties for clinical use. An alternative approach is to activate DCs *in situ* through the ligation of their cell surface receptors with monoclonal antibody conjugated to the antigen of interest, which has been shown to be an efficacious method of enhancing adaptive immune responses to pathogens [5].

Bacillus anthracis, the etiological agent of anthrax, is a Gram-positive spore-forming bacterium. The disease has three clinical presentations dependent on the route of inoculation, cutaneous, pulmonary and gastrointestinal anthrax. The sporulating nature of *B. anthracis* confers survival advantages in the environment and enables infection and persistence *in vivo*. Spores can exploit host cells to persist in niches and evade host immune responses capable of bacterial clearance, before germinating into vegetative cells. *B. anthracis* possesses two virulence plasmids: pXO1, encoding the proteins protective antigen (PA), lethal factor (LF) and edema factor (EF) which can form the binary toxins Lethal Toxin (LT) and Edema Toxin (ET) [6]; and pXO2, encoding the poly-D-glutamic acid capsule [6] required for immune evasion and intracellular survival [7].

Vaccines are an important strategy to protect at-risk individuals. Licensed anthrax vaccines such as Anthrax Vaccine Precipitate (AVP) and Anthrax Vaccine Adsorbed (AVA), together with next generation anthrax vaccines such as rPA and alum, require several priming doses followed by annual boosters. They protect against disease principally by inducing high titre antibody to PA, which neutralises anthrax toxins in the early stages of infection [8], [9], [10]. Despite the ability to induce a high titre antibody response, vaccines comprising alum as an adjuvant are generally poor inducers of cell-mediated immune (CMI) responses and enhanced CMI responses through DC vaccination may improve vaccine protective efficacy [11].

In this study we have explored the synergistic effects of passively administering specifically-activated DC at the same time as actively immunising mice with rPA and alum, to determine whether this will significantly reduce the time required to develop protective immunity against anthrax. In addition to survival, a key endpoint of this study was to determine whether this approach significantly enhanced bacterial clearance from the spleen in vaccinated and challenged mice and whether human DC would respond to activation in the same manner qualitatively and quantitatively as murine DC.

Results

Activation of DCs

The activation status of DCs was investigated prior to their use in transfusion. DCs were stimulated *ex vivo*, with vaccine antigens (rPA or heat-killed (HK) *B. anthracis* spores) or adjuvant (CpG) and the upregulation of costimulatory markers was assessed by flow cytometry. Pulsing of murine BMDC with rPA significantly upregulated (p<0.001) the expression of CD40, CD80, CD86 and MHCII, as effectively as pulsing with CpG. In contrast, HK *B. anthracis* caused the significant upregulation (p<0.05) of CD40 only on DC (Figure 1a).

In parallel with the studies on murine BMDC, *ex vivo* human DC, expanded from normal human peripheral blood mononuclear cells (PBMC), were pulsed with vaccine antigens and/or adjuvant, to determine the effect on their maturation and activation status. In these human studies, heat-killed *Bacillus cereus* was used in addition to HK *B. anthracis* as a positive control, since *B. cereus* is a related bacillus which causes gastrointestinal food-borne illness. Optimisation experiments to determine rPA (and *B. cereus*) doses demonstrated that similar to murine BMDC, pulsing of human DC with rPA significantly upregulated CD40 (p<0.01) and CD80 (p<0.001) (Figure 1b). Lymph-node homing marker CCR7 (upregulated on DC by maturation and activation) was also upregulated by rPA (p<0.001; Figure 1b). There was no change in expression of costimulatory markers CD83 or CD86 or in expression of receptors involved in DC recognition of bacteria or bacterial products (including Toll-like receptors 2 and 4; data not shown). Using an optimised rPA dose of 150 ng/ml for pulsing human DC, in combination with CpG, resulted in enhanced levels of CD40 and CD80 compared to rPA alone (Figure 1c), and the addition of HK *B. anthracis* to this combination enhanced expression even further (Figure 1d).

Cellular immune response to DC vaccination

The cellular immune response of mice transfused with BMDC pre-pulsed with rPA only (DC vaccine rPA only) or BMDC pre-pulsed with rPA, HK *B. anthracis* and CpG (DC vaccine), was characterised using an IFNγ ELISPOT to measure the recall response of their splenocytes *ex vivo* for rPA. Whilst an increase in the number of IFNγ SFC per 10^6 splenocytes was observed between sample days 7 (Figure 2a) and 14 (Figure 2b) for groups transfused with either unstimulated DC or either of the DC vaccines, this increase was not rPA-specific as there was no significant difference in number of IFNγ SFC between splenocyte samples which were rPA stimulated *ex vivo*, or unstimulated, at either time-point.

Pulsed human DC can activate naïve T-cells *ex vivo*

For comparison, *ex vivo* human DC pre- pulsed with either rPA or with *B. cereus* as a positive control, were cultured with naïve human T cells to determine if the latter could be specifically activated. Human naïve (CD45RO⁻) CD4⁺ blood T cells were enriched from normal PBMC and were CFSE- labelled prior to co-culture with rPA, HK *B.anthracis* (STI strain) and/or CpG-

pulsed DC, from the same donor in a syngeneic T cell stimulation assay. Human DC induced a dose-dependent proliferation of naïve CD4⁺ T cells in all cases. In initial experiments, rPA-pulsed DC stimulated a significantly enhanced proliferation of T cells compared with *B. cereus* or T cells stimulated by DC pulsed with medium only (p<0.05; Figure 2c). In later experiments, following optimisation of combination doses of vaccine antigens and adjuvant, the combination of rPA, CpG and HK *B. anthracis* (which we previously demonstrated induced the highest expression of costimulatory molecules on DC) was used to pulse DC and stimulated a significantly greater proliferation of naïve T cells (p< 0.001) than DC pulsed with adjuvant (CpG) only or CpG/rPA combined (Figure 2d).

Cytokine production by dividing human T-cells

Cytokine production by human T-cells dividing in response to a 5-day co-culture with syngeneic DC pulsed variously with rPA plus CpG, or rPA plus CpG plus HKSTI, was determined (Figure 3). No significant differences in T-cell cytokine production were seen upon stimulation with rPA-pulsed DC compared to medium only (Panel A), but T-cells stimulated with rPA/CpG/HK STI-pulsed DC produced significantly more TGFβ than those stimulated with rPA/CpG- or CpG only-pulsed DC (Panel B). There was no significant change in production of other cytokines studied (IL-10, IL-17 or IFNγ).

Cellular immune response to DC vaccination in combination with active immunisation

When splenocytes prepared from immunised mice were re-stimulated *ex vivo* with rPA, there was a significant increase in IFNγ⁺ SFC from mice actively immunised with rPA and alum compared to naïve mice at days 7 (p<0.05; Figure 4a) and 14 (p< 0.001; Figure 4b). The recall response to rPA at the earlier time point of 7 days post-immunisation, was even further enhanced in mice actively immunised with PA and alum together with transfusion of DC vaccine (p<0.001; Figure 4a). By day 14, both the actively immunised (rPA and alum) and the combined immunisation groups (rPA and alum and DC vaccine) had a significantly elevated (p<0.01 and p<0.001, respectively) recall response compared with mice given unstimulated DC, with no significant difference between the two immunised groups.

Anti-PA response to DC vaccination in combination with active immunisation

Analysis of day 14 sera from mice that had been transfused with DCs pre-pulsed with rPA, CpG and HK *B. anthracis* showed that they had developed a specific IgG response to PA (Figure 5). Mice which had been immunised with rPA and alum, or with rPA and alum and also transfused with the DC vaccine, had significantly elevated (p<0.05) anti-rPA IgG titres, when compared with mice receiving stimulated DCs alone (DC vaccine). In terms of antibody induction however, the combination of active immunisation with passive transfusion of pulsed DC, had no additive effect. In pilot studies we observed that the predominant IgG sub-class induced in mice either actively immunised with rPA & alum or adoptively transfused with rPA-pulsed DC, or both actively and passively immunised, was IgG1 (data not shown).

Post-challenge bacteriology and survival

Mice were challenged with 3×10^4 CFU *B. anthracis* STI i.p. (approximately 10 median lethal doses) 14 days post-immunisation. Mice treated with PBS only had a mean time to death of 3 days following challenge with 10MLD *B.anthracis* STI (data not

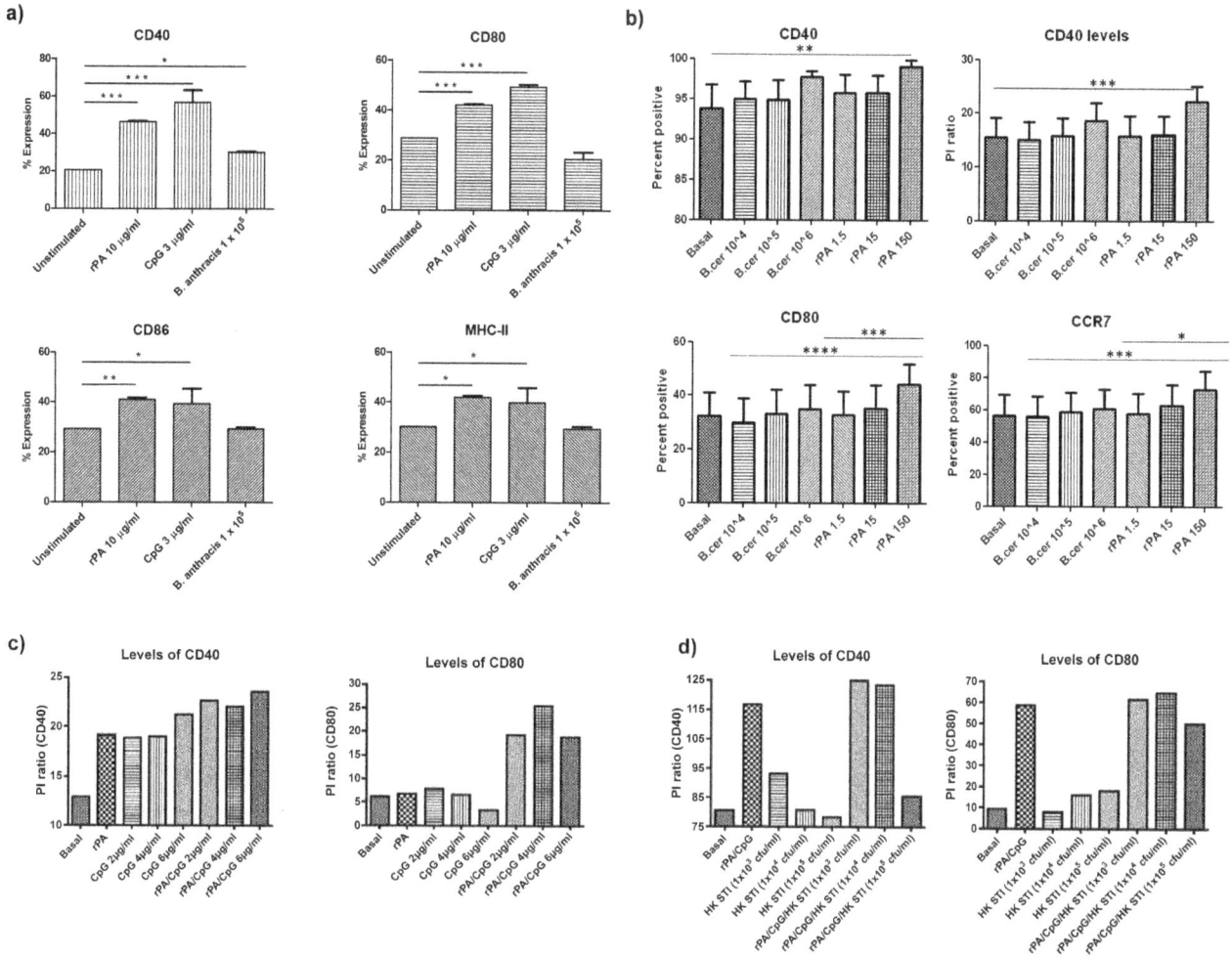

Figure 1. Co-stimulatory molecule expression on DC following antigen pulsing. a) Upregulation of MHC-II and co-stimulatory molecules on murine BMDCs. Costimulatory molecules on DCs were routinely upregulated by rPA and CpG following overnight co-culture whilst heat killed *B. anthracis* induced weak responses. Samples were analysed using a one-way-Anova with a Tukey post-hoc test (* p<0.05, ** p<0.01, *** p<0.001). **b)** Upregulation of CD40 and CD80 on human DC with rPA. Graphs represent mean±SEM proportion of DC expressing CD40 (n = 7), CD80 (n = 10) and CCR7 (n = 8). Levels of CD40 expression are also represented by mean±SEM positive intensity (PI) ratio (n = 7). One-way ANOVA (repeated measures) with ad-hoc Bonferroni corrections was applied (*p<0.05, **p<0.01, ***p<0.001, ****p<0.0001). **c)** Confirmatory experiments representing effects of rPA/CpG combined on levels of CD40 and CD80 expression, compared to rPA alone (and basal conditions/medium only). **d)** Confirmatory experiments representing effects of combination of vaccine antigens (rPA and HK *B. anthracis*) with CpG compared to rPA/CpG combination (n = 2).

shown). Two days post-challenge, a cohort of mice from each treatment group was culled with spleens taken to ascertain bacterial loads. Mice receiving unstimulated DCs together with alum showed limited survival (Figure 6) with all animals dead within 5 days and a splenic bacterial load significantly greater than all other groups (Figure 7). Mice receiving only the DC vaccine had 60% survival but a significantly (p<0.01) reduced bacterial load compared with the group receiving unstimulated DC with alum (negative controls), whilst mice immunised with rPA and alum showed 80% survival with a significantly (p<0.05) reduced bacterial load compared with negative controls. However, mice immunised with both rPA and alum and transfused with the DC vaccine had 100% survival and a highly significant reduction in bacterial load within 2 days of challenge, compared to the negative controls (p<0.001) and to the rPA and alum group (p<0.05).

There was a statistically significant difference in the survival curves for the negative control (alum+BMDC&CpG) group compared with the group actively immunised with rPA & alum

and also receiving rPA&HK *B.anthracis*-pulsed DC (p<0.002). Comparison of survival curves between the negative control (alum+BMDC&CpG) group and the group receiving rPA&HK *B.anthracis*-pulsed DC only, was also statistically significant (p< 0.01).

Discussion

Whilst there are currently licensed prophylactic vaccines for anthrax (e.g. Anthrax Vaccine Adsorbed, AVA and Anthrax Vaccine Precipitated, AVP) they have several limitations including a long primary schedule that requires multiple vaccinations (0, 3, 6 and 32 weeks currently for the UK AVP) to induce immunity, regular booster doses to maintain protective immunity and relatively poor development of CMI responses capable of clearing spores or vegetative bacteria. Furthermore, prophylactic antibiotic regimens require those suspected to have been exposed to take prolonged antibiotic courses (60 days) with the risk of residual

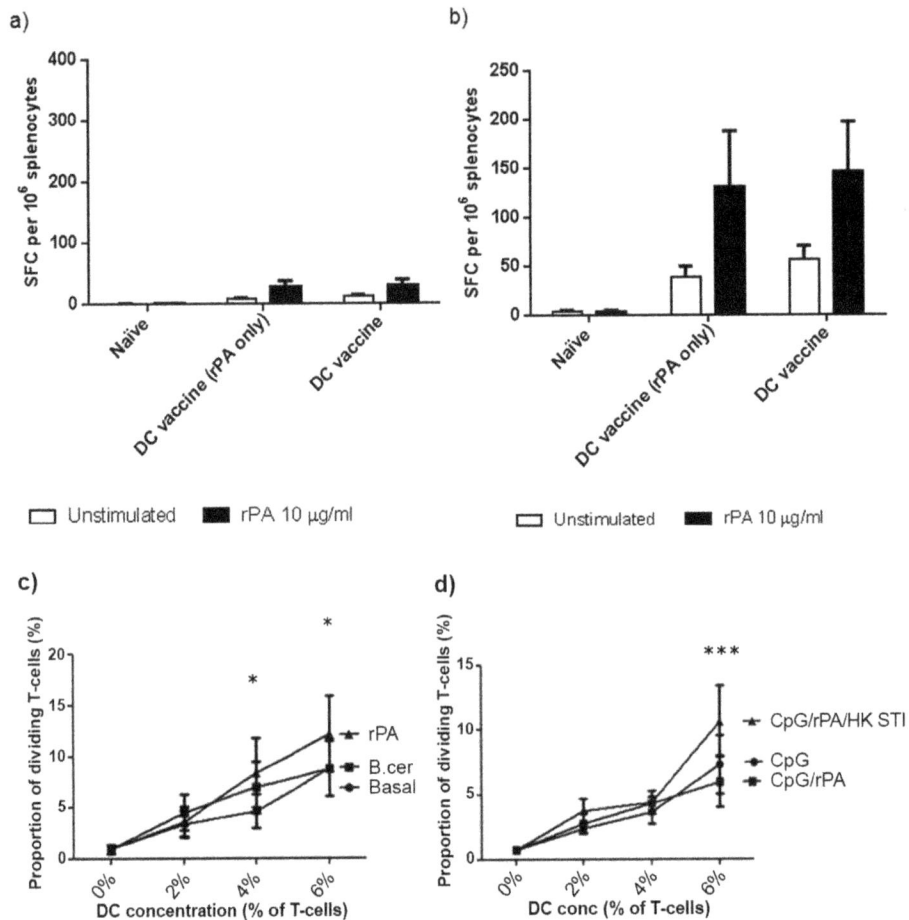

Figure 2. Stimulation of T cell responses. a and b) DCs were stimulated with rPA only (DC vaccine rPA only) or with PA, heat killed *B. anthracis* and CpG oligonucleotides (DC vaccine) and administered i.d. to A/J mice. Spleens were taken at 7 days (a) and 14 days (b) post- vaccination and restimulated *ex vivo* with rPA. A one-way Anova with Tukey multiple comparison post-hoc test was performed on the results (* $p < 0.05$, ** $p < 0.01$, *** $p < 0.001$). Error bars represent the standard error of the mean calculated from the means of three replicates from five animals. **c)** Proliferation of $CD4^+$ naive human T cells following 5-day co-culture with syngeneic human DC pulsed with medium only, *B. cereus* or rPA (n = 5). After 2-way ANOVA analysis with Bonferroni corrections, there were no significant differences between *B. cereus* and medium only (basal)-pulsed DC regarding stimulatory capacity but rPA-pulsed DC were significantly more stimulatory than basal conditions at 4% and 6% ($p < 0.05$ in both cases) and significantly more stimulatory than *B. cereus* pulsed DC at 6% ($p < 0.05$). **d)** $CD4^+$ naive human T-cell proliferation following 5-day co-culture with syngeneic DC pulsed with CpG only, rPA with CpG or combination of rPA, CpG and HK *B. anthracis* (n = 3). After 2-way ANOVA with Bonferroni corrections, there were no significant differences between CpG and rPA/CpG-pulsed human DC regarding stimulatory capacity but rPA/CpG/HK *B. anthracis*-pulsed human DC were significantly more stimulatory than both other conditions at 6% ($p < 0.001$ in both cases).

spores germinating after completion of the course and poor compliance to the regimen. Therefore a vaccine that can effectively induce CMI responses capable of reducing vegetative bacterial or spore burden is desirable, potentially by enhancing existing vaccines. In this study we examined the potential for DC transfusion to enhance conventional anthrax vaccination in terms of reducing the time required to develop protective immunity and enhancing the specific CMI response induced, with the rationale that this could significantly improve bacterial clearance post-exposure.

The *in vitro* co-stimulation of DCs with rPA, heat-killed *B. anthracis* and CpG resulted in the maturation of murine DCs with increased expression of MHC-II, CD80 and CD86 needed for presentation of antigen to $CD4^+$ T cells and of CD40, required for the co-stimulation of T and B cells. Similarly, human DC responded to rPA pulsing with enhanced CD40 and CD80 expression, which was further enhanced when CpG was added to

the rPA stimulus, and even further when both CpG and HK *B. anthracis* were added to rPA.

Although specifically activated, transfusion of these DC into mice did not induce an antigen-specific cellular immune response, as measured by IFNγ secretion following recall with rPA *ex vivo*, within 14 days of vaccination. This was not surprising, since previous studies have demonstrated that DC vaccination required 35 days to induce an antigen-specific anamnestic IFNγ response [12]. To determine if this time span could be reduced, active immunisation with rPA and alum was combined with DC vaccination. Mice receiving this combined immunisation had significantly enhanced CMI responses at only 7 days, as evidenced by a significant increase in the number of IFNγ+ spot-forming cells per 10^6 splenocytes on re-stimulation with rPA, compared to those immunised with rPA and alum alone, demonstrating that DC vaccination both accelerated and enhanced the response to conventional active immunisation.

a)

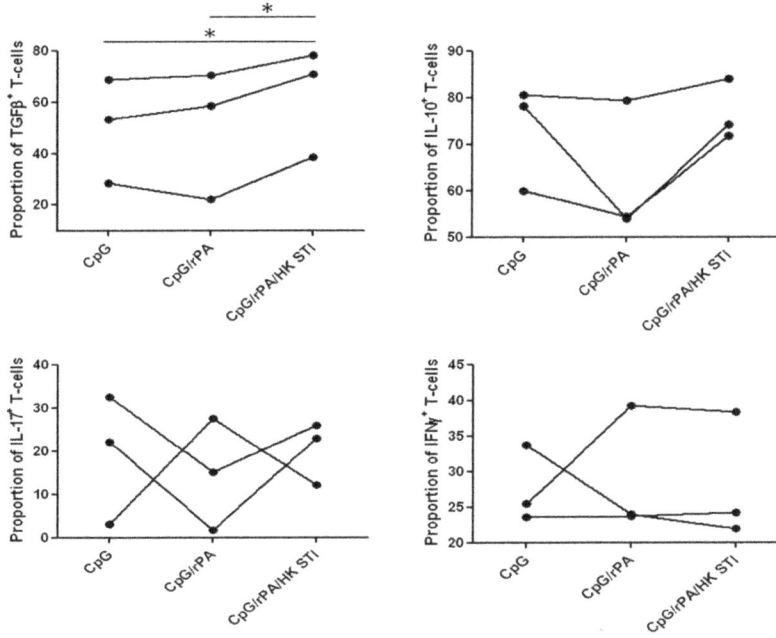

b)

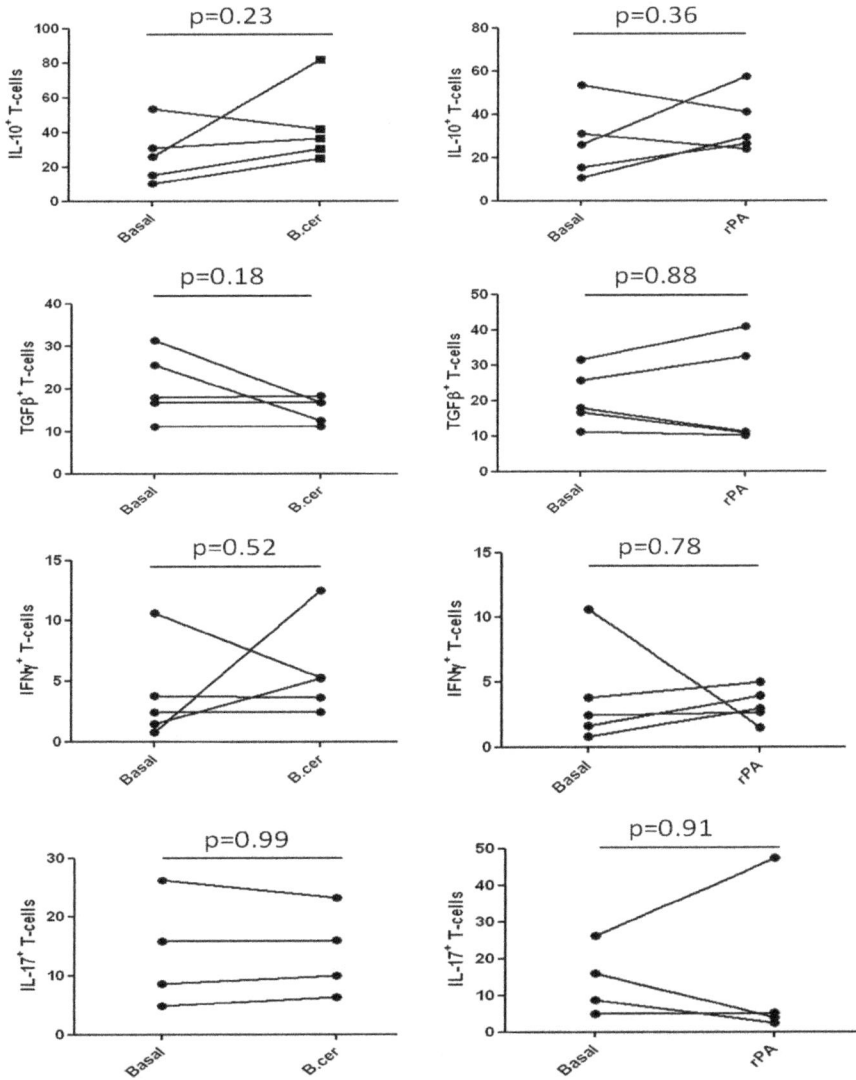

Figure 3. Cytokine production by human T-cells. Cytokine production by human T-cells stimulated by 6% medium (basal) or *B.cereus* or rPA-pulsed syngeneic DC (n = 5) (Panel A) or by 6% CpG-, rPA/CpG- or rPA/CpG/HK STI-pulsed syngeneic DC (n = 3) (Panel B) following 5-day co-culture. Paired t-test was applied, $p < 0.05$ was considered statistically significant (*$p < 0.05$, **$p < 0.01$, ***$p < 0.001$).

Furthermore human DC pulsed with rPA, caused a dose-related proliferative response in naïve human CD4+T-cells, which was further enhanced when DC were pulsed with CpG and HK *B. anthracis*, in addition to rPA and this was accompanied by a significantly enhanced secretion of TGFβ. The study of human DC-T cell interactions cannot exactly match the murine studies, since it is entirely based on *ex vivo* T-cell stimulation, however these concurrent human studies supported the murine data demonstrating that rPA, HK *B. anthracis* and CpG is an optimum activating combination for the DC. This allowed the optimum DC-activating combination of rPA+CpG+HKSTI to be deployed together with active immunisation in the mouse, to achieve accelerated T- cell mediated immune responses against *B. anthracis*.

The efficacy of the combined immunisation regimen was stringently tested by challenging mice with multiple lethal doses of *B. anthracis* only 14 days after immunisation. Whilst naïve mice rapidly succumbed to infection, 80% of those immunised with rPA and alum survived. The DC vaccine alone protected 60% of mice and this protection was attributed predominantly to the induction of a specific CMI response. By comparison, the DC vaccine, combined with rPA in alum immunisation, fully protected all the mice and these mice had a highly significant reduction in splenic bacteria as early as 2 days post-challenge. Mice receiving either the DC vaccine only, or rPA in alum only, had bacterial loads which although significantly reduced compared with naïve mice, were still elevated compared with the combined vaccine group.

This study provides proof-of-principle that a single transfusion of specifically activated DCs can augment the response to conventional active immunisation, with benefits in terms of accelerating time to immunity, specific CMI, survival and most significantly, clearance of *B. anthracis* in the murine model. Whilst these are significant findings, the passive transfusion of pre-stimulated DCs is not a pragmatic approach to mass vaccination in the clinic. We are pursuing alternative approaches to enhancing CMI through the *in situ* stimulation of DCs in the host, for example by targeting DCs with relevant antigens (such as PA and spore coat proteins) fused to an antibody directed at a DC surface receptor, such as DEC205, an approach that has been demonstrated successful in protecting against *Y. pestis* in mice [5]. Here, we have used activated DCs prophylactically to enhance CMI, but appropriately activated DCs could also be used in a post-exposure context to augment the CMI response in the early phase of infection. In conclusion, the *ex vivo* pulsing of DCs with pathogen-derived material and defined stimulatory antigens with CpG, has induced the maturation of DCs *ex vivo* and is able to direct the development of specific and efficacious T cell responses in an *in vivo* murine model of anthrax.

Materials and Methods

Ethics Statement

All animal procedures were performed in accordance with UK legislation as stated in the UK Animal (Scientific Procedures) Act

a)

b)

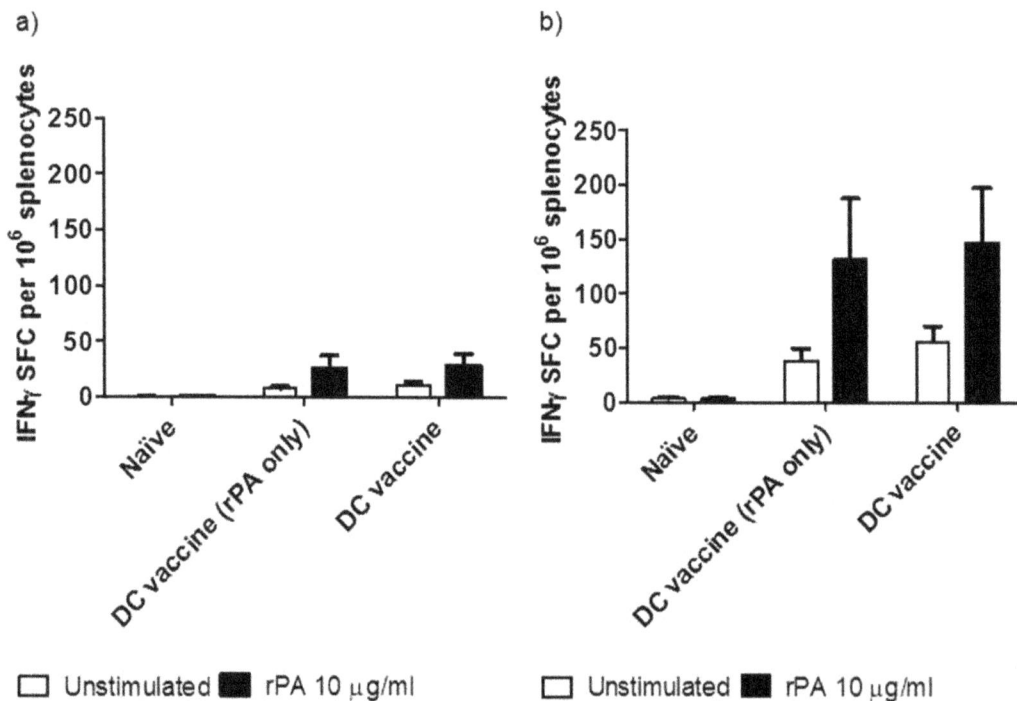

Figure 4. IFNγ spot- forming cells as measured by ELISPOT. DCs were stimulated with rPA, heat killed *B. anthracis* and CpG oligonucleotides and administered i.d. in combination with rPA and alum given i.m to A/J mice. Spleens were taken seven and fourteen days post vaccination and restimulated with rPA. A one-way Anova with Tukey multiple comparison post-hoc test was performed on the results (* $p < 0.05$, ** $p < 0.01$, *** $p < 0.001$). Error bars represent the standard error of the mean calculated from the means of three replicates from five animals.

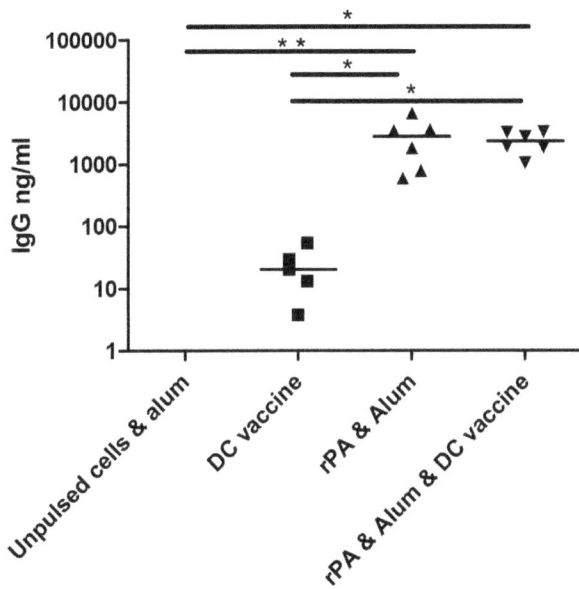

Figure 5. Antibody responses 14 days after either stimulated DCs, or rPA and alum, or both, were administered. Each point represents the mean of three replicates from five animals. A one-way Anova with Tukey multiple comparison post-hoc test was performed on the results (* $p < 0.05$, ** $p < 0.01$, *** $p < 0.001$).

1986. The Institutional Animal Care and Use Committee approved the Project licence (PPL 30/2488) which was granted on 02/11/2008.

All procedures with human blood samples were performed under Ethics Committee approval (reference 05/Q405/71 entitled 'Tissue specific immune regulation by dendritic cells in the intestine and other sites') from the Outer West London Research Ethics Committee (NHS) on 9 March 2010. An amendment to the protocol (Sub Study Version 1.0/dated 29 November 2010) was approved by the NHS on 14 February 2011. This protocol was reviewed by the U.S. Army Medical Research and Materiel Command (USAMRMC), Office of Research Protections (ORP), Human Research Protection Office (HRPO) and found to comply with applicable DOD, U.S. Army, and USAMRMC human subjects protection requirements. All human samples were obtained with written consent from the donor.

Mice

A/J mice were purchased from Charles River U.K. and held in specific pathogen -free facilities with free access to food and water and allowed to acclimatise for seven days prior to use. There is a positive correlation between the immunising dose of rPA and the protective antibody response when using A/J mice, making them a suitable model for anthrax infection studies [13]. Furthermore, A/J mice are deficient in the complement protein C5, making them susceptible to toxigenic *B. anthracis* [14]. Animals undergoing challenge were held in rigid isolators with both inflowing and out-flowing HEPA filtered air.

Murine DC culture method

DCs were prepared using a method modified from previous reports [15], [16]. Briefly, bone marrow was flushed from murine femurs and tibias and passed through a 40 μm cell sieve to create a single cell suspension. Bone marrow cells were washed in complete media (RPMI-1640 supplemented with 10% foetal calf serum, 1%

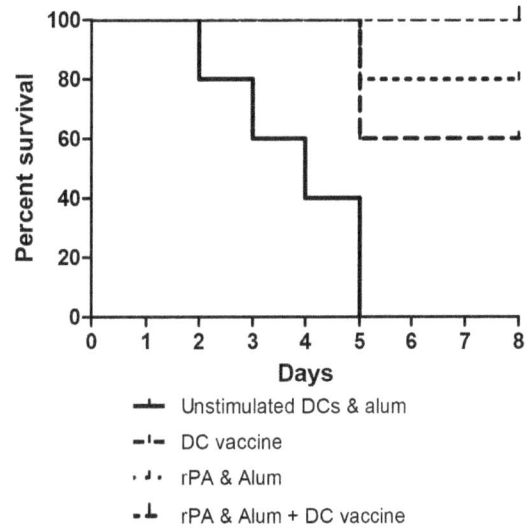

Figure 6. Post Challenge survival. Groups of 5 A/J mice immunised with a DC vaccine (comprising of DCs stimulated overnight with rPA, heat-killed *B. anthracis* and CpG), rPA in alum, or rPA in alum plus DC vaccine, or left naïve, were challenged at 14 days post-immunisation with 3×10^4 CFU *B. anthracis* STI (i.p.) and monitored for survival over the subsequent 8 days. There was a statistically significant difference in the survival curves for the negative control (alum+BMDC&CpG) group compared with the group actively immunised with rPA& alum and also receiving rPA&HK *B.anthracis*-pulsed DC ($p < 0.002$) by both the Mantel-Cox and Gehan-Breslow-Wilcoxon tests. Comparison of survival curves between the negative control (alum+BMDC&CpG) group and the group receiving rPA&HK *B.anthracis*-pulsed DC only, was also statistically significant ($p < 0.01$) when both tests were applied.

penicillin-streptomycin-glutamine and 50 μM 2-mercaptoethanol) and red cells lysed before being washed again. Cells were seeded at 1×10^6 cells mL and cultured in a fully humidified atmosphere at 37°C with 5% CO_2; complete media was supplemented with

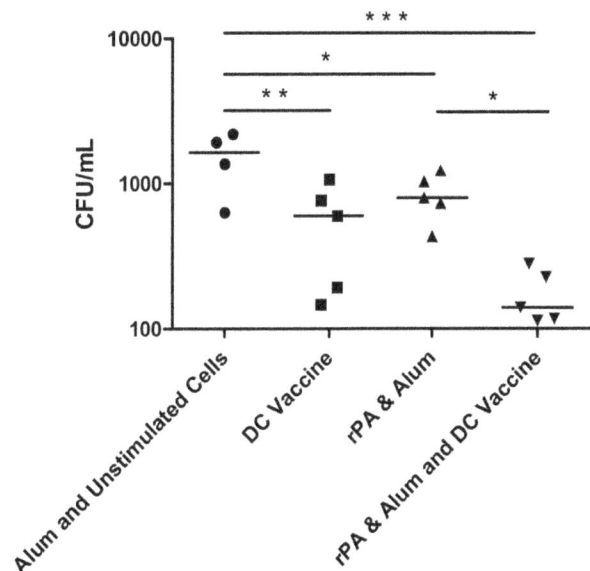

Figure 7. Enumeration of viable *B. anthracis* in the spleens of cohorts of mice two days post challenge. Each point represents the mean of three replicates from five animals, four from the naïve group due to an early death. A one-way Anova with Tukey multiple comparison post-hoc test was performed on the results (* $p < 0.05$, ** $p < 0.01$, *** $p < 0.001$).

20 ng/ml of GM-CSF. Media was replaced at day 3 and 5 before loosely adherent cells were harvested at day 8. Cells were confirmed to be >90% CD11c$^+$ by flow cytometry and used in stimulation assays.

Human DC characterisation method

Human blood was collected from healthy volunteers with no known autoimmune or inflammatory diseases, allergies or malignancies, following informed consent (EC number 05/Q0405/71). Peripheral blood mononuclear cells (PBMC) were obtained by centrifugation over Ficoll-Paque plus (Amersham Biosciences, Chalfont St. Giles, UK). Human low density cells (LDC) were obtained following Nycoprep centrifugation of 20 h.-cultured PBMC prior to antigenic pulsing or T-cell stimulation. Human DC were then identified as HLA-DR$^+$ lineage cocktail (CD3/CD14/CD16/CD19/CD34) live cells by flow cytometry for analysis of co-stimulatory molecules and cytokine production. LDC used as a DC source are 98–100% HLA-DR$^+$, with morphological characteristics of DC (both at optical and electron microscopy) and are potent stimulators of allogeneic naive T cells [17], [18].

Stimulation of dendritic cells

Human and murine DCs were stimulated with rPA, CpG ODN (Invivogen) and heat killed *B. anthracis* prepared using a method previously reported [19]. Briefly, *B. anthracis* (STI strain) spores were harvested and washed three times by centrifugation before being resuspended in PBS. The spore suspension was inactivated by incubation in a water bath for 2 h. at 90°C with occasional shaking. After inactivation the culture was checked for viability by inoculating 10 mL broths with heat-killed suspension and incubating at 37°C for one week. L-agar plates were subsequently inoculated with the entire broth and incubated for a further 7 days. An absence of growth indicated the spore suspension to be inactivated.

Flow cytometry to assess cellular activation

Murine antibodies with the following specificities and conjugations were purchased from Biolegend, CD11c-PeCy7, CD80-PE, CD86-APC, CD40-FITC, MHC-II PerCPCy5.5, together with appropriate isotype matched controls. After staining, cells were fixed with 1% paraformaldehyde in 0.85% saline and stored in the refrigerator prior to acquisition on the flow cytometer, within 48 hours.

Human monoclonal antibodies with the following specificities and conjugations were used: TLR2-FITC (TLR2.3), TLR4-FITC (HTA125), CD40-PE (LOB7/6), DC exclusion cocktail-PE-Cy5 (CD3 (S4.1), CD14 (TUK4), CD16 (3G8), CD19 (SJ25-C1), CD34 (581)) were purchased from AbD Serotec (Oxford, UK). CD83-PE (HB15e), CD80-FITC (L307.4), HLA-DR-FITC/APC (G46-6), CD86-FITC (24F), IL-10-APC (JES3-19F1), IL-12-PE (C11.5), IL-6-FITC (MQ2-13A5), IL-17-PE (SCPL1362), IFNγ-APC (25723.11), FoxP3-PE (259D/C7), CD4-PE (RPA-T4), CD3-PE/PeCy5/APC (UCHT1), CD8-APC (SK1), CD45RO-PE (UCHL1), CD45RA-PeCy5 (H1100) were purchased from BD Biosciences (Oxford, UK). CCR7-PE (150503) and TGFβ-PE (IC388P) were purchased from R&D Systems (Abingdon, UK). Appropriate isotype-matched control antibodies were purchased from the same manufacturers. After staining, cells were fixed with 1% paraformaldehyde in 0.85% saline and stored in the refrigerator prior to acquisition on the flow cytometer, within 48 hours.

Cytokine production by human DC

Intracellular cytokine production by DC was measured following antigenic pulsing of DC via comparison of monensin-treated DC (4 h.) and non-monensin-treated DC (incubated with medium only for 4 h.). Cells were then labelled for surface marker expression using monoclonal antibodies to identify DC as described above, fixed and permeabilised before labelling for cytokines prior to acquisition.

Enrichment of CD4$^+$ naive T cells for human DC stimulation assays

Blood from the same donor as the DC source was used to isolate human CD4$^+$ naive T cells. PBMC were depleted of CD14$^+$, CD19$^+$, HLA-DR$^+$, CD45RO$^+$ and CD8$^+$ cells using immuno-magnetic beads following the manufacturer's instructions. Flow cytometric analysis confirmed that >96% of these cells were CD45$^+$CD4$^+$ T cells (data not shown).

Human DC stimulation of T-cell assays

Human CD4$^+$ naive T cells were CFSE- labelled and incubated for 5 days with enriched syngeneic DC at 2, 4 and 6% (of total T-cell number), providing dose-dependent proliferation of T cells in all cases. Cells were recovered following 5d. culture and CFSE^{lo} proliferating cells were identified, analysed and quantified by flow cytometry.

Immunisations

DCs were prepared as above. For mouse immunisations, 2×10^6 DCs were stimulated with 10 μg/mL rPA, 6 μg/mL CpG and 10^4 CFU/mL heat-killed *B. anthracis* STI for 18 h. at 37°C. Cells were harvested and washed to remove excess antigen and resuspended in PBS. Mice, 5 per group, were immunised intradermally (i.d.) with 1×10^6 cells resuspended in 100 μl PBS on day 0 (the DC vaccine). Alternatively, mice were immunised with rPA and alum and received 10 μg rPA formulated in 100 μl of 0.26% v/v alum, intramuscularly (i.m.), on d.0. Mice receiving both DCs and rPA and alum, received these formulations at the same time on d 0.

ELISPOT

The number of rPA - specific IFNγ$^+$ splenocytes from naïve and immunised mice was assessed using an ELISPOT assay. Briefly, 7 or 14 d. post-immunisation mice were culled, spleens removed and macerated through a cell sieve. Cells were pelleted and red cells removed using lysis buffer before being washed, counted and seeded at 2×10^5 cells per well onto ELISPOT plates coated with anti-mouse IFNγ. Cells were stimulated with rPA, Con A or left unstimulated (media only), overnight in a humidified incubator at 37°C, 5% CO_2. Assay development occurred as per the manufacturer's instructions and plates read using an automated ELISPOT reader. Results are presented as the difference in spot-forming cells per 10^6 splenocytes, between treatment groups.

ELISA

The anti-PA antibody titre was determined as previously reported [20]. Briefly, microtitre plates were coated overnight at 4°C with 5 mg ml^{-1} rPA in PBS. Serum samples were double-diluted in PBS containing 1% w/v skimmed milk powder and incubated for 2 h. at 37°C. Binding of serum antibody was detected using horse-radish peroxidise conjugated goat anti-mouse IgG, diluted 1 in 2000 in PBS, and the substrate 2,20-Azinobis (3-ethylbenzthiazoline-sulfonic acid) (1.09 mM ABTS). Titres were presented as the end-point dilution, which gave an absorbance of

0.1 over background. Group means ± standard error of the mean were calculated.

Challenge

B. anthracis spores of the STI strain were diluted to an estimated challenge dose of 1×10^3 by serial dilution. *B. anthracis* STI is a pX01⁺, pX02⁻ unencapsulated toxigenic strain of *B. anthracis* that has been used previously as a live spore vaccine. Actual challenge dose was calculated by culturing the inoculum on nutrient agar plates for 48 h. Groups of ten mice were challenged intra-peritoneally (i.p.) and monitored, with those showing signs of severe illness humanely culled. Survivors were culled after 8d..

Bacteriology

Five mice per group were culled for bacteriology 2d. after challenge. Spleens were macerated through a wire mesh into sterile PBS. Splenocyte suspensions were serially diluted and 100 μL of each suspension added to nutrient agar in triplicate. Plates were incubated at 37°C for 48 h. before colony forming units (CFU) were enumerated.

Statistical analysis

Statistical analysis using paired and unpaired t-test, and one- and two-way Anova was performed using GraphPad Prism as stated in figure legends, with calculation of mean and standard error of the mean (SEM). Samples were analysed using a one-way-Anova with a Tukey post-hoc test (* p<0.05, ** p<0.01, *** p< 0.001). For comparison of survival curves, the log-rank Mantel-Cox and the Gehan-Breslow-Wilcoxon tests were applied.

Acknowledgments

The authors wish to thank PharmAthene Inc., Annapolis, MD 21401, United States, for permission to use their clinical grade rPA in these studies.

Author Contributions

Conceived and designed the experiments: IJTT ERM NRE SCK DW. Performed the experiments: IJTT ERM NRE MGS DW. Analyzed the data: IJTT ERM SCK DW. Contributed reagents/materials/analysis tools: NRE ERM IJTT. Wrote the paper: IJTT REM SCK DW.

References

1. Banchereau J, Briere F, Caux C, Davoust J, Lebecque S, et al. (2000) Immunobiology of dendritic cells. Annual Review of Immunology 18: 767-+.
2. Mahnke K, Guo M, Lee S, Sepulveda H, Swain SL, et al. (2000) The dendritic cell receptor for endocytosis, DEC-205, can recycle and enhance antigen presentation via major histocompatibility complex class II-positive lysosomal compartments. Journal of Cell Biology 151: 673–683.
3. Banchereau J, Steinman RM (1998) Dendritic cells and the control of immunity. Nature 392: 245–252.
4. Palucka K, Banchereau J (2012) Cancer immunotherapy via dendritic cells. Nature Reviews Cancer 12: 265–277.
5. Do Y, Koh H, Park CG, Dudziak D, Seo P, et al. (2010) Targeting of LcrV virulence protein from Yersinia pestis to dendritic cells protects mice against pneumonic plague. European Journal of Immunology 40: 2791–2796.
6. Okinaka R, Cloud K, Hampton O, Hoffmaster A, Hill K, et al. (1999) Sequence, assembly and analysis of pX01 and pX02. Journal of Applied Microbiology 87: 261–262.
7. Turnbull PCB (1991) Anthrax Vaccines - Past, Present and Future. Vaccine 9: 533–539.
8. Ivins BE, Welkos SL (1988) Recent Advances in the Development of An Improved, Human Anthrax Vaccine. European Journal of Epidemiology 4: 12–19.
9. Reuveny S, White MD, Adar YY, Kafri Y, Altboum Z, et al. (2001) Search for correlates of protective immunity conferred by anthrax vaccine. Infection and Immunity 69: 2888–2893.
10. Welkos S, Little S, Friedlander A, Fritz D, Fellows P (2001) The role of antibodies to Bacillus anthracis and anthrax toxin components in inhibiting the early stages of infection by anthrax spores. Microbiology-Sgm 147: 1677–1685.
11. Ivins BE, Welkos SL, Little SF, Crumrine MH, Nelson GO (1992) Immunization Against Anthrax with Bacillus-Anthracis Protective Antigen Combined with Adjuvants. Infection and Immunity 60: 662–668.
12. Elvin SJ, Healey GD, Westwood A, Knight SC, Eyles JE, et al. (2006) Protection against heterologous Burkholderia pseudomallei strains by dendritic cell immunization. Infection and Immunity 74: 1706–1711.
13. Welkos SL, Friedlander AM (1988) Pathogenesis and Genetic-Control of Resistance to the Sterne Strain of Bacillus-Anthracis. Microbial Pathogenesis 4: 53–69.
14. Welkos SL, Keener TJ, Gibbs PH (1986) Differences in Susceptibility of Inbred Mice to Bacillus-Anthracis. Infection and Immunity 51: 795–800.
15. Inaba K, Inaba M, Romani N, Aya H, Deguchi M, et al. (1992) Generation of Large Numbers of Dendritic Cells from Mouse Bone-Marrow Cultures Supplemented with Granulocyte Macrophage Colony-Stimulating Factor. Journal of Experimental Medicine 176: 1693–1702.
16. Lutz MB, Kukutsch N, Ogilvie ALJ, Rossner S, Koch F, et al. (1999) An advanced culture method for generating large quantities of highly pure dendritic cells from mouse bone marrow. Journal of Immunological Methods 223: 77–92.
17. Knight SC, Farrant J, Bryant A, Edwards AJ, Burman S, et al. (1986) Nonadherent, low-density cells from human peripheral-blood contain dendritic cells and monocytes, both with veiled morphology. Immunology 57: 595–603.
18. Holden NJ, Bedford PA, McCarthy NE, Marks NA, Ind PW, et al. (2008) Dendritic cells from control but not atopic donors respond to contact and respiratory sensitizer treatment in vitro with differential cytokine production and altered stimulatory capacity. Clinical and Experimental Allergy 38: 1148–1159.
19. Healey GD, Elvin SJ, Morton M, Williamson ED (2005) Humoral and cell-mediated adaptive immune responses are required for protection against Burkholderia pseudomallei challenge and bacterial clearance postinfection. Infection and Immunity 73: 5945–5951.
20. Flick-Smith HC, Waters EL, Walker NJ, Miller J, Stagg AJ, et al. (2005) Mouse model characterisation for anthrax vaccine development: comparison of one inbred and one outbred mouse strain. Microbial Pathogenesis 38: 33–40.

12

Elevated Soluble CD163 Plasma Levels Are Associated with Disease Severity in Patients with Hemorrhagic Fever with Renal Syndrome

Junning Wang[1], Weijuan Guo[2], Hong Du[1], Haitao Yu[1], Wei Jiang[1], Ting Zhu[1], Xuefan Bai[1]*, Pingzhong Wang[1]*

1 Department of Infectious Diseases, Tangdu Hospital, Fourth Military Medical University, Xi'an, Shaanxi Province, China, 2 Department of Obstetrics and Gynecology, Chang An Hospital, Xi'an, Shaanxi Province, China

Abstract

Background: Hantaan virus is a major zoonotic pathogen that causesing hemorrhagic fever with renal syndrome (HFRS). Although HFRS pathogenesis has not been entirely elucidated, the importance of host-related immune responses in HFRS pathogenesis has been widely recognized. CD163, a monocyte and macrophage-specific scavenger receptor that plays a vital function in the hosts can reduce inflammation, is shed during activation as soluble CD163 (sCD163). The aim of this study was to investigate the pathological significance of sCD163 in patients with HFRS.

Methods: Blood samples were collected from 81 hospitalized patients in Tangdu Hospital from October 2011 to January 2014 and from 15 healthy controls. The sCD163 plasma levels were measured using a sandwich ELISA, and the relationship between sCD163 and disease severity was analyzed. Furthermore, CD163 expression in 3 monocytes subset was analyzed by flow cytometry.

Results: The results demonstrated that sCD163 plasma levels during the HFRS acute phase were significantly higher in patients than during the convalescent stage and the levels in the healthy controls ($P<0.0001$). The sCD163 plasma levels in the severe/critical group were higher than those in the mild/moderate group during the acute ($P<0.0001$). A Spearman correlation analysis indicated that the sCD163 levels were positively correlated with white blood cell, serum creatine, blood urea nitrogen levels, while they were negatively correlated with blood platelet levels in the HFRS patients. The monocyte subsets were significantly altered during the acute stage. Though the CD163 expression levels within the monocyte subsets were increased during the acute stage, the highest CD163 expression level was observed in the CD14++CD16+ monocytes when compared with the other monocyte subsets.

Conclusion: sCD163 may be correlated with disease severity and the disease progression in HFRS patients; however, the underlying mechanisms should be explored further.

Editor: Jianming Qiu, University of Kansas Medical Center, United States of America

Funding: This work was supported by the National Basic Research Program of China (973 Program) (No. 2012CB518905) and National Natural Science Foundation of China (No. 81373118). The funders had no role in study design, data collection and analysis, decision to publish, or preparation of the manuscript.

Competing Interests: The authors have declared that no competing interests exist.

* Email: wangpz63@126.com (PZW); xfbai2011@163.com (XFB)

Introduction

Hantaviruses are negative-sense, single-stranded, ribonucleic acid (RNA) viruses that belong to the Bunyaviridae family [1]. These viruses cause two obvious syndromes in humans: hemorrhagic fever with renal syndrome (HFRS) in Europe and Asian and hantavirus pulmonary syndrome (HPS) in the Americas. Currently, there are as many as 150,000 cases of HFRS reported annually worldwide [2]. HFRS is endemic in all 33 provinces of the People's Republic of China, where it is a significant public health problem, in which 20,000–50,000 human cases are diagnosed annually [3]. Notably, Xi'an city, which is the central district of the Shaanxi province, had an increasing HFRS

incidence and mortality rate due to HFRS over the last three years [4]. There are five successive clinical phases in typical HFRS patients. These include the fever, hypotensive shock, oliguric, polyuric and convalescent phases. Additionally, some of these phases frequently overlap in severe cases, and several phases are frequently ignored in some mild cases of the disease [5]. The most remarkably pathological characteristics of HFRS are endothelial inflammation, loss of endothelial barrier function, immune cell migration and increased vascular permeability; however, HFRS pathogenesis is not entirely clear. Previous studies revealed that a "cytokine storm", increased immune responses, complement activation and platelet dysfunction might be involved in pathogenesis of HFRS [2,6]. Monocytes and macrophages bridging innate and adaptive immunity, high expression of cytokines activating monocytes and macrophages in the early phase of HFRS supports the immune-mediated pathogenesis [1].

Monocytes and macrophages constitute a significant component of the immune responses against viruses. These cells trigger inflammation as well as bridging innate and adaptive immunity following viral infections [7,8]. Monocytes in circulation represent a heterogeneous population. Three major subsets of monocytes have been identified based upon the relative expression of the lipopolysaccharide co-receptor, CD14 and the FcγRIII receptor, CD16. "Classical" monocytes (CD14++CD16−, Mon1) account for 80–90% of the monocytes in circulation, whereas the "intermediate" (CD14++CD16+, Mon2) and "non-classical" (CD14+CD16++, Mon3) monocyte subsets, of which the latter two subsets are summarized as CD16+ monocytes, account for 10 to 20% of the circulating monocytes [9,10]. The relative monocyte distribution that is observed in circulation is dynamic and changes as a function of the inflammatory and metabolic drivers that impact the differentiation between the subsets and their functions. CD16+ monocytes increase significantly in some inflammatory and immune disorders as well as in infectious conditions. These range from arthritis [11], inflammatory bowel disease [12], acute ischaemic heart failure [13], sepsis [14] to virus infections, such as HIV infection [15] and dengue fever [16].

CD163 is a specific scavenger receptor for hemoglobin/heme in vivo. It includes nine scavenger-receptor cysteine-rich domains that are located on the extracellular side of the monocytes and macrophages membrane [17]. One of its primary and well-described functions is the clearance of extracellular hemoglobin by a means of hemoglobin–haptoglobin complex endocytosis, which thus avoids the oxidative stress associated with free hemoglobin by liberating free iron, bilirubin, and carbon monoxide [18]. CD163 expression levels on monocytes down-regulation by inflammatory cytokines, such as tumor necrosis factor α (TNF-α) and granulocyte–macro-phage colony-stimulating factor (GM-CSF) [19,20]. A soluble form of CD163 is constituted by proteolytic cleavage of the extracellular part of the protein and is shed into circulation. Increased sCD163 levels are associated with both monocyte activation and proliferation during the course of infection or inflammation [21]. The shedding of CD163 is a constitutive process, but it can be increased by various stimuli, such as lipopolysaccharide (LPS), IL-6, and IL-10 [19]. Increased sCD163 serum concentrations have been reported in patients who suffer from various infectious and inflammatory diseases, such as sepsis, tuberculosis, diabetes, acquired immune deficiency syndrome, dengue fever, rheumatoid arthritis and hemophagocytosis [22,23]; however, the physiological role of sCD163 was unknown, until now.

This aims of this study were to observe the CD163 expression levels on peripheral blood monocyte subsets and the plasma sCD163 levels in HFRS patients and to further analyze the correlation among CD163, sCD163 and disease severity.

Methods

Ethics Statement

The study protocol conformed with the Declaration of Helsinki (2008 version) and was approved by the Ethics Committee of Tangdu Hospital, the Fourth Military Medical University. Written informed consent was obtained from all study participants.

Patients

Eighty-one hospitalized HFRS patients were enrolled in the study from October 2011 to January 2014 at Tangdu Hospital, the Fourth Military Medical University (Xi'an, China) (see Table 1). The clinical HFRS diagnosis was confirmed serologically by detection of IgM and IgG antibodies that were specific to the HTNV nucleocapsid protein [24]. Fifteen healthy volunteers were also included in the study as normal controls. Blood samples were collected from the patients during their hospitalization. All of the blood samples were separated into plasma and peripheral blood mononuclear cells (PBMC), then they were frozen at −80°C or liquid nitrogen until further use. The clinical parameters were collected during the patient hospitalizations, using routine hospital laboratory techniques.

According to the laboratory parameters and symptoms, such as body temperature, hemorrhage, edema, blood pressure and urine volume, the degree of HFRS disease severity was classified into the four clinical types, as formerly described [25]. These types were classified as: (1) mild, which included mild renal failure without an obvious oliguric stage and hypotension; (2) moderate, which included evident uremia, effusion (bulbar conjunctiva), hemorrhage (skin and mucous membrane) and acute renal failure with an obvious oliguric stage; (3) severe, which included severe uremia, effusion (bulbar conjunctiva and either pleura or peritoneum), hemorrhage (skin and mucous membrane), and acute renal failure with oliguria (a urine output of 100–500 ml/day) for ≤5 days or anuria (a urine output of <100 ml/day) for ≤2 days; and (4) critical, which were cases with one or more of the following symptoms compared with the severe patients: refractory shock (≥2 days), visceral hemorrhage, heart failure, pulmonary edema, brain edema, severe secondary infection and severe acute renal failure with oliguria (a urine output of 50–500 ml/day) for >5 days or anuria (a urine output of <100 ml/day) for >2 days, or a blood urea nitrogen level of >42.84 mmol/L. The exclusion criteria were: (1) any other kidney disease, (2) diabetes mellitus, (3) autoimmune disease, (4) hematological disease, (5) cardiovascular disease, (6) viral hepatitis (types A, B, C, D or E), and (7) any other liver disease. In addition, none received corticosteroids or other immunomodulatory drugs during the study period.

PBMC Isolation

PBMC from the healthy controls and HFRS patients were obtained from 20 ml of heparinized venous blood using density gradient centrifugation with lymphoprep 1.077 g/ml (d = 1.077 g/ml; Sigma-Aldrich, America). The PBMCs were harvested from the interface and washed twice in RPMI-1640. The PBMC viability was >95% after Trypan Blue exclusion. The PBMCs were then aliquoted and resuspended in 1 ml fetal calf serum and freeze media (10% DMSO in RPMI-1640) and stored initially at −70°C for 24 hours before introduction into liquid nitrogen cryopreservation for later analysis. All PBMC samples were obtained at the same time as the plasma samples that were used to measure sCD163.

Flow cytometry

Frozen PBMCs were quickly thawed in a 37°C water bath, until only a small crystal remained, and washed twice in 10 ml of heated RPMI with 10% fetal bovine serum. The thawed cells that were used for staining were incubated with 10% FCS at 37°C for 30 minutes prior to staining. The cells were then resuspended at a final concentration of 1×10^6 PBMCs/ml. A separate aliquot of cells were stained with a cocktail composed of 20 μl CD14 (anti-CD14-FITC, clone M5E2, BD Biosciences, San Jose, CA, USA), 5 μl CD16 (anti-CD16-APC, clone B73.1 BD Biosciences, San Jose, CA, USA), and 20 μl CD163 (anti-CD163-PE, clone GHI/61, BD Biosciences, San Jose, CA, USA). The cells were incubated in the dark for 30 min at 4°C. Following incubation, the cells were

Table 1. The HFRS Patient Clinical Characteristics.

	Mild	Moderate	Severe	Critical
Demographic characteristics				
Patient number	12	21	25	23
Sample number	19	39	49	38
Age (years)	40 (34–45)	41 (31–51)	44 (36–52)	39 (38–58)
Males (%)	63.6	70.8	70.0	82.6
The clinical parameters at acute stage				
sCD163 (mg/l)	2.07 (1.76–2.73)	3.31 (2.67–3.70)	3.93 (2.96–5.82)	5.03 (4.43–9.34)
WBC ($\times 10^3$/μL)	8.2 (5.5–13.3)	10.3 (8.8–18.7)	16.8 (10.9–22.4)	16.5 (12.8–35.2)
IFN-γ (pg/ml)	40.4 (24.7–54.8)	31.7 (22.2–77.3)	63.1 (41.8–118.1)	115.4 (32.6–180.1)
IL-6 (pg/ml)	24.5 (13.6–36.4)	30.5 (19.1–59.3)	48.8 (25.4–110.0)	114.5 (38.7–216.2)
PLT ($\times 10^3$/μL)	88.5 (62.7–103.5)	48.5 (34.3–98.3)	35.0 (23.5–44.5)	26.2 (16.3–60.2)
BUN (μmol/L)	5.5 (3.6–10.6)	15.1 (9.3–20.2)	22.7 (17.1–27.1)	16.6 (11.5–27.1)
Cr (μmol/L)	78 (69–219)	216 (135.5–299)	330 (243–544)	271 (189–398)
Monocyte ($\times 10^9$/L)	0.68 (0.48–2.12)	1.21 (0.88–1.88)	2.31 (1.51–2.96)	2.32 (1.34–3.91)

Values represent medians with their corresponding interquartile ranges. Acute stage include the febrile, hypotensive and oliguria phases.
Abbreviations: sCD163, soluble CD163; IL-6, Interleukin-6; IFN-γ, interferon–γ; WBC, white blood cells; PLT, platelet count; BUN, blood urea nitrogen; Scr, serum creatinine.

washed in 2 ml of cold PBS, pH 7.4. The flow cytometric analysis was performed within 1 hour using a FACS Aria II analyzer (BD Biosciences, San Jose, CA, USA). Monocytes were identified based on their forward and side scatter appearance. We recorded 100,000 events for each sample, CD14 and CD16 were used as monocyte markers, isotype-matched controls were used according to the manufacturer's recommendations, and the percentage of positive cells for each individual marker were obtained after monocyte gating. The percentage of CD163 positive monocytes out of the total monocyte population was recorded and analyzed. The data were analyzed with FlowJo software, version 7.6.1 (Oregon, USA).

ELISA assays

One hundred and forty-five plasma samples were obtained from 81 HFRS patients and 15 healthy control subjects and were stored at $-80°C$ until later use. The sCD163, IL-6 and IFN-γ concentration measurements were obtained by a double antibody sandwich ELISA (Human sCD163 ELISA Ready-SET Go! eBioscience Products, Catalog Number: 88-50360; IL-6 and IFN-γ, Mabtech Products, Catalog Number: 3424-1H-2, 3460-1H-2). In this study, duplicate wells were used to detect the plasma sCD163, IL-6 and IFN-γ concentrations. Each examination step was carried out strictly following the product manual.

Statistical analyses

The analyses were performed with the SPSS 17.0 (SPSS Inc, Chicago, IL, USA) and GraphPad Prism 5 software packages (GraphPad Software, San Diego CA). Medians and interquartile ranges were calculated for the continuous variables and numbers and percentages were calculated for the categorical variables. A Kruskal-Wallis test performed for analysis of variation among multiple groups. Mann–Whitney U tests were used to compare the sCD163 levels between the two independent groups. Correlations were compared with a Spearman's correlation analysis. All of the tests were two-sided and P values that were less than 0.05 were considered to be statistically significant.

Results

Clinical parameters and demographic conditions of HFRS patients

A total of 81 patients were confirmed to be HFRS following HTNV IgM and IgG specific antibody detection evaluations from the patients' serum specimens. From these patients, 145 plasma samples were collected during the febrile/hypotensive (Febr/Hypo), oliguric (Olig), diuretic (Diur), and convalescent (Conv) disease stages. On the basis of the clinical records and diagnostic criteria, 12, 21, 25, and 23 patients were classified as having mild, moderate, severe, and critical HFRS types, respectively. The clinical parameter specifics that were detected during the HFRS patient hospitalizations are summed in Table 1.

Changes in the soluble CD163 plasma level in the HFRS patients

The median sCD163 levels during the febrile/hypotensive, oliguric, diuretic, and convalescent stages, as well as in the normal controls, were 3.75 mg/l, 3.58 mg/l, 2.43 mg/l, 1.80 mg/l, and 0.81 mg/l, respectively. On the basis of the clinical disease course classification criteria, the acute phase comprised the febrile, hypotensive and oliguric stages, and the convalescent phase comprised the diuretic and convalescent stages [26]. During the acute phase, the sCD163 in the HFRS patient plasma samples was obviously higher than the levels observed in the normal controls (febrile/hypotensive or oliguric vs. NC, $P < 0.0001$). The plasma sCD163 level in the HFRS patients decreased during the convalescent phase (febrile/hypotensive vs. diuretic or convalescent, $P < 0.0001$; oliguric vs. convalescent, $P = 0.001$); however, it was still higher than the levels observed in the normal controls (diuretic vs. NC, $P = 0.004$) (Figure 1A). The plasma sCD163 levels in the patients with different disease severities displayed a similar change trend; however, a more distinct decline was observed in the severe/critical patient group (Figure 1B and 1D, $P<0.0001$). The sCD163 concentration in the acute phase was higher than the level that was observed during the convalescent phase in the HFRS patients (Figure 1C, $P<0.001$). The sCD163 concentration was also obviously higher during the acute and convalescent phases in the HFRS patients compared with those in the normal controls ($P<0.0001$), (Figure 1C and 1D). The sCD163 plasma levels in the severe/critical group were higher than those in the mild/moderate group during the acute ($P<0.0001$) (Figure 1E). The plasma sCD163 levels in the mild/moderate group were compared with those in the severe/critical group, and only 4 (13.7%) of the 29 mild/moderate group cases had plasma sCD163 levels that were over 4 mg/l, while 28 (60.8%) of the 46 severe/critical group cases had sCD163 levels that were over 4 mg/l (a 4.3-fold change between the high vs. mild/moderate groups). These results demonstrate that there was some kind of an association between the plasma sCD163 concentrations and the disease severity during the HFRS course.

The correlation between the sCD163 levels and clinical parameters

The relationships between the plasma sCD163 concentrations in the HFRS subjects and the key clinical parameters that can represent the disease severity were analyzed. A Spearman correlation analysis showed that the increased sCD163 concentration was positively correlated with the increased WBC (Figure 2A, r = 0.5322, $P<0.0001$), Crea (Figure 2C, r = 0.3718, $P<0.0001$), BUN (Figure 2D, r = 0.38, $P<0.0001$) levels, and negatively correlated with the decreased PLT counts (Figure 2B, r = −0.6109, $P<0.0001$) in the HFRS patients.

Monocyte subsets were altered in patients with HFRS

Monocytes and their subsets were identified by flow cytometry based on their forward and side scatter characteristics and by their CD14 and CD16 expression levels [27]. The gating strategy used to identify the classical (CD14++CD16−), intermediate (CD14++CD16+), and non-classical monocytes (CD14+CD16++) is shown in Figure 3C. Additionally, summary figures are displayed in Figures 3D, 3E, and 3F. The intermediate monocyte proportions (CD14++CD16+) were significantly increased during the patients of acute phase (median = 18.5%, interquartile range IQR = 15.3%–24.9%, $P<0.0001$) compared with the patients of convalescent phase (median = 6.5%, IQR = 5.1%–8.5%) and the healthy control (median = 5.0%, IQR = 3.3%–7.1%). However, no significant differences ($P> 0.05$) were observed between the convalescent phase and healthy control proportions, (Figures 3E). The classical (CD14++CD16−) and non-classical (CD14+CD16++) monocyte proportions were both significantly decreased during the acute phase (median = 68.4%, IQR = 61.8%–75.1%, and median = 1.6%, IQR = 1.1%–2.58%, $P<0.0001$) compared with those during the convalescent phase (median = 80.0%, IQR = 76.5%–81.6% and median = 3.6%, IQR = 2.5%–5.5%) and in the healthy controls (median = 83.0%, IQR = 80.1%–84.7% and median = 4.5%, IQR = 3.2%–6.1%); however no significant differences between both monocyte subsets ($P>0.05$) were observed between the patients of convalescent phase and the healthy controls, (Figures 3D and 3F).

The CD163 expression on the monocyte subsets

As is known, the CD163 expression on the monocyte subsets surface is different [15]. In this study, we confirmed that the CD163 expression on the CD14++CD16+ monocyte subset was most highly expressed compared with less expression on the CD14++CD16− monocyte subset and lower levels on the CD14+CD16++ monocyte subset (Figure 4B). CD163 expression on the CD14++CD16+ monocyte was more remarkable during the acute

phase (median = 64.2%, IQR = 38.8%–88.5%, $P<0.0001$) than during the convalescent phase (median = 17.3%, IQR = 11.3%–24.5%) in the HFRS patients and healthy controls (median = 16.3%, IQR = 9.4%–21.3%); however no significant ($P>0.05$) differences were observed during the convalescent phase and in the healthy controls. CD163 expression on the classical and non-classical monocytes were increased during the acute phase (median = 43.6%, IQR = 25.9%–68.8% and median = 30.0%, IQR = 22.4%–48.6%, $P<0.0001$) when compared with the convalescent phase (median = 14.0%, IQR = 8.1%–16.5% and median = 12.3%, IQR = 9.1%–21.1%) and healthy control findings (median = 11.6%, IQR = 8.3%–16.2% and median = 9.6%, IQR = 6.7%–15.4%); however, no significant differences ($P>0.05$) were observed in the convalescent phase and healthy control samples, (Figure 4B).

The sCD163 levels correlated with frequency of monocytes

There was a correlation between the sCD163 levels and the absolute monocyte counts, increased CD14++CD16+ monocyte percentage, and the CD163 expression on CD14++CD16+ monocyte. A Spearman correlation analysis demonstrated that the increasing sCD163 level was positively correlated with the increasing monocyte absolute counts (Figure 5A, r = 0.6673, $P<0.0001$), CD14++CD16+ monocytes (Figure 5B, r = 0.5779, $P<0.0001$) and the CD163 expression on CD14++CD16+ monocyte (Figure 5C, r = 0.6245, $P<0.0001$) in the HFRS patients.

The correlation between the sCD163 levels and cytokine

There was a correlation between the sCD163 plasma levels and IL-6 and IFN-γ plasma levels in the HFRS patients. A Spearman correlation analysis showed that the increased sCD163 concentration was positively correlated with the increased IL-6 (Figure 6A, r = 0.4837, $P<0.0001$), IFN-γ (Figure 6B, r = 0.4929, $P<0.0001$) concentration in the HFRS patients.

Discussion

Our study reports that the plasma levels of sCD163, a surface marker that is shed by monocytes, were significantly higher in HFRS patients during the acute phase than in the healthy controls and during patients of the convalescent stage. Importantly, the sCD163 plasma levels in the severe/critical group were higher than those in the mild/moderate group during the acute. The plasma sCD163 level elevation was also closely related to the clinical parameters in the present study. Additionally, we demonstrated that CD14++CD16+ monocyte ratio increased significantly during the acute phase. However, the CD14++CD16− and CD14+CD16++ monocyte ratios were reduced. Though the CD163 expression on the three monocyte subsets was increased during the acute stage, the CD163 expression on the CD14++CD16+ monocytes was the highest levels compared with the CD163 expression on the other monocyte subsets. This is consistent with research that evaluated HIV infection [15]. Additionally, the plasma sCD163 levels correlated with expansion of the CD14++CD16+ monocytes and increased CD163 expression on CD14++CD16+ monocyte. Overall, these results suggest that sCD163 is a novel marker for HFRS, and likely, the monocyte-mediated disease progression that is associated with Hantaviruses infection.

In our study, sCD163 levels were elevated during the acute stage; however, they fell gradually during the recovery stage. This is in agreement with a previous observation in malaria patients [28]. The sCD163 plasma levels in the severe/critical group were

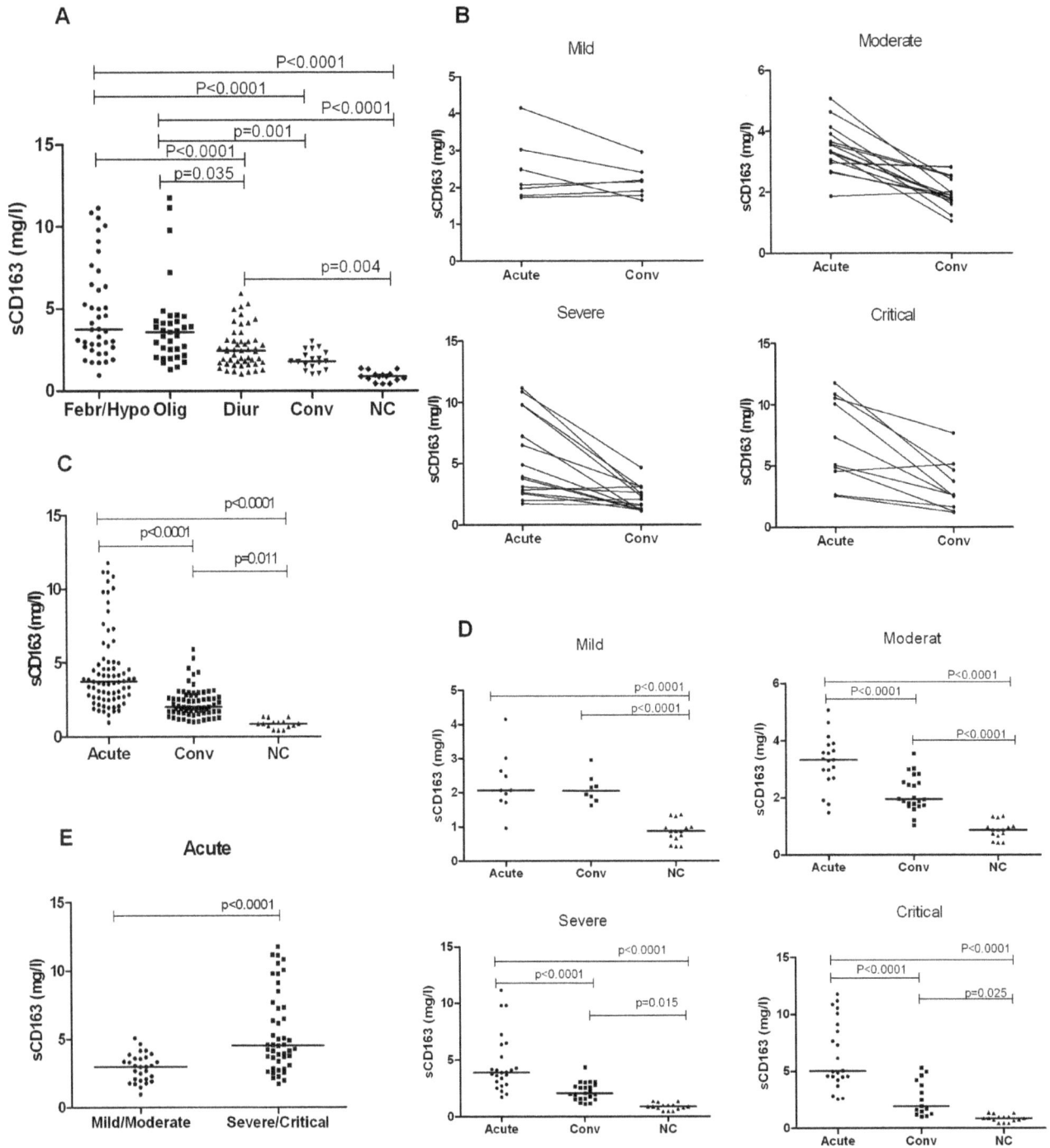

Figure 1. The obvious changes in the soluble CD163 (sCD163) plasma levels in the different HFRS severity patient groups. (A) Comparison of plasma sCD163 levels at the different HFRS stages in the patients. Data were obtained from 145 plasma samples that were collected during the febrile/hypotensive (Febr/Hypo), oliguric (Olig), diuretic (Diur), and convalescent (Conv) HFRS phases in the patients and from 15 healthy subject plasma samples that were used as normal controls (NC). Significant differences were observed between the following stage comparisons: febrile/hypotensive or oliguric vs. NC (P<0.0001); febrile/hypotensive vs. diuretic or convalescent (P<0.0001); oliguric vs. diuretic (P = 0.035), oliguric vs. convalescent (P = 0.001); and diuretic vs. NC (P = 0.004). (B) The plasma sCD163 level changes in the acute (which included the febrile, hypotensive, and oliguric stages) and convalescent phase samples (which included the diuretic and convalescent stages) of the same patient in the different disease severity groups are represented. (C) The changes in the patient sCD163 plasma levels of the acute and convalescent phases when compared with the normal controls. (D) The changes in the sCD163 plasma levels during the acute phase and convalescent phases when compare with the normal controls in the different disease severity groups. (E) Comparison of the acute phase sCD163 levels between the mild/moderate and the severe/critical groups. The significance of the differences among the multiple groups was determined with the Kruskal-Wallis test. The significance of the differences between the two groups was determined with the Mann–Whitney U test. Black lines represent medians and the P values are plotted in each graph.

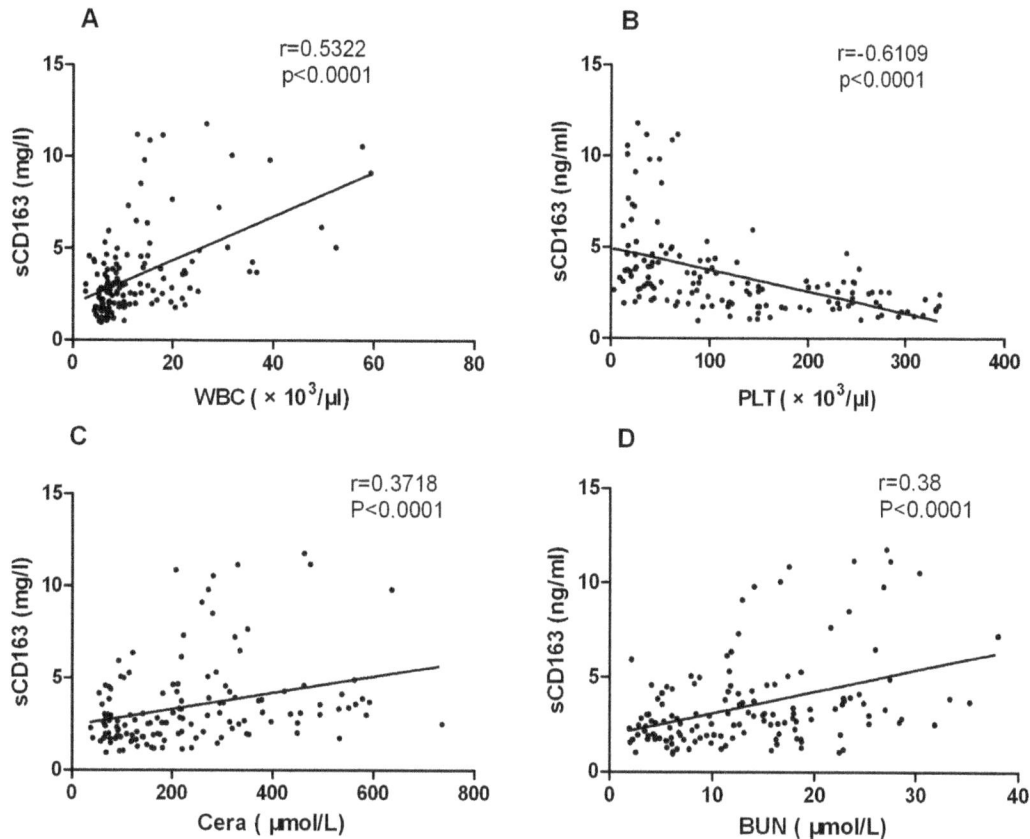

Figure 2. The relationship between elevated sCD163 plasma levels and the clinical parameters. The values are derived from the same blood sample from the HFRS subjects during hospitalization. The Spearman correlation test was used to test the correlation between the sCD163 levels and clinical parameters. The serum sCD163 concentrations were positively correlated with the white blood cells (WBC) (A), creatinine (Crea) (C), and the blood urea nitrogen (BUN) (D) levels for the entire group of subjects while they were negatively correlated with the platelet count (PLT) (B) levels. The r and P values are indicated in the graphs.

higher than those in the mild/moderate group during the acute, and interestingly, the mild/moderate group still had elevated sCD163, which suggested that monocyte activation occurs even with moderate disease during the acute stage, albeit to a lower extent. The sCD163, but not the membrane-bound form, might have anti-inflammatory functions because it inhibits T lymphocyte activation and proliferation in vitro [29]. The binding of Hb-Hp complexes to sCD163 has been shown to inhibit the supply of heme iron that is available for hemolysis that is caused by a bacterial infection [30]. Furthermore, during the innate immune response, CD163 plays a vital function in the hosts ability to reduce inflammation [31]. Interestingly, several inflammatory processes are associated with elevated sCD163 levels [31,32,33,34,35]. Because HFRS is associated with a higher inflammatory response and many inflammatory cytokines and chemokines are involved in the process, our research team [36] evaluated the serum TNF-α, IL-6, IL-4, IL-8,interferon (IFN)-γ, IP-10, and chemokine (C–C motif) ligand 5 levels in HFRS patients. The data showed that significant changes in serum TNF-α, IL-8, IFN-γ, IL-6, IP-10 and RANTES concentrations occurred in patients as they progressed through the different HFRS phases. In this experimental study, our found that increased sCD163 concentration was positively correlated with the increased IL-6 and IFN-γ. It seems that Hantaan virus infections induced over production of many inflammatory cytokines, known as a "cytokine storm" during the early stage. The increased sCD163 concentration

during the acute stage most likely serves as a counter regulatory mechanism against inflammation. These results could be interpreted together with previous reports to suggest that CD163 might have a key position in the infectious diseases [23]. The membrane-bound CD163 receptor itself has anti-inflammatory capabilities by scavenging plasma hemoglobin and the products formed from toxic heme decomposition [37].

There was also a positive correlation observed between elevated plasma sCD163 levels and BUN and Cr levels, which was previously shown to predict kidney dysfunction in HFRS patients [25]. This suggests that sCD163 might be involved in renal dysfunction. In fact, studies have shown that in PUUV infected patients, acute hantavirus infection was associated with immune reaction-induced renal tissue damage [38]. Sustained inflammation can lead to renal dysfunction, and vice-versa, renal dysfunction can fuel the inflammatory response; therefore, it is not surprising that sCD163 in our study kept rising in patients who developed kidney dysfunction. Elevated sCD163 levels have been reported in chronic kidney disease patients [39]. Hemolysis, disseminated intravascular coagulation (DIC), and bleeding are characteristic clinical manifestations for HFRS [1,24] and result in hemoglobin/heme release, which yields ferrous ions. At the same time, oxidation reduction reactions that catalyze hydrogen peroxide give rise to oxygen free radical release, which causes injury to the kidney and other organs [40]. Therefore, timely hemoglobin/heme clearance is required to avoid its excessive

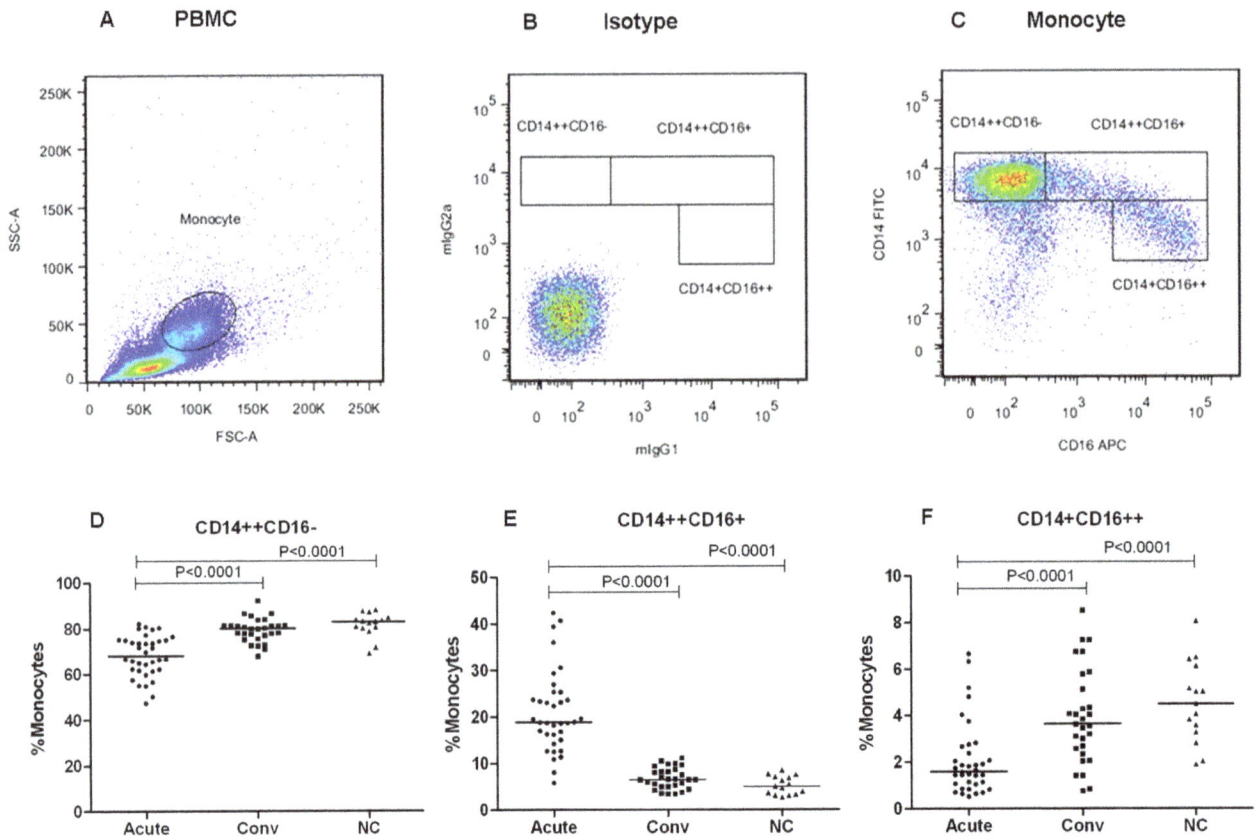

Figure 3. The monocyte subset proportions were altered in the HFRS subjects. A representative example of the monocyte subset analysis procedure is displayed (A, B, and C). (A) Monocytes from the total PBMC population were identified by forward (FSC) and side scatter (SSC) property analysis. (B) The isotypic negative control staining of CD14 and CD16 is displayed. (C) Using surface CD14 and CD16 expression, monocyte gated populations were further divided into three monocyte subsets, which were classic (CD14++CD16−), intermediate (CD14++CD16+) and non-classical monocytes (CD14+CD16++). A summary of the monocyte subset distribution analyses during the acute and convalescent HFRS phases and in the healthy subjects is displayed (D, E, and F). The significance of the differences among the multiple groups was determined by the Kruskal-Wallis test, Black lines represent medians and P values are plotted in each graph.

discharge into the blood and the outbreak of critical pathological responses. Hemoglobin/heme can only be cleared by monocyte/ macrophage phagocytes when combined with haptoglobin and CD163 recognition [18]. sCD163 is shed from monocyte surfaces and, for this reason, we speculate that plasma sCD163 is likely to be highly expressed during HFRS and reflects kidney injury during this disease. However, there are no reports regarding this issue.

In the acute stage, CD163 expression on monocyte subset was increased. We showed that CD163 is more highly expressed on CD14++CD16+ monocytes compared with CD14++CD16− and CD14+CD16++ monocytes. Additionally, we showed a significant correlation between plasma sCD163 levels and the percentage of CD14++CD16+ monocytes and CD163 expression on CD14++ CD16+ monocyte. This suggests that the sCD163 that is shed during Hantavirus infection is likely from CD14++CD16+ monocytes. These results may be support the hypothesis that CD14++CD16+ monocytes contribute to reduce inflammation reaction through anti-inflammatory mediator production that, in turn, inhibits T-cell differentiation and maturation. Other study found that CD14++CD16+ monocyte expansion also corresponded with disease progression in other diseases, including HIV infection [15], and in acute coronary syndrome [27]. Additionally, in the patients of convalescent phase, plasma sCD163 levels were

still higher than the normal control levels; however, the membrane-bound CD163 levels were not significantly different between the HFRS and normal control groups. Thus, it is possible that plasma sCD163 also comes from activated tissue macrophages [33]. Monocytes stay in circulation for only 1 to 3 days and then migrate to peripheral tissues either spontaneously or upon stimulation [41]. Monocytes are known to migrate to the vascular endothelium, secrete cytokines, and be involved in endothelial dysfunction, which leads to increased endothelial permeability [42]. There are several conflicting reports regarding CD163 protein expression on monocytes. Some studies have shown that during chronic inflammation, surface CD163 expression is decreased [32,43]. However, during acute inflammation, surface CD163 expression is increased [44,45]. Additionally, through CD163 shedding, decreased surface CD163 expression was followed by the recovery and induction of surface CD163 to higher levels [46]. We speculate that surface CD163 expression might vary according to different inflammatory states in patients and during different inflammation stages.

Although we obtained some significant results, the present study has limitations. It has to be emphasized that this study only shows associations without providing evidence for possible causal mechanisms. Additionally, there were a relatively small number of patients in this study. More research is needed, with a large

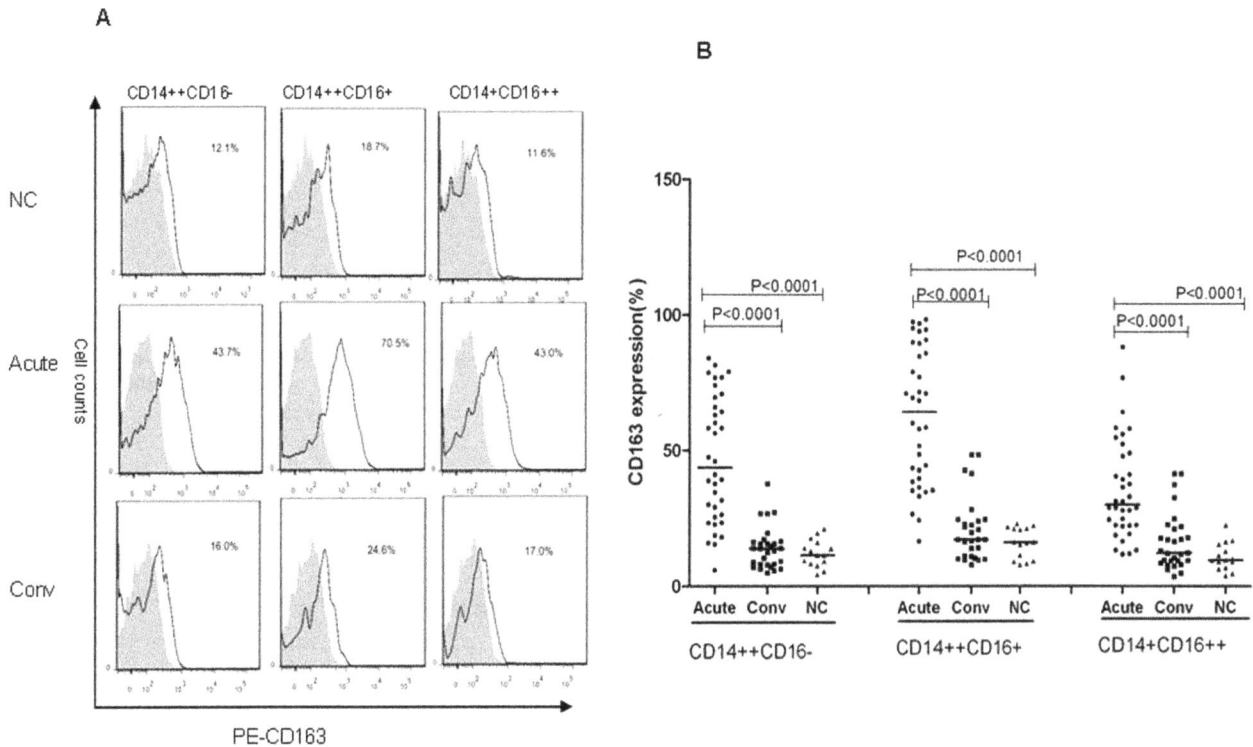

Figure 4. CD163 was differentially expressed on the monocyte subsets. (A) CD163 protein expression (black lines) in each monocyte subset is shown compared with the matched isotype control (shaded histograms) in the histograms. The data illustrate results from a representative experiment. (B) The CD163 expression summary data for the three monocyte subsets during the acute and convalescent phases and in the normal controls. The significance of the differences among the multiple groups was determined with the Kruskal-Wallis test. The black lines represent medians and *P* values are plotted for each graph.

sample and multi-center study, to improve our insight into the physiology and time course of sCD163 release and its relation with HFRS. This may be helpful for us to further understand the pathogenesis of the disease and to offer some useful information for HFRS prevention and treatment.

In conclusion, we have identified the presence of the protein marker, sCD163, in HFRS patients, which is shed from monocytes and macrophages and is related to monocyte expansion. Additionally, sCD163 levels may be useful in predicting

Hantavirus disease progression. This is the first observation that evaluated Hantaviruses infected patients with a plasma marker that is both exclusive to monocytes and an innate immune system activation marker that parallels severity and reflects the clinical parameters. Our findings indicate that sCD163 may serve as a useful biomarker for HFRS, but the underlying mechanisms should be explored further.

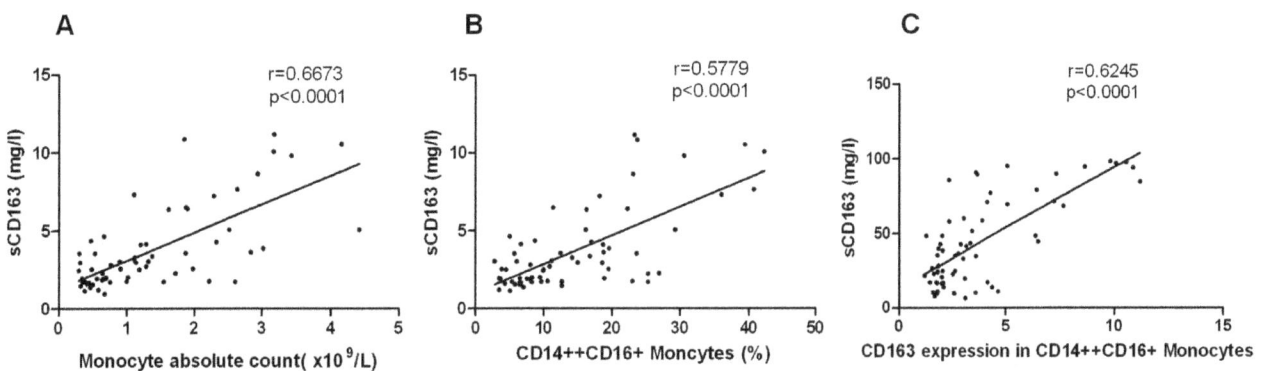

Figure 5. The sCD163 levels correlated with frequency of monocytes. Relationship between elevated plasma sCD163 levels and the absolute monocyte counts (A), intermediate (CD14++CD16+) monocyte percentage (B), and CD163 expression on the intermediate (CD14++CD16+) monocytes (C) evaluated by the Spearman correlation test, The values were derived from the same HFRS patient blood samples during their hospitalizations. The r and *P* values are indicated in the graphs.

A

B

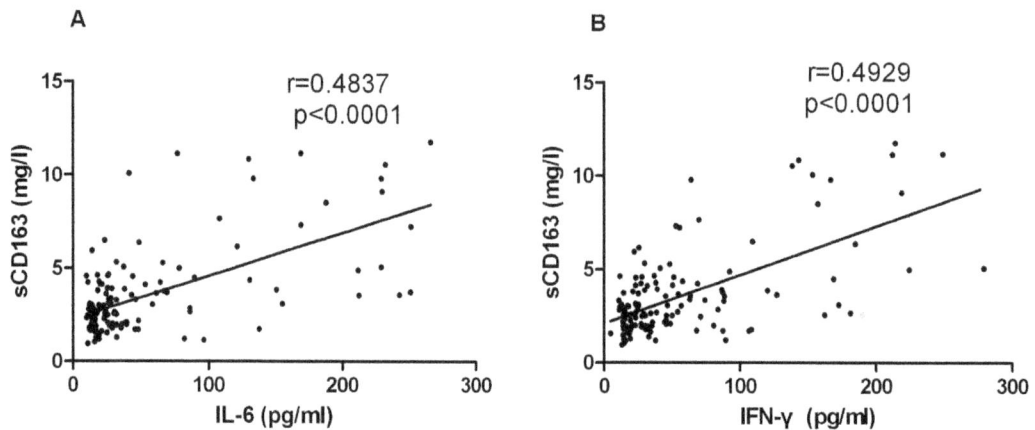

Figure 6. The sCD163 levels correlated with IL-6 and IFN-γ. Relationship between elevated plasma sCD163 levels and IL-6 (A) and IFN-γ (B) plasma levels evaluated by the Spearman correlation test. The values were derived from the same HFRS patient blood samples during their hospitalizations. The r and *P* values are indicated in the graphs.

Acknowledgments

The authors would like to express thanks to their colleagues from the Center of Infectious Diseases for their valuable support during this study.

References

1. Mustonen J, Makela S, Outinen T, Laine O, Jylhava J, et al. (2013) The pathogenesis of nephropathia epidemica: new knowledge and unanswered questions. Antiviral Res 100: 589–604.
2. Jonsson CB, Figueiredo LT, Vapalahti O (2010) A global perspective on hantavirus ecology, epidemiology, and disease. Clin Microbiol Rev 23: 412–441.
3. Zhang YH, Ge L, Liu L, Huo XX, Xiong HR, et al. (2014) The epidemic characteristics and changing trend of hemorrhagic Fever with renal syndrome in hubei province, china. PLoS One 9: e92700.
4. Du H, Li J, Jiang W, Yu H, Zhang Y, et al. (2014) Clinical study of critical patients with hemorrhagic fever with renal syndrome complicated by acute respiratory distress syndrome. PLoS One 9: e89740.
5. Schmaljohn C, Hjelle B (1997) Hantaviruses: a global disease problem. Emerg Infect Dis 3: 95–104.
6. Penttinen K, Lahdevirta J, Kekomaki R, Ziola B, Salmi A, et al. (1981) Circulating immune complexes, immunoconglutinins, and rheumatoid factors in nephropathia epidemica. J Infect Dis 143: 15–21.
7. Cassetta L, Cassol E, Poli G (2011) Macrophage polarization in health and disease. ScientificWorldJournal 11: 2391–2402.
8. Barbosa RR, Silva SP, Silva SL, Tendeiro R, Melo AC, et al. (2012) Monocyte activation is a feature of common variable immunodeficiency irrespective of plasma lipopolysaccharide levels. Clin Exp Immunol 169: 263–272.
9. Pedraza-Sanchez S, Hise AG, Ramachandra L, Arechavaleta-Velasco F, King CL (2013) Reduced frequency of a CD14+ CD16+ monocyte subset with high Toll-like receptor 4 expression in cord blood compared to adult blood contributes to lipopolysaccharide hyporesponsiveness in newborns. Clin Vaccine Immunol 20: 962–971.
10. Ghigliotti G, Barisione C, Garibaldi S, Brunelli C, Palmieri D, et al. (2013) CD16(+) monocyte subsets are increased in large abdominal aortic aneurysms and are differentially related with circulating and cell-associated biochemical and inflammatory biomarkers. Dis Markers 34: 131–142.
11. Coulthard LR, Geiler J, Mathews RJ, Church LD, Dickie LJ, et al. (2012) Differential effects of infliximab on absolute circulating blood leucocyte counts of innate immune cells in early and late rheumatoid arthritis patients. Clin Exp Immunol 170: 36–46.
12. Koch S, Kucharzik T, Heidemann J, Nusrat A, Luegering A (2010) Investigating the role of proinflammatory CD16+ monocytes in the pathogenesis of inflammatory bowel disease. Clin Exp Immunol 161: 332–341.
13. Wrigley BJ, Shantsila E, Tapp LD, Lip GY (2013) CD14++CD16+ monocytes in patients with acute ischaemic heart failure. Eur J Clin Invest 43: 121–130.
14. Zhang D, He J, Shen M, Wang R (2014) CD16 inhibition increases host survival in a murine model of severe sepsis. J Surg Res 187: 605–609.
15. Tippett E, Cheng WJ, Westhorpe C, Cameron PU, Brew BJ, et al. (2011) Differential expression of CD163 on monocyte subsets in healthy and HIV-1 infected individuals. PLoS One 6: e19968.
16. Azeredo EL, Neves-Souza PC, Alvarenga AR, Reis SR, Torrentes-Carvalho A, et al. (2010) Differential regulation of toll-like receptor-2, toll-like receptor-4,

CD16 and human leucocyte antigen-DR on peripheral blood monocytes during mild and severe dengue fever. Immunology 130: 202–216.
17. Moestrup SK, Moller HJ (2004) CD163: a regulated hemoglobin scavenger receptor with a role in the anti-inflammatory response. Ann Med 36: 347–354.
18. Van Gorp H, Delputte PL, Nauwynck HJ (2010) Scavenger receptor CD163, a Jack-of-all-trades and potential target for cell-directed therapy. Mol Immunol 47: 1650–1660.
19. Etzerodt A, Moestrup SK (2013) CD163 and inflammation: biological, diagnostic, and therapeutic aspects. Antioxid Redox Signal 18: 2352–2363.
20. Thomsen HH, Moller HJ, Trolle C, Groth KA, Skakkebaek A, et al. (2013) The macrophage low-grade inflammation marker sCD163 is modulated by exogenous sex steroids. Endocr Connect 2: 216–224.
21. Andersen MN, Abildgaard N, Maniecki MB, Moller HJ, Andersen NF (2014) Monocyte/macrophage-derived soluble CD163: a novel biomarker in multiple myeloma. Eur J Haematol.
22. Kjaergaard AG, Rodgaard-Hansen S, Dige A, Krog J, Moller HJ, et al. (2014) Monocyte Expression and Soluble Levels of the Haemoglobin Receptor (CD163/sCD163) and the Mannose Receptor (MR/sMR) in Septic and Critically Ill Non-Septic ICU Patients. PLoS One 9: e92331.
23. Buechler C, Eisinger K, Krautbauer S (2013) Diagnostic and prognostic potential of the macrophage specific receptor CD163 in inflammatory diseases. Inflamm Allergy Drug Targets 12: 391–402.
24. Manigold T, Vial P (2014) Human hantavirus infections: epidemiology, clinical features, pathogenesis and immunology. Swiss Med Wkly 144: w13937.
25. Du H, Wang PZ, Li J, Bai L, Li H, et al. (2014) Clinical characteristics and outcomes in critical patients with hemorrhagic fever with renal syndrome. BMC Infect Dis 14: 191.
26. Zhang Y, Liu B, Ma Y, Yi J, Zhang C, et al. (2014) Hantaan virus infection induces CXCL10 expression through TLR3, RIG-I, and MDA-5 pathways correlated with the disease severity. Mediators Inflamm 2014: 697837.
27. Funderburg NT, Zidar DA, Shive C, Lioi A, Mudd J, et al. (2012) Shared monocyte subset phenotypes in HIV-1 infection and in uninfected subjects with acute coronary syndrome. Blood 120: 4599–4608.
28. Mendonca VR, Luz NF, Santos NJ, Borges VM, Goncalves MS, et al. (2012) Association between the haptoglobin and heme oxygenase 1 genetic profiles and soluble CD163 in susceptibility to and severity of human malaria. Infect Immun 80: 1445–1454.
29. Frings W, Dreier J, Sorg C (2002) Only the soluble form of the scavenger receptor CD163 acts inhibitory on phorbol ester-activated T-lymphocytes, whereas membrane-bound protein has no effect. FEBS Lett 526: 93–96.
30. Weaver LK, Hintz-Goldstein KA, Pioli PA, Wardwell K, Qureshi N, et al. (2006) Pivotal advance: activation of cell surface Toll-like receptors causes shedding of the hemoglobin scavenger receptor CD163. J Leukoc Biol 80: 26–35.

Author Contributions

Conceived and designed the experiments: JNW HTY XFB. Performed the experiments: JNW TZ. Analyzed the data: JNW HD. Contributed reagents/materials/analysis tools: WJ. Wrote the paper: JNW WJG XFB PZW.

31. Etzerodt A, Rasmussen MR, Svendsen P, Chalaris A, Schwarz J, et al. (2014) Structural basis for inflammation-driven shedding of CD163 ectodomain and tumor necrosis factor-alpha in macrophages. J Biol Chem 289: 778–788.

32. Burdo TH, Lentz MR, Autissier P, Krishnan A, Halpern E, et al. (2011) Soluble CD163 made by monocyte/macrophages is a novel marker of HIV activity in early and chronic infection prior to and after anti-retroviral therapy. J Infect Dis 204: 154–163.

33. Burdo TH, Soulas C, Orzechowski K, Button J, Krishnan A, et al. (2010) Increased monocyte turnover from bone marrow correlates with severity of SIV encephalitis and CD163 levels in plasma. PLoS Pathog 6: e1000842.

34. Kazankov K, Barrera F, Moller HJ, Bibby BM, Vilstrup H, et al. (2014) Soluble CD163, a macrophage activation marker, is independently associated with fibrosis in patients with chronic viral hepatitis B and C. Hepatology.

35. Su L, Feng L, Song Q, Kang H, Zhang X, et al. (2013) Diagnostic value of dynamics serum sCD163, sTREM-1, PCT, and CRP in differentiating sepsis, severity assessment, and prognostic prediction. Mediators Inflamm 2013: 969875.

36. Wang PZ, Li ZD, Yu HT, Zhang Y, Wang W, et al. (2012) Elevated serum concentrations of inflammatory cytokines and chemokines in patients with haemorrhagic fever with renal syndrome. J Int Med Res 40: 648–656.

37. Possamai LA, Antoniades CG, Anstee QM, Quaglia A, Vergani D, et al. (2010) Role of monocytes and macrophages in experimental and human acute liver failure. World J Gastroenterol 16: 1811–1819.

38. Klingstrom J, Hardestam J, Stoltz M, Zuber B, Lundkvist A, et al. (2006) Loss of cell membrane integrity in puumala hantavirus-infected patients correlates with levels of epithelial cell apoptosis and perforin. J Virol 80: 8279–8282.

39. Simoni J, Simoni G, Griswold JA, Moeller JF, Tsikouris JP, et al. (2006) Role of free hemoglobin in 8-iso prostaglandin F2-alpha synthesis in chronic renal failure and its impact on CD163-Hb scavenger receptor and on coronary artery endothelium. ASAIO J 52: 652–661.

40. Nielsen MJ, Moestrup SK (2009) Receptor targeting of hemoglobin mediated by the haptoglobins: roles beyond heme scavenging. Blood 114: 764–771.

41. Geissmann F, Manz MG, Jung S, Sieweke MH, Merad M, et al. (2010) Development of monocytes, macrophages, and dendritic cells. Science 327: 656–661.

42. Kundumani-Sridharan V, Dyukova E, Hansen DR, Rao GN (2013) 12/15-Lipoxygenase mediates high-fat diet-induced endothelial tight junction disruption and monocyte transmigration: a new role for 15(S)-hydroxyeicosatetraenoic acid in endothelial cell dysfunction. J Biol Chem 288: 15830–15842.

43. Ye H, Wang LY, Zhao J, Wang K (2013) Increased CD163 expression is associated with acute-on-chronic hepatitis B liver failure. World J Gastroenterol 19: 2818–2825.

44. Kjaergaard AG, Rodgaard-Hansen S, Dige A, Krog J, Moller HJ, et al. (2014) Monocyte expression and soluble levels of the haemoglobin receptor (CD163/sCD163) and the mannose receptor (MR/sMR) in septic and critically ill non-septic ICU patients. PLoS One 9: e92331.

45. West SD, Goldberg D, Ziegler A, Krencicki M, Du Clos TW, et al. (2012) Transforming growth factor-beta, macrophage colony-stimulating factor and C-reactive protein levels correlate with CD14(high)CD16+ monocyte induction and activation in trauma patients. PLoS One 7: e52406.

46. Davis BH, Zarev PV (2005) Human monocyte CD163 expression inversely correlates with soluble CD163 plasma levels. Cytometry B Clin Cytom 63: 16–22.

13

Simplexide Induces CD1d-Dependent Cytokine and Chemokine Production from Human Monocytes

Stefania Loffredo[1], Rosaria I. Staiano[1], Francescopaolo Granata[1], Valeria Costantino[2], Francesco Borriello[1], Annunziata Frattini[1], Maria Teresa Lepore[1], Alfonso Mangoni[2], Gianni Marone[1]*, Massimo Triggiani[3]

1 Department of Translational Medical Sciences and Center for Basic and Clinical Immunology Research (CISI), University of Naples Federico II, Naples, Italy, 2 The NeaNAT group - Department of Pharmacy, University of Naples Federico II, Naples, Italy, 3 Division of Allergy and Clinical Immunology, University of Salerno, Salerno, Italy

Abstract

Monocytes are major effector cells of innate immunity and recognize several endogenous and exogenous molecules due to the expression of wide spectrum of receptors. Among them, the MHC class I-like molecule CD1d interacts with glycolipids and presents them to iNKT cells, mediating their activation. Simplexide belongs to a novel class of glycolipids isolated from marine sponges and is structurally distinct from other immunologically active glycolipids. In this study we have examined the effects of simplexide on cytokine and chemokine release from human monocytes. Simplexide induces a concentration- and time-dependent release of IL-6, CXCL8, TNF-α and IL-10 and increases the expression of *IL6*, *CXCL8* and *IL10* mRNA. Cytokine and chemokine release induced by simplexide from monocytes is dependent on CD1d since: i) a CD1d antagonist, 1,2-bis (diphenylphosphino) ethane [DPPE]- polyethylene glycolmonomethylether [PEG], specifically blocks simplexide-induced activation of monocytes; ii) CD1d knockdown inhibits monocyte activation by simplexide and iii) simplexide induces cytokine production from CD1d-transfected but not parental C1R cell line Finally, we have shown that simplexide also induces iNKT cell expansion *in vitro*. Our results demonstrate that simplexide, apart from activating iNKT cells, induces the production of cytokines and chemokines from human monocytes by direct interaction with CD1d.

Editor: Paul Proost, University of Leuven, Rega Institute, Belgium

Funding: This work was supported by grants from the Ministero dell'Università e della Ricerca (MT, and GM), the Regione Campania (GM), CISI Lab project, CRÈME project, TIMING project and European Union's Seventh Framework Programme FP7/2007–2013 under grant agreement n° 311848 (BlueGenics) (AM). The funders had no role in study design, data collection and analysis, decision to publish, or preparation of the manuscript.

Competing Interests: The authors have declared that no competing interests exist.

* Email: marone@unina.it

Introduction

Monocytes are a critical component of the mononuclear phagocyte system and play an important role in conditions as diverse as infections, cardiovascular diseases and cancer [1,2,3]. By expressing a wide spectrum of surface receptors, monocytes can recognize several chemically unrelated molecules (e.g. proteins and lipids) [4,5,6,7]. Glycolipids and glycosphingolipids are major components of several microorganisms, and are increasingly recognized as potent activators of immune cells [8,9]. These molecules can interact with the MHC class I-like molecule CD1d expressed on antigen presenting cells (APC), such as dendritic cells and monocytes [10,11].

Natural killer T cells with an invariant T cell receptor alpha chain (iNKT) recognize microbial glycolipids bound to and presented by CD1d [12,13,14]. α-Galactosylceramide (α-GalCer), a glycolipid extracted from the marine sponge *Agelas mauritiana* [15], stimulates NKT cells to rapidly produce both Th1 (IFN-γ) and Th2 (IL-4) cytokines in a CD1d-dependent manner [16,17]. Although it is well established that presentation of the CD1d-α-

GalCer complex by APC to iNKT cells results in their activation [17,18,19], it has been demonstrated that direct cross-linking of CD1d on human monocytes [20,21] and intestinal epithelial cells induces cytokine production [22,23].

Simplexide is the leading compound of a unique glycolipid class isolated from the sponge *Plakortis simplex* [24,25]. The lipid component of simplexide is unique among known classes of glycolipids, being a glycosylated long-chain secondary alcohol without further functional groups. The two lipophilic long alkyl chains are linked to a polar sugar head composed of the rare α-glucosyl-(1→4)-β-galactosyl disaccharide residue (Fig. 1). At least five different alkyl chain types are observed, and since there are two alkyl chains for molecule, up to 25 different molecular species may be present in natural simplexide. Although there is some early evidence that simplexide can modulate murine T cells [26], the effects of this molecule on human immune cells are unknown.

In this study we demonstrate that simplexide activates human monocytes and induces the production of cytokines and chemokines in a CD1d-dependent manner.

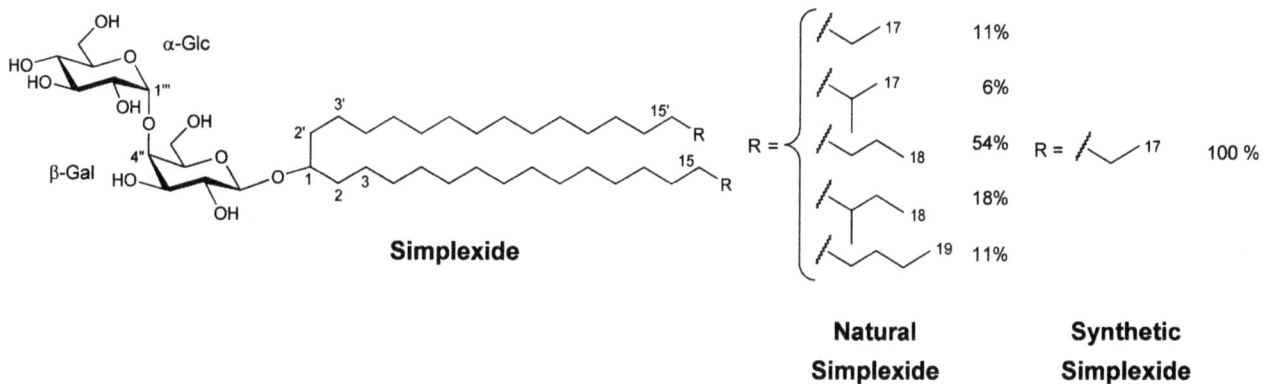

Figure 1. Chemical structure of simplexide. Simplexide is a glycolipid composed of long-chain secondary alcohols glycosylated by a disaccharide chain containing α-glucose and α-galactose. Natural simplexide is a mixture of homologues, with alkyl chains of different length (R) linked to the central CHOH group. In addition, a significant part of the alkyl chains has a methyl branch in the second-to-last or third-to-last carbon atoms. The percentage of each molecular species detected in natural simplexide is shown on the right. Synthetic simplexide was prepared as a chemically homogeneous compound.

Materials and Methods

Reagents

The following were purchased: lipopolysaccharide (LPS; from *Escherichia coli* serotype 026:B6), L-glutamine, ultraglutamine, antibiotic-antimycotic solution (10,000 IU/ml penicillin, 10 mg/ml streptomycin, and 25 µg/ml amphotericin B), MEM non essential amino acids solutions, Triton X-100, polymyxin B sulfate, Histopaque-1077, bovin serum albumin (BSA) and phorbol-12-myristate-13-acetate (PMA) (Sigma-Aldrich, St. Louis, MO); X-VIVO 15, Pen-Strep, and human AB serum (Lonza, Swiss); RPMI and fetal calf serum (FCS) (MP Biomedicals Europe, Illkirch, France). Human recombinant interleukin (IL)-2 (Peprotech, Italy). Mouse monoclonal IgG1 anti-human CD1d (Clone NOR3.2/13.17), goat polyclonal anti-human GAPDH, HRP-conjugated goat anti-mouse Ab, and HRP-conjugated rabbit anti-goat Ab were from Santa Cruz Biotechnology (Santa Cruz, CA). PE-anti-TCR Vα24 and PerCP-anti-CD3 were from Miltenyi Biotec (Bologna, Italy). FITC-anti-CD14, APC- and PE-anti-CD1d (Clone CD1d42) were from Becton Dickinson (San Jose, CA). 1,2-Bis(diphenylphosphino)ethane[DPPE]-polyethylene glycolmonomethylether[PEG] was from Avanti Polar Lipids (Alabaster, AL). Target-specific primers for *IL6*, *TNFα*, *IL10*, *CXCL8*, and *GAPDH* were designed using the Beacon Designer 3.0 (Biorad Laboratories, Milan, Italy) and produced and purified by Custom Primers (Life Technologies, Milan, Italy). All other reagents were from Carlo Erba (Milan, Italy).

Isolation and characterization of simplexide

Simplexide was isolated from Plakortis simplex at the Department of Pharmacy, University of Naples Federico II [26,27]. The structure and purity of the isolated glycolipids was confirmed by Proton Nuclear Magnetic Resonance (^{1}H-NMR) and mass spectrometry [26]. As with most glycolipids from sponges, each of the obtained glycolipids was an inseparable mixture of homologues, which are identical in the polar part of the molecule but slightly different in the length and branching of lipophilic chains. The relative amounts of branched and unbranched chains were evaluated by ^{1}H-NMR, while their length was determined by mass spectrometry. Both resulted to be very close to those reported in the original paper [24,27]. Structure reported in Figure 1 shows the relative amounts of homologues of natural simplexide. Stock solutions of glycolipid were prepared and stored in DMSO at a concentration of 3 mM unless otherwise specified and diluted to working concentration in RPMI immediately before the experiment. Synthetic simplexide was prepared from 1-octatecanol, 1-bromoheptane, methyl α-D-glucopyranose, and methyl β-D-galactopyranose (see Figure S1). Final purification of the synthetic compound was achieved using reversed-phase HPLC using an RP-18 column and MeOH as eluent. Natural α-GalCer was isolated from the marine sponge Agelas longissima using the same procedure as for simplexide. Synthetic α-GalCer (KRN7000) [28] was purchased from Cayman Chemical (Michigan, USA).

Cell isolation and purification

The study protocol involving the use of human blood cells was approved by the Ethical Committee of the University of Naples Federico II, and written informed consent was obtained from blood donors in according to the principles expressed in the Declaration of Helsinki. Monocytes were purified from buffy coats of healthy donors (HCV⁻, HBsAg⁻, HIV⁻) obtained from the Leukapheresis Unit. Peripheral blood mononuclear cells (PBMC) were obtained by centrifugation over Histopaque-1077. Monocytes were further purified by positive immunomagnetic selection using CD14 MicroBeads (Miltenyi Biotec, Bologna, Italy). This procedure yields a population of CD14⁺ monocytes with a purity greater than 99% as assessed by flow cytometry. Contaminating cells were predominantly CD3⁺ T cells. The presence of iNTK cells before and after immunomagnetic selection was assessed by flow cytometry using PE-anti-TCR Vα24 and PerCP-anti-CD3 antibodies. iNTK cells (identified as CD3⁺ Vα24⁺ cells) represented 0.1% of PBMC, whereas these cells were undetectable in monocyte preparations (Fig. 2).

The human C1R and stable CD1d-transfected C1R cell lines [29] were kindly donated by Prof. Vincenzo Cerundolo (Weatherall Institute of Molecular Medicine University of Oxford John Radcliffe Hospital). The cells were maintained in culture in RPMI supplemented with 10% FCS, 2 mmol/L L-glutamine, Pen-Strep and non essential amino acid. The expression of CD1d was assessed by flow cytometry using PE-conjugated anti-CD1d (Clone CD1d42; BD Pharmingen).

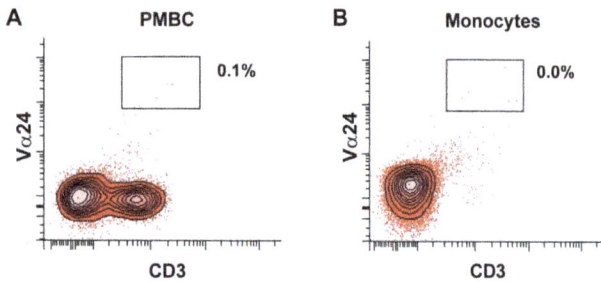

Figure 2. Flow cytometric analyses of iNKT cells among human PBMC and in highly purified monocytes. The percentage of iNKT cells in PBMC (A) and in monocytes (B) was analyzed by flow cytometry with anti-Vα24 and anti-CD3. The cells washed in PBS, were incubated at 4°C for 20 minutes with antibody mixes: PE-conjugated TCR Vα24 and PerCP-conjugated anti- CD3. For each sample 30,000 events were acquired on BD LSRFortessa. All flow cytometric analyses were performed using a BD FACSDiva software.

Flow cytometry

Cells were washed in staining buffer (phosphate buffered saline [PBS], 10% human AB serum, 0.05% NaN$_3$) and incubated at 4°C for 20 minutes with the following antibodies: PE-anti-TCR Vα24 (dilution 1:20), PerCP-anti-CD3 (dilution 1:20) and FITC-anti-CD14 (dilution 1:20). Then, cells were washed in washing buffer (PBS, 0.2% BSA, 0.05% NaN$_3$) and fixed in 2% paraformaldehyde before acquisition on a BD LSRFortessa. For each sample 30,000 events were acquired and analyzed with the BD FACSDIVA software system (Becton Dickinson).

Cell incubations

Monocytes were incubated (37°C, 2 to 24 h) in X-VIVO supplemented with 2 mM L-glutamine and various concentrations of simplexide (0.3–10 μM) or LPS (100 ng/ml). Simplexide preparations were routinely checked for LPS contamination (Limulus amebocyte Test, MP Biomedicals) and discarded if the LPS concentration was above the detection limit of the assay (0.125 EU/ml). In selected experiments simplexide (10 μM) and LPS (100 ng/ml) were preincubated (37°C, 30 min) with poly-myxin B (50 μg/ml) before addition to the cells. Since synthetic simplexide was remarkably less soluble in DMSO than natural simplexide, the experiments to compare natural and synthetic compound were done in polystyrene plates coated with various concentrations of glycolipids dissolved in methanol. Solvent was dried under nitrogen immediately before the addiction of cells. In another group of experiments, monocytes were preincubated with increasing concentrations of DPPE-PEG (1–30 μg/ml; 5 min) and then stimulated (37°C, 24 h) with simplexide (10 μM), α-GalCer (50 μM) or LPS (100 ng/ml). At the end of the experiment, the supernatant was removed, centrifuged (1,000 g, 4°C, 5 min) and stored at −80°C for subsequent determination of IL-6, TNF-α, IL-10, and CXCL8 release. The cells remaining in the plates were lysed with 0.1% Triton X-100 for total protein quantification by a Bradford-based assay (Biorad).

C1R and CD1d-transfected C1R were incubated (37°C, 24 h) in X-VIVO alone or with simplexide (10 μM), KRN7000 (1 μM) or PMA (100 ng/ml).

To assess iNKT expansion *in vitro*, PBMC were cultured in RPMI supplemented with 1% ultraglutamine, 1% antibiotic-antimycotic solution and 5% human AB serum and stimulated with simplexide (100 nM) or α-GalCer (100 nM). On day 2, IL-2 (100 U/ml) was added to each well. On day 7, cells were harvested

and the percentage of iNKT cells among CD3$^+$ cells was assessed by flow cytometry using PE-anti-TCR Vα24 and PerCP-anti-CD3 antibodies (Miltenyi Biotec).

RT-PCR for IL6, TNFα, IL10, and CXCL8

Monocytes ($5 \times 10^6/2$ ml) were incubated (37°C, 2 h) in X-VIVO in 12-well plates. The cells were then washed and incubated (37°C, 3–12 h) in the presence or the absence of simplexide (10 μM). At the end of the incubation, total RNA from monocytes was extracted by SV total RNA isolation system (Promega, Madison, WI), treated with RNase-free DNase I and suspended in DEPC water. RNA concentration were assessed by spectrophotometry. One μg of total RNA was reverse transcribed with oligo(dT) (50 μM) and Superscript III Reverse Transcriptase (200 U, Life Technologies) as described elsewhere [30]. Real-time quantitative PCR was performed on the iCycler (Biorad) using the Platinum SYBR Green qPCR kit (Life Technologies) and target-specific primers for IL6, TNFα, IL10, CXCL8, and GAPDH as previously reported [31]. PCR efficiency and specificity were evaluated by analyzing amplification curves with serial dilutions of the template cDNA and their dissociation curves. Each cDNA sample was analyzed in triplicate and the corresponding no-RT mRNA sample was included as a negative control. The data were analyzed with iCycler iQ analysis software (Biorad), the mRNA signals in each sample were normalized to that of the GAPDH mRNA, and the changes in IL6, TNFα, IL10 and CXCL8 mRNAs were expressed as fold increase in treated vs. unstimulated cells.

Cytokine Assay

The release of IL-6, TNF-α, IL-10 and CXCL8 in the culture supernatant was measured in duplicate determinations by commercially available ELISA kits (R&D, Minneapolis, MN USA) according to the manufacturer's instructions. Since the number of adherent monocytes can vary in each well and in different experiments, the results were normalized for the total protein content in each well, determined in the cell lysates (0.1% Triton X-100) by a Bradford based assay (Biorad).

Silencing of CD1d

Silencing of CD1d was performed with HyPerfect Transfection Kit (Qiagen, Italy) by using four different FlexiTube siRNAs (silencing RNAs) for CD1d (Qiagen, Hs_CD1D_1, Hs_CD1D_2, Hs_CD1D_4, Hs_CD1D_5), and the validated irrelevant Allstars siRNAs (Qiagen) used as negative control. Target sequences of the FlexiTube siRNAs were: Hs_CD1D_1 (siRNA-S1) = CCGGTT-GTGAAACCTACTGAA, Hs_CD1D_2 (siRNA-S2) = CAGAA-GTGCAAAGGTGTGCAA, Hs_CD1D_4 (siRNA-S4) = TGG-GCTTTACCTCCCGGTTTA, and Hs_CD1D_5 (siRNA-S5) = TGGGCTTTACCTCCCGGTTTA. The transfection protocol was as follows: adherent monocytes (10^6 per sample) were incubated (37°C, 18 h) in 6-well plates with OptiMEM (Life Technologies) supplemented with 12 μl of HyPerfect Transfection Reagent (Qiagen) and 750 ng/ml of each siRNA oligonucleotides. At the end of the incubation, the transfection medium was removed, replaced with RPMI containing 10% FCS, 2 mM L-glutamine and 1% antibiotic-antimycotic solution, and the cells were incubated (37°C) for additional 72 h. At the end of the transfection protocol the amount of CD1d was assessed by western blot. To this aim, the cells were lysed in lysis buffer (20 mM Tris pH 7.5, 5 mM EDTA, 1 mM PMSF, 2 mM benzamidine, 10 μg/ml leupeptin, 10 mM NaF, 150 mM NaCl, 1% Nonidet P-40 and 5% glycerol). Equal protein extracts (25 μg per sample) were separated on 4–12% Bis-Tris gels (NuPAGE®, Novex, Life

Technologies) and transferred to a nitrocellulose membrane (Schleicher & Schuell, Dassel, Germany). Membranes were then probed with the anti-CD1d (Clone NOR3.2/13.17), or anti-GAPDH Abs followed by HRP-conjugated secondary Abs. Membrane-bound Abs were visualized with the ECL detection system (GE Healthcare, Milan, Italy) and digitalized under the image analysis system ChemidocXRS (Biorad). Densitometric measurement of the signal intensity was performed with the Quantity One software (Biorad) and quantification of CD1d was obtained by calculating the ratio CD1d/GAPDH in each sample.

Statistical analysis

The data are expressed as mean values ± SE of the indicated number of experiments. Statistical analysis was performed by one-way analysis of variance (ANOVA) followed by Dunnett's test (when comparison was made against a control) or Bonferroni's test (when comparison was made between each pair of groups) by means of Analyse-it for Microsoft Excel, version 2.16 (Analyse-it Software, Ltd.). A p value of 0.05 or lower was considered to be significant.

Results

Simplexide induces the release of cytokines and chemokines from human monocytes

In a first group of experiments we examined the effects of simplexide on cytokine and chemokine production by human monocytes. Cells were incubated with increasing concentrations (0.1–10 µM) of simplexide and the release of cytokines and chemokines (IL-6, TNF-α, IL-10 and CXCL8) was determined. Simplexide induced a concentration-dependent release of IL-6, CXCL8 and, to a lesser extent, TNF-α and IL-10 (Fig. 3A–D). Simplexide was more potent in inducing the release of CXCL8 ($EC_{50}=0.4\pm0.07$ µM) than IL-6 ($EC_{50}=1.2\pm0.02$ µM), TNF-α ($EC_{50}=2.1\pm0.02$ µM) and IL-10 ($EC_{50}=2.2\pm0.04$ µM). The production of CXCL8 induced by simplexide was comparable to that of LPS (100 ng/ml), a well-characterized stimulus for these cells [32], whereas the release of IL-6, TNF-α and IL-10 was lower (Fig. 3A–D).

Although we used highly purified simplexide in these experiments, being of natural origin it may contain trace contaminants that could potentially activate monocytes. To exclude that the effect of simplexide could be due to LPS contamination, monocytes were stimulated with simplexide in the presence of polymyxin B (50 µg/ml), a potent inactivator of LPS [33]. Polymyxin B did not influence the capacity of simplexide to induce the release of IL-6, CXCL8 and TNF-α, whereas it almost completely suppressed the production of cytokines and chemokines induced by LPS (Table 1). To further exclude the possibility of monocyte activation due to trace contaminants other than LPS, we compared the effect of natural simplexide with that of its synthetic analogue. In these experiments, glycolipids were dissolved in methanol because synthetic simplexide was remarkably less soluble in DMSO than natural simplexide. This phenomenon can be explained by the different molecular species present in natural and synthetic simplexide. In fact, natural simplexide is a mixture of many homologous molecular species, whereas synthetic simplexide is chemically homogeneous. While the molecular heterogeneity of natural simplexide is unlikely to affect its biological properties, it could explain its higher solubility. In a recent paper [34], the chemical heterogeneity of some plant polysaccharides has been interpreted in terms of a reduced propensity to aggregation and, therefore, of increased solubility. Similarly, the heterogeneous natural simplexide is expected to be

more soluble than the chemically homogeneous synthetic compounds.

To avoid any effect due to different solubility, we precoated the plate with the glycolipids before the addition of the cells. Figure 4 shows that natural and synthetic simplexide induced similar release of both IL-6 (A) and CXCL8 (B) from monocytes. Under these experimental conditions, the amount of cytokines produced by monocytes is lower than that reported in Figure 3, when simplexide was added directly to the cell suspension. The comparable effects of the natural and synthetic simplexide confirm that activation of monocytes is directly due to the glycolipid and not to contaminants.

In the next group of experiments we examined the kinetics of IL-6, CXCL8, TNF-α and IL-10 release from monocytes stimulated with an optimal concentration of simplexide (10 µM). Figure 5 shows that production of CXCL8 began at 4 h and reached a plateau after 8 h, whereas IL-6 release progressively increased up to 24 h. Moreover, simplexide-induced release of TNF-α was rapid, reaching a maximum at 4 h and declining thereafter. Finally, the production of IL-10 was maximal between 8 and 12 h. Collectively, these results indicate that the release of cytokines/chemokines from human monocytes induced by simplexide follows distinct kinetics.

Simplexide increases cytokine and chemokine mRNA in monocytes

The kinetics of cytokine/chemokine production shown in Fig. 5 suggested that simplexide may differentially modulate their mRNA expression. Thus, we examined whether simplexide activates cytokine/chemokine gene expression in monocytes by real-time quantitative PCR. Simplexide significantly enhanced mRNA expression of IL6, CXCL8, and IL10. By contrast, simplexide did not influence the expression of TNFα at any time point examined. Again, the kinetics of induction were quite different, since IL6 mRNA progressively increased up to 12 hours (5.7±0.5, fold change over unstimulated cells) whereas CXCL8 and IL10 peaked at 6 hours (4.1±0.4 and 3.9±0.5 fold, respectively) and slightly declined after 12 hours (Fig. 6). These experiments confirm that different profiles of cytokine/chemokine production induced by simplexide are paralleled by different kinetics of mRNA expression. Interestingly, simplexide did not increase TNFα mRNA expression, suggesting that the release of this cytokine is due to secretion of preformed TNF-α from intracellular stores rather than de novo gene expression.

CD1d is required for monocyte activation induced by simplexide

Since CD1d is the main target of glycolipids, we hypothesize that it could be involved in simplexide-induced activation of human monocytes. Thus, we used three different experimental approaches to test this hyphotesis. First, we evaluated the effect of a sterically stabilized liposome composed of dipalmitoyl-phospha-tidylethanolamine covalently attached to polyethyleneglycol (DPPE-PEG). Previous studies have shown that DPPE-PEG is a potent CD1d antagonist and inhibits α-GalCer-induced activation of iNKT cells both in vivo and in vitro [35,36]. Figure 7 (A–B) shows that DPPE-PEG concentration-dependently inhibited simplexide-induced IL-6 and CXCL8 production from monocytes with similar IC_{50} (2.8 µg/ml and 7.2 µg/ml for IL-6 and CXCL8, respectively). The same pattern of response was observed when α-GalCer was used instead of simplexide (Fig. 7A–B). The specificity of the inhibitory effect of DPPE-PEG was supported by the observation that this compound had no effect on LPS-induced

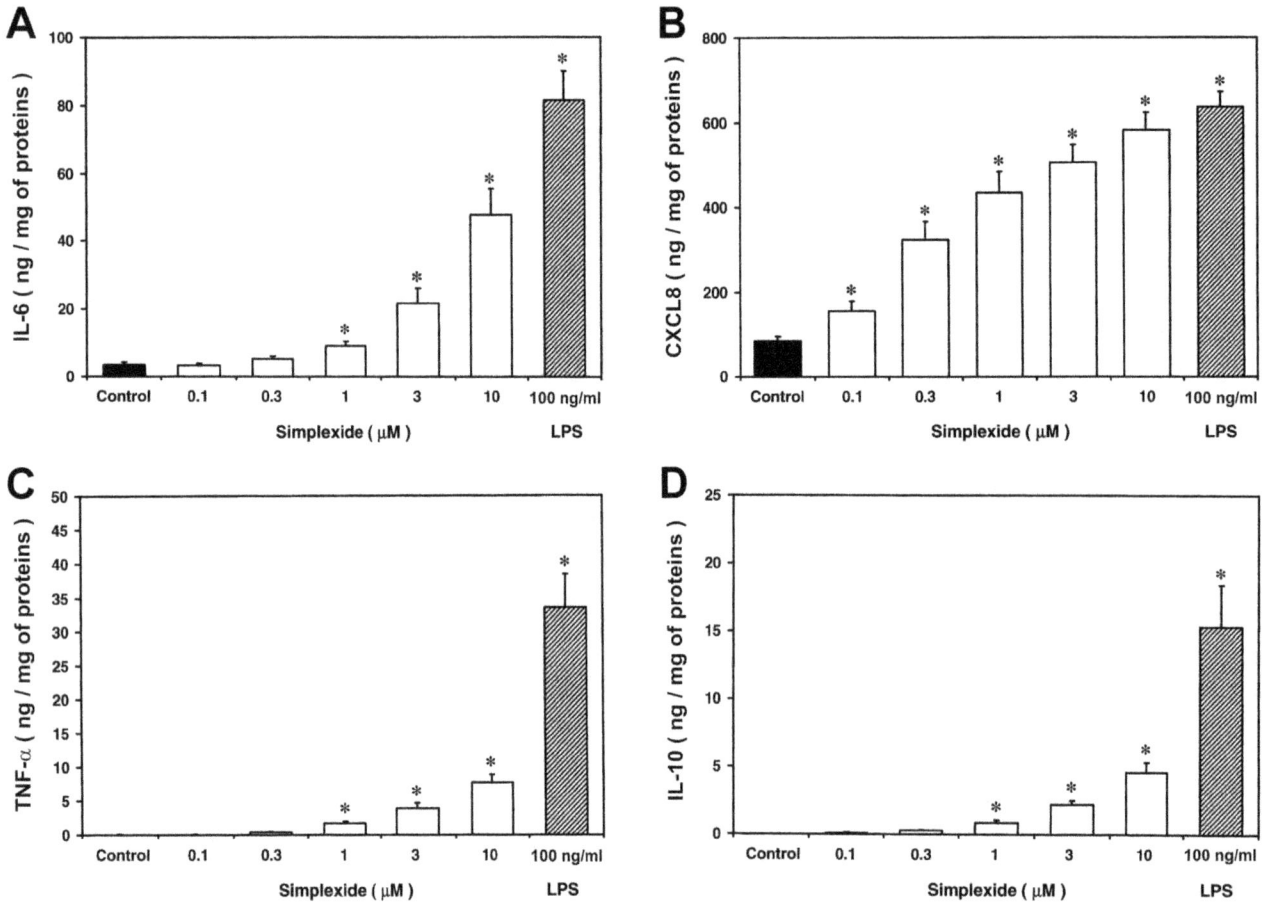

Figure 3. Effect of increasing concentrations of simplexide on IL-6 (panel A), CXCL8 (panel B), TNF-α (panel C) and IL-10 (panel D) release from monocytes. Monocytes were incubated (37°C, 8 h for TNF-α and IL-10 or 24 h for IL-6 and IL-8) with X-VIVO alone (control) or with the indicated concentrations of simplexide or LPS. At the end of incubation, the supernatant was collected and centrifuged (1000×g, 4°C, 5 min). Cytokines and chemokines were determined by ELISA. The values are expressed as ng of IL-6, CXCL8, TNF-α or IL-10 per mg of total proteins. Data are representative of ten independent experiments.

IL-6 and CXCL8 production (Fig. 7A–B). The maximum response (in ng/mg of proteins) of used stimuli was for IL-6: simplexide = 52.0±5.9; α-GalCer = 20.2±3.7; LPS = 81.5±8.3 vs. unstimulated cells 2.84±0.5; and for CXCL8: simplexide = 625.2±37.6 ng/mg of proteins; α-GalCer = 380.6±35.7; LPS = 637.5±55.6 vs. unstimulated cells 61.8±9.8.

In a second group of experiments, we silenced CD1d expression by using different siRNA oligonucleotides. Figure 8A shows a

representative experiment in which CD1d expression in transfected monocytes was evaluated by western blot. Two siRNA oligonucleotides (S1 and S5) markedly reduced CD1d protein in monocytes as compared to cells treated with irrelevant oligonucleotides (Sham). Two other siRNA oligonucleotides, S2 and S4, did not significantly reduce CD1d protein (data not shown). Densitometric analysis of three experiments showed that CD1d content was reduced by 60.5±6.5% and 67.9±7.6% with S1 and

Table 1. Effect of polymyxin B on simplexide- and LPS-induced release of IL-6, CXCL8 and TNF-α from monocytes.

	IL-6 (ng/mg of proteins)		CXCL8 (ng/mg of proteins)		TNF-α (ng/mg of proteins)	
	Control	+ polymyxin B	Control	+ polymyxin B	Control	+ polymyxin B
Untreated	3.5±0.7	3.4±0.7	112.9±11.6	113.±11.51	0.1±0.1	0.1±0.1
Simplexide	52.0±9.4*	54.3±9.4*	615.5±37.2*	600.9±26.9*	8.9±3.6*	9.2±4.1*
LPS	88.3±5.4*	14.9±0.3†	638.1±15.1*	29.8±0.7†	54.9±8.0*	3.5±0.9†

Monocytes were incubated for 8 h (TNF-α) or 24 h (IL-6 and CXCL8) with simplexide (10 μM) or LPS (100 ng/ml) either in the absence (Control) or the presence of polymyxin B (50 μg/ml). Data are the mean ± SE of three experiments.
* p<0.05 vs. respective untreated.
† p<0.05 vs. respective control.

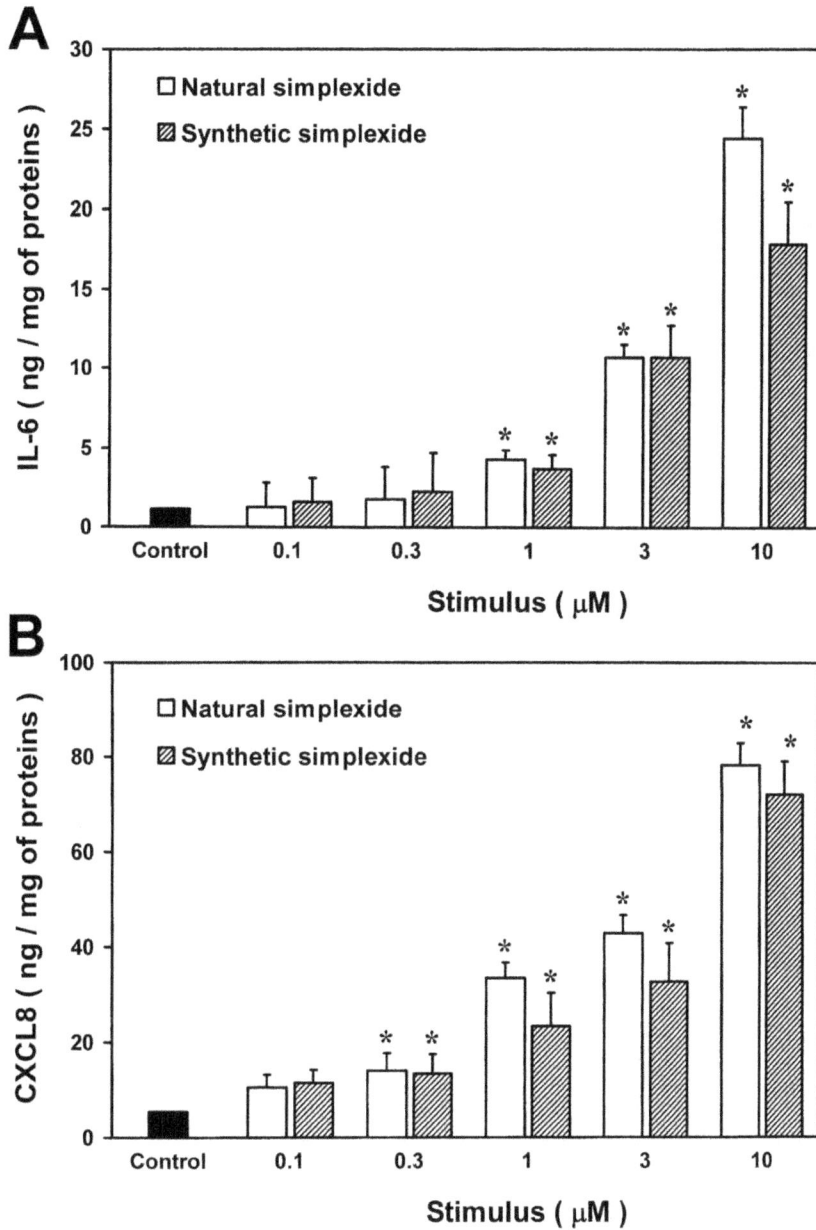

Figure 4. Effect of increasing concentrations of natural or synthetic simplexide on IL-6 (panel A) and CXCL8 (panel B) release from monocytes. Polystyrene plates were coated with indicated concentrations of glycolipids dissolved in methanol. Solvent was dried under nitrogen immediately before the addiction of cells. After 24 hours of incubation, the supernatant was collected and centrifuged ($1000 \times g$, 4°C, 5 min). Cytokines and chemokines were determined by ELISA. The values are expressed as ng of IL-6 or CXCL8 per mg of total proteins. Data are the mean ± SEM of six experiments. * $p<0.05$ *vs.* control.

S5, respectively ($p<0.05$ *vs.* sham), indicating that siRNA oligonucleotides successfully knocked down CD1d. Interestingly, CD1d knock down but not sham transfection significantly reduced CXCL8 release induced by simplexide (Fig. 8B), whilst monocyte production of CXCL8 in response to LPS was unaltered (data not shown).

To unambiguously confirm that CD1d was necessary for simplexide-induced cell activation, we employed a human lymphoblastoid cell line (C1R) stably transfected with CD1d. [29] Both transfected (C1R-CD1d) and parental (C1R) cells were stimulated with simplexide (10 µM), KRN7000 (1 µM), or PMA (100 ng/ml). Figure 9 shows that simplexide induced a significant

CXCL8 production by C1R-CD1d, but not C1R. Similar response was observed when C1R-CD1d and C1R were stimulated with the synthetic α-GalCer (KRN7000). By contrast PMA, which directly activates PKC [37], induced comparable release of CXCL8 in both cell lines.

Simplexide induce the expansion of human iNKT cells in vitro

As glycolipids presented by CD1d are recognized by and mediate the activation of iNKT, we asked whether simplexide could also induce iNKT cell expansion *in vitro*. To this aim, we incubated human PBMC with simplexide (100 nM) or α-GalCer

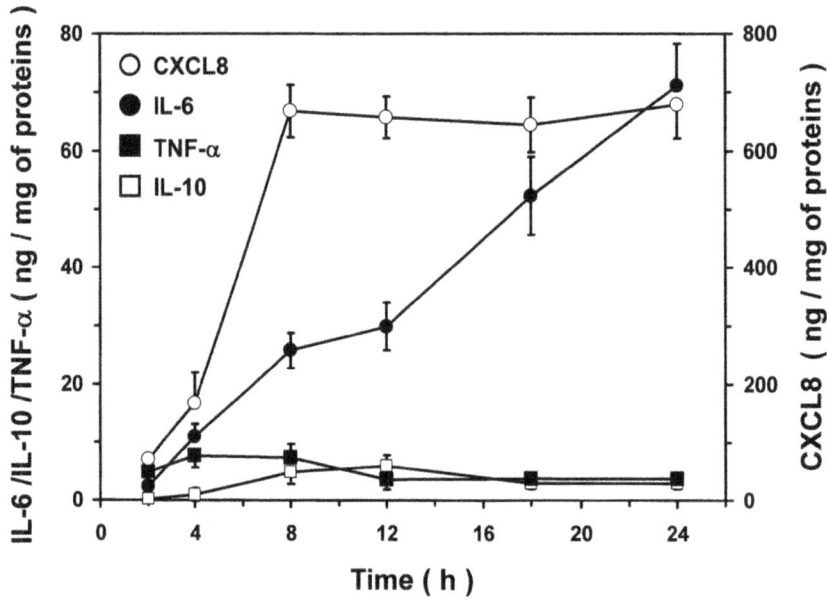

Figure 5. Kinetics of IL-6, CXCL8, TNF-α and IL-10 release from monocytes induced by simplexide. The cells were incubated (37°C, 3–24 h) with simplexide (10 μM). At the end of incubations, the supernatant was collected and centrifuged (1000×g, 4°C, 5 min). Cytokines and chemokines were determined by ELISA. The values are expressed as ng of IL-6, CXCL8, TNF-α or IL-10 per mg of total proteins. Data are the mean ± SEM of five experiments.

(100 nM) in the presence of IL-2 (100 U/ml) [38]. After 7 days, the percentage of CD3⁺Vα24⁺ cells was assessed by flow cytometry. Figure 10A illustrates the results of a typical experiment indicating that both α-GalCer and simplexide increased the percentage of iNKT cells. The results of four experiments summarized in Fig. 10B demonstrates that both α-GalCer and simplexide significantly induced an expansion of iNKT cells.

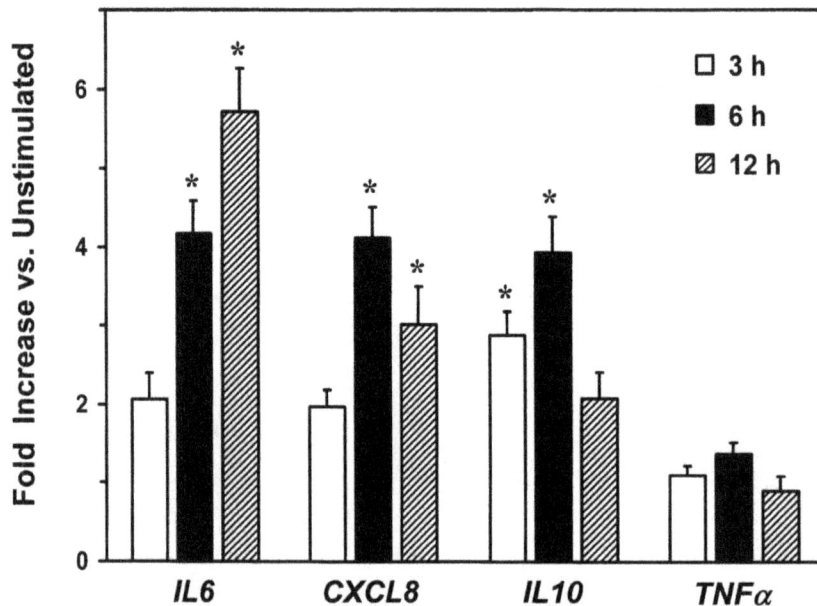

Figure 6. Effect of simplexide on IL-6, CXCL8, IL-10 and TNF-α mRNA expression in monocytes. The cells were incubated (37°C) for different time periods (3, 6, or 12 h) with simplexide (10 μM) or vehicle alone. mRNA levels for *IL6, CXCL8, IL10* and *TNFα* were quantitated by real-time PCR (see Methods). Expression of *IL6, CXCL8, IL10,* and *TNFα* (normalized for *GAPDH*) was expressed as fold changes *vs.* untreated cells. Data are the mean ± SE of five experiments. *p<0.05 *vs.* untreated.

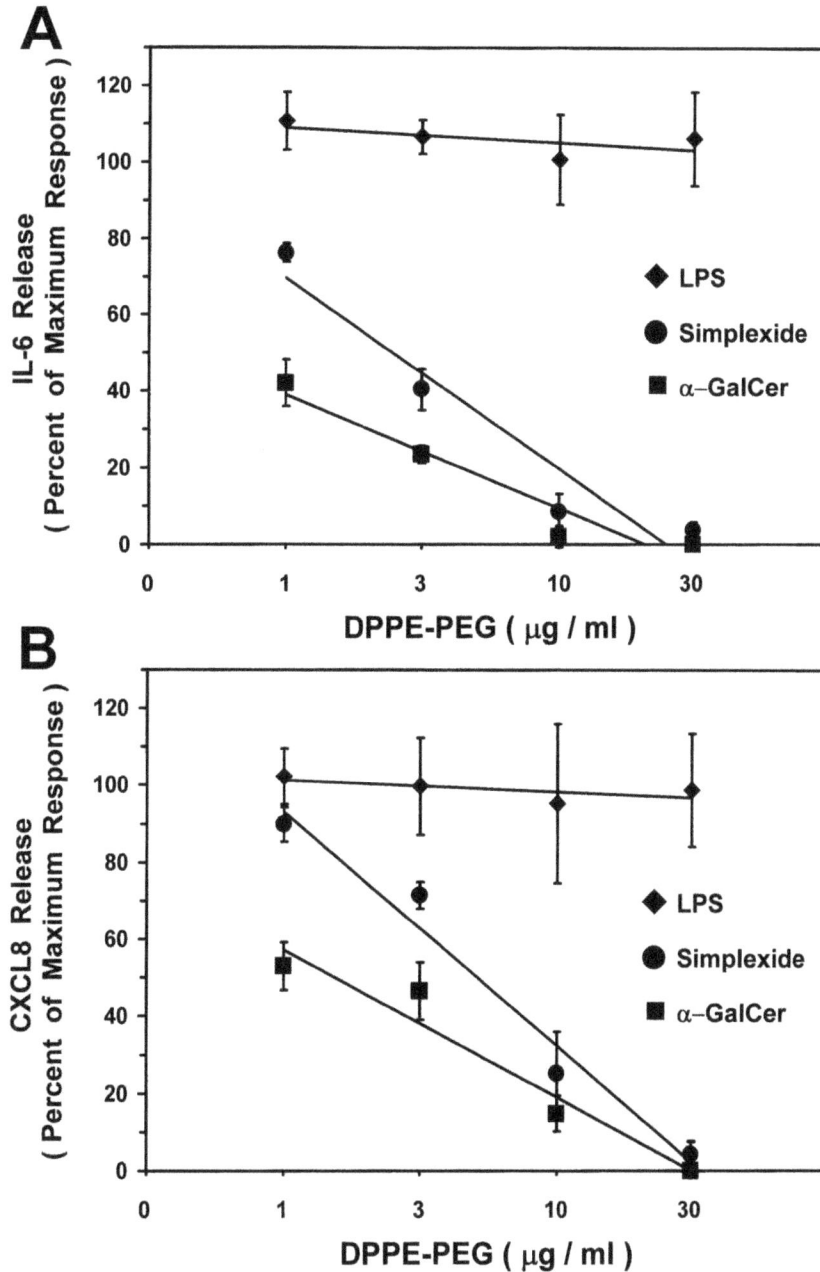

Figure 7. Effect of DPPE-PEG on simplexide-induced IL-6 (panel A) and CXCL8 (panel B) release from monocytes. Monocytes were preincubated (37°C, 5 min) with X-VIVO alone, or with the indicated concentrations of DPPE-PEG (1–30 µg/ml) and then stimulated (37°C, 24 h) with simplexide (●; 10 µM), α-GalCer (■; 50 µM) or LPS (♦; 1 µg/ml). At the end of incubation, the supernatant was collected and centrifuged (1000×g, 4°C, 5 min). Cytokines and chemokines were determined by ELISA. The values are expressed as ng of IL-6 or CXCL8 per mg of total proteins. Data are expressed as percent inhibition of the maximum response induced by simplexide or LPS alone calculated as $(R-R_b)/(R_{max}-R_b) \times 100$, where R is the release in samples treated with the agonists plus DPPE-PEG, R_b is the release in unstimulated samples and R_{max} is the release in samples stimulated with agonists alone. Data are the mean ± SEM of five experiments. The lines represent the best fit for inhibition of simplexide, α-GalCer or LPS.

Discussion

In this study we demonstrate that simplexide is a glycolipid that induces expression and release of cytokines and chemokines from human monocytes. Simplexide is almost as effective in inducing IL-6 and CXCL8 production as LPS. Natural and synthetic simplexide exert comparable effects, thus indicating that the stimulatory activity is due to the glycolipid molecule rather than trace contaminants. Simplexide activates the expression of IL6,

CXCL8 and IL10, but not TNFα mRNA a gene whose transcription is induced by LPS in monocytes [39]. However, a small albeit transient release of TNF-α is induced by simplexide. Interestingly, agonist-induced release of preformed TNF-α has been previously reported in immunologically activated human mast cells [40,41]. Our data suggest that preformed TNF-α is stored also in human monocytes and that simplexide activates the release of this cytokine independently of gene transcription. The effects of simplexide on cytokine and chemokine release are

A siRNA - Monocytes

B

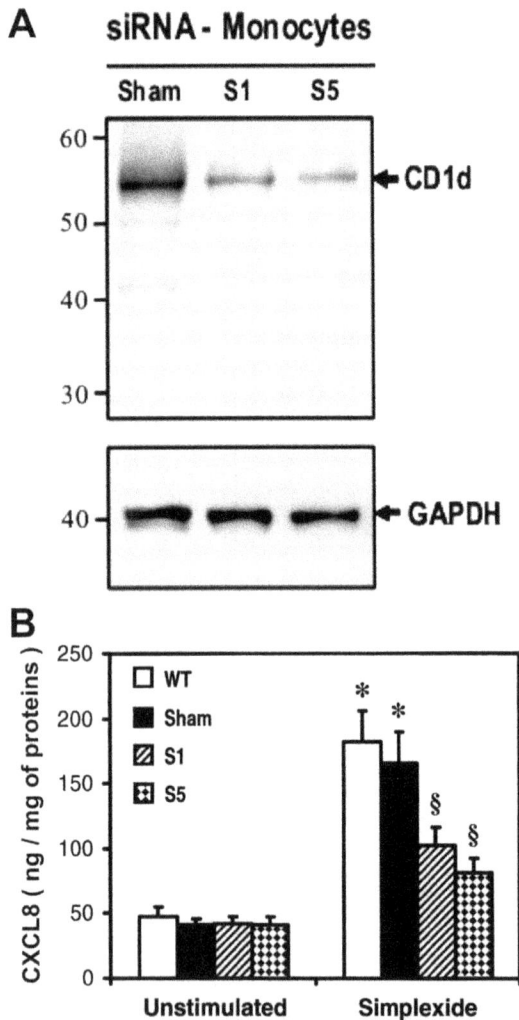

Figure 8. Effect of CD1d silencing on simplexide-induced release of CXCL8. Silencing of CD1d was performed as described in "Methods". (A) Western blot of monocytes transfected with two siRNA oligonucleotides (S1 and S5) or an irrelevant oligonucleotide (Sham). The immunoblot shown is representative of three different experiments. (B) Monocytes non-transfected (WT) or transfected with siRNA oligonucleotides (S1 and S5) or Sham were incubated (37°C, 24 h) with X-VIVO alone (unstimulated) or simplexide (10 µM). At the end of incubation, the supernatant was collected and centrifuged (1000×g, 4°C, 5 min). CXCL8 was determined by ELISA. The values are expressed as ng of CXCL8 per mg of total proteins. Data are the mean ± SEM of four experiments. * p<0.05 vs. the respective unstimulated. § p<0.05 vs. Sham.

mediated by CD1d expression on human monocytes. Finally, we show that simplexide expands iNKT cells in vitro to the same degree as α-GalCer.

According to the current hypothesis, stimulation of CD1d-expressing APC by glycolipids requires the concomitant presence of iNKT cells [17,18,19,42]. To discriminate whether the simultaneous presence of iNKT cells is mandatory for simplexide-induced cytokine production from monocytes, or this glycolipid can itself generate intracellular signals directly by interaction with CD1d, this study was performed with highly purified preparations of monocytes, where contaminant iNKT cells were 0.0%. The profile of cytokines/chemokines induced by simplexide in monocytes suggests that this glycolipid may potentially exert both proinflammatory and immu-

noregulatory activities. Both CXCL8 and TNF-α are potent mediators of inflammation and are involved in recruitment and activation of inflammatory cells. On the other hand, IL-6 and IL-10 are regulatory cytokines that can at least partially explain the immunosuppressive activity previously shown by simplexide in a murine model of T cell activation [27].

The results of our study support the hypothesis that simplexide-induced activation of monocytes is dependent on CD1d expressed by these cells. First, the aglycon of simplexide is a secondary alcohol without further functional groups, glycosylated by a disaccharide chain composed of an inner α-galactose and an outer glucose that possesses α anomeric configuration, similar to that involved in the immunoregulatory activity of α-GalCer [16]. Both molecules contain two long saturated alkyl chains that can fit into the CD1d lipid-binding groove. Thus, it is reasonable to hypothesize that simplexide binds to CD1d in a similar way as α-GalCer [13]. In addition, cytokine release induced by simplexide is suppressed by a CD1d antagonist, DPPE-PEG, and by CD1d knockdown. Finally, simplexide stimulates cytokine production by CD1d-transfected C1R cells whereas it has no effect on parental C1R cell line.

Two different groups have demonstrated that CD1d cross-linking by a monoclonal anti-CD1d antibody induces the release of cytokines from human monocytes [21] and intestinal epithelial cells [22]. The latter finding has been confirmed and extended by showing that CD1d crosslinking results in increased production of IL-10 in a model of inflammatory bowel disease [23]. We have confirmed that anti-CD1d induces IL-10 production from human monocytes provided that the anti-CD1d monoclonal antibody is bivalent and is able to cross-link CD1d molecules (Loffredo et al, in preparation). Although simplexide and anti-CD1d elicit similar responses, it is currently unknown whether simplexide interacts with CD1d on monocytes as a monovalent or bivalent agonist. The molecular interaction between simplexide and CD1d should be further investigated.

Naturally occurring glycolipids are increasingly recognized as modulators of innate and adaptive immunity [11,43]. Glycolipids can function as antigens primarily by interacting with CD1d expressed on APC [44]. Presentation of CD1d-bound glycolipids to NKT cells activates effector functions and cytokine production in NKT cells and subsequent transactivation of APC [18,19,20,45]. This canonical model of glycolipid-induced activation of immune responses has been largely investigated using α-GalCer and related molecules. We found that simplexide, akin to α-GalCer, induces the expansion of iNKT cells in vitro. It will be interesting to assess the cytokine profile expressed by iNKT cells in response to simplexide and whether this differ from that induced by α-GalCer.

Taken together, our findings demonstrate that simplexide can modulate the activity of different immune cells by inducing monocyte production of cytokines and chemokines in a CD1d-dependent manner and the expansion of iNKT in vitro. Further studies are required to understand the potential immunological applications of simplexide. Immunologically active glycosphingolipids, α-GalCer and its synthetic analog KRN7000, are currently being evaluated in cancer immunotherapy [46,47,48] and as vaccine adjuvants [49]. In addition, recent findings highlight the important role of CD1d in determining the host response to environmental stimuli [23]. The observation that simplexide is a novel activator of human monocytes and iNKT cells in vitro raises interesting perspectives on the therapeutic potential of this glycolipid.

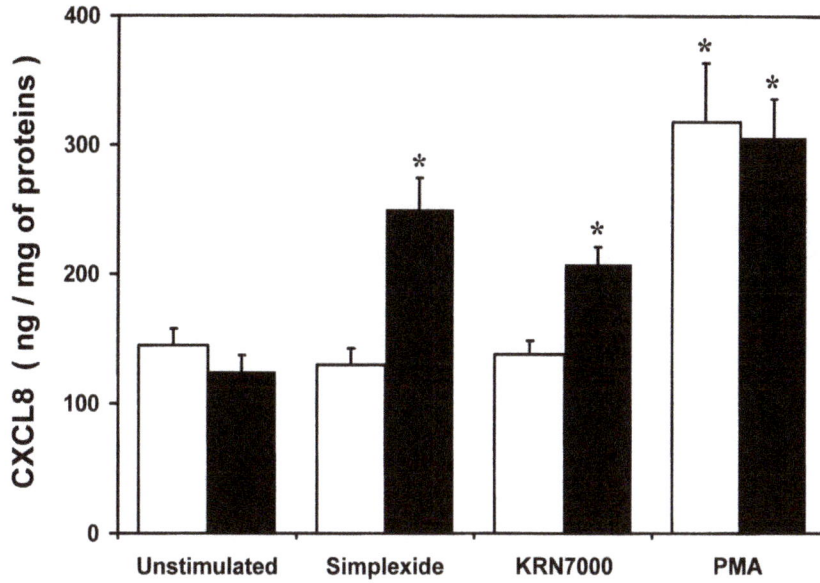

Figure 9. Effect of simplexide on C1R and C1R-CD1d cell lines. C1R and C1R-CD1d were incubated (37°C, 24 h) with X-VIVO alone (unstimulated), simplexide (10 μM), KRN7000 (1 μM) or PMA (100 ng/ml). At the end of incubation, the supernatant was collected and centrifuged (1000×g, 4°C, 5 min). CXCL8 was determined by ELISA. The values are expressed as pg of CXCL8 per mg of total proteins. Data are the mean ± SEM of six experiments. * p<0.05 vs. the respective unstimulated.

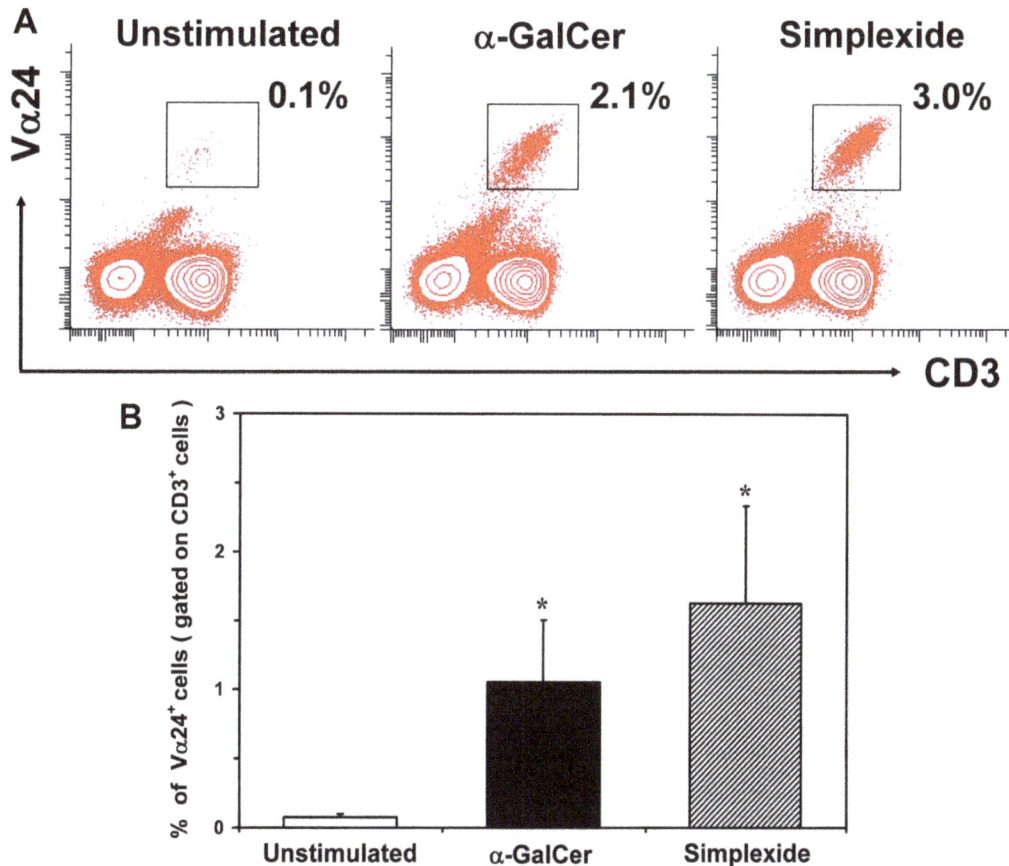

Figure 10. In vitro expansion of human iNKT cells. Human PBMC were stimulated with α-GalCer (100 nM) or simplexide (100 nM) for 7 days. iNKT expansion has been determined as percentage of Vα24+ cells among CD3+ lymphocytes. (A) Representative contour plots are shown. (B) Data are the mean ± SEM of four experiments. * p<0.05 vs. unstimulated.

Supporting Information

Figure S1 Reagents and conditions for preparation of synthetic simplexide. *a.* oxalyl chloride, DMSO, DCM, then Et$_3$N; *b.* Mg, Et$_2$O; *c.* Et$_2$O; *d.* BnBr, NaH, DMF; *e.* AcOH, HCl; *f.* CCl$_3$CN, Cs$_2$CO$_3$, DCM; *g.* PhCH(OCH$_3$)$_2$, TfOH, DMF; *h.* BnBr, NaH, DMF, TBAI; *i.* TES, TFA, DCM; *j.* TMSOTf, Et$_2$O; *k*: H$_2$, 20% Pd(OH)$_2$/C, EtOH, AcOH; *l*: Ac$_2$O, AcOH, H$_2$SO$_4$; *m.* NH$_2$NH$_2$·AcOH, DMF; *n.* CCl$_3$CN, Cs$_2$CO$_3$, DCM; *o.* TMSOTf, DCM; *p.* Et$_3$N, MeOH. Ac = acetyl, Bn = benzyl, DCM = dichloromethane, DMF = *N,N*-dimethylformamide, DMSO = dimethylsulfoxide, Et = ethyl, Ph = phenyl, TBAI = *tert*-butylammonium iodide, TES = trimethylsilane, Tf = trifluoromethanesulfonate, TFA = trifluoroacetic acid, TMS = trimethylsilyl.
(DOC)

Acknowledgments

Authors wish to dedicate this paper to the memory of Prof. Ernesto Fattorusso (1937–2012) who has inspired it.

Author Contributions

Conceived and designed the experiments: SL RIS MT AM. Performed the experiments: SL RIS FB VC AF MTL. Analyzed the data: SL FG. Contributed reagents/materials/analysis tools: SL RIS FB VC AM GM MT. Wrote the paper: SL GM AM MT.

References

1. Auffray C, Sieweke MH, Geissmann F (2009) Blood monocytes: development, heterogeneity, and relationship with dendritic cells. Annu Rev Immunol 27: 669–692.
2. Biswas SK, Mantovani A (2010) Macrophage plasticity and interaction with lymphocyte subsets: cancer as a paradigm. Nat Immunol 11: 889–896.
3. Hettinger J, Richards DM, Hansson J, Barra MM, Joschko AC, et al. (2013) Origin of monocytes and macrophages in a committed progenitor. Nat Immunol 14: 821–830.
4. Geissmann F, Manz MG, Jung S, Sieweke MH, Merad M, et al. (2010) Development of monocytes, macrophages, and dendritic cells. Science 327: 656–661.
5. Mildner A, Chapnik E, Manor O, Yona S, Kim KW, et al. (2013) Mononuclear phagocyte miRNome analysis identifies miR-142 as critical regulator of murine dendritic cell homeostasis. Blood 121: 1016–1027.
6. Serbina NV, Jia T, Hohl TM, Pamer EG (2008) Monocyte-mediated defense against microbial pathogens. Annu Rev Immunol 26: 421–452.
7. Strauss-Ayali D, Conrad SM, Mosser DM (2007) Monocyte subpopulations and their differentiation patterns during infection. J Leukoc Biol 82: 244–252.
8. Wu D, Fujio M, Wong CH (2008) Glycolipids as immunostimulating agents. Bioorg Med Chem 16: 1073–1083.
9. Wu D, Zajonc DM, Fujio M, Sullivan BA, Kinjo Y, et al. (2006) Design of natural killer T cell activators: structure and function of a microbial glycosphingolipid bound to mouse CD1d. Proc Natl Acad Sci U S A 103: 3972–3977.
10. Brigl M, Brenner MB (2004) CD1: antigen presentation and T cell function. Annu Rev Immunol 22: 817–890.
11. Brutkiewicz RR (2006) CD1d ligands: the good, the bad, and the ugly. J Immunol 177: 769–775.
12. Borg NA, Wun KS, Kjer-Nielsen L, Wilce MC, Pellicci DG, et al. (2007) CD1d-lipid-antigen recognition by the semi-invariant NKT T-cell receptor. Nature 448: 44–49.
13. Koch M, Stronge VS, Shepherd D, Gadola SD, Mathew B, et al. (2005) The crystal structure of human CD1d with and without alpha-galactosylceramide. Nat Immunol 6: 819–826.
14. Tyznik AJ, Farber E, Girardi E, Birkholz A, Li Y, et al. (2011) Glycolipids that elicit IFN-gamma-biased responses from natural killer T cells. Chem Biol 18: 1620–1630.
15. Morita M, Motoki K, Akimoto K, Natori T, Sakai T, et al. (1995) Structure-activity relationship of alpha-galactosylceramides against B16-bearing mice. J Med Chem 38: 2176–2187.
16. Kawano T, Cui J, Koezuka Y, Toura I, Kaneko Y, et al. (1997) CD1d-restricted and TCR-mediated activation of valpha14 NKT cells by glycosylceramides. Science 278: 1626–1629.
17. Kronenberg M (2005) Toward an understanding of NKT cell biology: progress and paradoxes. Annu Rev Immunol 23: 877–900.
18. Im JS, Arora P, Bricard G, Molano A, Venkataswamy MM, et al. (2009) Kinetics and cellular site of glycolipid loading control the outcome of natural killer T cell activation. Immunity 30: 888–898.
19. Salio M, Silk JD, Cerundolo V (2010) Recent advances in processing and presentation of CD1 bound lipid antigens. Curr Opin Immunol 22: 81–88.
20. Yue SC, Nowak M, Shaulov-Kask A, Wang R, Yue D, et al. (2010) Direct CD1d-mediated stimulation of APC IL-12 production and protective immune response to virus infection in vivo. J Immunol 184: 268–276.
21. Yue SC, Shaulov A, Wang R, Balk SP, Exley MA (2005) CD1d ligation on human monocytes directly signals rapid NF-kappaB activation and production of bioactive IL-12. Proc Natl Acad Sci U S A 102: 11811–11816.
22. Colgan SP, Hershberg RM, Furuta GT, Blumberg RS (1999) Ligation of intestinal epithelial CD1d induces bioactive IL-10: critical role of the cytoplasmic tail in autocrine signaling. Proc Natl Acad Sci U S A 96: 13938–13943.
23. Olszak T, Neves JF, Dowds CM, Baker K, Glickman J, et al. (2014) Protective mucosal immunity mediated by epithelial CD1d and IL-10. Nature.
24. Costantino V, Fattorusso E, Menna M, Taglialatela-Scafati O (2004) Chemical Diversity of Bioactive Marine Natural Products: An Illustrative Case Study Curr Med Chem 11: 1671–1692.
25. Fattorusso E, Mangoni A (1997) Marine glycolipids. Fortschr Chem Org Naturst 72: 215–301.
26. Costantino V, Fattorusso E, Mangoni A, Di Rosa M, Ianaro A (1999) Glycolipids from sponges. VII. Simplexides, novel immunosuppressive glycolipids from the Caribbean sponge Plakortis simplex. Bioorg Med Chem Lett 9: 271–276.
27. Costantino V, Fattorusso E, Mangoni A, Di Rosa M, Ianaro A, et al. (1996) Glycolipids from Sponges. IV. Immunomodulating Glycosyl Ceramides from the Marine Sponge Agelahs dispar. Tetrahedron 52: 1573–1578.
28. Banchet-Cadeddu A, Henon E, Dauchez M, Renault JH, Monneaux F, et al. (2011) The stimulating adventure of KRN 7000. Org Biomol Chem 9: 3080–3104.
29. Gadola SD, Dulphy N, Salio M, Cerundolo V (2002) Valpha24-JalphaQ-independent, CD1d-restricted recognition of alpha-galactosylceramide by human CD4(+) and CD8alphabeta(+) T lymphocytes. J Immunol 168: 5514–5520.
30. Granata F, Frattini A, Loffredo S, Staiano RI, Petraroli A, et al. (2010) Production of vascular endothelial growth factors from human lung macrophages induced by group IIA and group X secreted phospholipases A2. J Immunol 184: 5232–5241.
31. Triggiani M, Granata F, Petraroli A, Loffredo S, Frattini A, et al. (2009) Inhibition of secretory phospholipase A2-induced cytokine production in human lung macrophages by budesonide. Int Arch Allergy Immunol 150: 144–155.
32. Rossol M, Heine H, Meusch U, Quandt D, Klein C, et al. (2011) LPS-induced cytokine production in human monocytes and macrophages. Crit Rev Immunol 31: 379–446.
33. Bas S, Neff L, Vuillet M, Spenato U, Seya T, et al. (2008) The proinflammatory cytokine response to Chlamydia trachomatis elementary bodies in human macrophages is partly mediated by a lipoprotein, the macrophage infectivity potentiator, through TLR2/TLR1/TLR6 and CD14. J Immunol 180: 1158–1168.
34. Burton RA, Gidley MJ, Fincher GB (2010) Heterogeneity in the chemistry, structure and function of plant cell walls. Nat Chem Biol 6: 724–732.
35. Lombardi V, Stock P, Singh AK, Kerzerho J, Yang W, et al. (2010) A CD1d-dependent antagonist inhibits the activation of invariant NKT cells and prevents development of allergen-induced airway hyperreactivity. J Immunol 184: 2107–2115.
36. Nieuwenhuis EE, Gillessen S, Scheper RJ, Exley MA, Taniguchi M, et al. (2005) CD1d and CD1d-restricted iNKT-cells play a pivotal role in contact hypersensitivity. Exp Dermatol 14: 250–258.
37. Castagna M, Takai Y, Kaibuchi K, Sano K, Kikkawa U, et al. (1982) Direct activation of calcium-activated, phospholipid-dependent protein kinase by tumor-promoting phorbol esters. J Biol Chem 257: 7847–7851.
38. Tefit JN, Davies G, Serra V (2010) NKT cell responses to glycolipid activation. Methods Mol Biol 626: 149–167.
39. Guha M, Mackman N (2001) LPS induction of gene expression in human monocytes. Cell Signal 13: 85–94.
40. Gordon JR, Galli SJ (1990) Mast cells as a source of both preformed and immunologically inducible TNF-alpha/cachectin. Nature 346: 274–276.
41. Zhang B, Alysandratos KD, Angelidou A, Asadi S, Sismanopoulos N, et al. (2011) Human mast cell degranulation and preformed TNF secretion require mitochondrial translocation to exocytosis sites: relevance to atopic dermatitis. J Allergy Clin Immunol 127: 1522–1531 e1528.
42. Venkataswamy MM, Baena A, Goldberg MF, Bricard G, Im JS, et al. (2009) Incorporation of NKT cell-activating glycolipids enhances immunogenicity and vaccine efficacy of Mycobacterium bovis bacillus Calmette-Guerin. J Immunol 183: 1644–1656.
43. Barral DC, Brenner MB (2007) CD1 antigen presentation: how it works. Nat Rev Immunol 7: 929–941.

44. Mattner J, Debord KL, Ismail N, Goff RD, Cantu C 3rd, et al. (2005) Exogenous and endogenous glycolipid antigens activate NKT cells during microbial infections. Nature 434: 525–529.

45. Brigl M, Bry L, Kent SC, Gumperz JE, Brenner MB (2003) Mechanism of CD1d-restricted natural killer T cell activation during microbial infection. Nat Immunol 4: 1230–1237.

46. Motohashi S, Nagato K, Kunii N, Yamamoto H, Yamasaki K, et al. (2009) A phase I–II study of alpha-galactosylceramide-pulsed IL-2/GM-CSF-cultured peripheral blood mononuclear cells in patients with advanced and recurrent non-small cell lung cancer. J Immunol 182: 2492–2501.

47. Kobayashi E, Motoki K, Uchida T, Fukushima H, Koezuka Y (1995) KRN7000, a novel immunomodulator, and its antitumor activities. Oncol Res 7: 529–534.

48. Kunii N, Horiguchi S, Motohashi S, Yamamoto H, Ueno N, et al. (2009) Combination therapy of in vitro-expanded natural killer T cells and alpha-galactosylceramide-pulsed antigen-presenting cells in patients with recurrent head and neck carcinoma. Cancer Sci 100: 1092–1098.

49. Cerundolo V, Silk JD, Masri SH, Salio M (2009) Harnessing invariant NKT cells in vaccination strategies. Nat Rev Immunol 9: 28–38.

14

Proximal Tubule Epithelial Cell Specific Ablation of the Spermidine/Spermine N^1-Acetyltransferase Gene Reduces the Severity of Renal Ischemia/Reperfusion Injury

Kamyar Zahedi[1,4]*, **Sharon Barone**[1,4], **Yang Wang**[1], **Tracy Murray-Stewart**[2], **Prabir Roy-Chaudhury**[1], **Roger D. Smith**[3], **Robert A. Casero, Jr.**[2], **Manoocher Soleimani**[1,4]

1 Division of Nephrology and Hypertension, Department of Internal Medicine, University of Cincinnati College of Medicine, Cincinnati, Ohio, United States of America, 2 The Sidney Kimmel Comprehensive Cancer Center, Johns Hopkins University School of Medicine, Baltimore, Maryland, United States of America, 3 Department of Pathology and Laboratory Medicine, University of Cincinnati College of Medicine, Cincinnati, Ohio, United States of America, 4 Veterans Affair Medical Center, Cincinnati, Ohio, United States of America

Abstract

Background: Expression and activity of spermidine/spermine N^1-acetyltransferase (SSAT) increases in kidneys subjected to ischemia/reperfusion (I/R) injury, while its ablation reduces the severity of such injuries. These results suggest that increased SSAT levels contribute to organ injury; however, the role of SSAT specifically expressed in proximal tubule epithelial cells, which are the primary targets of I/R injury, in the mediation of renal damage remains unresolved.

Methods: Severity of I/R injury in wt and renal proximal tubule specific SSAT-ko mice (PT-SSAT-Cko) subjected to bilateral renal I/R injury was assessed using cellular and molecular biological approaches.

Results: Severity of the loss of kidney function and tubular damage are reduced in PT-SSAT-Cko- compared to wt-mice after I/R injury. In addition, animals treated with MDL72527, an inhibitor of polyamine oxidases, had less severe renal damage than their vehicle treated counter-parts. The renal expression of HMGB 1 and Toll like receptors (TLR) 2 and 4 were also reduced in PT-SSAT-Cko- compared to wt mice after I/R injury. Furthermore, infiltration of neutrophils, as well as expression of tumor necrosis factor-α (TNF-α), monocyte chemoattractant protein-1 (MCP-1) and interleukin-6 (IL-6) transcripts were lower in the kidneys of PT-SSAT-Cko compared to wt mice after I/R injury. Finally, the activation of caspase3 was more pronounced in the wt compared to PT-SSAT-Cko animals.

Conclusions: Enhanced SSAT expression by proximal tubule epithelial cells leads to tubular damage, and its deficiency reduces the severity of renal I/R injury through reduction of cellular damage and modulation of the innate immune response.

Editor: Prasun K. Datta, Temple University, United States of America

Funding: This work was supported by grants CA051085 and CA098454 (RAC) from National Institutes of Health and VA Merit Award (MS). These studies were supported in part by funds from the Center on Genetics of Transport and Epithelial Biology at the University of Cincinnati, funds from DCI and US Renal Care Inc. The funders had no role in study design, data collection and analysis, decision to publish, or preparation of the manuscript.

Competing Interests: This study was supported by funds from Dialysis Clinic Inc. and US Renal Care Inc. There are no patents, products in development or marketed products to declare.

* Email: zahedika@ucmail.uc.edu

Introduction

Polyamines (spermidine, Spd and spermine, Spm) are aliphatic cations that interact with nucleic acids and proteins. Through their interactions, polyamines play important roles in maintenance of nucleic acid structure, gene transcription, signal transduction and cell proliferation [1–5]. The cellular levels of polyamines are tightly regulated through their import, export, synthesis and catabolism. Polyamines are catabolized by back-conversion through their stepwise acetylation and oxidation by spermidine/

spermine N^1-acetyltransferase (SSAT) and N^1-acetylpolyamine oxidase (APAO), respectively, or oxidation of Spm by spermine oxidase (SMO). Oxidation of acetylated Spm and Spd by APAO generates H$_2$O$_2$ and 3-acetoaminopropanal, whereas oxidation of Spm by SMO generates H$_2$O$_2$, 3-aminopropanal. Both H$_2$O$_2$ and the respective aldehydes can lead to cell injury.

The expression and activity of SSAT increases in organs (e.g. liver, kidney and brain) subjected to ischemia/reperfusion (I/R), sepsis, toxic and traumatic injuries [6–10]. Transgenic animals that express high levels of SSAT develop skin lesions and pancreatitis [11–13]. *In vitro*, expression of SSAT causes oxidative stress, DNA damage, cell cycle arrest, and cell death [14–16]. These results suggest that elevated SSAT levels contribute to the onset of cell damage and tissue injury. Using SSAT-ko mice, we have shown that SSAT deficiency reduces the severity of sepsis and I/R induced injuries [6,17]. Although the aforementioned studies indicate that SSAT plays a maladaptive role in renal injuries, they do not identify the specific cells that are the source of this enzyme. We hypothesize that increased SSAT expression and activity in renal proximal tubule cells in response to renal I/R injury contributes to tubular damage and kidney dysfunction. In order to test this hypothesis, we generated proximal tubule cell-specific SSAT knockout (PT-SSAT-Cko) mice and determined the impact of cell specific ablation of the SSAT gene on the severity of kidney I/R injury.

Materials and Methods

Reagents

All chemicals were purchased from Sigma-Aldrich (St. Louis, MO) unless otherwise indicated. Oligonucleotides were purchased from Invitrogen (Carlsbad, CA). The following antibodies were used in this study: Rabbit anti-actin (Santa Cruz Biotech, Santa Cruz, CA), Rabbit anti-pro and cleaved Caspase 3 (H-277, Santa Cruz Biotech, Santa Cruz, CA), Rabbit anti-cleaved caspase 3 (Sigma-Aldrich, St Louis, MO), Rabbit anti-Poly (ADP-ribose) polymerase 1/2 (Santa Cruz Biotech, Santa Cruz, CA), Rabbit anti toll-like receprtor 2 (TLR2; Santa Cruz Biotech, Santa Cruz, CA) and 4 (TLR4; Santa Cruz Biotech, Santa Cruz, CA) and rabbit anti-HMGB1 (Novus Biologicals, Littelton, CO). All secondary antibodies were purchased from Invitrogen.

Generation and genotyping of PT-SSAT-Cko mice

LoxP-SSAT (C57BL6-SSAT-Cko$^{Neo-/Flp-}$) mice were generated in our laboratory [8]. Proximal tubule specific SSAT deficient (PT-SSAT-Cko) mice were generated by cross breeding of the C57BL6-SSAT-Cko$^{Neo-/Flp-}$ with C57BL6-Villin-promoter driven Cre-recombinase transgenic mice (Jackson Laboratories, Bar Harbor, ME). The Cre-recombinase mediated disruption of the SSAT gene was confirmed by comparing the genomic DNA from the tail and kidney as previously described [8]. Amplified DNA was examined for the presence of ~1450bp (wt) and ~240 bp (SSAT-Cko) products (**Fig. 1a**). The effect of SSAT gene ablation on the expression of its mRNA in the kidney was examined by northern-blot analysis (**Figs. 1b**).

Induction of renal I/R injury

Male PT-SSAT-Cko and wt mice (28–32 g) were used in these studies. Animals were provided with ample food and water and kept on a 12hr–12hr light–dark cycle at all times. In these studies, animals (n = 8/experimental group) were subjected to renal I/R injury through bilateral clamping of renal arteries for 30 minutes or sham operation as previously described [17]. Briefly, animals were anesthetized by intraperitoneal (i.p.) injection of Ketamine: Xylazine solution (100:10 µg/g body weight). This anesthetic regiment was used instead of inhaled gas since it is not associated with the induction of hypoxia. Once animals were unconscious the site of surgery (abdomen) was shaved and swabbed with betadine solution and ethanol. A medial incision was made, kidneys were exposed and animals were subjected to renal I/R injury through bilateral clamping of renal arteries for 30 minutes. As uninjured controls animals were subjected to sham operation (kidneys were not clamped). At timed intervals (12, 24, 48 and 72 hours), animals were sacrificed through administration of pentobarbital (100 mg/g

i.p.). Blood was collected by direct cardiac puncture and processed to obtain serum. Kidneys were harvested and either fixed in 4% paraformaldehyde, preserved in 70% ethanol and processed for histology and immunofluorescent studies, or snap-frozen in liquid nitrogen and used for RNA and protein extraction. Experiments assessing the effect of the inhibition of polyamine oxidases on the severity of renal I/R injury were performed as outlined above except wt animals (n = 5/group) were treated with vehicle (saline) or polyamine oxidase inhibitor, MDL72527 (100 mg/kg i.p.), 30 minutes after surgery. All studies involving animal were performed according to the standards in the "Guide for the Care and Use of Laboratory Animals" following a protocol approved by the University of Cincinnati Animal Care and Use Committee. All animal work complied with the National Institutes of Health guidelines.

Assessment of kidney histopathology

The histology of kidneys from injured and sham operated wt and PT-SSAT-Cko mice (minimum of 3 animals per group) was compared by light microscopic examination of H&E-stained sections in a blinded manner. Briefly, paraformaldehyde fixed/ethanol preserved tissue samples in were paraffin embedded. Tissue sections (5 µm) were cut, stained with H&E, slides were assigned random numerical codes for blinded evaluation and examined at 100 and 200X magnification. The extent of renal injury was assessed by examining the cortical and corticomedullary regions of the kidney for tubular dilatation, interstitial edema, cast formation and leukocyte infiltration. Kidneys were assigned an injury score of 0 to 3 (0, no injury; 1, mild injury; 2, moderate injury; 3, severe injury) to compare the severity of tissue damage.

Assessment of renal function

Serum creatinine and blood urea nitrogen (BUN) levels were measured using commercially available kits following the manufacturers (Bioassay Systems, Hayward, CA) instructions.

Measurement of tissue polyamine levels

Polyamine pools were analyzed chromatographically as described previously [18,19].

Cell culture studies

Human embryonic kidney cell line, HEK-293, capable of tetracycline inducible expression of SSAT was generated in our laboratory and has been described elsewhere [20]. In these studies cells treated with vehicle or tetracycline were examined for the integrity of their mitochondria using the MitoPT-JC1 mitochondrial staining kit (Immunochemistry Technologies, Bloomington, MN) or processed for protein extraction as described previously [16].

Northern blot analysis

RNA was extracted using the Tri-Reagent protocol (Molecular Research Center, Inc. Cincinnati, OH) and subjected to northern blot analysis as previously described [10]. Equal loading of RNA samples was confirmed by assessment of the ribosomal RNA (rRNA) band intensities.

Preparation of kidney and cell extracts

Flash frozen kidneys were pulverized, washed with ice-cold PBS and subjected to centriguation at 7,000 g for 5 min. Supernatants were discarded and 200 µl of extraction buffer (45 mM HEPES, 0.4 M KCl, 1 mM EDTA, 0.1 mM dithiothreitol, 10% glycerol, pH 7.8) was added to each pellet. Resulting suspensions were

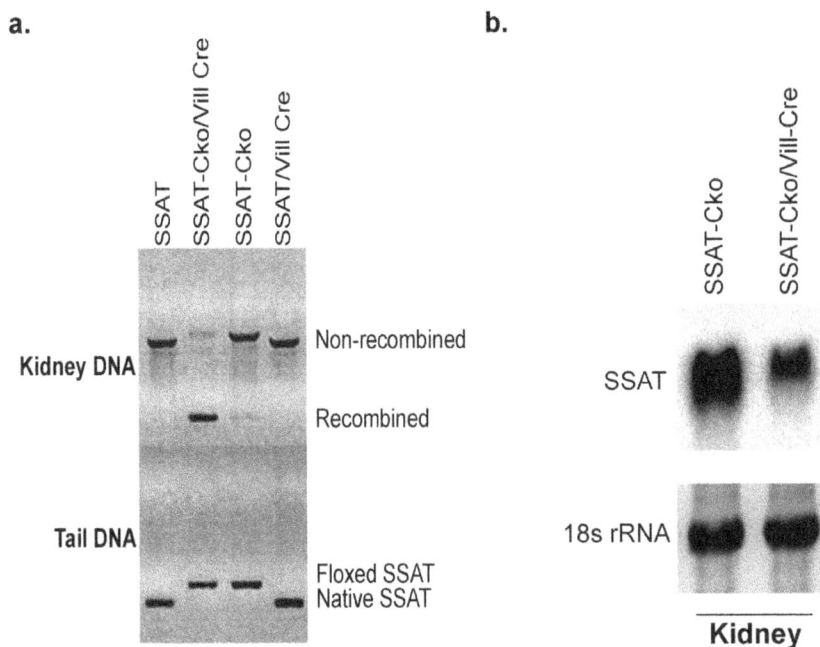

Figure 1. Characterization of proximal tubule cell specific SSAT knockout mice. a) Disruption of the SSAT gene was confirmed by examining the PCR amplification products of genomic DNA from the tail (bottom panel) and kidney (top panel) of SSAT-Cko/Vill-Cre (PT-SSAT-Cko) and their Cre-deficient (SSAT-Cko) littermates. b) Kidney RNA (30 µg/well) from PT-SSAT-Cko and wt mice was size fractionated and subjected to northern blot analysis in order to assess the effect of cre mediated ablation of the SSAT gene on the expression of its mRNA.

mixed vigorously, snap frozen in liquid nitrogen and immediately thawed. Next, 30 µl of 1% Triton X-100 in extraction buffer was added to a 100 µl aliquot of each sample. Samples were mixed vigorously and incubated for 5 min on ice. After centrifugation at 14,000 g for 5 min at 4°C to remove cellular debris, the supernatants were collected. Cell extracts were prepared by lysing the harvested cells in 1X RIPA buffer. All extraction buffers were supplemented with protease and phosphatase inhibitor cocktail (Thermo Scientific, Rockford, IL). The protein contents of kidney and cell extracts were determined by BCA assay (Thermo Scientific, Rockford, IL). For analysis of protein expression levels, 30 µg of each extract was size fractionated by polyacrylamide gel electrophoresis, transferred to nitrocellulose membrane and subjected to western blot analysis as previously described [16].

Measurement of renal cytokine levels

The expression levels of tumor necrosis-α (TNF-α), monocyte chemoattractant protein-1 (MCP-1) and interleukin-6 (IL-6) were assessed by northern blot analysis. The levels of these cytokines in kidney extracts of control and injured mice of both genotypes were measured using the appropriate ELISA kits following the manufacturers (eBioscience, San Diego, CA) instructions.

Immunofluorescent microscopic analysis of kidney sections

Kidney sections (5 µm) were processed for immunofluorescent detection of cleaved caspase 3, TLR2 and TLR4 as described previously [21].

Data analysis

Values are expressed as mean+/-SEM. The significance of differences between mean values of multiple samples was examined using ANOVA. A *"P"* value of less than 0.05 was considered statistically significant.

Results

Proximal tubule epithelium-specific ablation of the SSAT gene reduces the severity of renal I/R injury

The role of proximal tubule cell specific synthesis of SSAT in I/R injury has not been previously addressed. The severity of I/R injury was compared in wt and PT-SSAT-Cko mice in order to specifically determine the role of increased expression of SSAT in proximal tubule epithelial cells in the mediation of tubular damage and kidney dysfunction. Serum creatinine and BUN levels in all injured animals were significantly elevated compared to sham-operated animals (**Fig. 2a**). However, at 24 and 48 hours post I/R injury the serum creatinine and BUN levels were significantly ($p < 0.05$) lower in PT-SSAT-Cko compared to wt mice (**Fig. 2a**). Next, in order to confirm the results of the aforementioned functional studies, we examined the histology of kidneys in wt and PT-SSAT-Cko mice after sham operation or renal I/R injury. Examination of the superficial cortical (outer-cortex) and cortico-medullary (inner-cortex/outer-medulla) regions of the kidneys of sham-operated (non-ischemic) wt- and PT-SSAT-Cko mice did not reveal any histological abnormalities (**Table 1**; **Fig. 2b**). Comparison of the cortical histopathology of ischemic kidneys revealed that wt mice showed moderate tubular dilatation, interstitial edema, and cast formation, the PT-SSAT-Cko mice were protected against these changes and had reduced injury levels compared to their wt counterparts (**Fig. 2b**). Examination of the histology of corticomedullary region of animals subjected to I/R injury revealed that whereas wt animals have extensive tubular damage (e.g. severe tubular dilation and cast formation) the PT-SSAT-Cko mice display significant protection against structural

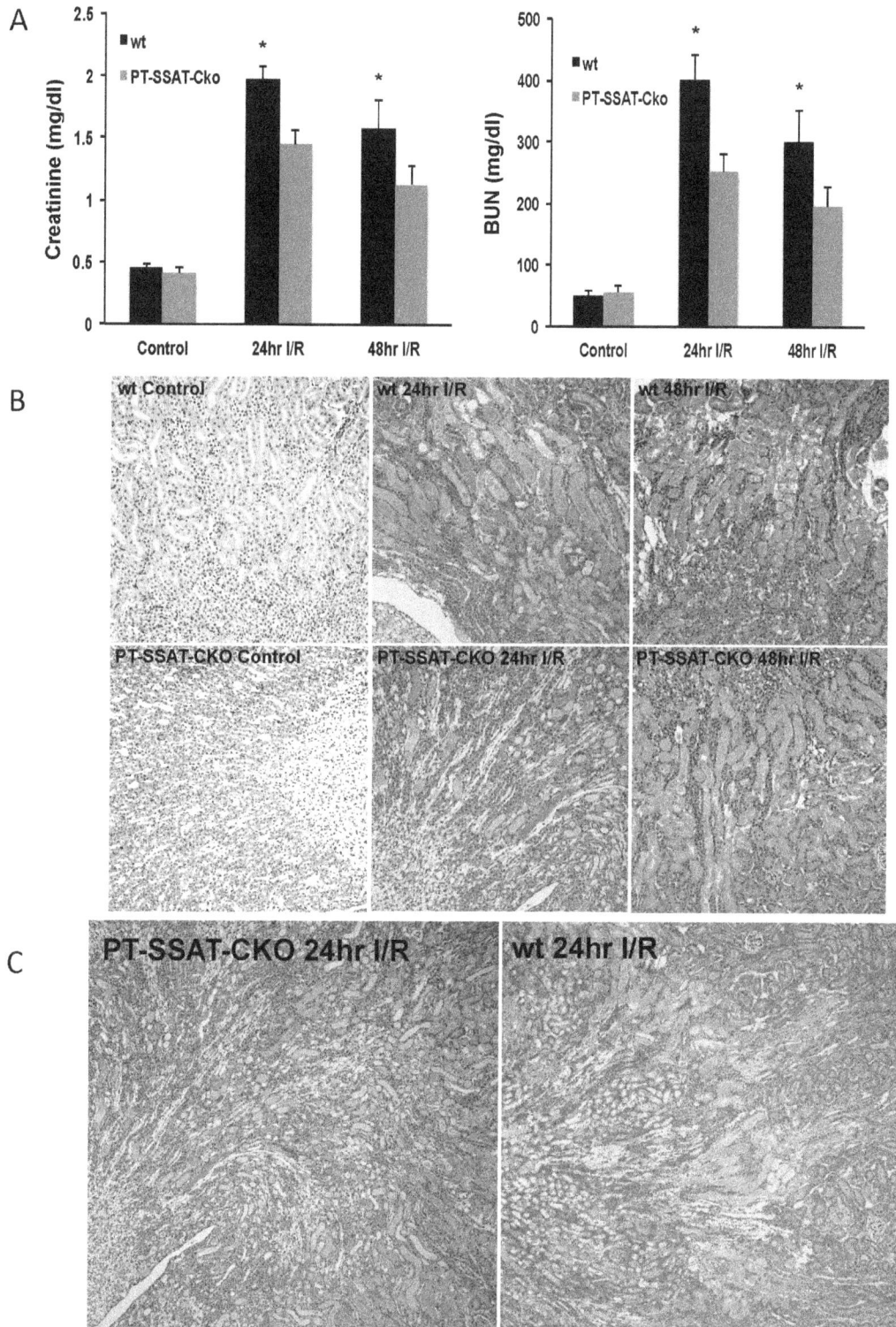

Figure 2. Assessing the effect of proximal tubule cell specific SSAT deficiency on the severity of renal I/R injury. Wt and PT-SSAT-Cko were subjected to Sham or I/R surgery. Animals (n = 8/experimental group) were sacrificed at timed intervals after treatment. a) Serum creatinine and BUN levels of sham operated and injured wt and PT-SSAT-Cko mice were compared following the protocol out lined in the Methods Section. Results are expressed as mean+/-SEM. A p<0.05 is considered significant. b) Kidney histology (Mag 200x) of sham operated and injured wt- and PT-SSAT-Cko- animals were compared. c) Kidney histology (Mag 100x) of injured wt- and PT-SSAT-Cko- animals was compared.

Table 1. Renal histopathology scores for wt and PT-SSAT-Cko mice subjected to sham surgery or renal I/R injury.

	Cortex					Inner cortex/ Outer medulla				
	Tubular Dilitation	Edema	Cast	Leukocyte Infiltration	Cumulative Score	Tubular Dilitation	Edema	Cast	Leukocyte Infiltration	Cumulative Score
Wild Type Sham (n = 2)	0.0+/−0.0	0.0+/−0.0	0.0+/−0.0	0.0+/−0.0	0.0+/−0.0	0.0+/−0.0	0.0+/−0.0	0.0+/−0.0	0.0+/−0.0	0.0+/−0.0
PT-SSAT-Cko Sham (n = 2)	0.0+/−0.0	0.0+/−0.0	0.0+/−0.0	0.0+/−0.0	0.0+/−0.0	0.0+/−0.0	0.0+/−0.0	0.0+/−0.0	0.0+/−0.0	0.0+/−0.0
Wild Type 24hr I/R (n = 3)	1.3+/−0.5	0.3+/−0.6	1.0+/−0.0	0.0+/−0.0	2.7+/−0.5*	3.0+/−0.0*	0.7+/−0.5	3.0+/−0.0*	1.3+/−0.5	8.0+/−0.8
PT-SSAT-Cko 24hr I/R (n = 3)	1.0+/−0.0	0.0+/−0.0	1.0+/−0.0	0.0+/−0.0	2.0+/−0.0	2.3+/−0.5	1.0+/−0.0	2.3+/−0.5	0.7+/−0.9	6.3+/−1.9
Wild Type 48hr I/R (n = 3)	1.0+/−0.0	0.0+/−0.0	0.7+/−0.5	0.0+/−0.0	1.7+/−0.5	2.3+/−0.5	0.7+/−0.5	3.0+/−0.0	1.0+/−0.0	7.0+/−0.8
PT-SSAT-Cko 48hr I/R (n = 3)	0.7+/−0.9	0.3+/−0.5	0.8+/−1.2	0.7+/−0.9	2.5+/−3.3	1.7+/−1.2	0.5+/−0.4	2.0+/−1.4	1.3+/−1.2	5.5+/−3.9

*$p < 0.05$.

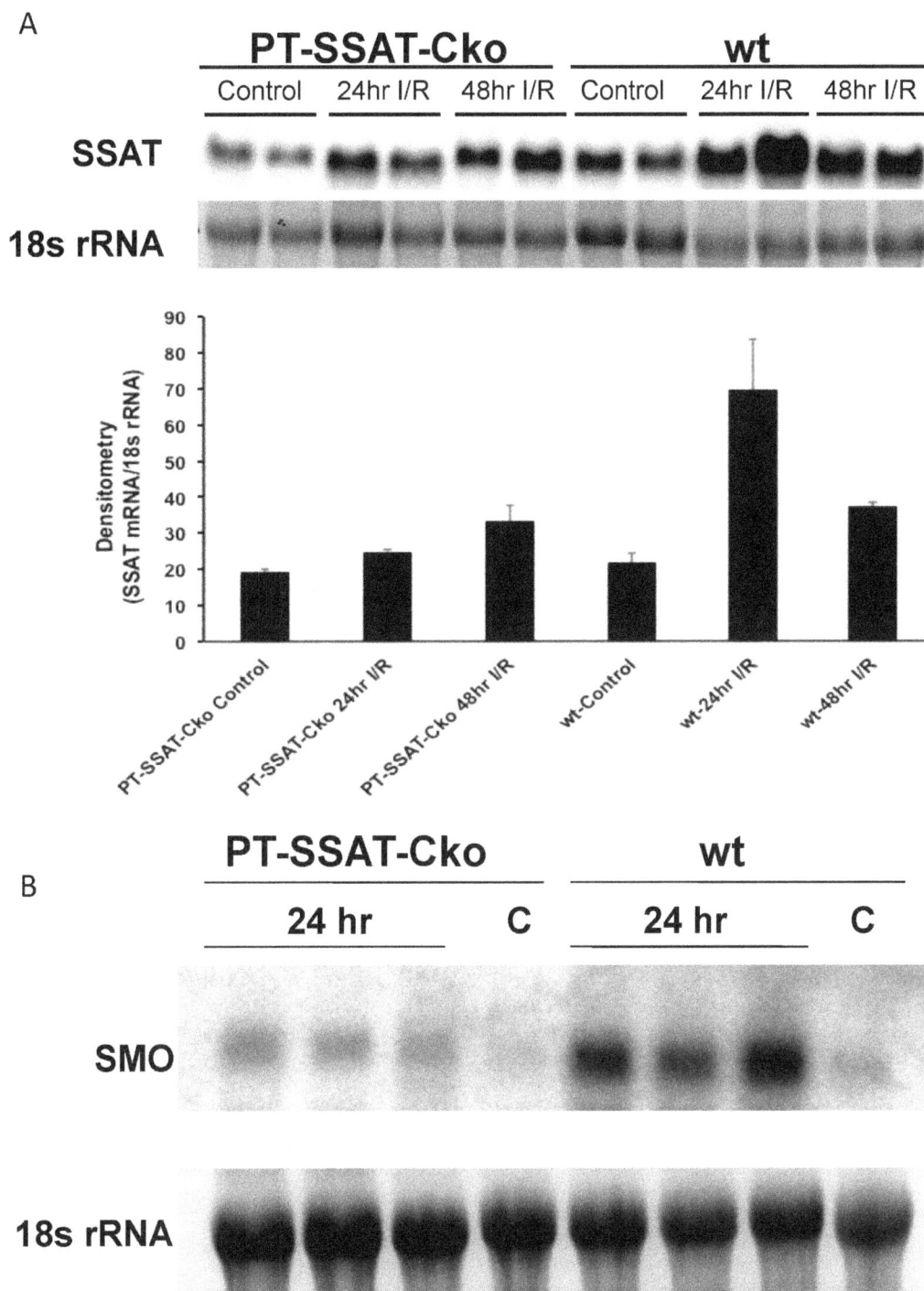

Figure 3. Comparison of the time course of expression of SSAT and SMO in the kidneys of sham operated and injured wt- and PT-SSAT-Cko-mice. a) Kidney RNA (30 μg/well) from sham operated and injured wt- and PT-SSAT-Cko-mice (n = 2) was size fractionated and subjected to northern blot analysis in order to compare the expression levels of SSAT transcripts. The intensity of SSAT mRNA and 18s rRNA bands were determined by densitometry. The intensity of SSAT bands were normalized against that of the corresponding 18s rRNA bands. The graph depicts the average normalized SSATmRNA/18s rRNA values. b) Kidney RNA (30 μg/well) from sham operated (n = 1) and injured wt and PT-SSAT-Cko mice (n = 3) was size fractionated and subjected to northern blot analysis in order to compare the SMO mRNA levels.

damage (e.g. moderate levels of tubular dilatation, cast formation and inflammatory cell infiltration) relative to their wt littermates (**Fig. 2b**). In general the SSAT-deficient animals exhibited less extensive and less severe ischemic injury compared to wt animals

(**Table 1, Fig. 2c**). Our results suggest that the severity of parenchymal damage is reduced in PT-SSAT-Cko animals. The reduction of the severity of kidney damage (i.e. renal histopathology) in PT-SSAT-Cko animals in addition to the data indicating

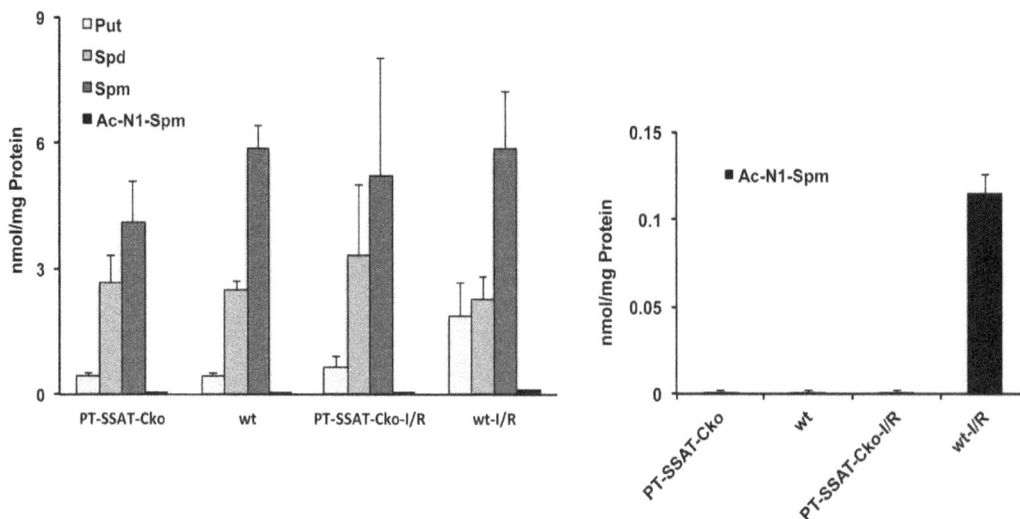

Figure 4. Measurement of polyamine levels in the kidneys of wt and PT-SSAT-Cko mice subjected to sham surgery or renal I/R injury. Kidney polyamine contents of wt and PT-SSAT-Cko mice were measured by HPLC. a) Kidney Put, Spd and Spm levels were determined at 24 hours post-sham or I/R surgery in wt and PT-SSAT-Cko animals. b) Acetyl-N^1-spermine levels in the kidneys of sham operated and injured wt and PT-SSAT-Cko mice were compared.

that these animals have better preserved renal function (i.e. serum creatinine and BUN levels) indicates that proximal tubule specific ablation of SSAT gene protects the kidneys against I/R injury. By extension, these studies suggest that enhanced SSAT expression and the attendant increase in polyamine back-conversion in proximal tubular epithelial cells plays a maladaptive role in the injury process in the kidneys subjected to I/R.

Next, we compared the expression of SSAT and SMO in sham-operated and injured wt and PT-SSAT-Cko mice. Our results indicate that SSAT mRNA expression increases in the kidneys of wt animals after I/R injury (24 hour post injury, **Fig. 3a**). In contrast, the renal expression of SSAT mRNA in PT-SSAT-Cko animals subjected to I/R injury did not significantly differ from that of their sham operated counterparts (**Fig. 3a**). While the expression of the SMO transcript was elevated in both genotypes after I/R injury, its levels were higher in the wt compared to PT-SSAT-Cko animals (**Fig. 3b**). Comparison of kidney polyamine levels at 24 hours post I/R or sham operation (**Fig. 4a**) indicate that Spd and Spm levels were similar in sham operated wt and PT-SSAT-Cko mice (2.48+/−0.23 and 5.86+/−0.56 and 2.68+/−0.63 and 4.12+/−0.95 nmol/mg protein, respectively) and did not change after I/R injury in either genotype (2.27+/−0.56 and 5.88+/−1.35 and 3.34+/−1.68 and 5.24+/−3.53 nmol/mg protein, respectively). The Put levels were similar in the kidneys of sham-operated wt and PT-SSAT-Cko mice (0.46+/−0.07 and 0.46+/−0.05 mol/mg protein). The kidney Put levels in injured PT-SSAT-Cko mice (0.67+/−0.26 nmol/mg protein) was not different from those of the sham-operated animals, while the renal Put content of wt mice after I/R injury (1.83+/−0.80) was higher than sham operated-mice of either genotype and injured PT-SSAT-Cko mice. As shown in **Fig. 4b**, acetylated polyamine levels were below detection limits in sham operated and injured PT-SSAT-Cko mice while acetylated-Spd and Spm levels were elevated in the kidneys of wt animals after I/R injury.

Reduced induction of SMO mRNA in the kidneys of PT-SSAT-Cko mice after I/R injury (**Fig. 3**) as well as the absence of acetylated polyamines that are generated via SSAT activity and

are degraded by APAO to generate H_2O_2 and aminoaldehydes suggest that oxidation of polyamines, through the activity of both SMO and APAO, plays a role in the reduction of severity of renal I/R injury in PT-SSAT-Cko animals. In order to address the role of polyamine oxidation in renal I/R injury, we examined the effect of inhibition of polyamine oxidases with MDL72527 on the severity of tissue damage in animals subjected to renal I/R injury. Our results indicate that serum creatinine levels (1.45+/−0.2 vs. 2.8+/−0.3 mg/dl) and the severity of tubular injury (i.e. tubular dilatation, cast formation and leukocyte infiltration) were significantly reduced in the MDL72527- compared to vehicle-treated animals at 24 hours post I/R injury (**Table 2** and **Fig. 5a and b**). These results indicate that polyamine oxidation contributes to the induction of tubular damage and the loss of renal function in I/R injury.

Increased expression of SSAT in cultured cells leads to mitochondrial damage and apoptosis

We have shown that increased expression of SSAT in cultured cells leads to aberrant cytoskeletal changes, DNA damage and growth arrest [16,20]. In order to elucidate the mechanistic basis of SSAT mediated cell injury, we examined the effect of its expression on the onset of apoptosis in HEK cells capable of inducible expression of SSAT. Our results indicate that induction of SSAT leads to the loss of mitochondrial membrane potential, activation of caspase 3, and cleavage of Poly (ADP-ribose) polymerase 1 (PARP1) (**Fig. 6a and b**). In addition, induction of SSAT expression led to increased production of high mobility group B1 (HMGB1) protein (**Fig. 6b**). These results suggest that enhanced expression of SSAT in cultured cells leads to the onset of apoptosis. Furthermore, enhanced levels of HMGB1 in cells that express high levels of SSAT can lead to the activation of the innate immune response, a known contributing factor to renal I/R injury [22].

Table 2. Renal histopathology scores for saline or MDL72527 treated mice subjected to Sham operation or renal I/R injury.

	Cortex					Inner cortex/Outer medulla				
	Tubular Dilitation	Edema	Cast	Leukocyte Infiltration	Cumulative Score	Tubular Dilitation	Edema	Cast	Leukocyte Infiltration	Cumulative Score
Saline Sham (n=2)	0.0+/−0.0	0.0+/−0.0	0.0+/−0.0	0.0+/−0.0	0.0+/−0.0	0.0+/−0.0	0.0+/−0.0	0.0+/−0.0	0.0+/−0.0	0.0+/−0.0
MDL72527 Sham (n=2)	0.0+/−0.0	0.0+/−0.0	0.0+/−0.0	0.0+/−0.0	0.0+/−0.0	0.0+/−0.0	0.0+/−0.0	0.0+/−0.0	0.0+/−0.0	0.0+/−0.0
Saline 24hr I/R (n=3)	1.4+/−0.5	0.6+/−0.8	1.3+/−0.4	0.0+/−0.0	3.2+/−1.5	2.8+/−0.4	0.6+/−0.5	3.0+/−0.0*	1.0+/−0.6*	7.2+/−1.2
MDL72527 24hr I/R (n=3)	1.3+/−0.4	0.2+/−0.4	0.8+/−0.4	0.0+/−0.0	2.3+/−0.9	1.8+/−0.6	0.8+/−0.4	2.1+/−0.8	0.0+/−0.0	4.8+/−1.9

*$p < 0.05$.

Proximal tubule epithelial cell specific ablation of the SSAT gene modulates the onset of the innate immune response and reduces the extent of apoptotic cell death

HMGB1 binding to TLR2 and 4 and activation of the innate immune response can lead to inflammation and apoptosis and play an important role in the mediation of renal I/R injury [22–26]. Based on increased expression of HMGB1 in SSAT expressing cells (**Fig. 6b**), and our *in vivo* results showing a reduction in leukocyte infiltration in PT-SSAT-Cko compared to wt animals (**Table 1**; **Fig. 2b and c**) we postulated that the lack of SSAT and reduced cell injury can modulate the onset of innate immunity and further reduce the severity of renal injury in PT-SSAT-Cko animals. In order to test this, we compared the onset of innate immune response (e.g. expression levels of HMGB1, TLR2 and TLR4) and apoptosis (cleaved caspase 3 levels) after I/R injury in wt and PT-SSAT-Cko mice. Although the renal expression of HMGB1, TLR2 and TLR4 increase in response to I/R injury in both groups, the expression of these molecules are reduced in PT-SSAT-Cko- compared to wt-animals (**Fig. 7 a and b**). The differences in the activation of innate immune response were further examined by comparing the extent of neutrophil infiltration and pro-inflammatory cytokine expression in the kidneys of wt and PT-SSAT-Cko animals after I/R injury. Examination of TNF-α, MCP-1 and IL-6 transcripts in the kidneys of injured animals revealed that the expression levels of these cytokines are reduced in PT-SSAT-Cko- compared to wt-mice after I/R injury (**Fig. 8a**). Assessment of the protein levels of the aforementioned cytokines also revealed that although the renal content of these cytokines is elevated in both wt- and PT-SSAT-Cko-mice, the former have a more robust response (**Fig. 8b**). Specifically, while the levels of all cytokines increased significantly in injured compared to control kidneys (sham operated animals) at 24 and 48 hours, the cytokine levels in the kidneys of wt animals compared to their PT-SSAT-Cko animals were significantly higher at 48 hrs post I/R injury (**Fig. 8b**). Additionally, chloroacetate esterase staining of the kidney sections revealed that compared to wt-mice the PT-SSAT-Cko animals have reduced levels of neutrophil infiltration (**Fig. 8c**).

Next, we examined the effect of SSAT deficiency on the onset of apoptosis, by comparing the levels of activated caspase 3 in wt and PT-SSAT-Cko animals. Activation of caspase 3 was evident in the proximal tubules of both injured wt and PT-SSAT-Cko animals. Comparison of the injured kidneys revealed that wt animals have increased levels of cleaved caspase 3 (**Fig. 9a**). Western blot analysis of kidney extracts from control and injured animals of both genotypes also confirmed the aforementioned results (**Fig. 9b Top panel, anti-pro and cleaved/activated caspase 3; middle panel, anti-cleaved/activated caspase 3**). These results indicate that the onset of innate immunity is modulated and the extent of renal tubule epithelial cell apoptosis is reduced in PT-SSAT-Cko animals compared to their wt littermates.

Discussion

The expression of SSAT increases dramatically in kidneys subjected to I/R injury [10]. Enhanced expression of SSAT in cultured cells leads to the depletion of polyamines, DNA damage and growth arrest [16,20]. Also, the extent of renal damage after I/R and bacterial lipopolysaccharide-induced renal injury is significantly reduced in SSAT-ko mice [6,17]. Although, these results suggest that increased SSAT expression and elevated polyamine back-conversion are critical in the mediation of I/R- and LPS-induced renal injuries, the role of increased expression of

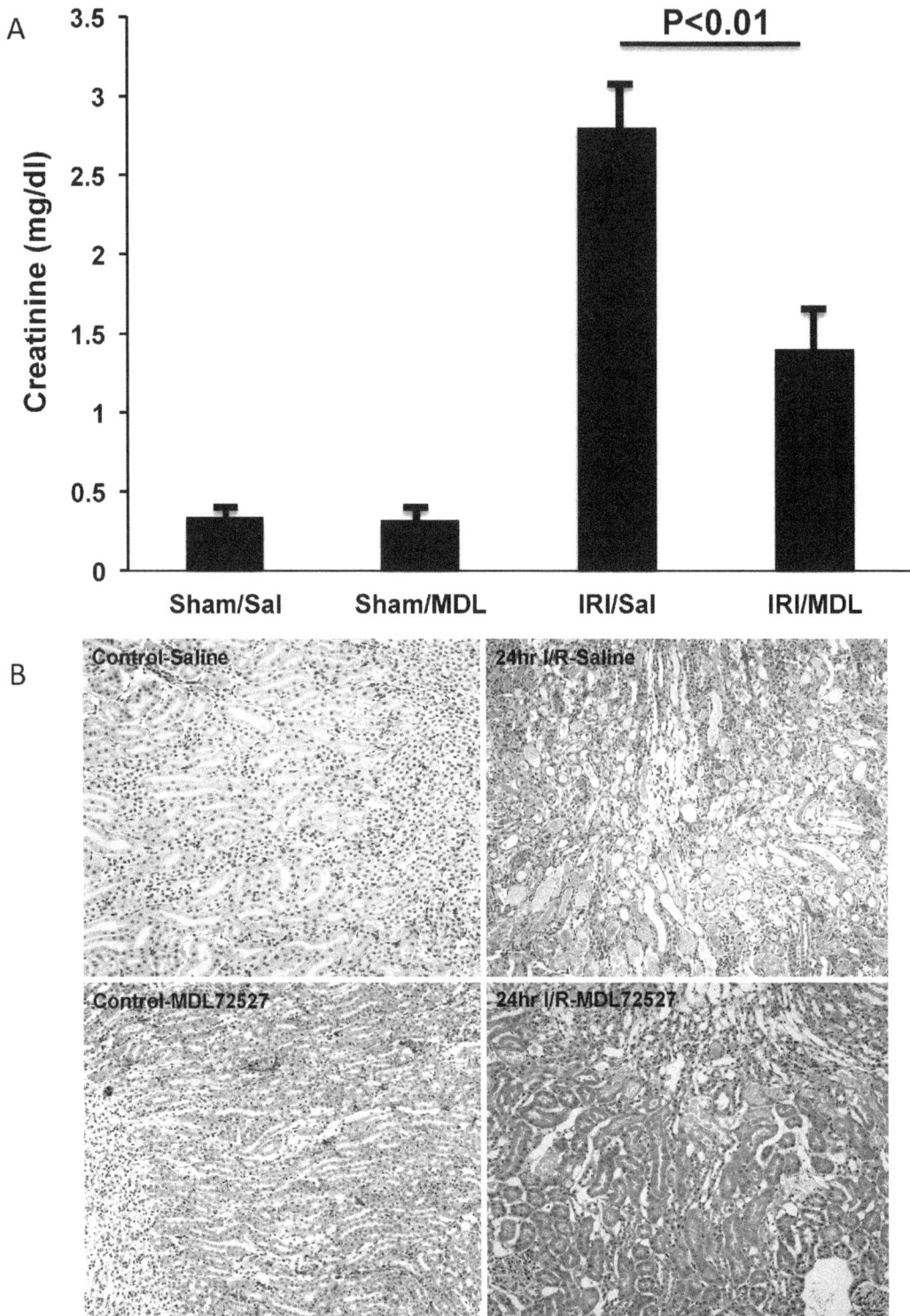

Figure 5. Assessing the effect of inhibition of polyamine oxidases on the severity of renal I/R injury. a) Serum creatinine levels of sham operated and injured mice injected with MDL72527 or vehicle (n = 5/experimental group) were compared following the protocol out lined in the Methods Section. Results are mean+/-SEM of three independent samples. A p<0.05 is considered significant. b) Kidney histology (Mag 200x) of control and injured animals from vehicle and MDL72527 treated groups were compared.

SSAT in proximal tubule epithelial cells, the primary targets of the aforementioned insults, in the mediation of tubular damage and renal dysfunction remains unclear. Our results indicate that the extent of tubular injury is reduced in PT-SSAT-Cko compared to wt mice (**Table 1; Fig. 2b and c**). The potential damaging role of SSAT expression by the parenchymal cells has been demonstrated in transgenic rats, where induction of SSAT in the pancreas leads to the onset of severe pancreatitis [11]; and in

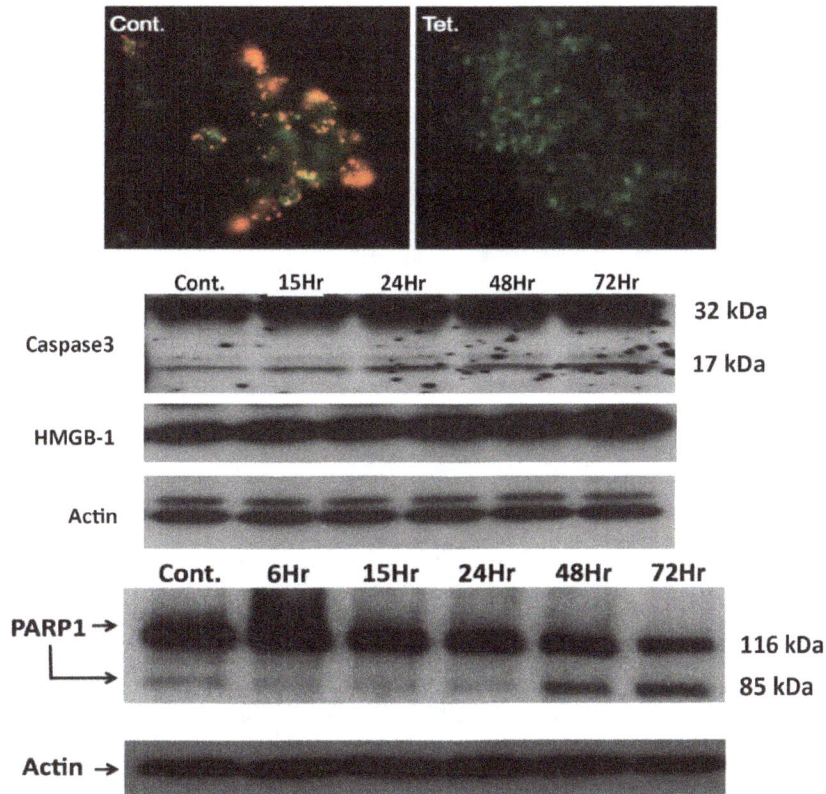

Figure 6. Determining the effect of SSAT expression in cultured çells. The effect of increased SSAT levels in HEK293 cells capable of tetracycline inducible expression of SSAT was examined. a) Effect of increased SSAT expression on mitochondrial integrity was compared in control (Cont.) and tetracycline-treated (Tet.), SSAT expressing, HEK293 cells by assessing the ability of these organelles to retain JC1 dye. JC1 dye is retained by non-depolarized-mitochondria (orange fluorescence) but not by depolarized-mitochondria. b) Cleavage of caspase 3 and PARP-1 (activation of apoptotic pathway), and expression of HMGB1 were examined in control (Cont.) and tetracyclin-treated, SSAT expressing, cells at timed intervals.

hepatocyte specific SSAT-ko mice, where deactivation of SSAT gene in hepatocytes reduces the severity of CCl_4-induced liver injury [8]. The results presented in this manuscript and studies cited above suggest that the increase in expression of SSAT by parenchymal cells and derangements in polyamine catabolism are important in the mediation of tissue damage and organ dysfunction.

In order to determine the role of SSAT mediated derangements in renal polyamine pools in I/R-mediated kidney injury the polyamine levels in the kidneys of sham-operated and injured wt and PT-SSAT-Cko mice were compared (**Fig. 4**). The only difference in polyamine levels, other than the expected absence of acetylated polyamines in the PT-SSAT-Cko mice, was the significant increase in Put levels in the kidneys of wt mice after I/R injury. The increase in Put levels in the wt but not PT-SSAT-Cko animals is similar to what we reported in our previous studies that examined the role of complete SSAT deficiency on the severity of hepatic and renal I/R injuries [17]. Interestingly, elevated Put levels were shown to reduce the viability of cultured hepatocytes [7]. The stability of renal content of Spd and Spm suggests that polyamine depletion per se may not be the driving force behind the tubular cell injury and renal dysfunction and that enhanced Put levels may play a role in the mediation of tissue injury. It should be noted that polyamine levels were measured in the whole kidney and therefore our results do not reflect the effect of their altered metabolism in a specific group of cells or

anatomical segment (e.g. epithelium of the S3 section of the renal proximal tubule that is the primary target of I/R induced injury) of the kidney.

Examination of the mRNA levels of SMO that is up regulated and plays an important role in the mediation of tissue injury [27,28], in control and injured wt and PT-SSAT-Cko mice revealed that its expression is significantly higher in the kidneys of injured wt compared to PT-SSAT-Cko animals (**Fig. 3b**). The increased expression of SMO in wt but not PT-SSAT-Cko animals as well as the potential cytotoxic effects of the products of polyamine oxidation (e.g. H_2O_2 and aminoldahydes) suggest that polyamine oxidation is important in the mediation of I/R induced renal tubular cell injury. The latter was confirmed when it was shown that MDL72527-treated mice had less severe kidney damage after renal I/R injury (**Table 2; Fig. 5**). These findings show that enhanced polyamine oxidation down stream of increased SSAT expression, most likely via increased expression of toxic metabolites such as H_2O_2 and aminoaldehydes, contributes to renal injury. The important role of polyamine oxidation in the mediation of tissue damage is further supported by previous studies which demonstrate that the inhibition of polyamine oxidases or neutralization of the products of their reaction reduces the extent of tissue damage in traumatic, toxic and septic injuries in brain, liver and kidney respectively [6–10,29–31].

In order to clarify the mechanism through which enhanced SSAT expression contributes to tissue damage we examined the

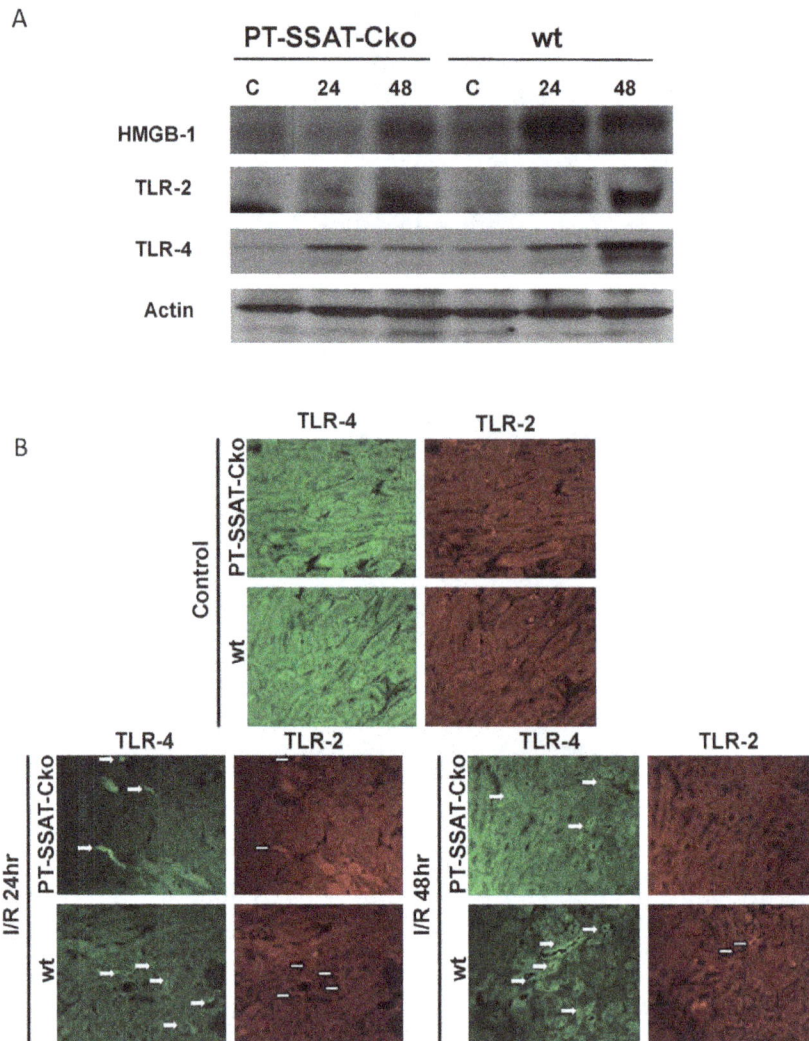

Figure 7. Proximal Tubule Epithelial Cell (PTEC) specific ablation of the SSAT gene dampens the onset of innate immune response and reduces the extent of I/R induced apoptotic cell death. The onset of innate immune response after I/R injury was compared in wt and PT-SSAT-Cko animals. a) Time course of the expression of HMGB1, TLR2 and 4 were compared in the kidneys of sham-operated and injured wt and PT-SSAT-Cko mice. The data are representative of three independent experiments. b) Expression of TLR2 and 4 were assessed by immunofluorescent microscopic examination of kidneys of wt and PT-SSAT-Cko mice after sham- or I/R surgery.

effect of its induction in cultured cells. We have previously shown that enhanced SSAT expression leads to DNA damage and cell cycle arrest [16]. Our current studies further demonstrate that increased expression of SSAT and up regulation of polyamine degradation lead to the activation of the intrinsic pathway of apoptosis. This data supports previous studies that show increased polyamine catabolism in cultured cells leads to the triggering of apoptosis [32,33].

The expression of HMGB1, a ligand involved in the activation of innate immune response [22,34], was also elevated in SSAT-expressing cells (**Fig. 6**). Increased expression of HMGB1 in cells that express high levels of SSAT, as well as reduction in inflammatory cell infiltration in the kidneys of PT-SSAT-Cko mice after I/R injury suggest that down regulation of polyamine catabolism through reduction of cell injury may dampen the activation of innate immune response, there by reducing the severity of organ damage. Therefore, we examined the effect of

proximal tubule specific deficiency of SSAT on the activation of innate immune response and onset of apoptosis. The expression of HMGB1, TLR2 and TLR4 were lower and more transient in the injured kidneys of PT-SSAT-Cko mice compared to their wt littermates (**Fig. 7**). Furthermore, leukocyte infiltration, and expression levels of IL-6, MCP-1 and TNF-α, cytokines known to contribute to I/R mediated renal injury [35–37], were also reduced in the kidneys of PT-SSAT-Cko- compared to wt-mice (**Fig. 8**). The activation/cleavage of caspase 3 was also lower in the injured kidneys of PT-SSAT-Cko-mice compared to their wt-littermates (**Fig. 9**). These results suggest that the activation of innate immune response and onset of apoptosis after renal I/R injury is less robust in PT-SSAT-Cko- compared to wt-animals. The role of HMGB1, TLR2, TLR4, activation of the innate immune response and onset of apoptosis in the pathogenesis of renal I/R injury are well established [22–26]. The expression of HMGB1, TLR2 and TLR4 increases in the kidneys of animals

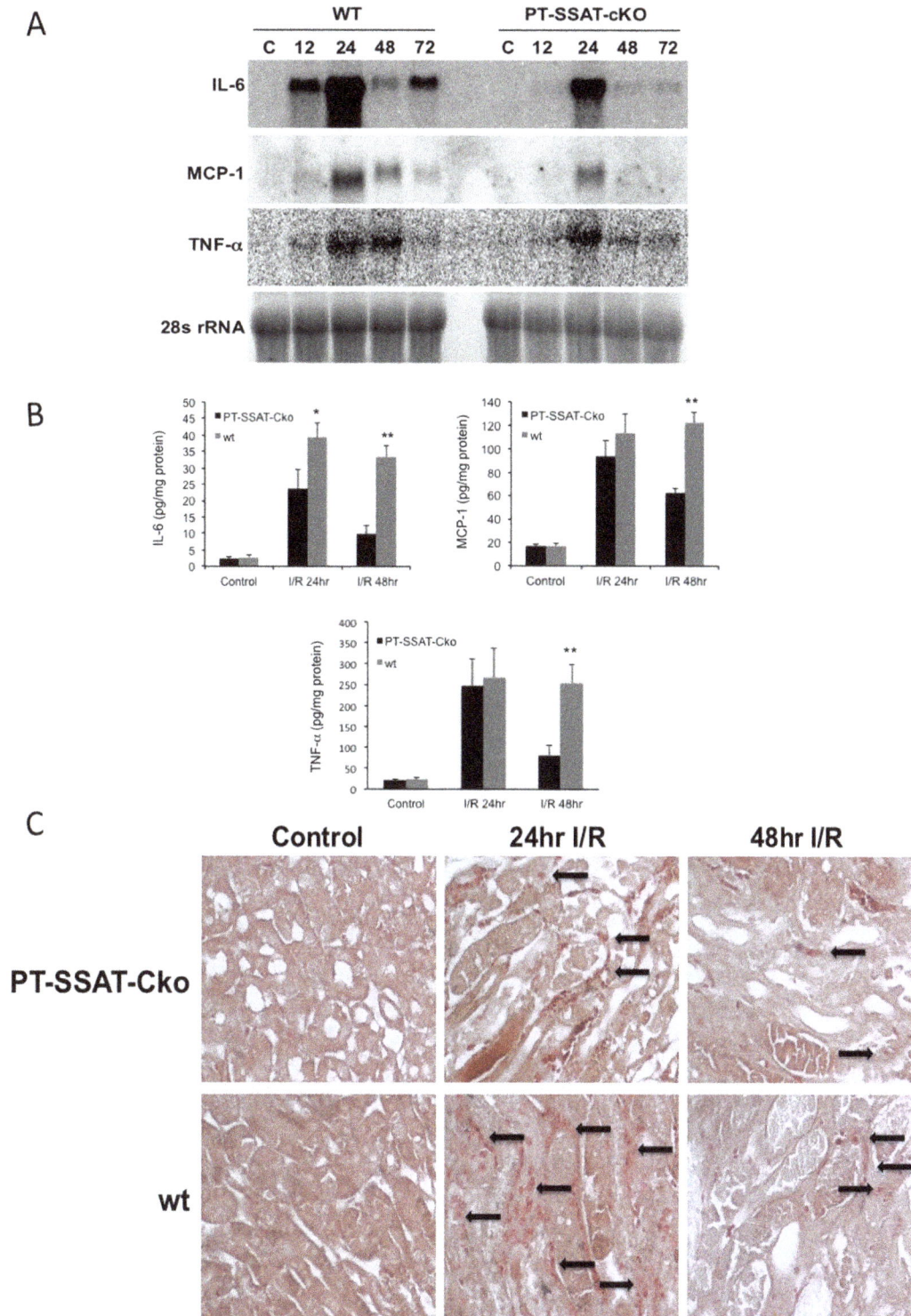

Figure 8. Expression of pro-inflammatory cytokines and neutrophil infiltration after I/R injury is reduced in the kidneys of PT-SSAT-Cko- compared to wt-mice. a) Kidney RNA (30 µg/well) from sham operated and injured wt and PT-SSAT-Cko mice was size fractionated and subjected to northern blot analysis in order to compare the expression levels of IL-6, MCP-1 and TNF-α transcripts. b) IL-6, MCP-1 and TNF-α levels in kidney extracts wt and PT-SSAT-Cko mice subjected to sham operation or renal I/R injury (n = 4 animals/genotype/treatment) were determined using ELISA. c) Kidney sections from sham operated and injured wt and PT-SSAT-Cko mice were subjected to chloroacetate esterase staining to examine the effect of SSAT ablation on the extent of neutrophil infiltration after renal I/R injury.

A

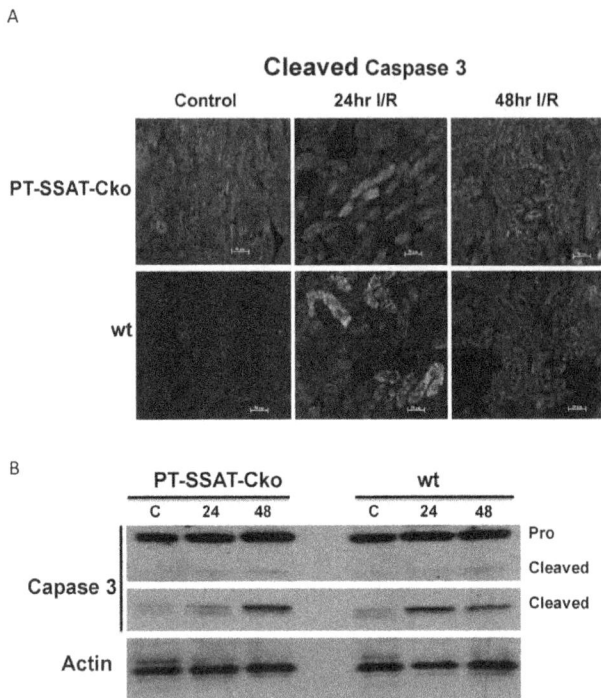

Cleaved Caspase 3

Control   24hr I/R   48hr I/R

PT-SSAT-Cko

wt

B

PT-SSAT-Cko   wt

C   24   48   C   24   48

Pro
Cleaved

Capase 3   Cleaved

Actin

Figure 9. Proximal Tubule Epithelial Cell (PTEC) specific ablation of the SSAT gene reduces the extent of I/R induced apoptotic cell death. a) Activated/cleaved caspase 3 levels in the kidneys of sham operated and injured wt and PT-SSAT-Cko mice were examined by immunofluorescent microscopy (Mag 200x). b) Pro- and cleaved-caspase 3 levels in the kidneys of sham operated and injured wt and PT-SSAT-Cko mice were examined by western blot analysis (top panel: anti-pro and cleaved caspase 3; middle panel: anti cleaved-caspase 3; bottom panel: anti-actin).

subjected to I/R injury [22–26]. In addition, blockade of HMGB1 or deficiency of TLR2 and 4 dampen the inflammatory response (i.e. reduce leukocyte infiltration, lower production of IL-6, MCP-

1 and TNF-α, and modulation of apoptotic response) and reduce the severity of renal I/R injury [22–26]. Based on our results (**Figs. 6–8**) we propose that the reduction in the severity of I/R induced kidney injury in PT-SSAT-Cko animals is partially due to the reduction in the initial cell injury which in turn dampens the onset of the innate immune response.

Our previous studies and the results presented here suggest that increased expression of SSAT and enhanced polyamine oxidation in proximal tubule epithelial cells contribute to tubular damage in renal I/R. Furthermore, our cell culture and animal studies suggest that the increase in polyamine catabolism at cellular level and the attendant alterations in cellular polyamine levels play an important role in the initial cell injury. The increased expression of oxidative stress and DNA damage markers, cell cycle arrest, onset of apoptosis and increased expression of HMGB1 in SSAT over-expressing HEK293 but not in un-induced HEK-293 cells supports this hypothesis (**Fig. 6** and reference 16). We also propose that short-circuiting of polyamine catabolism through ablation of SSAT in proximal tubule epithelial cells specifically reduces the severity of initial cellular damage in response to I/R and in turn dampens the activation of the innate immune response further reducing the extent of tubular damage and the severity of renal I/R injury. The latter is supported by our results that show when subjected to renal I/R injury PT-SSAT-Cko animals have reduced neutrophilia, and express reduced levels of HMGB1, TLR2, TLR4 and pro-inflammatory cytokines. The results presented here supports the hypothesis that polyamine back-conversion and oxidation in proximal tubule epithelial cells are important in the pathophysiology of renal I/R injury, and identify novel therapeutic targets and strategies for treatment of I/R induced kidney damage (i.e. SSAT-suppression and/or inhibition of polyamine oxidation).

Author Contributions

Conceived and designed the experiments: KZ MS. Performed the experiments: KZ SB YW TMS RDS. Analyzed the data: KZ RDS RAC MS. Contributed reagents/materials/analysis tools: KZ PRC RAC MS. Wrote the paper: KZ RDS MS.

References

1. Hasan R, Alam MK, Ali R (1995) Polyamine induced Z-conformation of native calf thymus DNA. FEBS Lett 368: 27–30.
2. Igarashi K, Kashiwagi K (2000) Polyamines: mysterious modulators of cellular functions. Biochem Biophys Res Commun 271: 559–564.
3. Janne J, Alhonen L, Leinonen P (1991) Polyamines: from molecular biology to clinical applications. Ann Med 23: 241–259.
4. Marton LJ, Pegg AE (1995) Polyamines as targets for therapeutic intervention. Annu Rev Pharmacol Toxicol 35: 55–91.
5. Casero RA Jr., Marton LJ (2007) Targeting polyamine metabolism and function in cancer and other hyperproliferative diseases. Nat Rev Drug Discov 6: 373–390.
6. Zahedi K, Barone SL, Kramer DL, Amlal H, Alhonen L, et al. (2010) The Role of Spermidine/Spermine-N1-Acetyltransferase in Endotoxin-Induced Acute Kidney Injury. Am J Physiol Cell Physiol 299: C164–174.
7. Barone S, Okaya T, Rudich S, Petrovic S, Tenrani K, et al. (2005) Distinct and sequential upregulation of genes regulating cell growth and cell cycle progression during hepatic ischemia-reperfusion injury. Am J Physiol Cell Physiol 289: C826–835.
8. Zahedi K, Barone SL, Xu J, Steinbergs N, Schuster R, et al. (2012) Hepatocyte-specific ablation of spermine/spermidine-N1-acetyltransferase gene reduces the severity of CCl4-induced acute liver injury. Am J Physiol Gastrointest Liver Physiol 303: G546–560.
9. Zahedi K, Huttinger F, Morrison R, Murray-Stewart T, Casero RA, et al. (2010) Polyamine catabolism is enhanced after traumatic brain injury. J Neurotrauma 27: 515–525.
10. Zahedi K, Wang Z, Barone S, Prada AE, Kelly CN, et al. (2003) Expression of SSAT, a novel biomarker of tubular cell damage, increases in kidney ischemia-reperfusion injury. Am J Physiol Renal Physiol 284: F1046–1055.

11. Alhonen L, Parkkinen JJ, Keinanen T, Sinervirta R, Herzig KH, et al. (2000) Activation of polyamine catabolism in transgenic rats induces acute pancreatitis. Proc Natl Acad Sci U S A 97: 8290–8295.
12. Pietila M, Alhonen L, Halmekyto M, Kanter P, Janne J, et al. (1997) Activation of polyamine catabolism profoundly alters tissue polyamine pools and affects hair growth and female fertility in transgenic mice overexpressing spermidine/spermine N1-acetyltransferase. J Biol Chem 272: 18746–18751.
13. Pietila M, Parkkinen JJ, Alhonen L, Janne J (2001) Relation of skin polyamines to the hairless phenotype in transgenic mice overexpressing spermidine/spermine N-acetyltransferase. J Invest Dermatol 116: 801–805.
14. Ha HC, Woster PM, Yager JD, Casero RA Jr. (1997) The role of polyamine catabolism in polyamine analogue-induced programmed cell death. Proc Natl Acad Sci U S A 94: 11557–11562.
15. Chen Y, Kramer DL, Diegelman P, Vujcic S, Porter CW (2001) Apoptotic signaling in polyamine analogue-treated SK-MEL-28 human melanoma cells. Cancer Res 61: 6437–6444.
16. Zahedi K, Bissler JJ, Wang Z, Josyula A, Lu L, et al. (2007) Spermidine/spermine N1-acetyltransferase overexpression in kidney epithelial cells disrupts polyamine homeostasis, leads to DNA damage, and causes G2 arrest. Am J Physiol Cell Physiol 292: C1204–1215.
17. Zahedi K, Lentsch AB, Okaya T, Barone S, Sakai N, et al. (2009) Spermidine/spermine-N1-acetyltransferase ablation protects against liver and kidney ischemia-reperfusion injury in mice. Am J Physiol Gastrointest Liver Physiol 296: G899–909.
18. Kramer D, Stanek J, Diegelman P, Regenass U, Schneider P, et al. (1995) Use of 4-fluoro-L-ornithine to monitor metabolic flux through the polyamine biosynthetic pathway. Biochem Pharmacol 50: 1433–1443.

19. Kramer DL, Diegelman P, Jell J, Vujcic S, Merali S, et al. (2008) Polyamine acetylation modulates polyamine metabolic flux, a prelude to broader metabolic consequences. J Biol Chem 283: 4241–4251.
20. Wang Z, Zahedi K, Barone S, Tehrani K, Rabb H, et al. (2004) Overexpression of SSAT in kidney cells recapitulates various phenotypic aspects of kidney ischemia-reperfusion injury. J Am Soc Nephrol 15: 1844–1852.
21. Zahedi K, Wang Z, Barone S, Tehrani K, Yokota N, et al. (2004) Identification of stathmin as a novel marker of cell proliferation in the recovery phase of acute ischemic renal failure. Am J Physiol Cell Physiol 286: C1203–1211.
22. Wu H, Ma J, Wang P, Corpuz TM, Panchapakesan U, et al. (2010) HMGB1 contributes to kidney ischemia reperfusion injury. J Am Soc Nephrol 21: 1878–1890.
23. Leemans JC, Stokman G, Claessen N, Rouschop KM, Teske GJ, et al. (2005) Renal-associated TLR2 mediates ischemia/reperfusion injury in the kidney. J Clin Invest 115: 2894–2903.
24. Rusai K, Sollinger D, Baumann M, Wagner B, Strobl M, et al. (2010) Toll-like receptors 2 and 4 in renal ischemia/reperfusion injury. Pediatr Nephrol 25: 853–860.
25. Shigeoka AA, Holscher TD, King AJ, Hall FW, Kiosses WB, et al. (2007) TLR2 is constitutively expressed within the kidney and participates in ischemic renal injury through both MyD88-dependent and -independent pathways. J Immunol 178: 6252–6258.
26. Wu H, Chen G, Wyburn KR, Yin J, Bertolino P, et al. (2007) TLR4 activation mediates kidney ischemia/reperfusion injury. J Clin Invest 117: 2847–2859.
27. Hong SK, Chaturvedi R, Piazuelo MB, Coburn LA, Williams CS, et al. (2010) Increased expression and cellular localization of spermine oxidase in ulcerative colitis and relationship to disease activity. Inflamm Bowel Dis 16: 1557–1566.
28. Xu H, Chaturvedi R, Cheng Y, Bussiere FI, Asim M, et al. (2004) Spermine oxidation induced by Helicobacter pylori results in apoptosis and DNA damage: implications for gastric carcinogenesis. Cancer Res 64: 8521–8525.
29. Ivanova S, Batliwalla F, Mocco J, Kiss S, Huang J, et al. (2002) Neuroprotection in cerebral ischemia by neutralization of 3-aminopropanal. Proc Natl Acad Sci U S A 99: 5579–5584.
30. Ivanova S, Botchkina GI, Al-Abed Y, Meistrell M 3rd, Batliwalla F, et al. (1998) Cerebral ischemia enhances polyamine oxidation: identification of enzymatically formed 3-aminopropanal as an endogenous mediator of neuronal and glial cell death. J Exp Med 188: 327–340.
31. Zhang W, Wang M, Xie HY, Zhou L, Meng XQ, et al. (2007) Role of reactive oxygen species in mediating hepatic ischemia-reperfusion injury and its therapeutic applications in liver transplantation. Transplant Proc 39: 1332–1337.
32. Hegardt C, Johannsson OT, Oredsson SM (2002) Rapid caspase-dependent cell death in cultured human breast cancer cells induced by the polyamine analogue N(1), N(11)-diethylnorspermine. Eur J Biochem 269: 1033–1039.
33. Vujcic S, Halmekyto M, Diegelman P, Gan G, Kramer DL, et al. (2000) Effects of conditional overexpression of spermidine/spermine N1-acetyltransferase on polyamine pool dynamics, cell growth, and sensitivity to polyamine analogs. J Biol Chem 275: 38319–38328.
34. Tsung A, Klune JR, Zhang X, Jeyabalan G, Cao Z, et al. (2007) HMGB1 release induced by liver ischemia involves Toll-like receptor 4 dependent reactive oxygen species production and calcium-mediated signaling. J Exp Med 204: 2913–2923.
35. Kielar ML, John R, Bennett M, Richardson JA, Shelton JM, et al. (2005) Maladaptive role of IL-6 in ischemic acute renal failure. J Am Soc Nephrol 16: 3315–3325.
36. Gao J, Zhang D, Yang X, Zhang Y, Li P, et al. (2011) Lysophosphatidic acid and lovastatin might protect kidney in renal I/R injury by downregulating MCP-1 in rat. Ren Fail 33: 805–810.
37. Grenz A, Kim JH, Bauerle JD, Tak E, Eltzschig HK, et al. (2012) Adora2b adenosine receptor signaling protects during acute kidney injury via inhibition of neutrophil-dependent TNF-alpha release. J Immunol 189: 4566–4573.

15

Topical Application of a Platelet Activating Factor Receptor Agonist Suppresses Phorbol Ester-Induced Acute and Chronic Inflammation and Has Cancer Chemopreventive Activity in Mouse Skin

Ravi P. Sahu[1,9], **Samin Rezania**[1,9], **Jesus A. Ocana**[2], **Sonia C. DaSilva-Arnold**[1,2], **Joshua R. Bradish**[1], **Justin D. Richey**[1], **Simon J. Warren**[1], **Badri Rashid**[1], **Jeffrey B. Travers**[2,3], **Raymond L. Konger**[1,2]*

1 Departments of Pathology & Laboratory Medicine, Indiana University School of Medicine, Indianapolis, IN, 46202, United States of America, **2** Department of Dermatology, Indiana University School of Medicine, Indianapolis, IN, 46202, United States of America, **3** Richard L. Roudebush Veterans Administration Medical Center, Indianapolis, IN, 46202, United States of America

Abstract

Platelet activating factor (PAF) has long been associated with acute edema and inflammatory responses. PAF acts by binding to a specific G-protein coupled receptor (PAF-R, *Ptafr*). However, the role of chronic PAF-R activation on sustained inflammatory responses has been largely ignored. We recently demonstrated that mice lacking the PAF-R (*Ptafr-/-* mice) exhibit increased cutaneous tumorigenesis in response to a two-stage chemical carcinogenesis protocol. *Ptafr-/-* mice also exhibited increased chronic inflammation in response to phorbol ester application. In this present study, we demonstrate that topical application of the non-hydrolysable PAF mimetic (carbamoyl-PAF (CPAF)), exerts a potent, dose-dependent, and short-lived edema response in WT mice, but not *Ptafr -/-* mice or mice deficient in c-Kit (c-*Kit*^W-sh/W-sh mice). Using an ear inflammation model, co-administration of topical CPAF treatment resulted in a paradoxical decrease in both acute ear thickness changes associated with a single PMA application, as well as the sustained inflammation associated with chronic repetitive PMA applications. Moreover, mice treated topically with CPAF also exhibited a significant reduction in chemical carcinogenesis. The ability of CPAF to suppress acute and chronic inflammatory changes in response to PMA application(s) was PAF-R dependent, as CPAF had no effect on basal or PMA-induced inflammation in *Ptafr-/-* mice. Moreover, c-Kit appears to be necessary for the anti-inflammatory effects of CPAF, as CPAF had no observable effect in c-*Kit*^W-sh/W-sh mice. These data provide additional evidence that PAF-R activation exerts complex immunomodulatory effects in a model of chronic inflammation that is relevant to neoplastic development.

Editor: Paul Proost, University of Leuven, Rega Institute, Belgium

Funding: This work was supported by the National Institutes of Health (www.nih.gov) (R01 HL062996, R21 ES017497, and R21 ES020965), the Veterans Administration (www.research.va.gov/funding)(VA Merit 510BX000853), and the Prevent Cancer Foundation (www.preventcancer.org). The funders had no role in study design, data collection and analysis, decision to publish, or preparation of the manuscript.

Competing Interests: The authors have declared that no competing interests exist.

* Email: rkonger@iupui.edu

9 These authors contributed equally to this work.

Introduction

Platelet activating factor (1-alkyl-2-acetyl glycerophosphocholine, PAF) is a bioactive lipid molecule produced by both enzymatic and non-enzymatic mechanisms [1]. Non-enzymatic production of PAF is dependent on free-radical mediated modification of the sn-2 polyunsaturated fatty acid of glycerophosphocholines to form PAF itself and other oxidized glycerophosphocholines (ox-GPCs) that exhibit the ability to activate the PAF receptor [1–5]. The biological activity of PAF is mediated by binding to a single G-protein coupled receptor (PAF-R) that is expressed on a wide variety of cells including keratinocytes [1,6,7]. Once produced, PAF elicits a variety of physiological and pathological effects that play a role in acute inflammation, wound healing, and angiogenesis. However, PAF is perhaps best known for its pro-inflammatory effects that mediate the systemic reaction

to shock, allergic reactions, and anaphylaxis [1]. In this role, PAF's actions are thought to be mediated by its ability to stimulate vasodilation and vascular permeability, platelet aggregation, bronchoconstriction, and alterations in leukocyte function [1]. These effects on leukocytes include the ability of PAF to stimulate mast cell activation and migration [8–10], mononuclear and neutrophilic phagocytosis [11–13], and M2 polarization of macrophages [14].

While it is clear that PAF acts to promote acute inflammatory effects, particularly those associated with anaphylaxis and shock, more recent evidence suggests that PAF may play a more complex role in immune function. PAF production through enzymatic and oxidative pathways appears to play a role in keratinocyte responses to genotoxic agents, such as ultraviolet B, cigarette smoke or chemotherapeutic agents [3,15–18]. Studies on the mechanisms of ultraviolet B (UVB)-induced systemic immunosuppression have demonstrated a requirement for PAF-R activation [3,10,19,20]. This UVB-induced systemic immunosuppression is characterized by an antigen-specific suppression of adaptive T-cell mediated immune responses [21,22]. In addition, we have recently demonstrated that *Ptafr-/-* mice exhibit an increase in cutaneous chemical carcinogenesis that is associated with a corresponding increase in phorbol ester (PMA)-induced cutaneous inflammation [7]. This data suggests that PAF-R activation may be also be important in regulating the innate immune system. However, the down-stream cellular mediators of this immunomodulatory activity are unknown.

The c-*Kit* gene codes for a receptor tyrosine kinase that binds the ligand, stem cell factor (SCF), and is important in [23]. The c-*Kit*$^{W-sh}$ (sash) mutation is an inversion of a 3.1 Mbp segment that disrupts the promoter region of the c-*Kit* gene [23]. Mice homozygous for the c-*Kit*$^{W-sh}$ mutation exhibit a profound loss of mast cells, but also lack melanocytes and interstitial cells of Cajal [23,24]. Thus, c-Kit$^{W-sh/W-sh}$ mice represent a common tool to assess mast cell function. Mast cells are tissue resident bone marrow derived cells, which like PAF, are well known mediators of allergic and anaphylactic reactions [25]. Mast cells are strategically localized in the subepithelial and submucosal spaces prone to environmental and infectious insults [25]. Moreover, the ability of PAF to promote anaphylactic responses is dependent on mast cell activation [8]. PAF is also a known activator and chemotactic agent for mast cells [9]. In addition to their role in promoting the wheel and flare reaction associated with type I hypersensitivity reactions, mast cells have also been shown to suppress chronic inflammation as well as adaptive immune responses [26-31]. Of particular relevance, mast cells act to limit murine models of contact hypersensitivity and chronic UVB-induced inflammation [32]. In addition, the role of the PAF-R in UVB-induced immunosuppression has been shown to result from PAF-R-dependent migration of mast cells to the lymph node, wherein they exert an interleukin (IL)-10-dependent immunosuppressive effect [10].

While we recently provided evidence that PAF has anti-inflammatory effects on chronic PMA-induced tumor promotion [7], it is possible that the effects of germ-line loss of the PAF-R could be due to compensatory embryonic or postnatal alterations in skin development [7]. Thus, a demonstration that PAF-R agonist treatment results in suppression of DMBA/PMA-induced carcinogenesis and inflammation would provide further support to the idea that the PAF-R has important anti-neoplastic and immunomodulatory effects. Our current studies examining the role of the PAF-R in PMA-induced inflammation adds to our previous report and reveals a complex immunomodulatory role for PAF-R signaling. Moreover, our findings using c-*Kit*$^{W-sh/W-sh}$ mice demonstrate a role for *c-Kit* and possibly mast cells in the immunomodulatory effects of PAF.

Methods

Ethics statement

The protocols were approved by the Committee on the Ethics of Animal Experiments of the Indiana University School of Medicine (Institutional Animal Care and Use Committee (IACUC) (Protocol Number: 3841 and 10639). Every attempt was made to minimize animal suffering.

Reagents and chemicals

Phorbol 12-myristate 13-acetate (PMA) was purchased from Promega, Madison, WI. 7,12-Dimethylbenz(a)anthracene (DM

BA) was obtained from Acros Organics, Fair Lawn, NJ. Carbamyl-PAF was obtained from Sigma-Aldrich (St. Louis, MO).

Animals

Ptafr knockout (*Ptafr-/-*) in the C57BL/6 background were originally obtained from Dr. Satoshi Ishii (Department of Biochemistry and Molecular Biology, Faculty of Medicine, The University of Tokyo), derived as previously described [33]. Age (8–12 week)-matched *Ptafr* +/+ C57BL/6 (WT) were used as controls (The Jackson Laboratories, Bar Harbor, ME). SKH-1 hairless, albino mice were obtained from Charles Rivers (Wilmington, MA). Mice containing the W-sash (W-sh) inversion mutation in the promoter region of the *c-kit* gene (*Kit*$^{W-sh}$) were obtained from the Jackson Laboratories in the C57Bl/6 background (B6.Cg-*Kit*$^{W-sh}$/HNihrJaeBsmGlliJ). Mice were housed under specific pathogen-free conditions at the Indiana University School of Medicine.

Ear thickness measurements

The left ear of each mouse was treated with 20 µl of cPAF (0.1, 0.3, or 1 mM in acetone). The right ear was treated with 20 µl of vehicle (acetone) alone. For PMA treatments, the left ear was treated with 10 µg of PMA in 20 µl of acetone, and the right ear was treated with vehicle (VEH) alone 3 times a week (arrows) for 16 days. For PMA and CPAF treatments, the mice were treated with PMA first, then 20 µl of 0.3 mM CPAF (in acetone) was added immediately after the PMA treatment. Ear thickness was measured at the indicated time points following treatment using a constant pressure analog thickness gauge (Peacock Model G, 0.4 N).

Epidermal thickness measurements

Mouse ears were treated for 18 days thrice weekly with vehicle, CPAF (6 nmole), PMA, or PMA and CPAF were formalin fixed and paraffin embedded (FFPE), and stained with hematoxylin & eosin (H&E). Epidermal thickness was measured by measuring the epidermal thickness 10 times in 5 consecutive 200 x fields, starting at the distal tip of the ear and moving proximally to the next adjacent field. Epidermal thickness was quantitated using an eyepiece reticle calibrated with a stage micrometer. All slides were blinded prior to measurement.

Tumorigenesis studies

For two stage chemical carcinogenesis studies, the dorsal skin of SKH-1 hairless mice were treated with once with DMBA, followed by repetitive treatments with PMA as previously described [7]. For tumor counting, only durable tumors >1 mm in greatest diameter were counted. After 25 weeks of PMA treatment, mice were sacrificed and tumor size (size at greatest dimension) was measured for each tumor. FFPE tumor sections from WT and *Ptafr -/-* mice were stained with H&E and the tumor type (Papilloma and microinvasive SCC (MISCC)) was assessed in blinded fashion by a board-certified dermatopathologist, as previously described [34]. For MPO activity, tumor-free areas of treated skin were removed and MPO activity levels were assessed as previously described [35].

PMA-induced inflammation in dorsal epidermis

The back skin of female WT or *Ptafr-/-* mice was shaved under anesthesia and was then treated with PMA or vehicle three times a week for 18 days as described above. Immediately after each PMA application, the mice were treated with vehicle or 100 µl of 0.3 mM CPAF (in acetone). On day 18, the mice were sacrificed and the treated dorsal epidermis was excised for skin thickness measurements, as previously described [35].

Mast cell counting

Mast cells were stained with toluidine blue in deparaffinized FFPE sections as described [36]. Four 200x images per biopsy specimen were captured sequentially along the length of the section using a Nikon Eclipse 80i. Nikon Elements Basic Research Image Analysis software (v. 4.13) was used to count the mast cells and measure the dermal area of interest. The total area and cell counts were then averaged [(mast cells/μm^2)x10^{-5}]. Given that mast cell counts differ at different body sites in mice, mast cell counts were performed in both the ears and the dorsal (back) epidermis.

Statistical analysis

Statistical significance was assessed by Prism 5.0 software (Graph Pad Software, San Diego CA) and significance was set as $p<0.05$.

Results

CPAF is topically active and results in a dose-dependent transient increase in ear thickness that is dependent on mast cells

In a previous study [7] and in Fig 1A, we show that a single topical application of increasing doses of the non-hydrolyzable PAF-R agonist, CPAF, results in a dose-dependent increase in ear thickness at two hours after application. In Fig 1B, a time course study demonstrates that CPAF-induced ear thickness changes occur rapidly, with significant increases in ear thickness noted by 1 hour after application and peak ear thickness was noted at 2 hrs. Importantly, following a single application of CPAF the changes in ear thickness were transient and declined to near baseline by 8 hours after application. The rapid and transient nature of the response strongly suggests that changes in vascular permeability leading to edema formation are largely responsible for the changes in ear thickness. This is consistent with the well-known ability of PAF to induce vasodilation and vascular permeability [37]. To rule out PAF-R independent effects [38], mice with germline loss of the *Ptafr* gene (*Ptafr-/-* mice) were also treated with CPAF. At all doses studied, topical CPAF application failed to elicit an inflammatory reaction in *Ptafr-/-* mice (Figs 1A&B), verifying the specificity of the pharmacological effect.

Finally, the ability of CPAF to induce rapid edema reactions has been linked to mast cell activation [8,9]. We therefore determined whether the ability of CPAF to induce an early edema reaction at 2 hrs could be blocked in mice lacking mast cells (c-Kit$^{W-sh/W-sh}$ mice). In Fig 2 we verify that mast cells are indeed required for the early increase in ear thickness mediated by CPAF application.

Topical CPAF protects against cutaneous chemical carcinogenesis

The studies in Fig 1 demonstrate that CPAF exhibits specific dose-dependent pharmacologic activity following topical application. The use of a topical delivery approach also avoids potential toxicities associated with systemic PAF-R agonist treatment [37]. In addition, the PAF-R is prone to the phenomenon of ligand-induced down-regulation and desensitization [1,39]; this regulatory feature is characteristic of G-protein coupled receptors and can lead to a paradoxical loss of receptor activation by subsequent ligand binding [1,40]. Thus, given that carcinogenesis studies would require long-term repetitive application of CPAF, we utilized the 0.3 mM concentration of CPAF which induced an intermediate, but significant increase in ear thickness measurements (Fig 1A). For these studies, CPAF was applied immediately after DMBA or PMA application for the duration of the study.

Consistent with our previous study that demonstrated that *Ptafr-/-* mice exhibit increased DMBA/PMA-induced tumor formation, in Fig 3A we show that topical treatment of CPAF resulted in a significant reduction in DMBA/PMA-induced tumor burden. CPAF treatment also demonstrated a modest, but significant protective effect on tumor incidence (Fig 3B). Moreover, while *Ptafr-/-* mice exhibited a significant increase in the frequency of larger tumors [7], mice treated with topical CPAF exhibited a significant increase in smaller tumor sizes (Fig 3C). In addition, we previously demonstrated that *Ptafr-/-* mice exhibit an increase in SCC formation relative to WT mice [7]. However, in this current study, no frank SCCs were observed and mice treated topically failed to exhibit a significant change in the proportion of grade 1–3 papillomas or microinvasive SCCs (Figure S1 in File S1). Finally, tumor-free areas of skin treated with CPAF exhibited a marked reduction in DMBA/PMA-induced inflammation, as assessed using myeloperoxidase (MPO activity), a marker of granulocytic cell infiltrates (Fig 3D) [41]. This is consistent with our previous results in -/- mice, which exhibited an augmentation of MPO activity following chronic, repetitive PMA treatments [7].

Topical CPAF treatment suppresses inflammation induced by repeated applications of the tumor promoter PMA

In our previous report [7], we showed that a first PMA application induced a significant increase in ear thickness in WT mice 2 days after application. A second PMA application resulted in a further increase in ear thickness that partially resolved. Thereafter, subsequent PMA applications failed to elicit further increases in ear thickness. In contrast, a significant and persistent increase in ear thickness was observed during the 18 days of PMA treatments (sustained chronic inflammatory phase). As in our previous study, loss of the PAF-R resulted in a blunting of the peak ear thickness observed after the second PMA application, but a higher level of sustained chronic inflammation after continued thrice weekly PMA applications (Figure S2 in File S1 and [7]). We therefore examined whether topical CPAF administration would have the opposite effect and suppress the sustained chronic inflammation induced by PMA treatment. In Fig 4A we show that the application of topical CPAF immediately after each application of PMA results in a significant reduction in both the peak inflammatory response noted on day 4, as well as a reduction of the sustained inflammatory response that was noted throughout the period of PMA application (18 days). Interestingly, at these later time points, CPAF had no effect on ear thickness measurements in WT mice not treated with PMA, suggesting that topical CPAF is ineffective in inducing a significant sustained inflammatory response at the dose tested (0.3 mM). Finally, we next demonstrated that the effect of CPAF was entirely dependent on the PAF-R, as CPAF and Veh applications showed nearly identical ear thickness measurements at all time points following PMA application to *Ptafr-/-* mice (Fig 4B). While CPAF significantly blocked PMA-induced ear thickness in WT mice (Fig 4A), this response was completely lost in *Ptafr-/-* mice treated with PMA (Fig 4B). Finally, in Fig 4C, we show that the ability of CPAF to suppress PMA-induced skin thickness changes was not dependent on anatomic site. CPAF significantly suppressed PMA-induced increases in dorsal back skin thickness after 18 days of thrice weekly treatment.

A.

B.

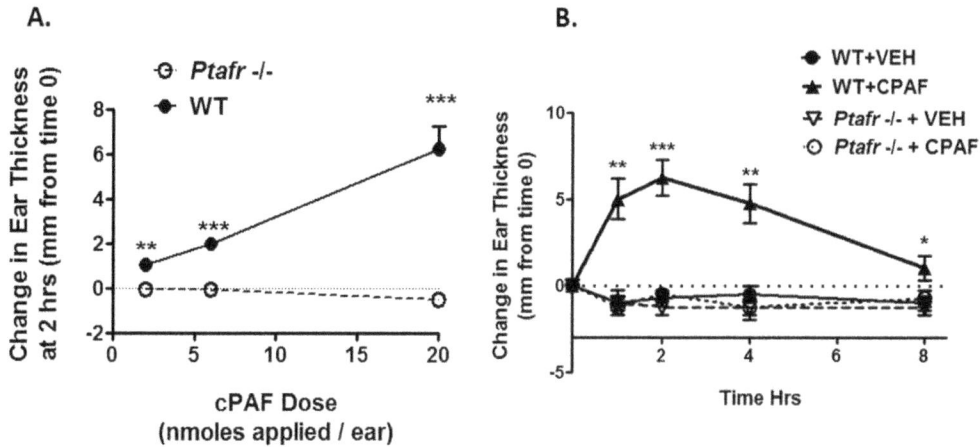

Figure 1. Dose and time related acute ear inflammation changes in response to topical CPAF. *1A. Topical CPAF dose-dependently induces rapid inflammatory responses as measured by ear thickness measurements.* One ear of WT and *Ptafr* (-/-) were treated with one of three doses of CPAF (20 µl of a 0.1, 0.3, and 1.0 mM solution for a total treatment dose of 2, 6, or 20 nmole CPAF per ear). The contralateral ear was treated with acetone alone (VEH). Ear thickness was measured prior to treatment and 2 hours after treatment. After the pretreatment ear thickness values were subtracted, the mean and SEM were plotted (n = 4 for 20 nmole and n = 8 for 2 & 6 nmole CPAF & VEH treated mouse ears). *1B. Topical CPAF treatment induces a rapid, but transient increase in inflammation as measured by ear thickness changes.* One ear of wildtype (WT) and *Ptafr* (-/-) mice was treated with 20 µl of CPAF (20 nmoles of a 0.1 mM solution in acetone) and 20 µl of acetone (VEH) was applied to the contralateral ear. Ear thickness was measured just prior to reagent application and at 1, 2, 4, and 8 hours after application. Results represent the mean and SEM (n = 4 mice) after subtracting the pretreatment ear thickness. CPAF induced a significant increase in ear thickness in WT mice relative to the WT+VEH treated ears. *, $p < 0.05$; **, $p < 0.01$; ***; $p < 0.001$; 2-tailed t-test.

We next determined the histopathologic changes in ear skin that result from multiple PMA applications with or without CPAF treatments. Multiple PMA applications to mouse skin are known to induce epidermal hyperplasia and leukocyte infiltration [42,43]. In Fig 5A–I, we show that multiple PMA applications to WT mouse ears results in a clear increase in ear thickness accompanied by dermal expansion, leukocyte infiltration and epidermal

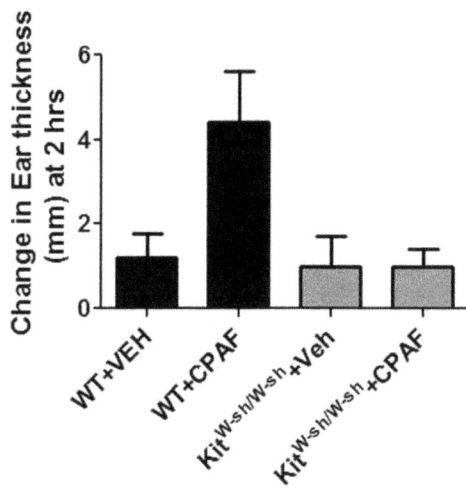

Figure 2. CPAF induces transient ear thickness changes are blocked in c-Kit$^{W-sh/W-sh}$ mast cell deficient mice. WT and c-Kit$^{W-sh/W-sh}$ mice were treated with vehicle (VEH) alone on one ear, and 20 ml of 0.3 mM CPAF (6 nmole) on the contralateral ear. Ear thickness was measured both prior to and 2 hrs after reagent application. After subtraction of the ear thickness at time 0, the mean and SEM were plotted (n = 5 for WT mice, n = 4 for Kit$^{W-sh/W-sh}$ mice). *, $p < 0.05$; 2-tailed t-test.

hyperplasia. Moreover, co-treatment of WT mice ears with CPAF resulted in a reduction in PMA-induced leukocyte infiltrates while *Ptafr-/-* mice exhibited a marked increase in ear thickness, dermal expansion, inflammatory cell infiltrates, and epidermal hyperplasia (Fig 5A–H). Relative to WT mice, *Ptafr-/-* mice exhibited a marked increase in granulocytic infiltrates following chronic PMA treatments (Fig 5 and Figure S3 in File S1). Moreover, CPAF treatment suppressed the observed PMA-induced inflammatory infiltrates in WT, but not *Ptafr-/-* mice. This data is in agreement with our previous study demonstrating that *Ptafr-/-* mice exhibit a marked increase in MPO activity following PMA treatment [7], as well as our data in Fig 3D that shows that CPAF treatment suppresses MPO activity in DMBA/PMA treated mice. Since neutrophils are shown to play an important role in mouse skin photocarcinogenesis [35], this reduction in granulocytic infiltrates could play an important role in the observed anti-tumor effects of topical CPAF treatment in chemical carcinogenesis (Fig 3A&B). Given that the degree of chronic inflammation is commonly associated with epidermal hyperplasia, it is somewhat surprising that while CPAF treatment suppressed PMA-induced granulocytic inflammation in WT mice, CPAF treatment did not alter PMA-induced epidermal hyperplasia in either WT or *Ptafr-/-* mice (Fig 5I).

PAF exerts complex effects on the initial inflammatory response to PMA application

The pro-inflammatory tumor promoter PMA is known to induce a rapid edema reaction in mouse ears [42,43]. This is followed by a gradual rise in leukocyte infiltration as measured by MPO and/or N-acetylglucosaminidase (NAF) activity that peaks at around 24 hrs [42,43]. Given that PAF is a potent vasoactive lipid mediator that promotes rapid edema reactions [37], we next examined how CPAF would affect early inflammatory changes following the first PMA application in WT and *Ptafr-/-* mice. As seen in Fig 6A, PMA treatment induces a rapid increase in ear

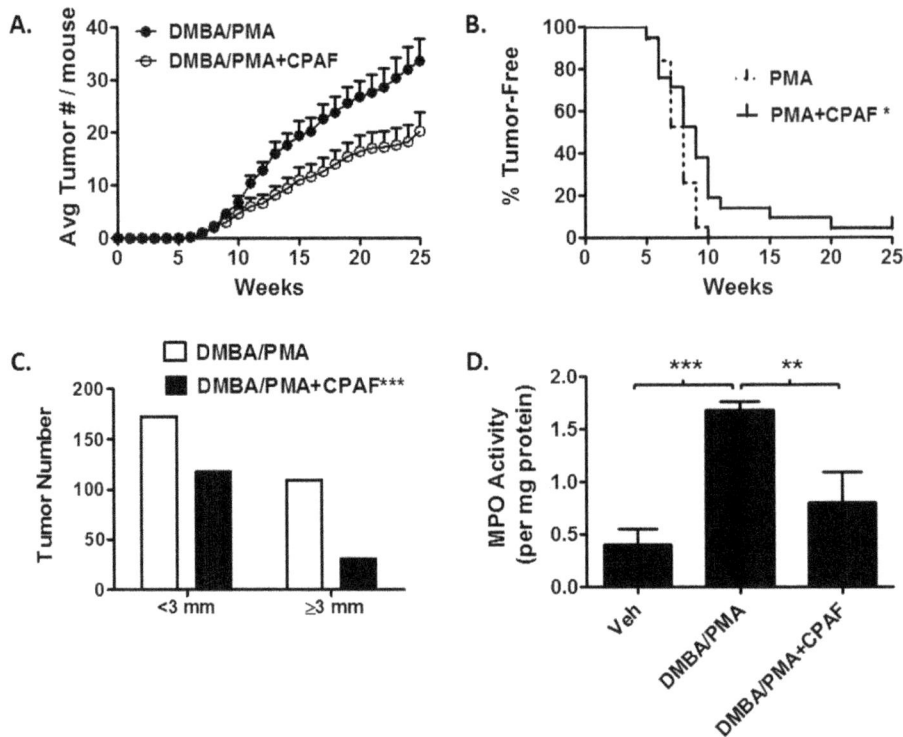

Figure 3. Topical application of CPAF suppresses DMBA/PMA-induced tumorigenesis. *3A. Topical treatment with CPAF suppresses DMBA/ PMA-induced tumor multiplicity.* SKH-1 mice were treated once with DMBA+/- CPAF, then with PMA or PMA+CPAF for 25 weeks. Durable tumors were counted on a weekly basis. Tumor multiplicity (Avg tumor number per mouse was plotted at each week. Results represent the mean and SEM for n = 19–20 mice/group. $p < 0.05$ for weeks 9–12,14–25; $p < 0.01$ for week 13; Mann-Whitney U test. *3B. Topical CPAF delayed tumor incidence in mice treated with DMBA/PMA.* The percent of mice remaining tumor free over the 25 week chemical tumorigenesis study were plotted using a survival curve. The treatment with CPAF resulted in a significant change in the tumor incidence, with a median time until first tumor occurrence of 8 weeks for DMBA/PMA treated and 9 weeks for DMBA/PMA+CPAF treated mice. *, $p < 0.05$; Log-rank (Mantel-Cox) Test. *3C. Topical CPAF treatment results in a smaller number of large tumors (≥3 mm in greatest diameter) after 25 weeks of treatment.* Tumor size distribution was plotted as the number of tumors in each size distribution for each treatment group. Histopathologic exam showed no significant difference in the rates of papilloma and SCC formation between the treatment groups (not shown). ***, $p = 0.0001$ Fisher's exact test. *3D. DMBA/PMA-induced MPO activity is suppressed by CPAF.* After the mice were euthanized following 25 weeks of DMBA/PMA +/- CPAF treatment, tumor free areas of skin were excised and MPO activity was assessed in tissue lysates. After normalization to total protein, MPO activity was plotted as the mean and SEM (n = 5–9 mice per group). **, $p < 0.05$; ***, $p < 0.001$; 2-tailed t-test.

thickness that was first observed two hours after application. Ear thickness changes peaked at approximately 24 to 48 hrs. In contrast, *Ptafr-/-* mice exhibited a reduction in the initial ear thickness changes noted at 2 & 8 hrs, suggesting that PMA-induced edema responses were PAF-dependent. It was therefore surprising to find that WT mice treated with CPAF immediately after PMA application also exhibited an approximately 50% loss of PMA-induced early ear thickness changes observed at 2 hrs (Fig 6B). This suggests a complex role for the PAF-R in regulating initial vasoactive edema changes in response to PMA.

While the above data suggests a complex role for the PAF-R in regulating initial PMA-induced inflammation, similar results were seen at 24 and 48 hrs, which represent the period in which inflammation is heavily dependent on inflammatory cell infiltrates. As with the 2 & 8 hr time points, *Ptafr-/-* mice exhibited reductions in PMA-induced ear thickness changes at 24 & 48 hrs. However, topical CPAF was also significantly suppressed the PMA-induced increases in ear thickness that occurred at 24 & 48 hrs (Fig 6B). That these effects are PAF-R dependent are seen by the complete loss of activity of CPAF in *Ptafr-/-* mice (Fig 6B). Thus, topical CPAF exerted complex, but PAF-R-dependent

effects on PMA-induced edema and early inflammatory changes in mouse ears.

Topical CPAF has no effect on PMA-induced inflammation in c-KitW-sh/W-sh mice

While mast cells are known mediators of PAF-induced edema reactions, PMA is also known to induce mast cell degranulation and mast cell deficient mice exhibit a marked decrease in both PMA-induced edema reactions and leukocyte infiltration [43–45]. Thus, we sought to determine whether CPAF would have any effect on PMA-induced inflammation in c-$Kit^{W-sh/W-sh}$ mice. In Fig 7A, we show that c-$Kit^{W-sh/W-sh}$ mice exhibit an impaired PMA-induced ear inflammation response at 2 and 8 hrs, consistent with a role in regulating early edema reactions. As in previous studies [43], this data suggests an important role for mast cells in the acute inflammatory effects of PMA on mouse skin. Given that loss of the PAF-R resulted in a similar loss in PMA-induced acute inflammatory effects, we determined whether c-$Kit^{W-sh/W-sh}$ mice were susceptible to CPAF-induced effects on inflammation. In Fig 7B, we show that the ability of topical CPAF to suppress PMA-induced ear thickness was absent in $Kit^{W-sh/W-sh}$

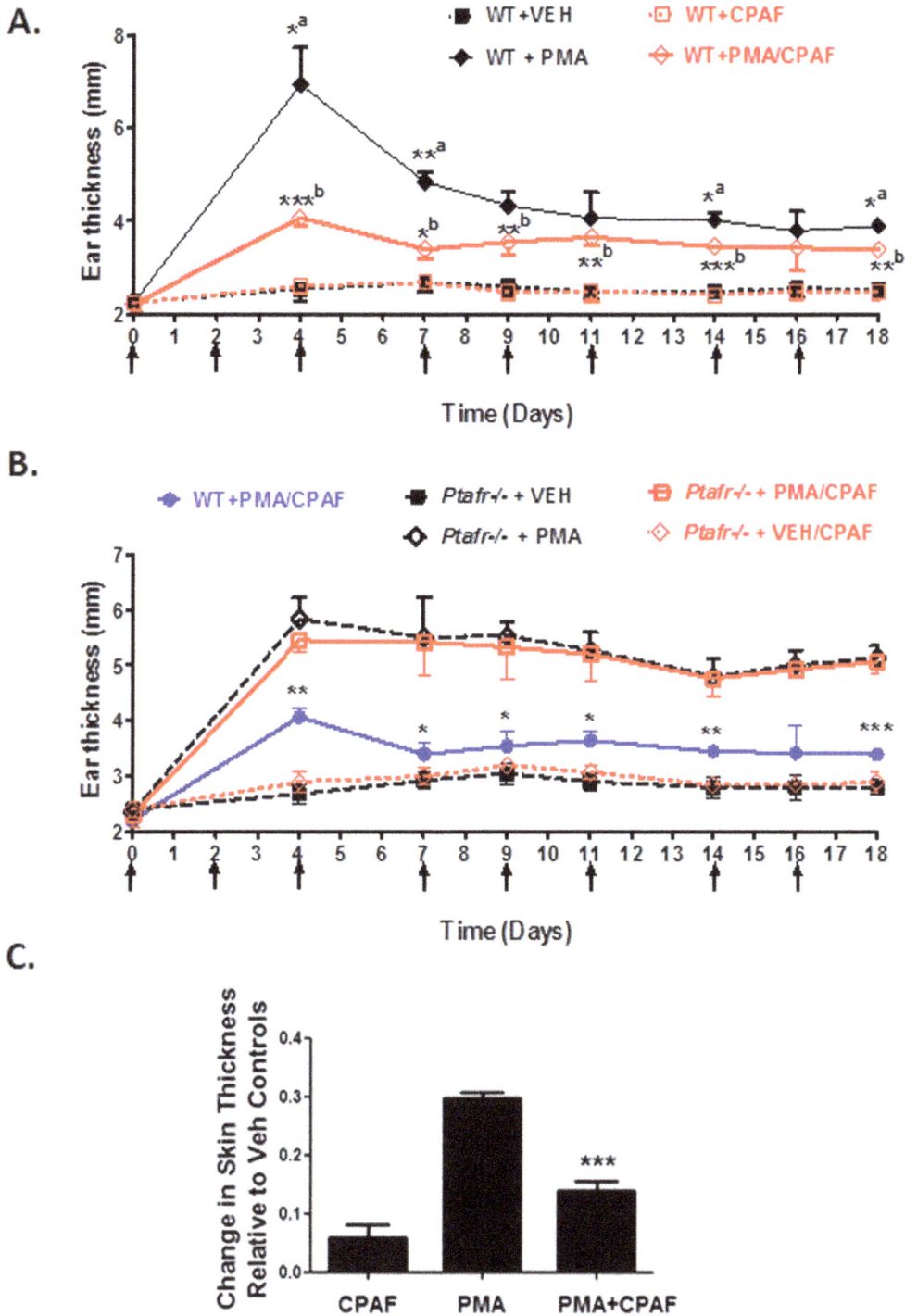

Figure 4. Effect of CPAF treatment on ear thickness changes over an 18 day course of thrice weekly PMA applications in WT and *Ptafr-/-* **mice.** *4A. Topical CPAF treatment suppresses PMA-induced changes in ear thickness in WT mice.* CPAF (6 nmoles) alone or PMA +/- CPAF were applied to WT mouse ears thrice weekly for 18 days. Skin thickness measurements were taken at time 0 and just prior to each reagent application. After subtraction of the time 0 ear thickness, ear thickness changes were plotted as the mean and SEM (n = 4–5 mice per group). PMA relative to PMA+CPAF ([a]), PMA+CPAF relative to CPAF([b]); *, $p < 0.05$; **, $p < 0.01$; ***, $p < 0.001$; 2-tailed *t*-test. *4B. Topical CPAF treatment is ineffective in altering PMA-induced ear thickness changes in Ptafr-/- mice. Ptafr-/-* mice were treated and assessed as in 4A above. For the sake of comparison, the data for the PMA + CPAF treatment in WT mice is included. (mean and SEM; n = 4–5 mice per group). WT mice treated with PMA + CPAF exhibit a significant decrease in ear thickness measurements relative to *Ptafr-/-* mice treated with PMA + CPAF (*, $p < 0.05$; **, $p < 0.01$; ***, $p < 0.001$; 2-tailed *t*-test). *4C. Topical CPAF treatment suppresses PMA-induced skin thickness increases in dorsal epidermis following 18 days of treatment.* The dorsal epidermis of SKH-1 mice was treated thrice weekly with vehicle, CPAF, PMA, or PMA + CPAF. Doses of PMA and CPAF were the same as that used for the tumorigenesis studies in Fig 3. ***, $p < 0.05$ relative to PMA treated skin; 2-tailed *t*-test (n = 3 per group).

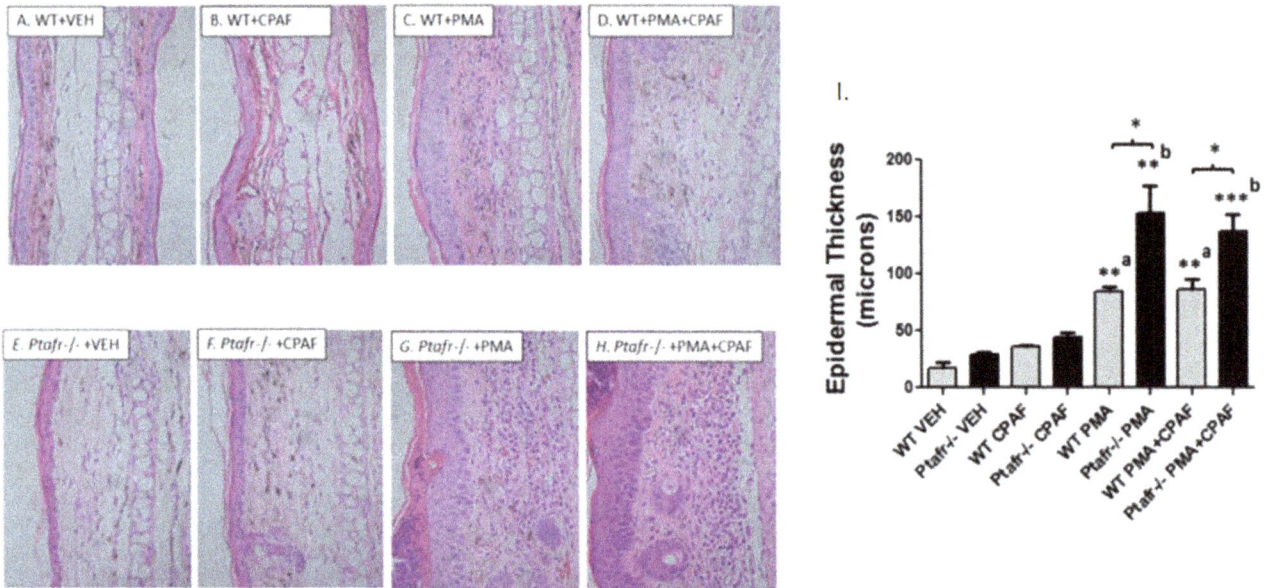

Figure 5. Inflammatory infiltrates and epidermal thickness in WT and *Ptafr-/-* mouse ears treated chronically with CPAF, PMA or PMA + CPAF. *5A–H. Inflammatory infiltrates are increased in Ptafr-/- mice treated with PMA, while CPAF suppresses inflammatory cell infiltrates in PMA treated WT mice.* After treating WT and *Ptafr-/-* mouse ears for 18 days with VEH, CPAF, PMA, or PMA + CPAF as described in Fig 4, mice were sacrificed and the ears excised for formalin fixation, paraffin embedding and hematoxylin & eosin (H&E) staining. Photomicrographs taken at 400x magnification are shown. *5I. PMA-induced epidermal thickness is augmented in Ptafr-/- mice, while CPAF has no effect on PMA-induced epidermal thickness in either WT or Ptafr-/- mice.* Epidermal thickness was measured in WT and *Ptafr-/-* mice treated for 18 days with VEH, CPAF, PMA, and PMA + CPAF as described in Fig 4A&B. Epidermal thickness in mm is expressed in the mean and SEM for 3–4 ears per experimental group. Significantly different from WT VEH control ([a]), significantly different from the *Ptafr-/-* VEH control ([b]). *, $p < 0.05$; **, $p < 0.01$; ***, $p < 0.001$; 2-tailed *t*-test.

mice at all time points up to 48 hrs. Moreover, in the model of repetitive PMA applications (Fig 7C), $Kit^{W-sh/W-sh}$ mice exhibit a phenotype that mimics the phenotype seen in *Ptafr-/-* mice (see Figure S2 in File S1). Again, topical CPAF had no effect on PMA-induced chronic inflammation in c-$Kit^{W-sh/W-sh}$ mice (Fig 7C).

Finally, to verify that the changes in *Ptafr-/-* mice were not simply due to a loss of dermal mast cells, we next counted dermal mast cells in the ear skin of *Ptafr-/-* mice following 18 days of treatment with vehicle or PMA (Figure S4 in File S1). There was no significant difference in dermal mast cells in *Ptafr-/-* mice

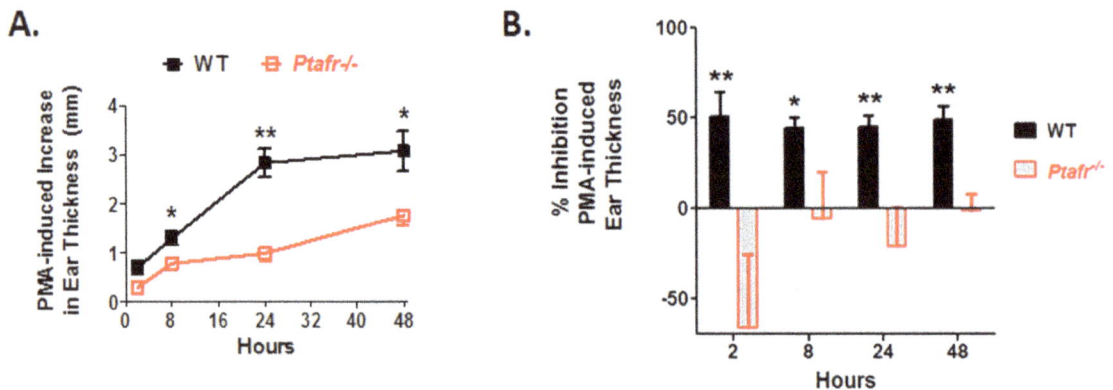

Figure 6. Following a single application of PMA, *Ptafr-/-* mice exhibit a reduction in PMA-induced ear thickness while CPAF treatment also induces a paradoxical PAF-R dependent decrease in PMA-induced ear thickness. For all studies in Figs 6, WT and *Ptafr-/-* mice were treated with VEH, PMA, CPAF (6 nmole) or PMA + CPAF as described in Fig 4A&B. Ear thickness measurements were made just prior to reagent application as well as at the indicated time points up to 48 hrs. *6A. Ptafr-/- mice exhibit a reduction in early and delayed ear thickness increases following a single PMA application.* Ear thickness plots for WT and *Ptafr-/-* mice treated with and without PMA are shown. Statistically significant changes are noted to WT mice treated with PMA relative to *Ptafr-/-* mice treated with PMA. Results represent the mean and SEM of ear thickness after subtracting the ear thickness at time 0 (n = 4–12 mice per group). *, $p < 0.05$; **, $p < 0.01$; *t*-test. *6B. Coadministration of topical CPAF blocks PMA-induced increases in ear thickness at all time points (2–48 hrs).* PMA-induced ear thickness changes were assessed in WT or *Ptafr-/-* mice treated with PMA or PMA + CPAF. After subtracting the ear thickness at time 0, the ability of CPAF to suppress PMA-induced ear thickness changes was calculated as a percentage inhibition of PMA-induced ear thickness increases. CPAF treatment resulted in a significant inhibition of PMA-induced ear thickness changes at all time points ($p < 0.01$–0.05; % inhibition significantly different from no inhibition, Wilcoxon Signed Rank Test). CPAF treatment had no significant effect on PMA-induced ear thickness changes in *Ptafr-/-* mice (One sample analysis, Wilcoxon Signed Rank Test). The percent inhibition of PMA-induced ear thickness changes by CPAF in WT mice was also significantly different than that seen in *Ptafr-/-* mice (*, $p < 0.05$; **, $p < 0.01$; *t*-test).

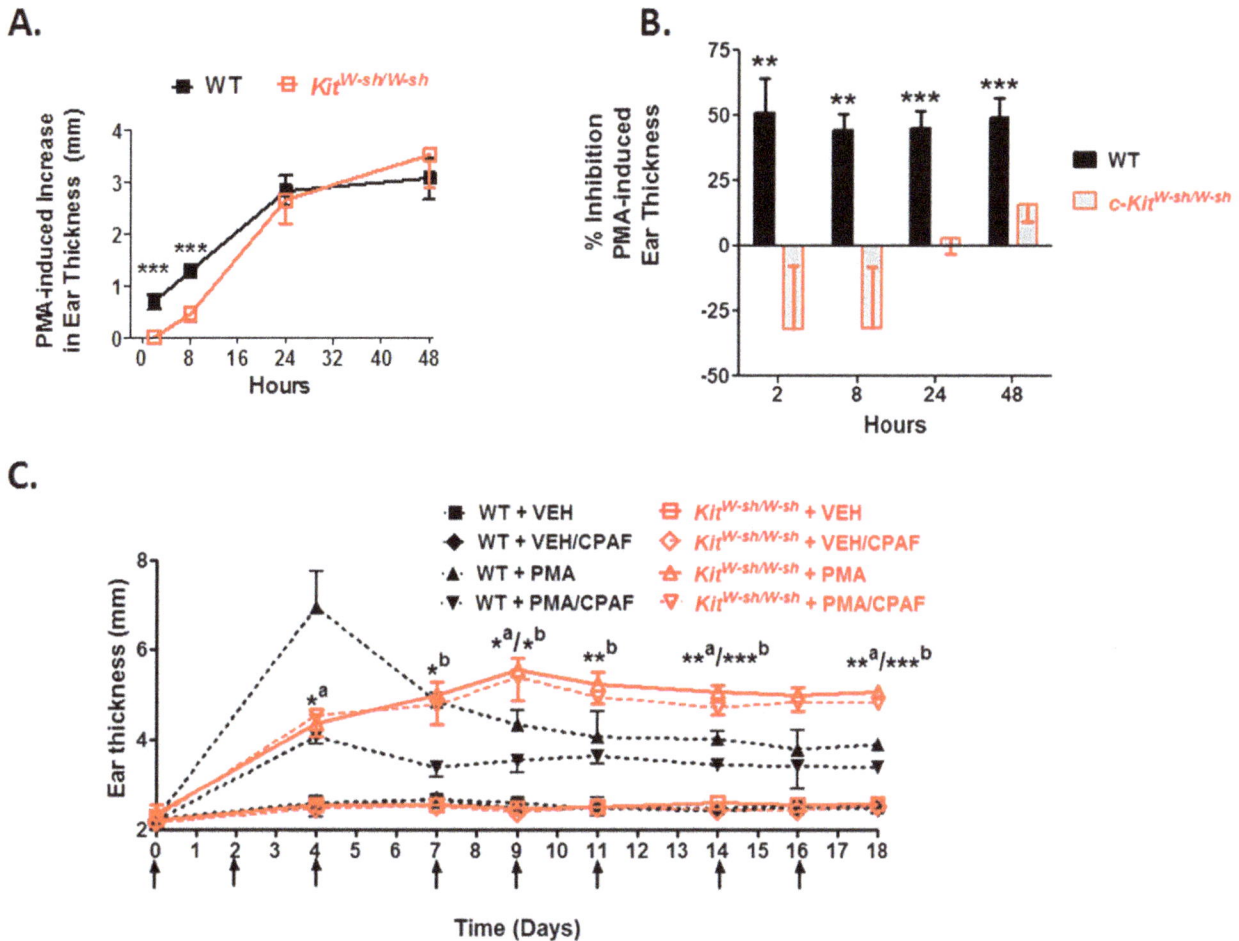

Figure 7. Kit^W-sh/W-sh mice exhibit a reduction in PMA-induced acute inflammation but an augmented chronic or sustained inflammatory response to multiple PMA applications. For all experiments in Fig 7A–C, ear thickness measurements were made just prior to reagent application as well as at the indicated time points up to 18 days. Results represent the mean and SEM of ear thickness (n = 4–14 mice per group). *, $p < 0.05$; **, $p < 0.01$; ***, $p < 0.01$; 2-tailed t-test. *7A. Mast cell deficient mice have a blunted initial inflammatory response to a single application of PMA.* WT and c-Kit^W-sh/W-sh mice were treated with VEH or PMA as described in Fig 4A&B. After subtracting the ear thickness at time 0 prior to PMA application, ear thickness changes were plotted (n = 12–14 mice/group). Ear thickness changes were significantly reduced in c-Kit^W-sh/W-sh mice treated with PMA relative to WT + PMA mice at 2 and 8 hrs following PMA application. ***, $p < 0.001$. *7B. Following a single application of PMA, topical CPAF treatment has no effect on PMA-induced ear thickness changes in c-Kit^W-sh/W-sh mice.* PMA-induced ear thickness changes were assessed in WT or c-Kit^W-sh/W-sh mice treated with PMA or PMA + CPAF. After subtracting the ear thickness at time 0, the ability of CPAF to suppress PMA-induced ear thickness changes was calculated as a percentage inhibition of PMA-induced ear thickness increases. CPAF treatment resulted in a significant inhibition of PMA-induced ear thickness changes at all time points (see also fig 6B). CPAF treatment had no significant effect on PMA-induced ear thickness changes in c-Kit^W-sh/W-sh mice (Wilcoxon Signed Rank Test). The percent inhibition of PMA-induced ear thickness changes by CPAF in WT mice was also significantly different than that seen in c-Kit^W-sh/W-sh mice (**, $p < 0.01$, ***, $p < 0.001$; t-test). *7C. Topical CPAF is inactive in Kit^W-sh/W-sh mice while these mice also exhibit a reduction in acute inflammatory ear thickness changes observed in the first 4 days, but exhibit a significant increase in chronic sustained ear thickness changes.* Significant differences were noted at the indicated time points in WT mice treated with PMA relative to Kit^W-sh/W-sh mice treated with PMA ([a]) as well as in WT mice treated with PMA/CPAF relative to Kit^W-sh/W-sh mice treated with PMA/CPAF ([b]).

relative to WT mice in ears. This is in agreement with a recent study by another group [10]. However, PMA failed to induce a significant increase in mast cell numbers as previously reported [46]. This difference may be due to the fact that we used a shorter time period of PMA-induced inflammation than this previous report.

Discussion

In this current study, we show that topical CPAF is pharmacologically active as it elicits a modest dose-dependent transient increase in ear thickness. Ear thickness changes peak at 2 hrs and are largely normalized at 8 hrs, consistent with transient edema formation. This is consistent with the well-known effects of PAF as a pro-inflammatory mediator. This pharmacological activity is further shown to be dependent on the PAF-R and is lost in c-Kit^W-sh/W-sh mice, suggesting a dependence on c-Kit as well. A major finding of our earlier study was that the sustained inflammation that occurs in response to repetitive PMA applications was increased in *Ptafr-/-* mice. While the pro-inflammatory effects of PAF are well known, this data suggests a counter regulatory role for the PAF-R in limiting the chronic or sustained inflammation associated with repeated PMA exposures. Consistent with this idea, our new studies demonstrate that co-administration of topical

CPAF along with PMA results in a suppression of the sustained inflammatory response elicited by repetitive tumor promoter application. Since chronic inflammation is thought to promote carcinogenesis [35,47–49], we previously suggested that the increased susceptibility to chemical carcinogenesis observed in *Ptafr-/-* mice may be due to anti-inflammatory effects. This is supported by our observations that topical CPAF suppresses DMBA/PMA-induced carcinogenesis, and that this chemopreventive activity correlates with a reduction in MPO activity.

In contrast to the effects of PAF-R activation on the sustained inflammatory response to multiple PMA applications, PAF-R signaling appears to exert complex pro-inflammatory and anti-inflammatory effects during the initial PMA-induced edema and inflammatory response observed in the first 48 hrs after a single PMA application. *Ptafr-/-* mice exhibited a reduction in ear thickness changes during the first 48 hrs following an initial PMA application. This would be consistent with PAF-R activation serving as a downstream mediator of PMA-induced acute inflammatory responses. This is indeed consistent with the known pro-inflammatory effects of PAF in regulating both edema and leukocyte recruitment [42,43]. However, in our studies, topical CPAF is shown to consistently induce a paradoxical suppression of PMA-induced ear thickness at all time points following either a single PMA application and at later time points following multiple PMA treatments. The possibility that effects of exogenous CPAF are not PAF-R dependent is highly unlikely, as CPAF had no significant effect on PMA-induced inflammation at any time point in *Ptafr-/-* mice.

It is unclear how CPAF application (PAF-R activation) and loss of PAF signaling both result in reductions in PMA-induced edema &/or leukocyte infiltration at early time points following a single PMA application. This could indicate that exogenous CPAF exerts a supraphysiologic response at the receptor level that suppresses PMA-induced inflammatory signaling. It is known that some G-protein coupled receptors, particularly those coupled to Gi-alpha subunit signaling, can also activate Gbeta/gamma subunit signaling when receptors are activated at a higher molar level [50,51]. Alternatively, it is possible that CPAF exerts effects on inflammation through a complex interplay between multiple cell types with counter-regulatory functions.

A second major finding of our study is that c-Kit is likely critical for our observed effects of CPAF on PMA-induced inflammation. Topical CPAF failed to elicit a response in c-$Kit^{W-sh/W-sh}$ mice at all time points following PMA application(s). Like PAF, mast cells have long been known to be pro-inflammatory mediators of type I hypersensitivity reactions [52]. More recent data indicates that mast cells exert complex effects on both innate and adaptive immune responses [26–28]. The resistance of mast cell deficient mice to the initial PMA-induced edema and inflammatory response is consistent with previous studies demonstrating that mast cell deficient mice exhibit a marked decrease in both PMA-induced edema reactions and leukocyte infiltration [43–45]. Moreover, our data suggests that mast cells may be necessary for the ability of CPAF to suppress the sustained inflammation observed following multiple PMA applications. It might be noted that a similar observation was noted in mice exposed to contact allergen or chronic low dose ultraviolet B [32]. In this study, mast cells limited the leukocyte infiltration, necrosis and epidermal hyperplasia that were associated with these insults [32]. Since mast cells can produce both pro-inflammatory and anti-inflammatory mediators [29,31], it is possible that initially pro-inflammatory mast cells alter their secretory phenotype under conditions of repetitive chronic inflammatory stimuli resulting in a switch to anti-inflammatory mediator release. This idea is supported by our

data that shows that c-$Kit^{W-sh/W-sh}$ mice exhibit a reduction in the initial PMA-induced inflammation, but exhibit enhanced sustained chronic inflammation with chronic repetitive PMA applications. The weak edema response noted by topical CPAF administration is consistent with data indicating that PAF fails to elicit histamine secretion from dermal mast cells from humans [8,53], although PAF is a potent activator of histamine release from mast cells derived from peripheral blood or lung tissue [8]. In contrast, the ability of mast cells to promote immune suppression following UVB irradiation depends on a PAF-dependent mast cell migration to lymph nodes [10]. Finally, it should be noted that melanocytes are absent in c-$Kit^{W-sh/W-sh}$ mice. Moreover, c-$Kit^{W-sh/W-sh}$ mice also exhibit increased numbers of immature granulocytic myeloid derived suppressor cells (MDSCs) within the spleen [23]. Thus, it is possible that some or all of the effects that we observed in c-$Kit^{W-sh/W-sh}$ mice are independent of mast cells or require mast cell interaction with melanocytes or MDSCs.

While our findings demonstrate that c-$Kit^{W-sh/W-sh}$ mice exhibit enhanced inflammation following repeated PMA applications, a recent study demonstrated that Kit^{W}/Kit^{W-v} mice exhibited a decrease in inflammatory cell accumulation over a 7 week period following DMBA treatment and repeated PMA applications [54]. It is possible that this discrepancy could be accounted for by the absence of DMBA treatment in our studies. More likely, this report is consistent with the known reduction in differentiated bone marrow derived cells in Kit^{W}/Kit^{W-v} mice that is not observed in c-$Kit^{W-sh/W-sh}$ mice [24]. In support of this idea, Kit^{W}/Kit^{W-v} mice also exhibited a reduction in total CD45^{+}, CD8^{+}, F4/80^{+}, and Gr-1^{+} cells prior to treatment [54].

While topical CPAF suppressed not only PMA-induced inflammation, it also suppressed NMSC formation following chemical carcinogenesis. Moreover, *Ptafr-/-* mice exhibit enhanced DMBA/PMA-induced tumorigenesis [7]. Given that c-*Kit* appears to be critical to the effects of PAF on PMA-induced inflammation, it would be of interest to perform future studies to determine whether c-$Kit^{W-sh/W-sh}$ mice exhibit increased tumorigenesis in response to chemical carcinogens or UVB treatments. It has been proposed that mast cells should promote skin cancer formation through multiple mechanisms, particularly their ability to suppress anti-tumor adaptive immune responses [29,30]. In studies in which mast cells have been directly assessed in tumor models, mast cells are associated with both pro-tumor and anti-tumor activity in lymphoma and models of adenocarcinoma [55–60]. Given the above discussion, it should be noted that a recent study demonstrated that Kit^{W}/Kit^{W-v} mice exhibit a pronounced increase in DMBA/PMA induced tumor formation [54]. Since these mice exhibit changes in other bone marrow derived cell types, it is important to note that this tumor phenotype was reversed by mast cell reconstitution of the treated skin [54].

It has been proposed that PAF should promote skin cancer formation secondary to its ability to induce a systemic T-cell immunosuppression [61]. Similarly, our studies have shown that PAF-induced immunosuppression promotes the growth of syngeneic tumors in mice [19]. Thus, the ability of topical CPAF to suppress chemical carcinogenesis in mice would run counter to previous thoughts regarding the role of PAF in tumorigenesis. It is possible that both mast cells and PAF-R activation act to promote tumor formation via loss of immune surveillance mechanisms, but this is countered by their ability to suppress the promoting aspects of cutaneous inflammation. Thus, it may be that a tissue or context dependent balance between adaptive and innate immune system immunoregulation may determine the ultimate role of PAF in tumorigenesis. Alternatively, relatively high UVB doses are required to induce systemic immunosuppression [62]. This implies that relatively high systemic concentrations of PAF are necessary to induce systemic immunosuppression. Thus, it is possible that our relatively low doses of topical CPAF administration may readily elicit a suppression of local inflammation, but have minimal effects on systemic immunosuppression. The use of higher topical doses or systemic administration of CPAF in our current model may prove informative in future studies to address this idea. Finally, chronic repetitive PMA and/or CPAF applications could act to promote a change in specific mast cell mediator release, to promote an altered balance of phenotypically distinct mast cells (MMC or CTMC), or alter the microenvironmental cues that drive mast cell function. In any case, future studies are necessary to better address the relative role of PAF in altering both adaptive and innate immune responses in cutaneous carcinogenesis. Further work is also necessary to determine whether PAF-R signaling acts to suppress tumor formation in the more clinically relevant photocarcinogenesis model.

Supporting Information

File S1   Contains Figs S1-S4.
(PDF)

Acknowledgments

The authors gratefully acknowledge Danielle Jernigan and Kellie Clay Martel for their work in maintaining the mouse colony used for these studies.

Author Contributions

Conceived and designed the experiments: RLK. Performed the experiments: SR RPS JAO SCD JRB SJW BR JDR. Analyzed the data: RLK SR RPS. Contributed reagents/materials/analysis tools: RLK JBT. Wrote the paper: RLK.

References

1. Stafforini DM, McIntyre TM, Zimmerman GA, Prescott SM (2003) Platelet-activating factor, a pleiotrophic mediator of physiological and pathological processes. Crit Rev Cl Lab Sci 40: 643–672.
2. Yao Y, Wolverton JE, Zhang Q, Marathe GK, Al-Hassani M, et al. (2009) Ultraviolet B Radiation Generated Platelet-Activating Factor Receptor Agonist Formation Involves EGF-R-Mediated Reactive Oxygen Species. J Immunol 182: 2842–2848.
3. Sahu RP, Petrache I, Van Demark MJ, Rashid BM, Ocana JA, et al. (2013) Cigarette Smoke Exposure Inhibits Contact Hypersensitivity via the Generation of Platelet-Activating Factor Agonists. The Journal of Immunology 190: 2447–2454.
4. Konger RL, Marathe GK, Yao Y, Zhang Q, Travers JB (2008) Oxidized glycerophosphocholines as biologically active mediators for ultraviolet radiation-mediated effects. Prostaglandins & Other Lipid Mediators 87: 1–8.
5. Marathe GK, Harrison KA, Murphy RC, Prescott SM, Zimmerman GA, et al. (2000) Bioactive phospholipid oxidation products. Free Radical Biology & Medicine 28: 1762–1770.
6. Travers JB, Huff JC, Rola-Pleszczynski M, Gelfand EW, Morelli JG, et al. (1995) Identification of functional platelet-activating factor receptors on human keratinocytes. Journal of Investigative Dermatology 105: 816–823.
7. Sahu RP, Kozman A, Yao Y, DaSilva SC, Rezania S, et al. (2012) Loss of the Platelet Activating Factor Receptor in mice augments PMA-induced inflammation and cutaneous chemical carcinogenesis. Carcinogenesis 33: 694–701.
8. Kajiwara N, Sasaki T, Bradding P, Cruse G, Sagara H, et al. (2010) Activation of human mast cells through the platelet-activating factor receptor. Journal of Allergy and Clinical Immunology 125: 1137–1145.e1136.
9. Nilsson G, Metcalfe DD, Taub DD (2000) Demonstration that platelet-activating factor is capable of activating mast cells and inducing a chemotactic response. Immunology 99: 314–319.
10. Chacón-Salinas R, Chen L, Chávez-Blanco AD, Limón-Flores AY, Ma Y, et al. (2013) An essential role for platelet-activating factor in activating mast cell migration following ultraviolet irradiation. Journal of Leukocyte Biology.
11. Muehlmann LA, Michelotto PV Jr., Nunes EA, Grando FCC, da Silva FT, et al. (2012) PAF increases phagocytic capacity and superoxide anion production in equine alveolar macrophages and blood neutrophils. Research in Veterinary Science 93: 393–397.
12. Rios FJO, Gidlund M, Jancar S (2011) Pivotal role for platelet-activating factor receptor in CD36 expression and oxLDL uptake by human monocytes/macrophages. Cellular Physiology & Biochemistry 27: 363–372.
13. de Oliveira SI, Fernandes PD, Amarante Mendes JGP, Jancar S (2006) Phagocytosis of apoptotic and necrotic thymocytes is inhibited by PAF-receptor antagonists and affects LPS-induced COX-2 expression in murine macrophages. Prostaglandins & other lipid mediators 80: 62–73.
14. Rios FJ, Koga MM, Pecenin M, Ferracini M, Gidlund M, et al. (2013) Oxidized LDL Induces Alternative Macrophage Phenotype through Activation of CD36 and PAFR. Mediators of Inflammation 2013: 8.
15. Darst M, Al-Hassani M, Li T, Yi Q, Travers JM, et al. (2004) Augmentation of Chemotherapy-Induced Cytokine Production by Expression of the Platelet-Activating Factor Receptor in a Human Epithelial Carcinoma Cell Line. The Journal of Immunology 172: 6330–6335.
16. Dy LC, Pei Y, Travers JB (1999) Augmentation of ultraviolet B radiation-induced tumor necrosis factor production by the epidermal platelet-activating factor receptor. J Biol Chem 274: 26917–26921.
17. Li T, Southall MD, Yi Q, Pei Y, Lewis D, et al. (2003) The epidermal platelet-activating factor receptor augments chemotherapy-induced apoptosis in human carcinoma cell lines. Journal of Biological Chemistry 278: 16614–16621.
18. Marathe GK, Johnson C, Billings SD, Southall MD, Pei Y, et al. (2005) Ultraviolet B Radiation Generates Platelet-activating Factor-like Phospholipids underlying Cutaneous Damage. Journal of Biological Chemistry 280: 35448–35457.
19. Sahu RP, Turner MJ, DaSilva SC, Rashid BM, Ocana JA, et al. (2012) The environmental stressor ultraviolet B radiation inhibits murine antitumor immunity through its ability to generate platelet-activating factor agonists. Carcinogenesis 33: 1360–1367.
20. Zhang Q, Yao Y, Konger RL, Sinn A, Cai S, et al. (2008) UVB radiation-mediated inhibition of contact hypersensitivity reactions is dependent on the platelet-activating factor system. J Invest Dermatol 128: 1780–1787.
21. Norval M (2006) The mechanisms and consequences of ultraviolet-induced immunosuppression. Progress Biophys Mol Biol 92: 108–118.
22. Kripke ML (2013) Reflections on the Field of Photoimmunology. J Invest Dermatol 133: 27–30.
23. Michel A, Schuler A, Friedrich P, Doner F, Bopp T, et al. (2013) Mast cell-deficient Kit(W-sh) "Sash" mutant mice display aberrant myelopoiesis leading to the accumulation of splenocytes that act as myeloid-derived suppressor cells. Journal of Immunology 190: 5534–5544.
24. Grimbaldeston MA, Chen C-C, Piliponsky AM, Tsai M, Tam S-Y, et al. (2005) Mast Cell-Deficient W-sash c-kit Mutant KitW-sh/W-sh Mice as a Model for Investigating Mast Cell Biology in Vivo. The American journal of pathology 167: 835–848.
25. Collington SJ, Williams TJ, Weller CL (2011) Mechanisms underlying the localisation of mast cells in tissues. Trends in Immunology 32: 478–485.
26. de Vries VC, Noelle RJ (2010) Mast cell mediators in tolerance. Current Opinion in Immunology 22: 643–648.
27. Frenzel L, Hermine O (2013) Mast cells and inflammation. Joint, Bone, Spine: Revue du Rhumatisme 80: 141–145.
28. Galli SJ, Tsai M (2010) Mast cells in allergy and infection: versatile effector and regulatory cells in innate and adaptive immunity. European Journal of Immunology 40: 1843–1851.
29. Ch'ng S, Wallis RA, Yuan L, Davis PF, Tan ST (2005) Mast cells and cutaneous malignancies. Mod Pathol 19: 149–159.
30. Sarchio SNE, Kok L-F, O'Sullivan C, Halliday GM, Byrne SN (2012) Dermal mast cells affect the development of sunlight-induced skin tumours. Experimental Dermatology 21: 241–248.
31. St John AL, Abraham SN (2013) Innate immunity and its regulation by mast cells. Journal of Immunology 190: 4458–4463.
32. Grimbaldeston MA, Nakae S, Kalesnikoff J, Tsai M, Galli SJ (2007) Mast cell-derived interleukin 10 limits skin pathology in contact dermatitis and chronic irradiation with ultraviolet B. Nat Immunol 8: 1095–1104.
33. Zhang Q, Mousdicas N, Yi Q, Al-Hassani M, Billings SD, et al. (2005) Staphylococcal lipoteichoic acid inhibits delayed-type hypersensitivity reactions via the platelet-activating factor receptor. The Journal of Clinical Investigation 115: 2855–2861.
34. Sahu RP, DaSilva SC, Rashid B, Martel KC, Jernigan D, et al. (2012) Mice lacking epidermal PPARγ exhibit a marked augmentation in photocarcinogenesis associated with increased UVB-induced apoptosis, inflammation and barrier dysfunction. Int J Cancer 131: E1055–E1066.
35. Hatton JL, Parent A, Tober KL, Hoppes T, Wulff BC, et al. (2007) Depletion of CD4+ Cells Exacerbates the Cutaneous Response to Acute and Chronic UVB Exposure. J Invest Dermatol 127: 1507–1515.
36. Churukian CJ, Schenk EA (1981) A toluidine blue method for demonstrating mast cells. J Histotechnology 4: 85–86.
37. Bulger EM, Maier RV (2000) Lipid mediators in the pathophysiology of critical illness. Critical Care Medicine 28: N27–36.
38. Dyer KD, Percopo CM, Xie Z, Yang Z, Kim JD, et al. (2010) Mouse and Human Eosinophils Degranulate in Response to Platelet-Activating Factor (PAF)

and LysoPAF via a PAF-Receptor–Independent Mechanism: Evidence for a Novel Receptor. The Journal of Immunology 184: 6327–6334.

39. Dupré DJ, Chen Z, Le Gouill C, Thériault C, Parent J-L, et al. (2003) Trafficking, Ubiquitination, and Down-regulation of the Human Platelet-activating Factor Receptor. Journal of Biological Chemistry 278: 48228–48235.

40. Konger RL, Scott GA, Landt Y, Ladenson JH, Pentland AP (2002) Loss of the EP2 prostaglandin E2 receptor in immortalized human keratinocytes results in increased invasiveness and decreased paxillin expression. American Journal of Pathology 161: 2065–2078.

41. Klebanoff SJ (2005) Myeloperoxidase: friend and foe. Journal of Leukocyte Biology 77: 598–625.

42. Young LM, Kheifets JB, Ballaron SJ, Young JM (1989) Edema and cell infiltration in the phorbol ester-treated mouse ear are temporally separate and can be differentially modulated by pharmacologic agents. Agents and Actions 26: 335–341.

43. Rao T, Currie J, Shaffer A, Isakson P (1993) Comparative evaluation of arachidonic acid (AA)- and tetradecanoylphorbol acetate (TPA)-induced dermal inflammation. Inflammation 17: 723–741.

44. Heiman AS, Crews FT (1985) Characterization of the effects of phorbol esters on rat mast cell secretion. Journal of Immunology 134: 548–555.

45. Cantwell ME, Foreman JC (1987) Phorbol esters induce a slow, non-cytotoxic release of histamine from rat peritoneal mast cells. Agents & Actions 20: 165–168.

46. Waskow C, Bartels S, Schlenner SM, Costa C, Rodewald H-R (2007) Kit is essential for PMA-inflammation–induced mast-cell accumulation in the skin. Blood 109: 5363–5370.

47. Gebhardt C, Riehl A, Durchdewald M, Németh J, Fürstenberger G, et al. (2008) RAGE signaling sustains inflammation and promotes tumor development. J Exp Med 205: 275–285.

48. Dougan M, Dranoff G (2008) Inciting inflammation: the RAGE about tumor promotion. The Journal of Experimental Medicine 205: 267–270.

49. Hanahan D, Weinberg Robert A (2011) Hallmarks of Cancer: The Next Generation. Cell 144: 646–674.

50. Boyer JL, Graber SG, Waldo GL, Harden TK, Garrison JC (1994) Selective activation of phospholipase C by recombinant G-protein alpha- and beta gamma-subunits. Journal of Biological Chemistry 269: 2814–2819.

51. Park D, Jhon DY, Lee CW, Lee KH, Rhee SG (1993) Activation of phospholipase C beta gamma subunits. Journal of Biological Chemistry 268: 4573–4576.

52. Amin K (2012) The role of mast cells in allergic inflammation. Respiratory Medicine 106: 9–14.

53. Krause K, Gimenez-Arnau A, Martinez-Escala E, Farre-Albadalejo M, Abajian M, et al. (2013) Platelet-activating factor (PAF) induces wheal and flare skin reactions independent of mast cell degranulation. Allergy 68: 256–258.

54. Siebenhaar F, Metz M, Maurer M (2014) Mast cells protect from skin tumor development and limit tumor growth during cutaneous de novo carcinogenesis in a Kit-dependent mouse model. Experimental Dermatology 23: 159–164.

55. Gounaris E, Erdman SE, Restaino C, Gurish MF, Friend DS, et al. (2007) Mast cells are an essential hematopoietic component for polyp development. Proceedings of the National Academy of Sciences 104: 19977–19982.

56. Sinnamon MJ, Carter KJ, Sims LP, LaFleur B, Fingleton B, et al. (2008) A protective role of mast cells in intestinal tumorigenesis. Carcinogenesis 29: 880–886.

57. Chang DZ, Ma Y, Ji B, Wang H, Deng D, et al. (2011) Mast cells in tumor microenvironment promotes the in vivo growth of pancreatic ductal adenocarcinoma. Clinical Cancer Research 17: 7015–7023.

58. Rabenhorst A, Schlaak M, Heukamp LC, Forster A, Theurich S, et al. (2012) Mast cells play a protumorigenic role in primary cutaneous lymphoma. Blood 120: 2042–2054.

59. Tanaka T, Ishikawa H (2013) Mast cells and inflammation-associated colorectal carcinogenesis. Seminars In Immunopathology 35: 245–254.

60. Tanooka H, Kitamura Y, Sado T, Tanaka K, Nagase M, et al. (1982) Evidence for involvement of mast cells in tumor suppression in mice. Journal of the National Cancer Institute 69: 1305–1309.

61. Sreevidya CS, Khaskhely NM, Fukunaga A, Khaskina P, Ullrich SE (2008) Inhibition of Photocarcinogenesis by Platelet-Activating Factor or Serotonin Receptor Antagonists. Cancer Res 68: 3978–3984.

62. Sahu RP, Yao Y, Konger RL, Travers JB (2012) Platelet-activating Factor Does Not Mediate UVB-induced Local Immune Suppression. Photochemistry and Photobiology 88: 490–493.

16

Evolution of an Expanded Mannose Receptor Gene Family

Karen Staines, Lawrence G. Hunt, John R. Young, Colin Butter*

The Pirbright Institute, Compton, United Kingdom

Abstract

Sequences of peptides from a protein specifically immunoprecipitated by an antibody, KUL01, that recognises chicken macrophages, identified a homologue of the mammalian mannose receptor, MRC1, which we called MRC1L-B. Inspection of the genomic environment of the chicken gene revealed an array of five paralogous genes, MRC1L-A to MRC1L-E, located between conserved flanking genes found either side of the single MRC1 gene in mammals. Transcripts of all five genes were detected in RNA from a macrophage cell line and other RNAs, whose sequences allowed the precise definition of spliced exons, confirming or correcting existing bioinformatic annotation. The confirmed gene structures were used to locate orthologues of all five genes in the genomes of two other avian species and of the painted turtle, all with intact coding sequences. The lizard genome had only three genes, one orthologue of MRC1L-A and two orthologues of the MRC1L-B antigen gene resulting from a recent duplication. The Xenopus genome, like that of most mammals, had only a single MRC1-like gene at the corresponding locus. MRC1L-A and MRC1L-B genes had similar cytoplasmic regions that may be indicative of similar subcellular migration and functions. Cytoplasmic regions of the other three genes were very divergent, possibly indicating the evolution of a new functional repertoire for this family of molecules, which might include novel interactions with pathogens.

Editor: Michelle L. Baker, CSIRO, Australia

Funding: This work was funded by the BBSRC (Biotechnology and Biological Sciences Research Council) under grant number BBS/E/I/00001423 as part of the Institute Strategic Programme Grant to the Avian Viral Diseases Programme at the Pirbright Institute. The funders had no role in study design, data collection and analysis, decision to publish, or preparation of the manuscript.

Competing Interests: The authors have declared that no competing interests exist.

* Email: colin.butter@avianimmunology.org

Introduction

Recent evolution of the repertoire of molecules involved in the function of the immune system has resulted in substantial divergence in the composition and functions of the gene families to which these molecules belong. Even among mammals, different families of molecules may carry out equivalent functions in different species [1]. While the functions of many molecules in immunity are well conserved between mammalian and avian species, in other cases there is extensive divergence in molecular repertoires, with cytokines and chemokines providing examples [2]. These differences often involve gene duplication followed by functional diversification [3]. Thus evolution has led to variety in molecular details in spite of more conserved underlying mechanisms in solutions to the problems of infection. Variation in molecular repertoires may underlie some of the differences between species in host-pathogen interactions. An understanding of these differences will be essential to optimise approaches to immune protection.

The mannose receptor C-type 1 gene (*MRC1, CD206*) is the eponymous member of the mannose receptor family. Their gene products are type I transmembrane glycoproteins containing arrays of C-type lectin domains (CTLDs). The family also includes DEC205 (CD205), MRC2 (Endo180, CD280) and Phospholipase A_2 receptor (PLA$_2$R), each having important functions in immunity [4]. These receptors all have an N-terminal cysteine-rich domain (CysR) followed by a single fibronectin type II domain

(FNII), then either 8 (MRC1, MRC2 and PLA$_2$R) or 10 (DEC205) CTLDs separated by linker regions. They have a transmembrane domain and a short cytoplasmic tail containing motifs that signal endocytosis. In mammals, *DEC205* and *PLA$_2$R* genes are arranged in tandem on one chromosome, while the others are unlinked. In the three genes encoding 8 CTLDs, the 30 exon gene structure and the splicing phases of all introns are completely conserved. The CTLDs fall into two groups, one having an extra pair of cysteine residues at the N-terminal end of the domain (domains 2, 3, 4, 6, 8) [5]. While individual CTLDs generally have low affinities for carbohydrate ligands, the molecules can exhibit high affinities for complex carbohydrate by cooperative binding [6]. Only the fourth CTLD of human MRC1 retains strong enough binding to have lectin activity on its own [7].

The mannose receptor is a recycling endocytosis receptor, rapidly internalised via clathrin-coated vesicles and delivered to early endosomes, with the majority of the receptors in the intracellular location in the steady state [8]. Endocytosis of bound molecules underlies the primary function of the mannose receptor in the recognition of pathogen associated molecular patterns and their consequent uptake for engulfment and for antigen presentation [9]. A soluble form of the mammalian mannose receptor, produced by proteolytic cleavage [10], may also function in the delivery of antigens to lymphoid follicles [11]. Clearance by binding to the mannose receptor may also be involved in the regulation of levels of some hormones [12]. In chickens, the orthologue of mammalian PLA$_2$R acts as an Fc receptor (FcRY), the functional equivalent of mammalian FcRn, extending the range of its endocytic targets to immune complexes [13].

Binding of the mannose receptor by a virus may elicit immunomodulatory responses [14]. It may also facilitate viral entry in a cell either indirectly, as with HIV [15], or directly, as with Dengue [16]. In the mouse, binding of influenza virus by the mannose receptor, in addition to its more widespread binding to sialic acid, is important for virus entry into macrophages [17]. The virus replicates inside infected macropahges, but they do not release infective virus. Instead, the infection enhances the presentation of influenza virus antigens and stimulates the generation of pro-inflammatory cytokines. Thus the participation of the mannose receptor in allowing infection of macrophages contributes to innate and eventually to adaptive protection [18]. Reciprocally driven evolution of the virus and the mannose receptor in different species may thus be a significant contributor to differences in host-pathogen interactions.

Employing mass spectrometry of immunoprecipitated antigen, we identified a molecule recognised by a macrophage marker antibody, KUL01 [19], as a chicken homologue of MRC1. Inspection of neighbouring avian genome sequence revealed that the locus contained five tandemly repeated genes encoding similar molecules that are likely to have arisen through duplication, of a single ancestral MRC1 gene, in the avian lineage. Very different cytoplasmic sequences and differences in relative transcript levels in tissues indicate diversification of function among the duplicated genes.

Results

The KUL01 antibody recognises a homologue of the macrophage mannose receptor MRC1

KUL01 antibody bound to agarose beads was used to adsorb proteins from a lysate of the transformed chicken macrophage cell line HD11, which were analysed by SDS PAGE after elution at low pH. Specific bands, obtained from beads coated with KUL01 but not from those coated with control antibody, were excised, digested with trypsin and analysed my mass spectroscopy. The major specifically recognised molecule was a (doublet) band with an apparent molecular weight of 180 kDa (figure 1). By Mascot search of the NCBI non-redundant chicken proteins in the IPI database, a sufficient number of peptides from the tryptic digest of this band were identified as being derivable from the sequence IPI00814304 to unequivocally identify it as the source of antigen specifically adsorbed by KUL01 (figure S1 and table S1). It was annotated as being a chicken homologue of MRC1.

Genomic context of chicken MRC1 orthologues

The genomic context of the gene for the KUL01 antigen was inspected to see whether additional evidence from conserved gene order would support its identification as the orthologue of MRC1. Inspection of the region between orthologues of the highly conserved genes, *SLC39A12* and *STAM*, that flank *MRC1* in mammals, revealed multiple segments with similarity to the *MRC1* gene. Existing annotation and EST data, together with manual examination, allowed the definition of five potential *MRC1L* genes. For convenience, these were labelled *MRC1L-A to E* in sequence in the direction of their transcription (which is inverse to the genome map). Annotations of this gene array from different sources varied widely, in detailed exon composition, splicing sites and numbers of genes. To evaluate the predicted gene models, a series of PCR primers were designed for amplification of segments of the predicted transcripts from RNA. PCR products were amplified from RNA from the HD11

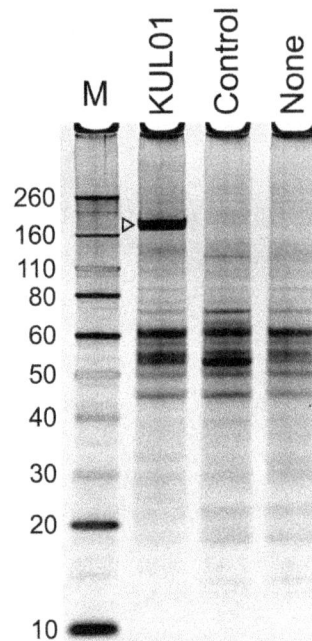

Figure 1. KUL01 specifically precipitates a molecule with apparent molecular weight 180 kDa. Track M contains molecular weight standards. The other tracks contain materials absorbed from a precleared lysate of the HD11 macrophage cell line, by agarose beads to which were attached either KUL01, an isotype matched control antibody, or no antibody, and eluted at low pH. The open arrowhead points to the band(s) specifically absorbed by the KUL01 antibody, which were analysed by mass spectroscopy.

transformed macrophage cell line, and from a cDNA library from RPRL Line 0 chicken spleen.

All predicted exons were amplified from spliced transcripts from the Line 0 chicken cDNA. All the transcript sequences confirmed in this way contained intact reading frames for MRC1-like proteins. These were submitted to the ENA database and received accession numbers HF569039, HF566127, HF569040, HF569041, HF569042, in order *MRC1L-(A to E)* and are provided in figure S2, together with their genomic locations. The *MRC1L-B* and *–C* genes are now correctly annotated in the ENSEMBL database (ENSGALT00000043091, ENSGALT00000014059). Annotation of the other genes is currently inaccurate, with errors as described in file S1 and are liable to change in subsequent database versions. Differences from the corresponding red jungle fowl genomic sequences are enumerated in table S2. The exon structures of the genes and their coding content are compared in figure 2. All encoded eight CTLDs. All except D also contained the exons encoding CysR and FNII receptor domains. That exception apart, the 30-exon structures are identical to that of the mammalian MRC1 genes, with all splice phases conserved and very similar exon lengths for all except the terminal exons.

One alternative splice acceptor site, for exon 8 of the MRC1L-E gene, resulting in the insertion of six amino acids, was found in a minority of the sequenced clones from Line 0 cDNA. While that was the only variant transcript in the Line 0 cDNAs, in the HD11 RNA, more frequent alternatively spliced transcripts were detected for *MRC1L-E*, most of which resulted in interruption of the open reading frame, so that no intact open reading frame for *MRC1L-E* was found in the HD11 cDNA. Thus it is possible the alternative splicing seen in HD11 was an artefact of the transformation of

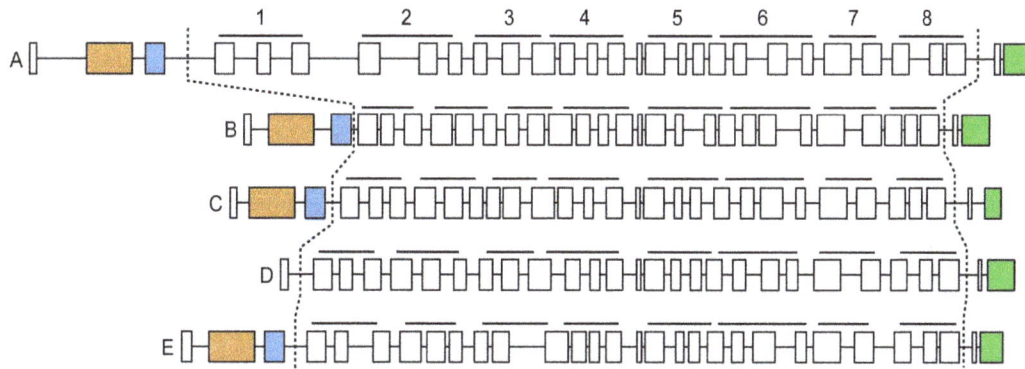

Figure 2. Structure of paralogous *MRC1* genes in the chicken genome. Exons are shown to scale as rectangles. Introns are drawn to 1/10 of the exon scale, except for the shortest which are expanded for visibility. Orange and blue exons are the CysR and FNII domains in all genes except D. The terminal green exon contains transmembrane and cytoplasmic regions. The central array of exons encodes the eight CTLDs indicated by the black bars above each gene.

these cells. The alternative spliced transcripts are illustrated in figure S3.

The locations of conserved features in the CTLDs of the chicken MRC1L genes are shown in figure 3. The tryptophan/ hydrophobic/glycine/hydrophobic (WIGL) motif characteristic of the family [20] is present in all these domains of all genes, with minor variations. Four cysteine residues are also conserved in all these domains, an outer pair forming the disulphide bond spanning most of the domain, and an inner pair forming the disulphide bond stabilising the β3–β4 hairpin [21].

MRC1L genes in other species

The UCSC genome browser BLAT search [22,23] with individual and concatenated chicken genes was used to locate orthologous genes in genomes of other birds (turkey and zebrafinch), painted turtle, lizard and Xenopus (sequences in figure S4 and locations in figure S2). In all cases, the alignments with the highest scoring similarities were found between a pair of highly conserved orthologues of the same flanking genes, *SLC39A12* and *STAM*. Exons missing from these BLAT alignments were easily identified by manual inspection. The arrangements of these genes are compared with the orthologous region of the mouse genome in figure 4. The genes in the three birds are very similar, in structure and size of all five genes. The two gaps between the coding sequences of genes C, D and E are small compared with those between the upstream genes. The turtle appears to have a very similar set of five genes, although they occupy a segment of genome twice the length of that in the birds. The lizard genome contains only three genes, while the Xenopus genome, like the mammalian, contains only one *MRC1L* gene. The mouse genome, like that of other mammals, contains an additional gene, *TMEM236*, between the shared flanking genes.

Phylogenetic trees were constructed using a variety of sequence subsets and methods. The great majority of the results had similar topology to the tree depicted in figure 5. Several of the genes identified in other species were missing all or parts of exons in gaps in the genome assemblies. Some signal peptide exons were uncertain, and gene D lacked CysR and FNII domain exons. To avoid bias by these omissions, the tree shown was constructed using just those parts of the CTLDs that were available from all of the genes involved. All species had a single gene that was placed in the same clade as the mammalian *MRC1* gene in 100% of bootstrapped trees. For the avian and turtle genes, the same pattern of species was found for each gene, implying that these

arose by duplication before the divergence of these species. In contrast, the lizard lacked orthologues of genes C, D and E, but appeared to have two relatively similar genes of the gene represented in chickens by the KUL01 antigen. Thus the simplest consistent history of this gene family would be an original duplication of the ancestral MRC1 gene, giving rise to the *MRC1L-B* gene, followed in the shared avian and turtle ancestor by further duplications producing genes *C, D* and *E*, and in the lizard lineage by a second duplication of the *MRC1L-B* gene. Trees constructed using all the separated CTLDs generally gave the same pattern of species within a clade representing each domain, providing no evidence for domain reassortment. The majority produced the same topology as the tree shown, although bootstrap values were lower. Where the topologies differed, the bootstrap values were insufficient to support any contrary implications. A minority of alternative tree construction methods failed to place the lizard genes 2 and 3 in the MRC1L-B clade.

The cytoplasmic regions of the *MRC1L* gene products are compared in figure 6. The pattern of similarities between sequences are consistent with the evolutionary history that was implied by phylogenetic analysis. This part of the protein is highly conserved between the single mammalian *MRC1* gene and the other genes assigned to the same clade by analysis of the CTLDs. In these molecules, it contains potential motifs involved in targeting to the endocytic pathway, φxNxxY [24,25] and (DE)xxxLZ [25,26]. These motifs are shared by the genes that fall into the MRC1L-B clade that includes the KUL01 antigen, except for the replacement of tyrosine by histidine in the second of the two lizard genes in this clade. The group of genes including mammalian MRC1 also has a di-aromatic motif (YF) that may be involved in endosome sorting [27]. Although the latter is absent from the MRC1L-B orthologues, there are several other residues conserved between these two groups of proteins. In contrast, the cytoplasmic regions of the three downstream genes, found only in the bird and turtle genomes, are highly divergent between paralogues, although well conserved among orthologues. The product of MRC1L-C has only very short cytoplasmic sequences beyond the positively charged region expected to lie immediately inside the plasma membrane. Products of genes D and E have cytoplasmic sequences quite different from each other as well as from those of the MRC1L-A and MRC1L-B molecules. None of the downstream genes contain the endocytosis motifs conserved in the two upstream genes, although the MRC1L-D genes do have a β   α   α   β2   L1   L2   L3   L4   β3   β4   β5

Ω   Φ θ C   θ   θ O E   Ωθ   ΦθGθ   Φ Ω G Ω Ω W   P   EOCθ Ω   G WND C   Ω C

```
M1  LTGILYQINSKSAL---TWHQARASCKQQNADLLSVTEIHEQMYLTGLTSSL-------SSGLWIGLNSLSVRSGWQWAGGSPFRYLNWLPGSP--------------SSEPGKS-CVSL---NPGKNAKWENLECVQKLGYICK
A1  LTNVQYQINSESAL---TWHQARKSCQQQKAELLSITELHEQTYLAGLTGKL-------SSALWFGLNSLNFDSGWQWVGGAPFRYLNWVPGHP--------------SPEPGKI-CAAL---NPGKVAKWENWECNQKLGYICK
B1  LTETHYQINSNSLL---TWHQAKRSCQQQNAELLSVTNPHEEMFLLGLTSDLG-F----DAKLWTGLVRR-LDSSWEWTEGSPLRYLNWAPGNP--------------SVELLKM-CGTF---Q-CRNGKWENVACNQKLGYICQ
C1  LRNAHYQINSESAL---TWHQARKSCQQQNAELLSITDIHEQTYLKELTEST-------DSALWIGLNRLDLKSGWEWIGGTPFQYLNWAPGSP--------------SPESGKL-CVVL---NPETKAKWQNWECDQKLGYICK
D1  STGVLYQINSESAL---TWHQARKSCQEQNAELLSITEIHEQEYVGELIKKF-------SFALWIGLNTLNFNSGWQWAGGSPFRYLNWAPGSP--------------FPAPGKI-CGTM---NPRQNAKWENQACNQRFGYICK
E1  LTGTFYQINFQSAL---TWHQARHSCKQEQNAELLSVTEIEHEQEYVRDLIDSN-----RSPLWIGLNSLNLHSGWQWSGGTPFRYFNWAPGSP--------------SPEPDKL-CAVL---NPRTDAKWENRPCEQKVGYICK
```

```
M2  YAGHCYRIHREEKK---IQKYALQACRKEGGDLASIHSIEEFDFIFSQLGYP------NDELWIGLNDIKIQMYFEWSDGTPVFTKWLPGEP--------------SHENNRQEDCVVM----KGKDGYWADRACEQPLGYICK
A2  YAGHCYIIHRDPK----IWKDALTSCRKEDGDLASIHNVEEYSFVISQLGYQP-----DDELWIGLNDLKVQMYFEWSDGTPVTYAKWLRGEP--------------THANNRQEDCVVM----KGKDGFWADHSCEKKIGYICK
B2  YAGHCYRIYRTPK----IWKQAQSSCRKEDGDLTSIHNVEEYSFIVSQLGYKP-----DDELWIGLNDFRFQMYFEWSDGTPVTYTKWQQRQP-------------THTPN-KADCIVM----NGEDGFWADSTCERKLGYICK
C2  YVDHCYKIFRETK----GWQEALTSCQNAGSHLASIONFEEHSFIVSGLGYKP-----TDKLWIGLNDHKFQMFFEWSDGTPVTYTKWHLGEP--------------SSTNNRPEDCVVMI---KGQDGYFADSNCEKKAGYVCK
D2  YASHCYSIQRESK----AWKDALTSCKRQGGDLASVHSITEYSFLVSQLGYMP-----TEELWLGLNDLKTHFYFEWSDGTPVTFTTWQRRHP-------------TYRNG-LEDCVVM----KGQDGYWATDVCDKQFGYICK
E2  YAGHCYSIHREPR----AWKDALMSCNESNGNLASIHNSEEHAFILSQLGYKA-----TDDLWIGMNDFSTQMYFEWSDETPVTYKWLPGEP--------------THAVSGQEDCVVM----AGEDGYWADSDCDRKLGYICR
```

```
M3  HGFVCYLIGSTLS----TFTDANHTCTNEKAYLTTVEDRYEQAFLTSLVGLRP-----EKYFWTGLSDVQNKGTFRWTVDEQVQFTHWNADMP----------GRKAGCV--AMKTGVACGLWDVLSCEEKAKFVCK
A3  HGFVCYFIGSTFV----TFSQANQTCERHQAYLATVQDRYEQAYLTSLVGLKT-----ERYFWIGLSDVEEKGTFKWANGEYVLFTHWNSEMP----------GRKPGCV--AMRTGTAGGLWDVIKCEEKAKFLCK
B3  HGFVCYSIGQLPA----TFSEAKLICEENKAHLATVRDRYEQAFLTSIIGFKP-----VKYFWIGLSDMEEQGTFRWAGGDPVIFTHWNMGMP---------GREPGCV--AMRTGTSAGLWDILNCEEKNLFLCK
C3  YGTYCYFIGHVPA----TFSEANNTCKGEKGYLATVESRYEQAYLTSLVGLRP-----ERYFWLGLSDMEDQGTFRWSSGEDVSFTHWGAAIP---------GSKPGCV--AMRTGTAAGLWDVLDCESKQKYICK
D3  YGFHCYLVGSALA----TFSDANKTCEQSKAYLATVETRNEQAFLISLTGLRS-----GKYFWLGLSDTEKRGMFKWTSGETPSFTHWNSAMP----------GKEQGCV--AMGTGVSAGLWDVISCQETANFLCK
E3  HGSVCYLVGRAPV----TFSEAVKTCERIGGYLTTIEDRYEQAYLTSFVGLSS-----EKCFWIGLSNTEEQEIFKWETGEGVFYTNWNSAMP----------GKEVGCV--ALRTGSAAGLWDVQNCELKAKFLCK
```

```
M4  KTSMCFKLYAKGKHEKKTWFESRDFCKAIGGELAISKSKDEQQVIWRLITSSGSY---HELFWLGLTYGSPSEGFTWSDGSPVSYENWAYGEP-----------NNYQNVEYCGELKGDP---GMSWNDINCEHLNNWICQ
A4  RISFCFKPFSKGE-QKKTWLESQEFCRTIGGDLASISGKDEQQVIWRSIANNGFY---HQHFWMGLYYLNPDDGFAWSDGSPVRYENWGFGEP-----------NNYQGIELCAEISGDS---SMLWNDRHCDYLYGWICQ
B4  QSSFCFKIFQRGREKMQTWIGARDFCRAIGGDLACIHSEEEQKLISS--LNKDYR---HVSYWMGLNALGSDGGFTWCDGSPVNFQKWANGEP----------NNYDGNEKCGVFYGYN---DMKWNDMFCEHMQDYVCQ
C4  DATSCYKFCRSDIKKKSWIEARDFCRQIGGDLATINNEEEKKMISR--GNSHCR----FERVWLGIFSLNPDEGFAWSDGSPVRYTGWS-DHP---------RSSGGHMFCGVIDGRTF--SGQWLLLPCEEQHDWVCQ
D4  HADSCFKFFVRDKNLKKNWFEAEEFCREIGGNLVTINSKEDQVLIWQLALEKGLQ---TQGFWMGLFLLNPSDGFTWIDGSPVIYENWDEDEP----------NNDKGIEHCVMFNRSP---QMRWNDLYCEYLLNWICE
E4  STNSCFRTFVREKNHKKTWFEARDFCREIGGDLAAINSEEEQRVIEDLITKKLPS---SQLFWIGLQRLDPDGGLSWSDRSPVSYM---KTTP-----------FYDDPLENCGAISKEH---SISWINMHCEYSLDWICE
```

```
M5  YKDQYQYYFSKEK----ETMDNARAFCKKNFGDLATIKSESEKKFLWKYINKNG-----GQSPYFIGMLIS-MDKKFIWMDGSKVDFVAWATGEP--------NFANDDENCVTMYTNS----GFWNDINCGYPNNFICQ
A5  NEDRHYYFSTES----VPMEKGREFCKKNFGDLVVIDSETERKFLWRYILKNG-----KEDAYFIGLQLS-VDQRTSWMDGTPVNYLAWAPHEP---------NFANNDENCVVMYKNL----GFWNDINCGYPNPYICE
B5  YNHKEYYFSKEE----MPMEKAREYCKKNGGDLAIIENESERTFLWKY----TFYKD-RGNNFFIGLTVS-LDKTFRWIDGSTVNYVAWAPNEP---------NFANNDENCVVMYTQT----GTWNDLNCCSVFICK
C5  YKDKLYYISKEQ----VSMEEAQEFCRMNSADLAVISSNSERRFIQRALIKNDKYRT-ESEQYFIGLKIS-LDKTFSWIDGTPVTYVAWAPNEP---------NFANNEEHCVVMFSKQ----GLWNDVNCGTTNRFVCE
D5  YEDKQYYFSRER----VPMEEARRICQRNFADLVVIEDESERQFIWKYINRKRSGVFFQEESYFIGLFVS-SDQKLSWLGKTPVNYVAWAPGEP--------NYSHNDENCVVMKEDF----GFWNDINCGLKNTFICE
E5  KGDKQYFFSTES----TSMEKARTFCKNHRGDLAIIGDNNQRIFLWKYILKNG-----KLHSYLIGLILN-ADRQFRWVDGSTLHYAPWAQGEP---------NFASAQEHCVVLDKKY----GLWNDVSCGHSHGFICE
```

```
M6  YKNKCFKIFGFANEEKKSWQDARQACKGLKGNLVSIENAQEQAFVTYHMRDST------FN-AWTGLNDINAEHMFLWTAGQGVHYTNWKGYP----------GGRRSSLSYEDADCVVVIGGNSREAGTWMDDTCDSKQGYICQ
A6  FQNKCYKIFGSTEDERVTWHAARTACMNLGGNLATIPNEQVQAFLTFHMKDFL------TD-TWIGLNDINHELHFLWTDGTGVHYTNWAKGFP----------SGHLGSYSYNG-QADCVVMRNNPVKEAGKWADESCDNNRGYICQ
B6  FDNKCFKAFGLNENYTLTWHAARNNCITSGGNLATISKKENQAFLMSLLKNTA------TD-AWIGLNDINHEHTYLWTDGSPVYYTNWAK--------------GSRSYYS-KDDCVYMKKNPIEQAGKWKDGDCKASKSYICQ
C6  FNNKCFKIFASNTTRKLAWHDAREVCIDLGGNLASVANEHAQAFVYYHLKDAT------TN-VWIGMNDINRESTFLWADGSTVSYTNWVEGAPETKQSFFDYYEYELLEDNTVETDCVFMTKSD---GKWRRDDSCDNERGYICQ
D6  FQNKCYKIVGSREEERLTWYSARSACIEQGGNLASIHNAQVQAFLTFHLKDVT------DE-TWIGLNDK---HSYIWTDGSPYDYACWARGFP----------LGKYNRVGWKTDCIAMMIRSVNEAGKWENTDCHHNKSYICQ
E6  FKNQCYKFFGSQFQY---WYTANRDCISLGGHLATIQNEQVQAFLTYHLKDVL------YN-PWIGLNDIISELNFVWADGNTVSYTNWAPDSPKLYEPILYDSLHPEDGHNRMQYDCVSLK-TDYTDIGKWSDESCSKSSGYICQ
```

```
M7  YGKSSYSLMKLK----LPWHEAETYCKDHTSLLASILDPYSNAFAW-MKMHPF-----NVPIWIALNSNLTNNEYTWTDRWRVRYTNWGADEP--------------KLKSACV--YMD---VDGYWRTSYCNESFYFLCK
A7  YGNSSYLFIRTK----MNWEDARENCKRDQFDLSSILDPYSHSFLW-LKILKY-----GVPIWIGLNSNVTNGRYEWIDNWRMKYTKWAEGEP--------------KQKIGCV--YLD---ISGAWKTGSCNESYFSVCK
B7  YDDDRYAVINYK----MNWEEAQKNCKDQHADLASILDPYVEAYLW-LQTLKH-----GEPVWIGLNSNTTHGLYMWSDRRRSRYHNWASGEP--------------NKNAACA--YLD---LDGFWKTTSCNETFLSLCK
C7  YGDSSYLIVSSK----MQWEEARKNCQEQRAELASILDAYIHSFLW-IQMQKY-----GKPVWIGLKSNITRSYYKWTDNWKTRFTKWAAEEP--------------KKKNACV--YLD---LDGTWKTAPCKEMYFSVCK
D7  YGNSSYLIIPSK----MSWEEARKACREKSSELASISDYYSNIFLL-LQAAQY-----GEPLWIGINSNLSYGYYRWSDKRKIDFSNWHYEEP--------------KEKIACV--FLE---LSGEWKTAPCNEKHFSVCK
E7  SDGISYSVIHSK----MNWEEAQQSCNSNASELASILDPYSQSLLF-LIAQEY-----GQPMWIGLNSYMTEGKYRWIDRWRLVYSKWSSGEP--------------KQTLACV--YLD---TDGTWKTASCKEKLFSICK
```

```
M8  FYGHCYYFESSFT---RSWGQASLECLRMGASLVSIETAAESSFLSYRVEPLKSK----TN-FWIGMFRN-VEGKWLWLNDNPSFVFNWKTGDP--------------SGERNDCVVLASSS----GLWNNIHCSSYKGFICK
A8  FRGHCYYVESSST---RNWAQASLECLRLGASLVSVEDSAEASLFTYIIEPLEGK----TSTFWTGMYRN-VDGKFLWLNDTAVNFVNWNTGEP--------------SPQQNEHCVEMYANS----GYWNNIYCTSYKGYVCK
B8  FRGHCYYVHTTSE---ASWPAASMMCIQMGASLVSIEDPAEMNFLLLYLSPFASD----NRKFWLGLFKN-IEGEWMMWSDRSVVEFVNWEKGEP-------------TVMYDKHCVHMDVSS----GAWRNYYCSVDRNFICK
C8  YHGHCYYIEASAA---TSWAQASLKCTHLGATLVSVENVDESDFLIHTTQLLGNK----VGGFWIGLYRN-VDDQWLWLDNAVMDFVNWEEKE--------------SDEKHHCVEMTAPS----GYWDNTDCSSEKGFICK
D8  FRSHCYYFNPS-E---MSWVQSVTQCIQSGGMLTSVVDLAESNFLEEHADLYTSK----TSGFWIGLYRN-INGQLLWQDNSVLDFVNWGEAEP-------------LEEQHENEYCVQLSASS----GSWNSIPCSSRKGFICK
E8  FHGHCYHFEAVRK---KRWSQAHEECARLAADLLSVGDYTEANFVAETIKILHGK----SPNFWIGLKRD-DREQWVWTDKSELDFVNWQIGEP--------------ANRMHKDCGEVCALT----GFWNTNVCSFRKGYICK
```

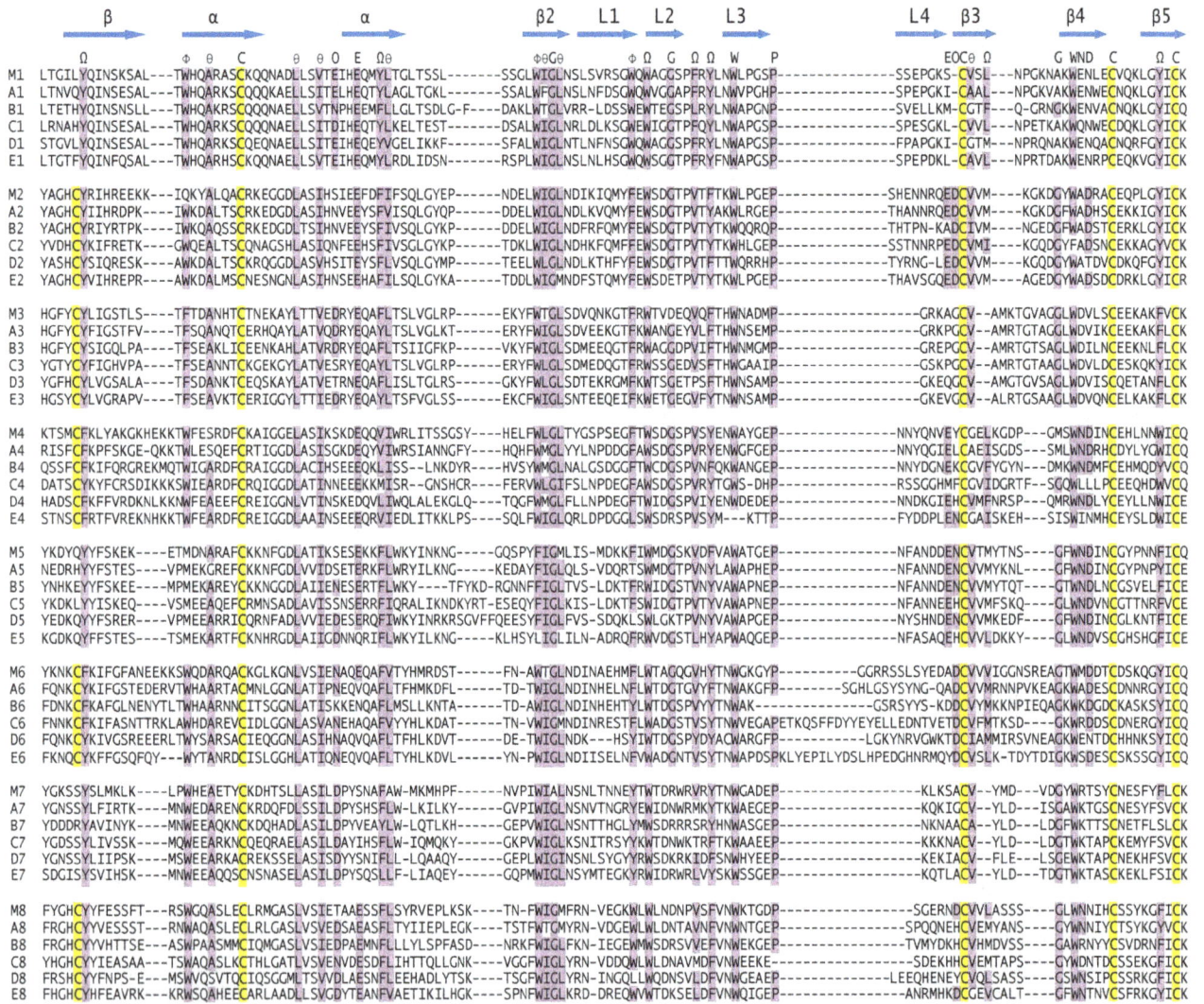

Figure 3. C type lectin domains of the avian MRC1 orthologue gene products. Sequences are labelled on the left, M being the mouse MRC1 sequence while the chicken genes are labelled A to E in genome order in the direction of their transcription, with sequential numbers to indicate the domains in order. Dashes indicate missing residues in the alignment. The short linker peptides between domains are omitted from this figure. Residues reported [20,51] to be conserved throughout the mannose receptor family are indicated above the sequences using the symbols Ω, aromatic or aliphatic; φ, aromatic; θ, aliphatic; C, E, G, P, W, N, D the standard amino acid codes; O, carbonyl oxygen containing (DNEQ). The corresponding residues in the sequences are shaded, yellow for cysteine and purple for the others. Additional cysteine residues in domains 2, 3, 4, 6 and 8 are also shaded. Likely locations of secondary structural features in the mouse sequence [52] are indicated by blue arrows above the sequence; β, beta strand; α alpha helix; L loop.

potential alternative endocytic pathway targeting motif YxxZ (FxxZ in the turtle) [28].

Transcription in tissues

Amplification of the spliced cDNAs for all five genes from the HD11 cell line suggested that all five genes might be transcribed in macrophages. PCR products were also obtained for all the genes from a spleen cDNA library. To obtain a more general picture of the pattern of transcript levels from these genes, quantitative PCR assays were developed for each and applied to compare levels of mRNA for each gene in different normal tissues. The mRNA levels, relative to 28S rRNA, found in various tissues from six Line 0 birds are shown in figure 7.

Exceptionally, the level of *MRC1L-A* transcript was highest in the liver whilst the level in the skin was highest for the other four

genes, though only marginally so for *MRC1L-B*. Genes *C*, *D* and *E* had remarkably similar patterns of transcript levels in tissues, possibly indicating coordinated regulation. There was some variation between genes in the levels in different parts of the gut, although duodenum always had lower levels than distal regions of the digestive tract. Within the lymphoid tissues the highest level was always seen in the spleen. Relative transcript levels of all the genes were lowest in either kidney or liver. These assays are not calibrated to compare transcript levels between different genes.

The same assay was used to compare levels of expression, relative to 28S RNA, in several transformed cell lines (figure S5). Expression was clearly highest in the two macrophage cell lines, HD11 and MQ. Much lower levels of MRC1L-A were detected in some of the T cell derived cell lines.

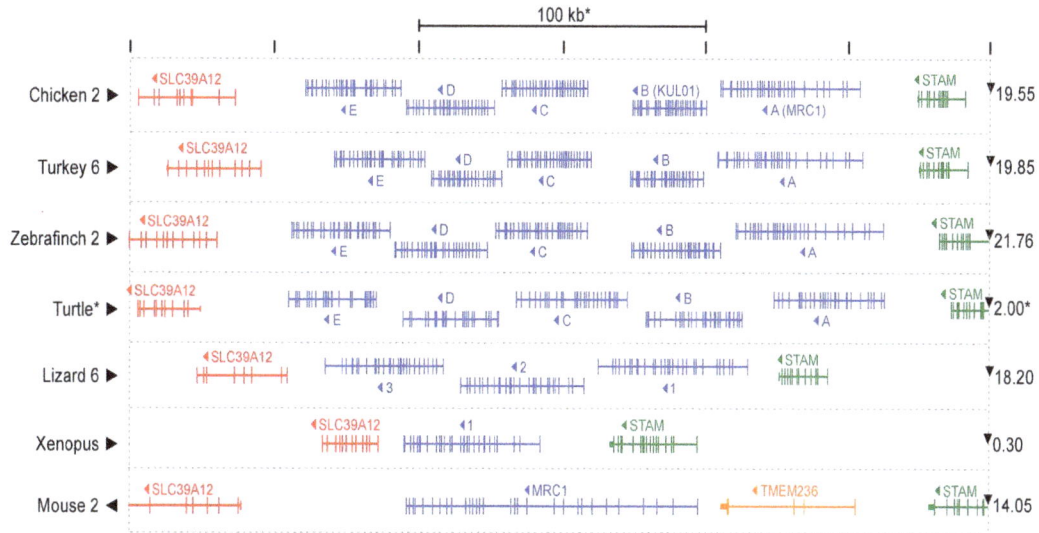

Figure 4. Arrangement the MRC1 orthologue locus in different species. Species are labelled at the left, with a numeral indicating the chromosome where that is known. Black arrowheads indicate the relative orientations of the reference genome maps. The conserved flanking genes SLC39A12 and STAM are indicated in red and green respectively. An additional gene TMEM236, found only in mammalian genomes, is coloured yellow. Predicted MRC1 paralogues are shown in blue. Vertical lines represent the exons of each gene. All the genomes are represented at the same scale, so that the region between vertical dotted lines is 300 kilobase pairs, except in the case of the Painted Turtle, where it represents 600 kilobase pairs. The location in megabase pairs of the right hand end of the map in the chromosome, or other map segment, is indicated at the right. The coding sequences of all genes shown run from right to left in this map, as indicated by arrowheads.

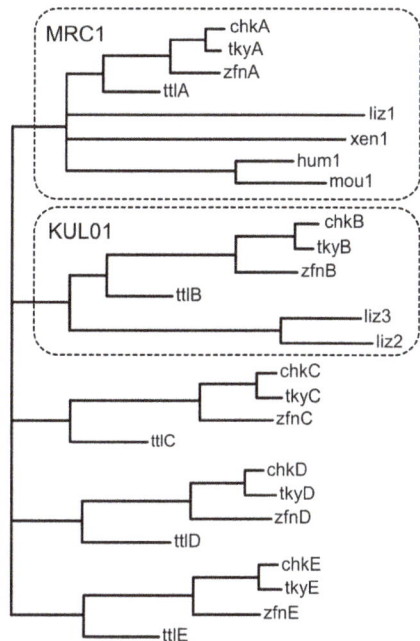

Figure 5. Evolutionary relationships of avian MRC1L genes. A maximum likelihood phylogenetic tree was constructed from predicted exons encoding all the CTLDs, using the Tamura-Nei model in the MEGA software, with 100 bootstrap datasets. All nodes with bootstrap values less than 100 were coalesced into multifurcations. Leaves are labelled with a three letter species code (chk, chicken (*Gallus gallus*); tky, turkey (*Maleagris gallopavo*); zfn, zebrafinch (*Taeniopygia guttata*); ttl, painted turtle (*Chrysemys picta bellii*); liz, lizard (*Anolis carolinensis*); xen, *Xenopus tropicalis*; hum, human (*Homo sapiens*); mou, mouse (*Mus musculus*); followed by either a letter or a number indicating the order of the genes in the direction of transcription. Clades representing orthologues of the MRC1 (human) and KUL01 (chicken) genes are surrounded by dotted lines.

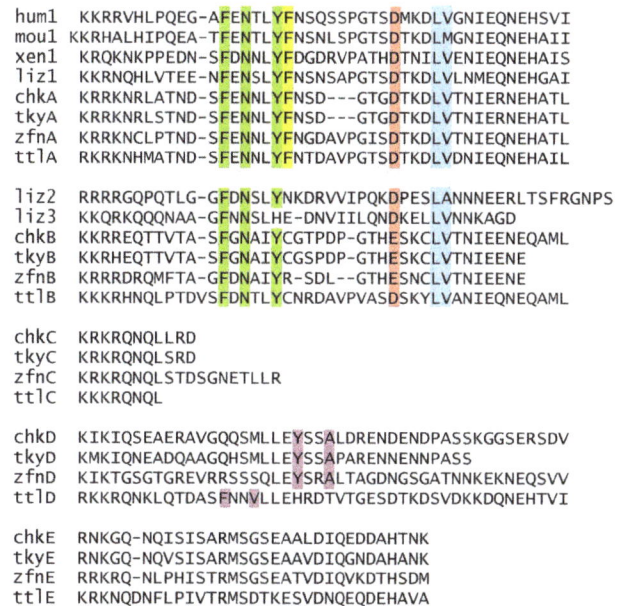

Figure 6. Alignments of cytoplasmic regions of MRC-like genes from various species. Gene names are as described in the legend to figure 5. Shaded residues show the locations of peptide motifs that may be involved in targeting to the endocytic pathway; green for the φxNxxY, red and blue for the (DE)xxxLZ motif, and purple for YxxZ (φ indicating a bulky hydrophobic residue and Z indicating a hydophobic residue). Light green shading indicates an overlapping potential di-aromatic endosome sorting motif in the MRC1 and MRC1L-A sequences.

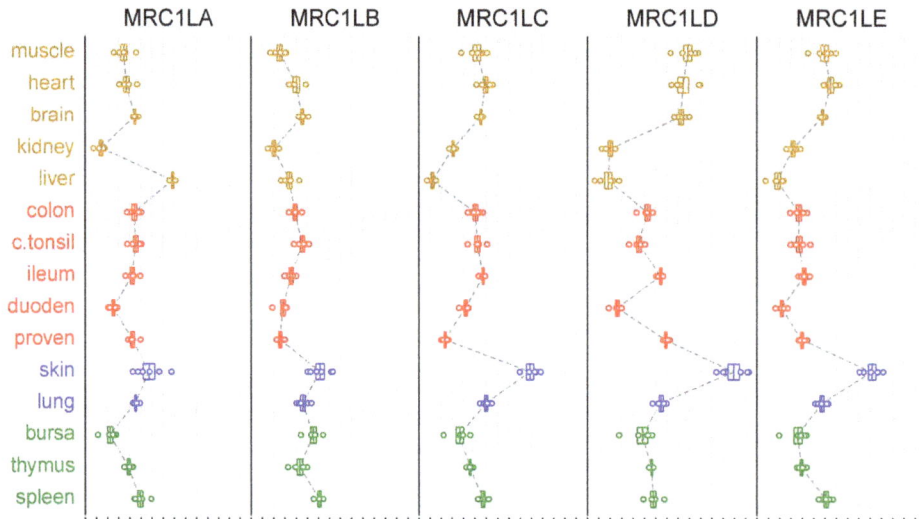

Figure 7. Relative levels of each MRC1 orthologue mRNA in different tissues, measured by quantitative PCR. Tissues, as labelled at the left, are grouped according to preponderance of immune function. For each gene, relative levels of mRNAs are plotted horizontally using a logarithmic scale with arbitrary origins. Circles are individual measurements from each of six birds. Boxes are centered on the means, and their ends indicate the standard errors of those means. All measurements were normalised relative to a constant level of 28S rRNA in each sample and adjusted to the log2 scale using the measured PCR efficiency of standard dilution series, before calculation of means and standard errors. Grey vertical lines and small scale bars at the bottom indicate two-fold differences in relative mRNA measurements.

Discussion

In the human genome, the region of chromosome 10 between the flanking markers *SLC39A12* and *STAM* is annotated as containing a tandemly repeated region, each repeat containing the genes *TMEM236* and *MRC1*. The repeated genes are part of a duplicated segment of about 200 kB with greater than 99% identity, separated by a large gap. There are only two BAC end pairs spanning the gap. In contrast all other mammals that we examined, including other primates, have only one copy of the *TMEM236* and *MRC1* genes between the same flanking marker orthologues, without the gap. While a very recent duplication in humans cannot be ruled out, it seems much more likely that this is a mis-assembled region in the human genome and thus that all mammals carry only a single *MRC1* gene. In species from other classes of terrestrial vertebrate, examination of the region of the genomes between the most highly similar homologues of the flanking markers revealed that some of these contained multiple, tandemly arranged diverged paralogues of *MRC1*. *Xenopus tropicalis* genomes contained only a single gene, the lizard *Anolis carolinensis* had three, while three birds and the painted turtle had five. This indicated duplication of the ancestral *MRC1* gene in the avian lineage and its precursors. The most likely sequence of events would have been an initial duplication producing the ancestors of chicken *MRC1L-A* and *MRC1L-B* genes, followed by a much more recent duplication of the latter in the lizard, and by further early duplications in the common ancestor of birds and turtles. In this context, it is of note that the phylogenetic position of the turtle has been the subject of much debate over a number of decades. Whilst a recent report based on an analysis of microRNAs suggested that turtles form a clade with lizards [29], subsequent reports place them in the archosaur lineage with birds and the crocodylia [30,31]. The more recent proposal is compatible with the simplest possible history of the MRC1 genes described in the present report.

Chicken orthologues of the adjacent *DEC205* [32] and *PLA₂R* genes, and of the *MRC2* gene, are found elsewhere in the genome.

The additional genes in the *MRC1* locus are therefore not relocated orthologues of these genes.

All the identified genes in all the species examined had intact reading frames coding for proteins with the CTLD structure normally found in members of the mannose receptor family. All were found as spliced mRNAs in the chicken. Thus it is unlikely that any of the duplicated genes is a pseudogene, although differently spliced variants of the genes *D* and *E* transcripts were found in HD11 cDNA that had interrupted reading frames. The physical distances between the genes *C, D* and *E* were small, and the pattern of variation of their transcript levels in tissues was very similar. It may be that the transcription of these three genes is co-ordinately regulated by a shared set of upstream *cis*-acting elements. Indeed, the PCR amplifications used to confirm splice junctions would not have detected splicing between exons in different genes, so that the existence of splice variants that combine segments of the three genes, in a manner similar to the TWEPRIL transcripts from the TWEAK-APRIL genes in mouse [33], is not excluded.

The HD11 cell line contained mRNA for all five *MRC1L* genes, but peptides from protein immunoadsorbed by KUL01 included only those from MRC1L-B. This would be consistent with the KUL01 epitope being exclusive to MRC1L-B. However, the similarities between the MRC1L paralogues, while low, are sufficient that we could not exclude the possibility of recognition of the product of one or more of the other genes in the context where KUL01 is applied as a macrophage marker. To test this possibility we conducted two further experiments. As shown in figure S6, treatment of HD11 cells with transfection reagents including a small interfering RNA (siRNA) with 25/25 nucleotide identity to *MRC1L-B* cDNA sequence, caused 90% reduction in the median level of binding of fluorescently labelled KUL01 antibody, compared with the identical levels observed after the same treatment with either a control siRNA without or with no siRNA. The maximum similarity of the effective siRNA with the other *MRC1L* cDNA sequences, in either orientation, were 15/18 (A), 15/23 (C), 16/20 (D) and 17/22 (E). These are similar to the maximum similarity of the control siRNA with MRC1L-B cDNA (16/25), and would not generally be expected to be sufficient for cross-interference. However, since off-target interference effects have been reported with lower similarities, this observation does not completely exclude the possibility of cross reaction with the product of another MRC1L gene. In a second experiment, figure S7, we observed that that the KUL01 antibody only identified MRC1-B when expression plasmids coding for potential extracellular regions of all five MRCIL genes, as fusion proteins, were transfected into COS-7 cells. This provides compelling evidence that the KUL01 anybody binds the product of the MRC1L-B gene and not the remaining paralogues. Whilst the qRT-PCR analysis of MRC1L-B transcripts is consistent with the observed staining patterns reported with KUL01 across a number of immune-related tissues [19] it is not possible from the present data to infer the cellular distribution of the expression of the remaining MRC1L molecules, although, except for MRC1L-A in the liver, the similarity of the transcript profiles would be consistent with their predominant expression in the same cells as MRC1L-B.

In mammals, MRC1 is a multi-functional molecule. Being a pathogen-associated pattern recognition receptor, its involvements in uptake of antigen for presentation are important functions in innate and adaptive immune responses [9,34], but it also has roles in the clearance of hormones [12] and the regulation of circulating cytokine levels [35–37]. Cellular expression of the molecule is not restricted to macrophage alone but is also present on immature dendritic cells, reflecting its role in antigen capture [38].

The information presented here does not tell us whether a shared ancestor of birds and mammals had multiple MRC1L genes, with subsequent gene loss in the mammalian lineage, or whether it had a single gene that was subsequently duplicated only in the avian lineage. The former possibility would allow the hypothesis that the modern functions of mammalian MRC1 might have been distributed between the original paralogous genes. The latter model would have allowed the evolution of novel functional roles for the newly duplicated genes. The similarities between the cytoplasmic domains of MRC1L-A and MRC1L-B, especially with regard to trafficking signals, suggest biological functions similar to the mammalian MRC1, with the possibility of functional redundancy between these molecules. The very different cytoplasmic sequences of the other genes might reflect substantial functional divergence of these from the mammalian MRC1 genes.

The immune functions of MRC1 in the macrophage have given it an important role in determining the effectiveness of the response to influenza virus infection, at least in the lungs of mice. This presents a single interaction that is likely to be an effective target for evolution of viral virulence. If the additional genes in birds have similar functions in avian macrophages, then there is scope for redundant interactions with the virus that might be harder to evade. Expression of all these genes in macrophages is suggestive of conservation of these interactions. It will therefore be important to investigate whether these molecules have suitable carbohydrate binding activities, whether they are involved in endocytosis and phagocytosis, and whether modulation of their expression affects the susceptibility and response to influenza infection of avian macrophages. We have observed abortive replication of influenza in an avian macrophage cell line (KS and CB, Unpublished observations), which would allow a similar protective role for the MRC1L genes to that of MRC1 in the mouse, in generating effective responses. The involvement of multiple molecules, increasing redundancy in virus receptors, could increase the robustness of this immune mechanism in birds.

The known interaction of the mannose receptor with influenza virus in mice allows the hypothesis that a similar situation occurs in birds, facilitating infection of macrophages but leading to a protective innate immune response [18]. There are other enveloped avian viruses, including Marek's Disease Virus, Infectious Bronchitis Virus and Newcastle Disease Virus, that might be supposed to induce IFN-α by interaction with the mannose receptor [14].

Examples in which the mannose receptor acts as an innate pattern recognition molecule include the internalization of the yeast cell-wall particle zymosan [39], the phagocytosis of Pneumocystis by human alveolar macrophages [40] and Mycobacterium tuberculosis by the monocytic human cell line THP-1 [41]. The mannose receptor also appears to play a role in modulating the adaptive immune response through a role in myeloid plasticity [42]. However, the full repertoire of host-pathogen interactions allowed by the mannose receptor, and particularly the relevance of an expanded Mannose Receptor gene family, remains to be elucidated.

Materials and Methods

Ethics statement

All animal procedures were performed in accordance with the UK Animals (Scientific Procedures) Act 1986 [43]. This study was approved by the Pirbright Institute Ethical Review Panel and the UK Home Office under project licence 30/2683.

Experimental animals

RPRL (Regional Poultry Research Laboratory, East Lansing, MI.) Line O birds were obtained from the Compton specific pathogen free breeding facility, from parents negative for antibodies to specified pathogens, and were kept in controlled-environment isolation rooms with food and water provided *ad libitum*. For RNA preparations, tissue sections (approximately 500 mg), from birds between 4 and 5 weeks old, were collected into RNA Later stabilization fluid (Ambion, UK).

Antibodies, cells and cell lines

KUL01 is a monoclonal IgG1 antibody that recognises an antigen present on the surface of at least a subset of macrophages in chickens [19]. Purified antibody was purchased from Southern Biotech (Alabama).

The retrovirus-transformed macrophage-like cell line HD11 [44] was cultured in RPMI 1640 medium (Invitrogen), 10% FCS. Lines used in figure S5 are described in the figure legend.

Immunoprecipitation

Five to seven million HD11 cells pelleted at 200×g for 5 min were washed 3 times in PBS and resuspended in 500 μl of ice cold lysis buffer consisting of 20 mM TrisHCl, 100 mM NaCl, 0.5% v/v NP40 pH 7.6 to which 10 μl/ml HALT protease inhibitor cocktail and 10 μl/ml EDTA (Pierce Thermo product 87786) had been added. After vigorous mixing and incubation on ice for 30 minutes, Cell debris was then removed by centrifugation at 17,000×g for 15 minutes at 4°C and the lysate was stored at −80C.

Immunoprecipitations were carried out using a Thermo Scientific Pierce Immunoprecipitation kit (product number 1859011), following the manufacturer's instructions. Three hundred μg of antibody (Southern Biotech) was coupled to 100 μl AminoLink Plus Coupling Resin. Lysates were pre-cleared by two overnight incubations, mixing end over end at 4°C with agarose resin (Thermo Scientific) previously washed in lysis buffer, and then incubated for 2.5 hours with the immobilized antibody. After washing three times with 400 μl lysis buffer, bound proteins were eluted using five 100 μl aliquots of 0.1 M glycine. HCl, pH 2.8 including 0.5% (v/v) NP-40. Proteins were recovered from the pooled eluates by addition of trichloroacetic acid to 10% (w/v) and incubated on ice over night before pelleting in a microfuge at 17,000×g for 20 min at 4°C. Pellets were washed with 1 ml of ice cold 90% (v/v) acetone in water, then dried in a speed vac before resuspension and heating to ≥80°C in PAGE sample buffer including DTT for 10 min. PAGE was performed using 4–12% polyacrylamide Tris-Tricine gels in MES buffer and proteins visualised by rinsing the gels in water then incubating for 1–2 hours in Imperial stain (Thermo Scientific) followed by de-staining in water.

Peptide analysis

Bands of interest were excised from PAGE gels, cut into 1 mm cubes and individually placed in a covex 96 well microtitre plate. Reduction with DTT, alkylation with iodoacetamide and digestion using trypsin (Promega V511A) were all performed using a Hewlett Packard MassPREP robot. Digested extracts were transferred into low volume glass sample vials (Chromocol), dried in a speedvac then resuspended in 10 μl of 3% acetonitrile with 0.1% TFA. Liquid chromatography was carried out using a Waters NanoAquity UPLC system which supplied solvents A (0.1% formic acid in water) and B (0.1% formic acid in acetonitrile) to a 1.7 μm, 75 μm ×250 mm, BEH 130 C18 column (Waters) (HPLC solvents were all LC-MS grade from Fisher Scientific). Sample was concentrated onto a 180 μm ×20 mm, 5 μm Symmetry C18 trap (Waters) for 3 minutes at 15 μl/min, and separated at 250 nl/min using a gradient which ramped initially from 3–10% B over 1 minute then to 50% B over 41 minutes and to 85% B in 3 minutes followed by a wash step at this concentration for 2 minutes before re-equilibration at 3% B. Ionised peptides were analysed by a quadrupole time of flight (Q-ToF) Premier mass spectrometer (Waters) in data-dependent acquisition mode where a MS survey scan was used to automatically select multicharged peptides for further MS/MS fragmentation. From each survey scan up to four peptides were selected for fragmentation. MS/MS collision energy was dependent on precursor ions mass and charge state. A reference spectrum was collected every 10 seconds from Glu-fibrinopeptide B(785.8426 m/z), introduced *via* a reference sprayer. Raw MS/MS specta were processed using ProtenLynx Global Server (Waters) and were searched against the NCBInr database using the Mascot search algorithm.

RNA and quantitative PCR

RNA was extracted from 100 mg samples, of fifteen tissues from six birds of the same inbred line, using the Trizol Plus RNA Purification kit (Life Technologies), according to the manufacturer's instructions. Homogenisation was performed using a Mixer Mill MM300 (Retsch) and 3 mm stainless steel cone balls (Retsch). An on-column DNase digestion step was included (Purelink DNAse, Life Technologies). The majority of samples were diluted to have A_{260} approximately 1.0. Some samples with low RNA yields were used at up to ten-fold lower A_{260}.

Primers and probes for real-time quantitative PCR assay of 28S rRNA [45] and of the five predicted chicken macrophage mannose receptor mRNAs are detailed in table S3. The *MRC1L* cDNA primers and probes were designed so that the primers were entirely in different exons and the probe was approximately centred on an intron-exon boundary. *MRC1L* gene primers and probes were designed using Genscript primer design software (https://www.genscript.com/ssl-bin/app/primer) and Primer Express (Applied Biosystems, Foster City, California, USA). These

primers gave no detectable signal after 40 cycles with 2.5 ng chicken genomic DNA in the standard assay conditions.

Probes incorporated 5-carboxyfluorescein (FAM) at the 5′ end and N,N,N,N′ tetramethyl-6-carboxyrhodamine (TAMRA) at the 3′ end. Assays were carried out using the Superscript III platinum one-step qRT-PCR kit (Invitrogen). Amplification and detection of specific products were carried out with the 7500 Fast Real Time System (Taqman; Applied Biosystems) with the following cycle profile: 50°C for 5 min, 95°C for 2 min and then 40 cycles of 95°C for 3 sec and 60°C for 30sec.

To measure the PCR efficiencies, six 10-fold dilutions, of the highest expressing tissue for each MRC1-L assay, and of HD11 RNA for the 28S assay, were used in triplicate measurements. All *MRC1L* gene mRNA measurements were normalised to the levels of 28S ribosomal RNA in the samples using the equation $X_t = C_t - s(C_t' - Q)/s'$ where Ct is the gene-specific threshold cycle, Ct′ is the threshold cycle for the 28S ribosomal RNA assay (on a constant dilution of the sample), s and s′ are slopes of linear regressions of threshold cycles (C_T) against $\log_{10}(RNA)$ for target gene and 28S assays respectively. All sample Ct values were within the range of the standard plots. Details of the normalisation calculations and of statistical analyses confirming differential expression between tissues are provided in document S1 and document S2.

Sequencing and bioinformatics

Primers listed in table S4 were designed to amplify overlapping segments of the five predicted transcripts. Preparative PCR amplifications were carried out using methods described elsewhere [32], using templates of a line 0 chicken spleen cDNA library [46], freshly prepared total RNA from line 0 chicken spleen and total RNA from the cell line HD11. Amplified products excised from agarose gels were cloned into the pGEM-T-Easy vector (Promega). DNA prepared using the Qiagen QIAprep spin miniprep kit were used for sequencing. Sequencing reactions were performed by GATC Biotech. Sequence data were analysed using STADEN [47]. Multiple clones of PCR products were sequenced from each amplification to obtain the consensus sequence and to identify clones free from PCR errors.

Extensive use was made of the ClustalW [48]. The UCSC genome browser (http://genome.ucsc.edu; [49]) during the manual refinement of gene structures and in the preparation of figure 4. Assembly versions used were chicken, WUGSC 2.1/galGal3; turkey, TGC Turkey_2.01/melGal1; zebra finch, WUGSC 3.2.4/taeGut1; lizard, Broad AnoCar2.0/anoCar2; painted turtle, v3.0.1/chrPic1; Xenopus tropicalis, JGI 4.2/xenTro3; mouse, GRCm38/mm10; human, GRCh/hq19. Phylogenetic analyses were carried out using the MEGA package [50].

Supporting Information

Figure S1 Peptide sequences from MRC1L-B found in trypic digest of KUL01-adsorbed material.
(PDF)

Figure S2 Chicken MRC1L cDNA sequences and genomic locations of orthologues.
(FASTA)

Figure S3 Alternative splicing in MRC1L-E cDNA.
(PDF)

Figure S4 Predicted sequences of MRC1L orthologues in other species.
(TXT)

Figure S5 Relative mRNA levels of MRC1L genes in chicken cell lines.
(PDF)

Figure S6 Suppression of KUL01 antigen expression by MRC1L-B specic siRNA.
(PDF)

Figure S7 KUL01 specifically recognises the MRC1L-B gene product in transfected COS cells.
(PDF)

Table S1 List of peptides from tryptyic digest of KUL01-adsorbed material.
(PDF)

Table S2 Differences between Line 0 cDNA sequence and genomic jungle fowl sequence.
(PDF)

Table S3 Primers and probes for TaqMan quantitative PCR.
(PDF)

Table S4 Primers used in amplifying chicken MRC1L cDNAs.
(PDF)

Document S1 Statistical analysis of qPCR data for MRC1L genes in different tissues.
(DOCX)

Document S2 Statistical test for differences in MRC1L transcripts between tissues.
(PDF)

File S1 Chicken MRC1L genes: Links to ENSEMBL identifiers & Errors in release 75.
(RTF)

Acknowledgments

The authors would like to thank Dr John Hammond, for advice pertaining to phylogenetic analysis, and the dedicated staff of the Institute's animal services.

Author Contributions

Conceived and designed the experiments: KS LGH JRY CB. Performed the experiments: KS LGH JRY CB. Analyzed the data: KS LGH JRY CB. Contributed reagents/materials/analysis tools: JRY. Wrote the paper: KS LGH JRY CB.

References

1. Barten R, Torkar M, Haude A, Trowsdale J, Wilson MJ (2001) Divergent and convergent evolution of NK-cell receptors. Trends in Immunology 22: 52–57.
2. Kaiser P, Poh TY, Rothwell L, Avery S, Balu S, et al. (2005) A genomic analysis of chicken cytokines and chemokines. Journal of Interferon and Cytokine Research 25: 467–484.
3. Hughes AL (1994) The Evolution of Functionally Novel Proteins after Gene Duplication. Proceedings of the Royal Society B-Biological Sciences 256: 119–124.
4. Weis WI, Taylor ME, Drickamer K (1998) The C-type lectin superfamily in the immune system. Immunological Reviews 163: 19–34.
5. Taylor ME, Conary JT, Lennartz MR, Stahl PD, Drickamer K (1990) Primary Structure of the Mannose Receptor Contains Multiple Motifs Resembling Carbohydrate-Recognition Domains. Journal of Biological Chemistry 265: 12156–12162.
6. Taylor ME, Drickamer K (1993) Structural Requirements for High-Affinity Binding of Complex Ligands by the Macrophage Mannose Receptor. Journal of Biological Chemistry 268: 399–404.
7. Taylor ME, Bezouska K, Drickamer K (1992) Contribution to Ligand-Binding by Multiple Carbohydrate-Recognition Domains in the Macrophage Mannose Receptor. Journal of Biological Chemistry 267: 1719–1726.
8. Tietze C, Schlesinger P, Stahl P (1982) Mannose-Specific Endocytosis Receptor of Alveolar Macrophages - Demonstration of 2 Functionally Distinct Intracellular Pools of Receptor and Their Roles in Receptor Recycling. Journal of Cell Biology 92: 417–424.
9. Stahl PD, Ezekowitz RAB (1998) The mannose receptor is a pattern recognition receptor involved in host defense. Current Opinion in Immunology 10: 50–55.
10. Martinez-Pomares L, Mahoney JA, Kaposzta R, Linehan SA, Stahl PD, et al. (1998) A functional soluble form of the murine mannose receptor is produced by macrophages in vitro and is present in mouse serum. Journal of Biological Chemistry 273: 23376–23380.
11. Martinez-Pomares L, Gordon S (1999) Potential role of the mannose receptor in antigen transport. Immunology Letters 65: 9–13.
12. Fiete DJ, Beranek MC, Baenziger JU (1998) A cysteine-rich domain of the "mannose" receptor mediates GalNAc-4-SO4 binding. Proceedings of the National Academy of Sciences of the United States of America 95: 2089–2093.
13. Tesar DB, Cheung EJ, Bjorkman PJ (2008) The chicken yolk sac IgY receptor, a mammalian mannose receptor family member, transcytoses IgY across polarized epithelial cells. Molecular Biology of the Cell 19: 1587–1593.
14. Milone MC, Fitzgerald-Bocarsly P (1998) The mannose receptor mediates induction of IFN-alpha in peripheral blood dendritic cells by enveloped RNA and DNA viruses. Journal of Immunology 161: 2391–2399.
15. Nguyen DG, Hildreth JEK (2003) Involvement of macrophage mannose receptor in the binding and transmission of HIV by macrophages. European Journal of Immunology 33: 483–493.
16. Miller JL, Dewet BJM, Martinez-Pomares L, Radcliffe CM, Dwek RA, et al. (2008) The mannose receptor mediates dengue virus infection of macrophages. Plos Pathogens 4.
17. Reading PC, Miller JL, Anders EM (2000) Involvement of the mannose receptor in infection of macrophages by influenza virus. J Virol 74: 5190–5197.
18. Upham JP, Pickett D, Irimura T, Anders EM, Reading PC (2010) Macrophage Receptors for Influenza A Virus: Role of the Macrophage Galactose-Type Lectin and Mannose Receptor in Viral Entry. Journal of Virology 84: 3730–3737.
19. Mast J, Goddeeris BM, Peeters K, Vandesande F, Berghman LR (1998) Characterisation of chicken monocytes, macrophages and interdigitating cells by the monoclonal antibody KUL01. Veterinary Immunology and Immunopathology 61: 343–357.
20. Weis WI, Kahn R, Fourme R, Drickamer K, Hendrickson WA (1991) Structure of the Calcium-Dependent Lectin Domain from a Rat Mannose-Binding Protein Determined by Mad Phasing. Science 254: 1608–1615.
21. Zelensky AN, Gready JE (2003) Comparative analysis of structural properties of the C-type-lectin-like domain (CTLD). Proteins-Structure Function and Genetics 52: 466–477.
22. Kent WJ (2002) BLAT - The BLAST-like alignment tool. Genome Research 12: 656–664.
23. Kent WJ, Sugnet CW, Furey TS, Roskin KM, Pringle TH, et al. (2002) The human genome browser at UCSC. Genome Research 12: 996–1006.
24. East L, Isacke CM (2002) The mannose receptor family. Biochimica Et Biophysica Acta-General Subjects 1572: 364–386.
25. Mellman I (1996) Endocytosis and molecular sorting. Annual Review of Cell and Developmental Biology 12: 575–625.
26. Pond L, Kuhn LA, Teyton L, Schutze MP, Tainer JA, et al. (1995) A Role for Acidic Residues in Di-Leucine Motif-Based Targeting to the Endocytic Pathway. Journal of Biological Chemistry 270: 19989–19997.
27. Schweizer A, Stahl PD, Rohrer J (2000) A di-aromatic motif in the cytosolic tail of the mannose receptor mediates endosomal sorting. Journal of Biological Chemistry 275: 29694–29700.
28. Sandoval IV, Bakke O (1994) Targeting of membrane proteins to endosomes and lysosomes. Trends Cell Biol 4: 292–297.
29. Hedges SB (2012) Amniote phylogeny and the position of turtles. Bmc Biology 10.
30. Chiari Y, Cahais V, Galtier N, Delsuc F (2012) Phylogenomic analyses support the position of turtles as the sister group of birds and crocodiles (Archosauria). Bmc Biology 10.
31. Crawford NG, Faircloth BC, McCormack JE, Brumfield RT, Winker K, et al. (2012) More than 1000 ultraconserved elements provide evidence that turtles are the sister group of archosaurs. Biology Letters 8: 783–786.
32. Staines K, Young JR, Butter C (2013) Expression of Chicken DEC205 Reflects the Unique Structure and Function of the Avian Immune System. PLoS One 8: e51799.
33. Pradet-Balade B, Medema JP, Lopez-Fraga M, Lozano JC, Kolfschoten GM, et al. (2002) An endogenous hybrid mRNA encodes TWE-PRIL, a functional cell surface TWEAK-APRIL fusion protein. Embo Journal 21: 5711–5720.
34. Prigozy TI, Sieling PA, Clemens D, Stewart PL, Behar SM, et al. (1997) The mannose receptor delivers lipoglycan antigens to endosomes for presentation to T cells by CD1b molecules. Immunity 6: 187–197.
35. Shibata Y, Metzger WJ, Myrvik QN (1997) Chitin particle-induced cell-mediated immunity is inhibited by soluble mannan - Mannose receptor-mediated phagocytosis initiates IL-12 production. Journal of Immunology 159: 2462–2467.
36. Vautier S, MacCallum DM, Brown GD (2012) C-type lectin receptors and cytokines in fungal immunity. Cytokine 58: 89–99.

37. Yamamoto Y, Klein TW, Friedman H (1997) Involvement of mannose receptor in cytokine interleukin-1 beta (IL-1 beta), IL-6, and granulocyte-macrophage colony-stimulating factor responses, but not in chemokine macrophage inflammatory protein 1 beta (MIP-1 beta), MIP-2, and KC responses, caused by attachment of Candida albicans to macrophages. Infection and Immunity 65: 1077–1082.

38. Sallusto F, Cella M, Danieli C, Lanzavecchia A (1995) Dendritic cells use macropinocytosis and the mannose receptor to concentrate macromolecules in the major histocompatibility complex class II compartment: downregulation by cytokines and bacterial products. J Exp Med 182: 389–400.

39. Underhill DM, Ozinsky A, Hajjar AM, Stevens A, Wilson CB, et al. (1999) The Toll-like receptor 2 is recruited to macrophage phagosomes and discriminates between pathogens. Nature 401: 811–815.

40. Zhang JM, Zhu JP, Bu X, Cushion M, Kinane TB, et al. (2005) Cdc42 and RhoB activation are required for mannose receptor-mediated phagocytosis by human alveolar macrophages. Molecular Biology of the Cell 16: 824–834.

41. Diaz-Silvestre H, Espinosa-Cueto P, Sanchez-Gonzalez A, Esparza-Ceron MA, Pereira-Suarez AL, et al. (2005) The 19-kDa antigen of Mycobacterium tuberculosis is a major adhesin that binds the mannose receptor of THP-1 monocytic cells and promotes phagocytosis of mycobacteria. Microbial Pathogenesis 39: 97–107.

42. Mishra PK, Morris EG, Garcia JA, Cardona AE, Teale JM (2013) Increased Accumulation of Regulatory Granulocytic Myeloid Cells in Mannose Receptor C Type 1-Deficient Mice Correlates with Protection in a Mouse Model of Neurocysticercosis. Infection and Immunity 81: 1052–1063.

43. UK Home Office (1986) Guidance on the Operation of the Animals (Scientific Procedures) Act.

44. Beug H vKA, Doderlein G, Conscience J-F, Graf T (1979) Chicken hematopoietic cells transformed by seven strains of defective avian leukemia viruses display three distinct phenotypes of differentiation. Cell 18: 375–390.

45. Moody A, Sellers S, Bumstead N (2000) Measuring infectious bursal disease virus RNA in blood by multiplex real-time quantitative RT-PCR. J Virol Methods 85: 55–64.

46. Tregaskes CA, Bumstead N, Davison TF, Young JR (1996) Chicken B-cell marker chB6 (Bu-1) is a highly glycosylated protein of unique structure. Immunogenetics 44: 212–217.

47. Staden R (1996) The Staden sequence analysis package. Molecular Biotechnology 5: 233–241.

48. Larkin MA, Blackshields G, Brown NP, Chenna R, McGettigan PA, et al. (2007) Clustal W and clustal X version 2.0. Bioinformatics 23: 2947–2948.

49. Meyer LR ZA, Hinrichs AS, Karolchik D, Kuhn RM, Wong M, et al. (2012) The UCSC Genome Browser database: extensions and updates 2013. Nucleic Acids Res Nov 15.

50. Tamura K, Peterson D, Peterson N, Stecher G, Nei M, et al. (2011) MEGA5: Molecular Evolutionary Genetics Analysis Using Maximum Likelihood, Evolutionary Distance, and Maximum Parsimony Methods. Molecular Biology and Evolution 28: 2731–2739.

51. Kim SJ, Ruiz N, Bezouska K, Drickamer K (1992) Organization of the Gene Encoding the Human Macrophage Mannose Receptor (Mrc1). Genomics 14: 721–727.

52. Harris N, Super M, Rits M, Chang G, Ezekowitz RAB (1992) Characterization of the Murine Macrophage Mannose Receptor - Demonstration That the down-Regulation of Receptor Expression Mediated by Interferon-Gamma Occurs at the Level of Transcription. Blood 80: 2363–2373.

17

PIM Kinases as Potential Therapeutic Targets in a Subset of Peripheral T Cell Lymphoma Cases

Esperanza Martín-Sánchez[1,2], **Lina Odqvist**[1], **Socorro M. Rodríguez-Pinilla**[3], **Margarita Sánchez-Beato**[4], **Giovanna Roncador**[5], **Beatriz Domínguez-González**[1], **Carmen Blanco-Aparicio**[6], **Ana M. García Collazo**[6], **Esther González Cantalapiedra**[6], **Joaquín Pastor Fernández**[6], **Soraya Curiel del Olmo**[2], **Helena Pisonero**[2], **Rebeca Madureira**[2], **Carmen Almaraz**[2], **Manuela Mollejo**[7], **F. Javier Alves**[8], **Javier Menárguez**[9], **Fernando González-Palacios**[10], **José Luis Rodríguez-Peralto**[11], **Pablo L. Ortiz-Romero**[12], **Francisco X. Real**[1], **Juan F. García**[13], **James R. Bischoff**[6], **Miguel A. Piris**[1,2]*

1 Molecular Pathology Programme, Spanish National Cancer Research Centre (CNIO), Madrid, Spain, 2 Cancer Genomics Group, Marqués de Valdecilla Research Institute (IDIVAL) & Pathology Department, Hospital Universitario Marqués de Valdecilla, Santander, Spain, 3 Pathology Department, Fundación Jiménez Díaz, Madrid, Spain, 4 Onco-hematology Area, Instituto de Investigación Sanitaria Hospital Universitario Puerta de Hierro - Majadahonda, Madrid, Spain, 5 Monoclonal Antibodies Core Unit, Spanish National Cancer Research Centre (CNIO), Madrid, Spain, 6 Experimental Therapeutics Programme, Spanish National Cancer Research Centre (CNIO), Madrid, Spain, 7 Pathology Department, Hospital Virgen de la Salud, Toledo, Spain, 8 Pathology Department, Hospital La Paz, Madrid, Spain, 9 Pathology Department, Hospital Gregorio Marañón, Madrid, Spain, 10 Pathology Department, Hospital Ramón y Cajal, Madrid, Spain, 11 Pathology Department, 12 de Octubre University Hospital, Medical School Universidad Complutense, Instituto i+12, Madrid, Spain, 12 Dermatology Department, 12 de Octubre University Hospital, Medical School Universidad Complutense, Instituto i+12, Madrid, Spain, 13 Translational Research Laboratory, M. D. Anderson Cancer Center Madrid, Madrid, Spain

Abstract

Currently, there is no efficient therapy for patients with peripheral T cell lymphoma (PTCL). The Proviral Integration site of Moloney murine leukemia virus (PIM) kinases are important mediators of cell survival. We aimed to determine the therapeutic value of PIM kinases because they are overexpressed in PTCL patients, T cell lines and primary tumoral T cells. PIM kinases were inhibited genetically (using small interfering and short hairpin RNAs) and pharmacologically (mainly with the pan-PIM inhibitor (PIMi) ETP-39010) in a panel of 8 PTCL cell lines. Effects on cell viability, apoptosis, cell cycle, key proteins and gene expression were evaluated. Individual inhibition of each of the PIM genes did not affect PTCL cell survival, partially because of a compensatory mechanism among the three PIM genes. In contrast, pharmacological inhibition of all PIM kinases strongly induced apoptosis in all PTCL cell lines, without cell cycle arrest, in part through the induction of DNA damage. Therefore, pan-PIMi synergized with Cisplatin. Importantly, pharmacological inhibition of PIM reduced primary tumoral T cell viability without affecting normal T cells *ex vivo*. Since anaplastic large cell lymphoma (ALK+ ALCL) cell lines were the most sensitive to the pan-PIMi, we tested the simultaneous inhibition of ALK and PIM kinases and found a strong synergistic effect in ALK+ ALCL cell lines. Our findings suggest that PIM kinase inhibition could be of therapeutic value in a subset of PTCL, especially when combined with ALK inhibitors, and might be clinically beneficial in ALK+ ALCL.

Editor: Jose Angel Martinez Climent, University of Navarra, Center for Applied Medical Research , Spain

Funding: This work was supported by grants from the Asociación Española Contra el Cáncer, Fondo de Investigaciones Sanitarias (PI051623, PI052800 and FIS 11/1759), RTICC (RD06/0020/0107) and Ministerio de Ciencia e Innovación (SAF2008-0387-1). EMS was supported by a grant from the Department of Education, Universities and Research of the Basque Government (BFI08.207). MSB was supported by a Contract Miguel Servet from Fondo de Investigaciones Sanitarias (CP11/00018). The funders had no role in study design, data collection and analysis, decision to publish, or preparation of the manuscript.

Competing Interests: The authors have declared that no competing interests exist.

* Email: mapiris@humv.es

Introduction

Peripheral T cell lymphomas (PTCL) are a very aggressive and heterogeneous group of hematological malignancies [1,2]. Very little is known about their molecular biology, and consequently, the search for efficient therapies that would improve the outcome of these patients remains challenging [3]. Several factors are responsible for our limited knowledge, such as the low incidence of PTCL, the heterogeneity of its subtypes and the few representative models (cell lines or mouse models) available. It is worth to note that majority of the available cell lines cover very few PTCL subtypes, and are mostly derived from cutaneous T cell lymphomas, including its two most prevalent forms: Sézary Syndrome and Mycosis Fungoides [4].

Among the different PTCL subtypes, PTCL-Not Otherwise Specified (PTCL-NOS), Angioimmunoblastic T-cell Lymphoma (AITL) and Anaplastic Large Cell Lymphoma (ALCL) are the most frequent ones. Within the ALCL group, there are two subgroups, depending on the presence or absence of the chromosomal translocation t(2; 5) (p23; q35), which involves the *ALK* and *NPM1* genes and leads to the overexpression of the fusion protein NPM-ALK [3]. This is considered to be the main oncogenic force in ALK+ ALCL, because it activates the Jak/STAT pathway [5,6]. The ALK+ ALCL is the only PTCL subgroup with a relatively good prognosis [7], however, around

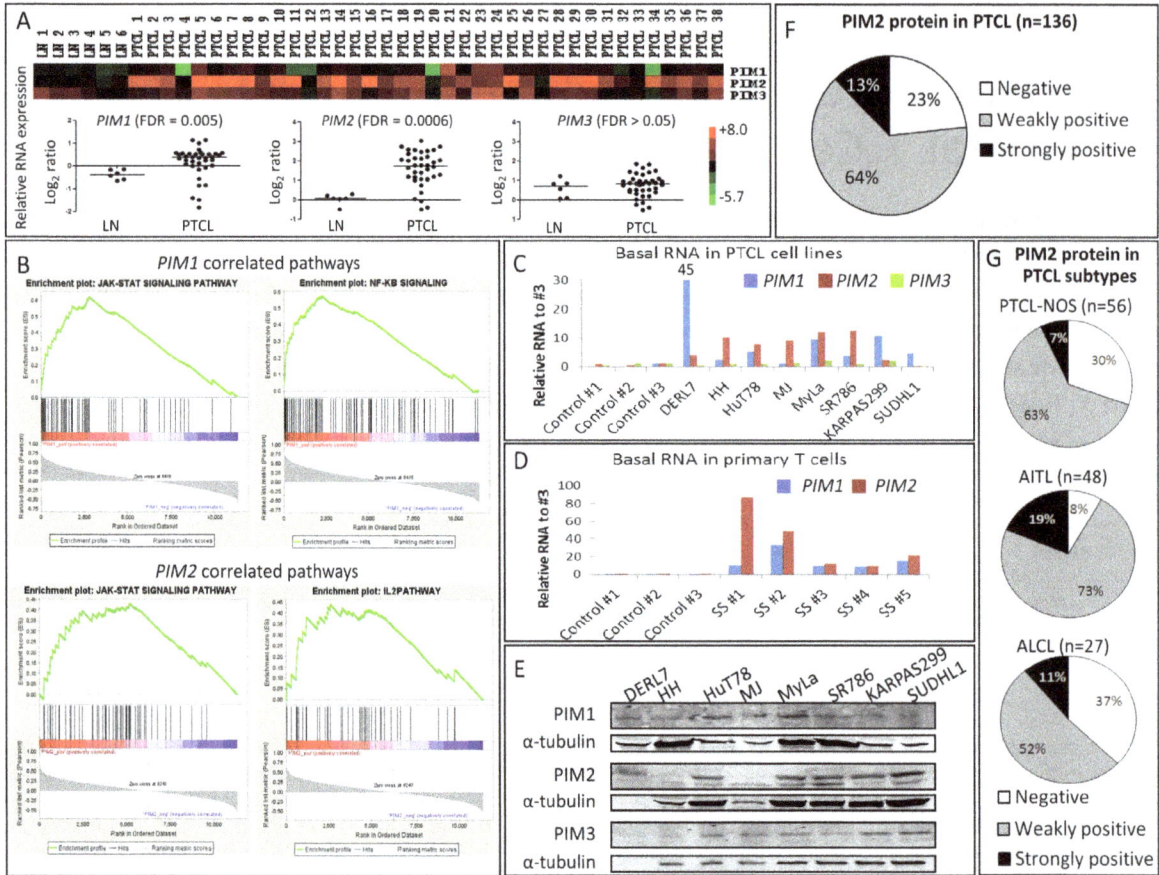

Figure 1. PIM kinases as potential therapeutic targets in PTCL. (A) Gene expression profiling of tumoral samples from 38 human PTCL patients compared with 6 reactive lymph nodes (LN) by microarrays revealed a significantly increased expression of *PIM1* and *PIM2* genes (FDR<0.05), but not *PIM3*. The heatmap is shown in the upper panel, and the relative quantification (Log$_2$ ratio) comparing PIM expression in PTCL *versus* LN is shown in the lower panel. (B) GSEA ranked all significantly altered genes between PTCL and LN according to its correlation with *PIM1* or *PIM2* expression and displayed them in the red-to-blue bar. Each gene belonging to every pathway was interrogated whether it appeared positively (in the red region of the bar) or negatively (in the blue side) correlated. Using this approach GSEA identified a positive and significant correlation between *PIM1* and *PIM2* expression and Jak/STAT, NF-κB and IL-2 signaling pathways in the PTCL molecular signature (FDR<0.25). (C) PIM family genes mRNA level was measured by RT-qPCR in eight PTCL cell lines and (D) primary tumoral T cells from 5 Sézary Syndrome patients (SS #1–5), and compared with normal T cells isolated from 3 healthy donors (Control #1–3). The relative RNA amount of PIM has been calculated as a relative quantification, as described in the Methods section (RQ = $2^{-\Delta Ct}$), normalized with non-tumoral cells: RQ in PTCL/RQ in healthy #3. In both settings, *PIM1*, and especially *PIM2*, but not *PIM3* expression was found to be increased in PTCL. (E) PIM kinase protein basal levels in PTCL cell lines measured by Western blot. PIM1 and PIM2 isoforms are also shown. (F) Distribution of PIM2 protein in a series of tumoral samples from 136 PTCL patients measured by immunohistochemistry. Negative, weakly positive and strongly positive samples were defined by the presence of <5%, 5–20% and >20% positive cells. (G) Distribution of PIM2 protein in the most common PTCL subtypes measured by immunohistochemistry.

40% of ALK+ ALCL patients fail to be cured using standard therapeutic approaches [3]. New drugs, such as the ALK inhibitor Crizotinib, seem to improve the survival in these patients in early clinical trials [8].

Although different histological subtypes of PTCL have been identified, the treatment approach has been essentially based on the application of anthracycline-based combination chemotherapy, resulting in poor outcomes [9]. To date, only 3 agents have been recently approved by the FDA for the treatment of relapsed or refractory PTCL: pralatrexate, romidepsin and brentuximab vedotin [9,10]. Nevertheless, the development of new, efficiently targeted therapies is of great importance to PTCL patients [9,11,12].

The Proviral Integration site of the Moloney murine leukemia virus (PIM) family is an important mediator of cell survival, comprising three ubiquitously expressed serine/threonine kinases (PIM1, PIM2 and PIM3) with a broad range of cellular substrates

that promote cell growth, proliferation and drug resistance. They are overexpressed in a number of human cancers and frequently associated with poor prognosis in most hematological malignancies [13]. PIM kinases are typically induced by the activation of transcription factors downstream of growth factors, cytokines and mitogenic stimuli signaling pathways, such as the Jak/STAT and NF-κB [13,14], and are also protected from proteasomal degradation by HSP-70 and HSP-90 [15]. Their activities are mediated through the phosphorylation of a number of proteins, including regulators of transcription (MYC, MYB, RUNX1, RUNX3), cell cycle (p21, p27, CDC25A, CDC25C), protein translation (EIF4E, 4E-BP1), apoptosis (BAD, BCL2, ASK1), signaling intermediates (SOCS1, SOCS3, MAP3K5, mTOR, AKT), and drug resistance proteins (ABC transporters) [13,14,15].

Studies using transgenic mice have shown that PIM kinases cooperated with important genes involved in B- and T-cell lymphomagenesis, such as, c-Myc, BCL6 and E2A–PBX1 [14].

On the other hand, triple *PIM1-PIM2-PIM3* knockout mice have been reported to be viable, fertile, and just smaller compared with wild type littermates [13,14,15]. Very recently, an abnormal hematopoiesis has been described in these triple-knockout mice [16]. These findings indicate that PIM kinases are important for lymphomagenesis and their absence is well tolerated, suggesting that selective PIM kinase inhibitors might have a low toxicity profile [13]. Based on this, along with some differences in the structural conformation of the ATP-binding pocket in the active site compared with other kinases, PIM kinases have been proposed as promising therapeutic targets for pharmacological inhibition. So far, a number of small molecule inhibitors have been tested *in vitro*, but clinical data are only available for a handful of them. One of the most promising PIM inhibitors (PIMi) was SGI-1776, a compound with activity against PIM1, PIM2 and PIM3 at nanomolar concentrations [13,14,15], which induced apoptosis at micromolar doses in chronic lymphocytic leukemia [17], mantle cell lymphoma [18], and acute myeloid leukemia [19]. Unfortunately, the phase I clinical trial of this compound was discontinued in November 2010 because of a strong cardiotoxic effect that impaired its further development [15,20].

This study aimed to determine the efficiency of PIM kinase inhibition in PTCL, to explore the molecular response of PTCL cells to pharmacological pan-PIM inhibition and to identify those PTCL subgroups that are more susceptible to PIM inhibition.

Materials and Methods

Ethics statement

The research was approved by the Hospital Universitario Marqués de Valdecilla ethics committee (Santander, Spain).

All the human samples used in this study have been procured from the Spanish CNIO Biobank, located in the Spanish National Cancer Research Centre (Madrid, Spain) (https://www.cnio.es/ing/servicios/biobanco/index.asp), and according to the Spanish legal framework regarding written informed consent and sample anonymization.

Additionally, some samples used here were also previously used in [15].

Bioinformatics analysis in the PTCL patient series

The gene expression profiles of frozen tumoral samples from 38 PTCL patients and 6 reactive lymph nodes were compared using microarrays. Briefly, differentially expressed genes between PTCL and reactive lymph nodes were identified using a t-test. Then, Gene Set Enrichment Analysis (GSEA) ranked them according to its correlation with *PIM1* or *PIM2* expression. More details are provided in the Supplementary Information (Methods S1). All raw microarray data regarding the PTCL patient series are available at the Gene Expression Omnibus under accession number GSE36172.

Cell lines, primary samples and reagents

Eight human PTCL cell lines were used in this study. HH (cutaneous T cell lymphoma) and MJ (HTLV1+ PTCL) were obtained from the American Type Cell Collection (ATCC, Rockville, MD); MyLa (Mycosis Fungoides) and HuT78 (Sézary Syndrome) were obtained from the European Collection of Cell Cultures (ECACC, Salisbury, UK); DERL7 (hepatosplenic gamma-delta T cell lymphoma) and SR786, KARPAS-299 and SU-DHL-1 (ALK+ ALCL) were obtained from the German Collection of Microorganisms and Cell Cultures (DSMZ, Braunschweig, Germany). All of them except MJ were cultured in RPMI 1640 medium (IMDM medium for MJ cells) supplemented with 10%

heat-inactivated fetal bovine serum (FBS) and 1% penicillin/streptomycin (all from Life Technologies, Carlsbad, CA) in a humidified atmosphere at 37°C and 5% CO_2. The DERL7 cell line was supplemented with 20% FBS and 20 ng/ml human IL-2 (PeproTech, Rocky Hill, NJ). Cell lines were previously authenticated by DSMZ (year 2010–2011).

Human primary samples were used to measure the basal *PIM1*, *PIM2* and *PIM3* mRNA levels. Tumoral and normal T cells were respectively isolated from the peripheral blood of 5 Sézary Syndrome patients and 3 healthy donors, through negative selection using the RosetteSep kit (StemCell Technologies, Grenoble, France). Sample purity was checked by flow cytometry, and an enrichment of >90% of CD3+ cells was ensured in all samples. Additionally, the PIM inhibitor sensitivity of primary T cells from 8 PTCL patients (5 Sézary Syndrome and 3 Mycosis Fungoides) and 5 healthy donors was tested.

The pan-PIM inhibitors ETP-39010 [21], ETP-47652, ETP-47551 and ETP-46638 were developed by the Experimental Therapeutics Programme of the Spanish National Cancer Research Centre (Madrid, Spain). The chemical structure of these compounds has been published in [22] under publication number WO 2011/080510. (http://www.wipo.int/portal/index.html.en). The ALK inhibitor (ALKi) Crizotinib was obtained from Selleck Chemicals (Houston, TX). All inhibitors were dissolved in DMSO and the stocks were kept at −20°C. They were diluted in culture medium at desired concentrations immediately before use. For the controls DMSO concentration in the medium was lower than 0.2%.

PIM genetic silencing experiments

Transient genetic silencing was performed in PTCL cell lines as follows: HH, SR786, SU-DHL-1 and MyLa cell lines were electroporated with specific small interference RNAs (siRNAs) against *PIM1*, *PIM2* and *PIM3* genes, using the Neon Transfection System (Life Technologies) and following the manufacturer's instructions, as previously described [23]. Briefly, cells were incubated without antibiotics overnight and resuspended in R buffer at a density of 500,000 cells/ml. Then, siPIM1 (s10527), siPIM2 (s21749), siPIM3 (HSS140560) and the Non-Template Control (NTC, AM4635) (all from Life Technologies) were added to the cells at several concentrations (25–100 nM). Microporation conditions were set up for each cell line (900 V, 30 ms and 2 pulses for HH, SR786 and SU-DHL-1; 1300 V, 20 ms and 2 pulses for MyLa), aiming for the highest transfection efficiency with the minimum loss of cell viability. Cells were then electroporated under these conditions to allow for the entry of the siRNAs into the cell and 100 μl of the suspension were seeded in 2 ml for 24, 48, 72 and 96 h.

In addition, a stable PIM knockdown was carried out in PTCL cell lines using the MISSION product line from Sigma-Aldrich (St Louis, MO) according to the manufacturer's instructions. The base vector (pLKO.1-puro) contains the Puromycin resistance gene for mammalian cells selection. Thus, sensitivity to Puromycin was first tested in several PTCL cell lines, and optimal concentrations were chosen from a wide range. Then, the optimal amount of lentiviral particles was assessed using the control transduction particles, both the negative (Non-targeting shRNA, SHC016V) and the positive (Turbo-GFP, SHC003V) lentiviruses (Sigma-Aldrich). MyLa was the only used cell line showing high infection efficiency, and therefore, was the best model to test PIM stable knockdown. Briefly, MyLa cells were infected with MISSION lentiviral transduction particles containing specific short-hairpin RNA (shRNA) against *PIM1* (SHCLNV-NM_002648), *PIM2* (SHCLNV-NM_006875) and *PIM3*

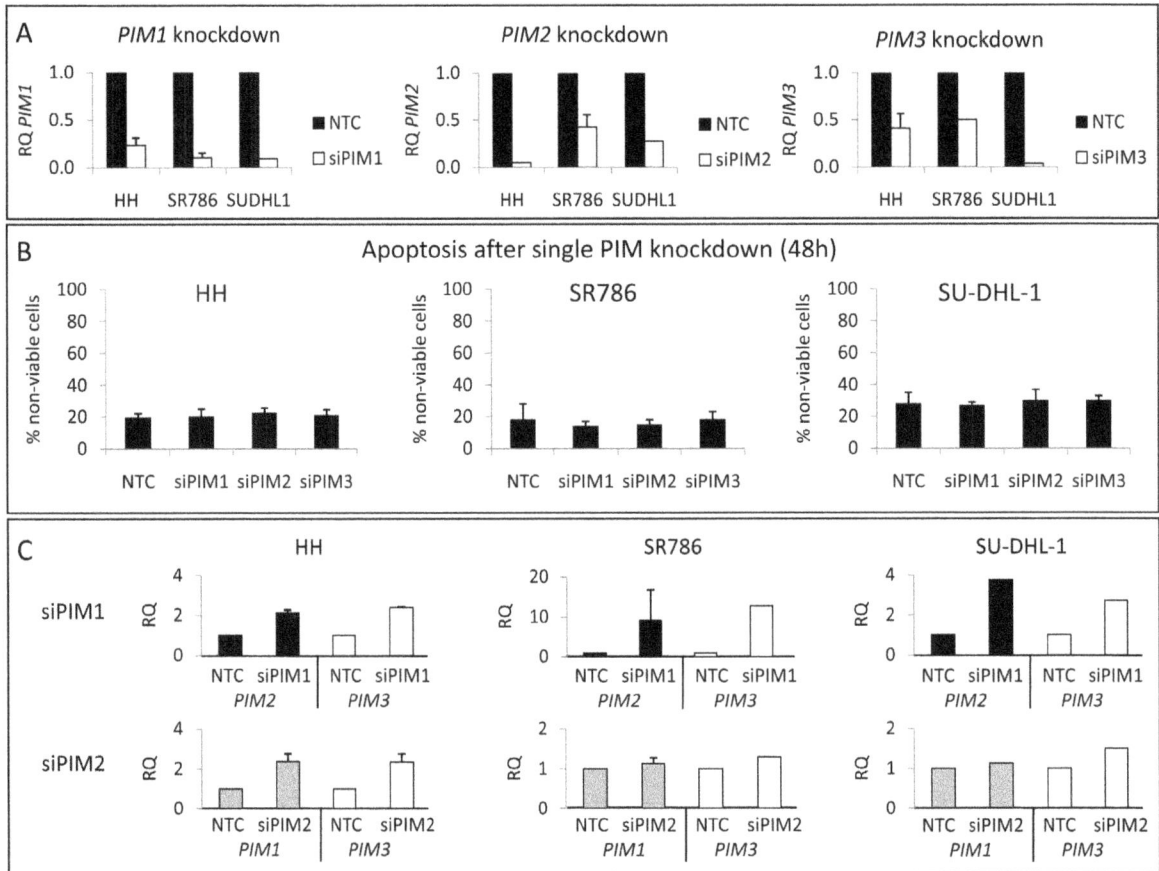

Figure 2. Individual *PIM1*, *PIM2* and *PIM3* genetic silencing in PTCL cell lines by siRNA. (A) All three PIM family genes were silenced in HH, SR786 and SU-DHL-1 cell lines, using several siRNA doses (25–100 nM) and times (24–72 h). Knockdown efficiency was measured by RT-qPCR and compared with the Non-Template Control (NTC). Graphs show the silencing 24 h after the addition of 100 nM siRNA. RQ, relative quantification, has been calculated as described in the Methods section (RQ = $2^{-\Delta\Delta Ct}$). (B) Single PIM gene silencing did not induce apoptosis in any PTCL cell lines. Graphs show data from 48 h silencing. The percentage of non-viable cells was calculated as Annexin V+/PI- plus Annexin V+/PI+ cells. (C) RT-qPCR showing a compensatory mechanism among the PIM family genes: when one PIM gene was silenced, the other PIM genes became upregulated. RQ, relative quantification, has been calculated as described in the Methods section (RQ = $2^{-\Delta\Delta Ct}$).

(SHCLNV-NM_001001852) (all from Sigma-Aldrich) using Poly-brene (hexadimethrine bromide) as a transduction enhancer (8 µg/ml). After 24 h post-infection, lentiviral particles were removed and Puromycin (4 µg/ml) was added to culture media. Green fluorescence was checked for 15 days using a Nikon Ti Epi-Fluorescence microscope and the imaging software NIS-Elements (Nikon, Amsterdam, Netherlands) and flow cytometry.

Cell viability assay

For drug cytotoxicity experiments, PTCL cell lines and primary tumoral and normal T cells were seeded in 96-well plates at a density of 10,000 cells per well, and pan-PIM inhibitors, ALKi, Cisplatin or combinations were added at a range of doses for 48 h (for primary cells) and 72 h (for cell lines), using DMSO as control. Cell viability was measured as the intracellular ATP content using CellTiter-Glo Luminescent Cell Viability Assay (Promega, Madison, WI), following the manufacturer's instructions.

For drug combination experiments, cells were treated with a wide range of doses and cell viability was measured as explained above. The combination index (CI) was calculated using CalcuSyn software (Biosoft, Ferguson, MO) following the Chou & Talalay method [24], where values of CI<1, ≈1 and >1 indicate synergism, an additive effect and antagonism, respectively.

Flow cytometry analysis

The distribution of cells during the phases of the cell cycle and induction of apoptosis were evaluated by flow cytometry using propidium iodide (PI, Sigma-Aldrich, St Louis, MO) staining and the APC-Annexin V (Beckton Dickinson, BD, Franklin Lakes, NJ) binding assay, respectively. Data from 10,000 cells were detected on a FACS Calibur flow cytometer (BD) and analyzed using CellQuest Pro software (BD).

RNA extraction and quantitative RT-PCR

Total RNA was extracted and purified using RNeasy Mini-Kit (Qiagen, Valencia, CA) following the manufacturer's instructions in order to check the PIM genes' knockdown efficiency, to understand the molecular response to the pan-PIMi and to measure basal mRNA levels of these genes in PTCL cell lines and primary tumoral and normal T cells.

The expression of *PIM1, PIM2, PIM3, ERCC8, XRCC2* and *XRCC5* genes was measured by quantitative RT-PCR. Briefly, total RNA was retrotranscribed using the SuperScript enzyme (Life Technologies) (10 min at 25°C, 60 min at 42°C and 15 min at 70°C). Two µl of the resulting cDNA were placed in a 384-well plate with 0.75 µl Taqman probes (*PIM1* Hs01065494_g1, *PIM2* Hs00179139_m1, *PIM3* Hs00420511_g1, *ERCC8*

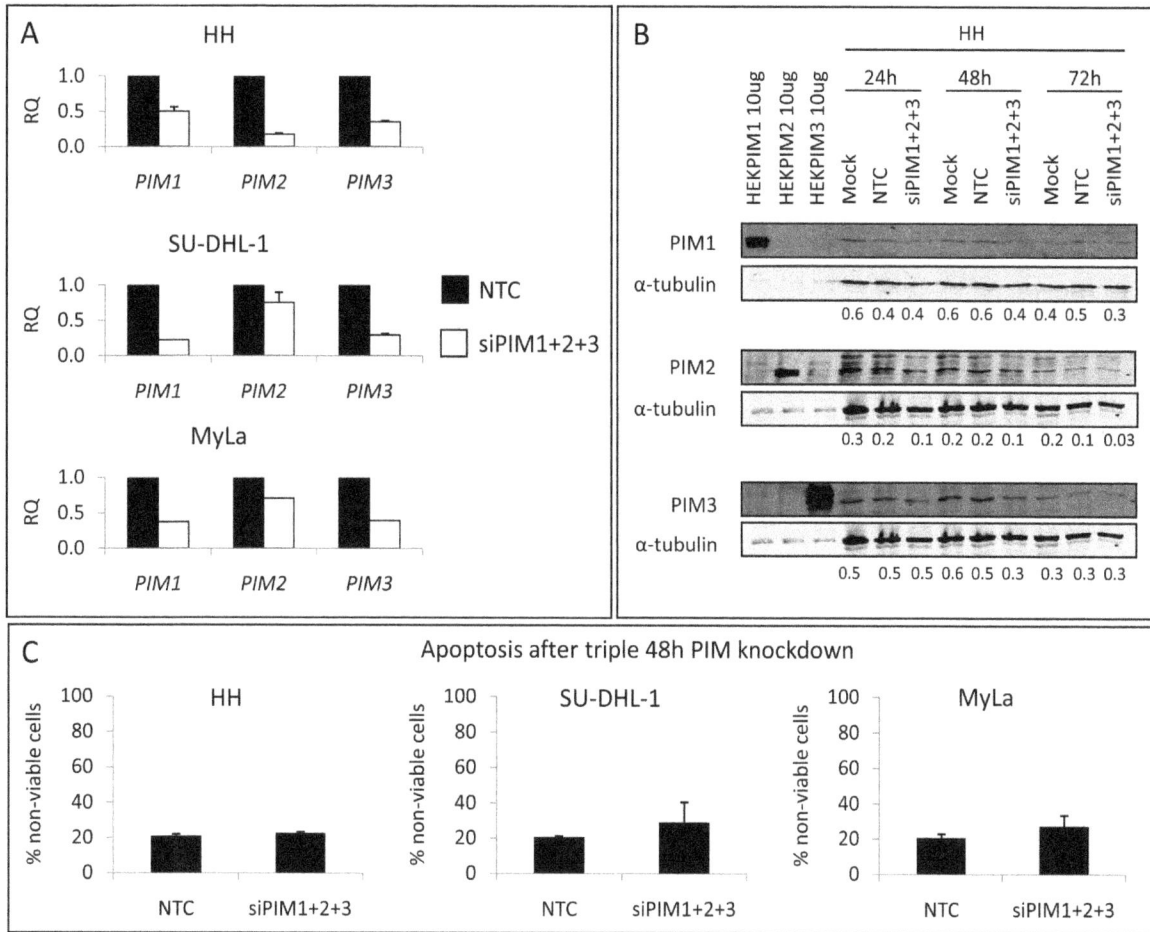

Figure 3. Simultaneous *PIM1+ PIM2+ PIM3* genetic silencing in PTCL cell lines by siRNA. (A) The triple knockdown was carried out in the HH, SU-DHL-1 and MyLa cell lines, using 33 nM siPIM1+33 nM siPIM2+33 nM siPIM3 for 24–72 h. As an average for the 3 PIM genes, the knockdown efficiency, measured by RT-qPCR, was around 70% at the mRNA level 24 h after the microporation (RQ, relative quantification, calculated as in Figure 2), and (B) around 50% at the protein level after 48 h, compared with the Non-Template Control (NTC). Numbers presented are PIM/tubulin ratios. (C) These knockdown conditions did not induce apoptosis in any PTCL cell lines. The percentage of non-viable cells was calculated as Annexin V+/PI− plus Annexin V+/PI+ cells.

Hs00163958_m1, *XRCC2* Hs03044154_m1, *XRCC5* Hs00897854_m1, and the endogenous control *RN18S1* Hs03928990_g1; all from Life Technologies) in a final volume of 15 µl. PCR amplification was performed in using the Applied Biosystems Prism 7900HT Sequence Detection System (Life Technologies) under the following thermal cycler conditions: 2 min at 50°C, 10 min at 95°C and 30 cycles (15 s at 95°C and 1 min at 60°C).

Relative Quantification (RQ) was calculated following the ΔCt method: $RQ = 2^{-\Delta Ct}$, where ΔCt is the difference between the Ct of the gene of interest and the Ct of the endogenous gene control *RN18S1*. In addition, in knockdown experiments RQ was normalized as $RQ = 2^{-\Delta\Delta Ct}$, where $\Delta\Delta$Ct is the difference between the ΔCt in knockdown cells and the ΔCt in control cells.

Microarray hybridization and data analysis

The molecular response of PTCL cells to the pan-PIMi ETP-39010 was explored through gene expression analysis. DERL7, HuT78, MyLa and SR786 cells were treated with 10 µM pan-PIMi for 0, 2, 4, 6, 10 and 24 h. At each time, DMSO- and pan-PIMi-treated cells were harvested and total RNA extracted as described above, and the quality assessed in a 1% agarose-gel.

Samples were hybridized onto 4×44 K microarray slides (Whole Human Genome, Agilent Technologies, Inc., Santa Clara, CA), as described in the Supplementary Information (Methods S1). Short Time-series Expression Miner (STEM) [25] identified differentially expressed genes under each condition, and Gene Ontology (GO) categories were used to recognize functional groups. A False Discovery Rate (FDR) <0.05 was considered significant. All raw microarray data regarding the molecular response to pan-PIMi in PTCL are available at the Gene Expression Omnibus under accession number GSE42595.

Immunofluorescence and immunohistochemistry

After treatment with 10 µM of the pan-PIMi ETP-39010 for 24 h, γH2A.X was measured in MyLa cells by immunofluorescence. Immunohistochemical staining of PIM2 was carried out in a series of formalin-fixed and paraffin-embedded tumoral samples from 136 PTCL patients (Table S1) in a Bond Max automatic immunostainer (Leica Microsystems, Wetzlar, Germany). Details are provided in the Supplementary Information (Methods S1).

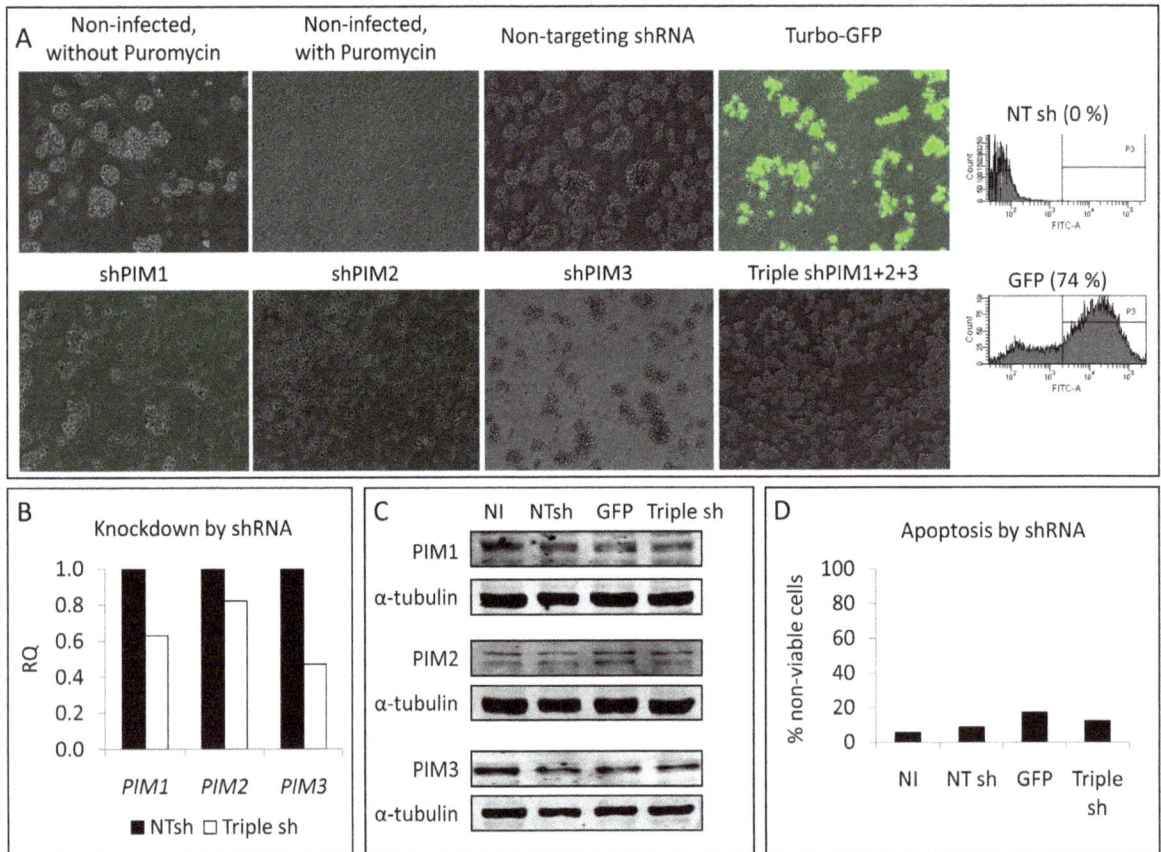

Figure 4. PIM genetic silencing in PTCL by shRNA. (A) MyLa cells were infected with lentiviral particles containing the pLKO.1-puro vector with a non-targeting shRNA, the Turbo-GFP gene, or shRNAs for each of the PIM family genes. Cells were maintained under Puromycin selection for 3 weeks. Images were obtained 8 days post-infection with a Nikon Ti Epi-Fluorescence microscope (10X magnification). Green fluorescence was also assessed in the negative (NT sh) and the positive controls by flow cytometry, and percentages of green cells are indicated in the histograms. (B) Triple knockdown efficiency was measured by RT-qPCR and compared with the Non-Targeting shRNA (NTsh). Graphs show the silencing at the mRNA level 15 days after the lentiviral infection. RQ, relative quantification, has been calculated as described in the Methods section (RQ = $2^{-\Delta\Delta Ct}$). (C) Western blots showing the effect of the triple lentiviral infection on PIM protein levels 15 days post-infection (NI, non-infected cells; NTsh, cells infected with the non-targeting shRNA; GFP, cells infected with Turbo-GFP; Triple sh, cells infected with shPIM1+ shPIM2+ shPIM3). (D) These knockdown conditions did not affect cell viability. The percentage of non-viable cells was calculated as Annexin V+/7AAD− plus Annexin V+/7AAD+ cells: (NI, non-infected cells; NTsh, cells infected with the non-targeting shRNA; GFP, cells infected with Turbo-GFP; Triple sh, cells infected with shPIM1+ shPIM2+ shPIM3).

Statistical analysis

Unless otherwise specified, all experiments were done three times and all numerical data were expressed as the average of the values ± the standard error of the mean. Statistical significance of differences between groups was established by Student's independent samples t-test (SPSS v17.0). p-values <0.05 were considered significant.

Results

PIM kinases as potential therapeutic targets in PTCL

First, using microarrays, *PIM1* and especially *PIM2* genes, but not *PIM3*, were found to be significantly overexpressed (FDR< 0.05) in tumoral samples from 38 PTCL patients compared with 6 reactive lymph nodes (Figure 1A). *PIM1* and *PIM2* expression was significantly correlated with Jak/STAT, NF-κB and IL-2 pathways in our PTCL patient series (Figure 1B), indicating a strong relationship between these pathways and the expression of PIM kinases in PTCL. Furthermore, *PIM1* and, again, especially *PIM2*, but not *PIM3* expression was increased in a panel of 8

PTCL cell lines (Figure 1C) and primary tumoral T cells from 5 Sézary Syndrome patients (Figure 1D) relative to normal T cells from 3 healthy donors. Similarly, PIM protein levels were also detected by Western blot in all PTCL cell lines, with slight differences in the most expressed PIM2 isoform (Figure 1E).

Since *PIM2* was the most upregulated PIM kinase in PTCL (both patients and cell lines) at the mRNA and protein levels, we explored the expression of the PIM2 protein by immunohistochemistry in a series of 136 PTCL patients. We found that 77% of these samples were positive for PIM2 expression (Figure 1F and Figure S1), and that the trend was largely maintained in the most common PTCL subtypes, with a slight predominance in the AITL subtype (Figure 1G). Although our series was limited, a preliminary significant association was found between PIM2 expression and a shorter overall survival only in the ALCL subtype, both ALK+ and ALK− cases, but not in other PTCL subtypes (Figure S2).

These findings suggest that PIM kinases could be of potential therapeutic value in PTCL.

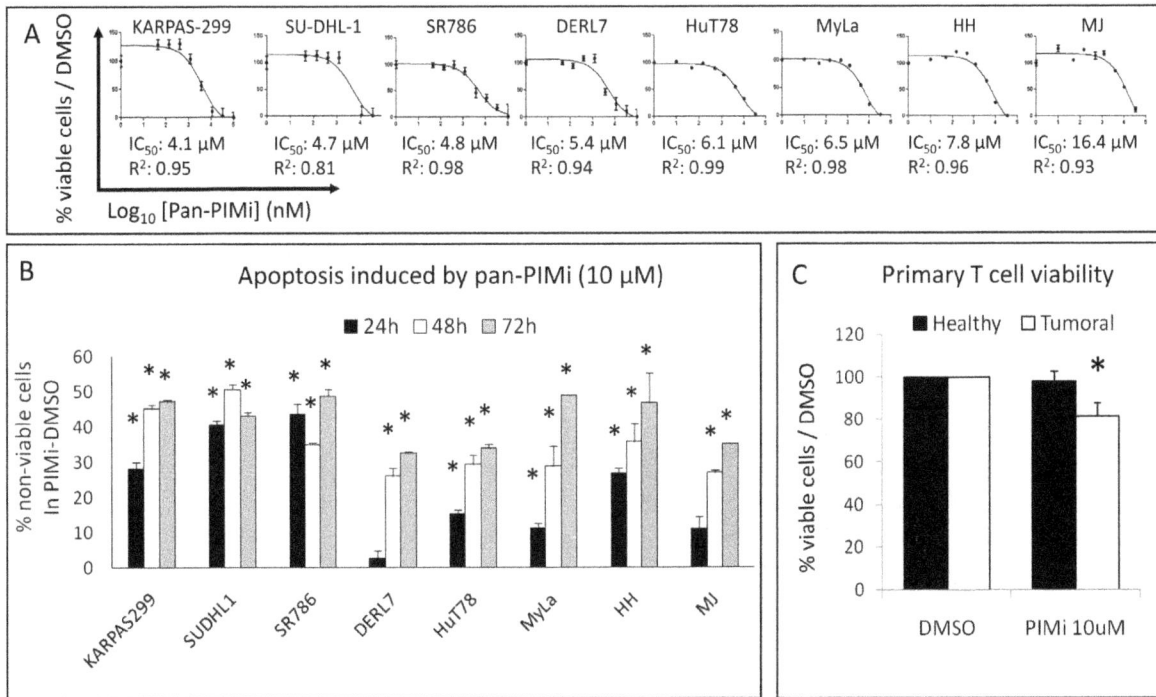

Figure 5. Pharmacological pan-PIM kinase inhibition in PTCL cell lines. (A) The pan-PIMi ETP-39010 reduced cell viability in all PTCL cell lines (IC_{50} values calculated after 72 h of treatment are shown). (B) The pan-PIMi ETP-39010 strongly induced apoptosis in a time-dependent manner in all PTCL cell lines (*, $p < 0.05$, from comparison with DMSO-treated cells). The percentage of non-viable cells was calculated as Annexin V+/PI− plus Annexin V+/PI+ cells in the PIMi-treated condition minus the DMSO-treated control. (C) The pan-PIMi ETP-39010 (10 µM for 48 h) slightly but significantly reduced cell viability only in tumoral T cells from 8 PTCL patients (Mycosis Fungoides and Sézary Syndrome), but did not affect normal T cells from 5 healthy donors (*, $p < 0.05$ compared with DMSO).

PIM kinase genetic silencing in PTCL

To test this hypothesis, genetic silencing experiments with siRNAs were performed specifically to abolish the expression of *PIM1*, *PIM2* or *PIM3* genes in PTCL cell lines. Knockdown efficiency differed with the cell line and time point, varying from around 70 to 95% in the *PIM1* or *PIM2* mRNA, and lower for *PIM3* (Figure 2A). However, no significant effects on cell survival were observed, either with respect to apoptosis induction (Figure 2B and Table S2) or cell cycle arrest (Figure S3). These results indicated that the remaining protein or other untargeted genes were responsible for triggering survival.

As PIM genes belong to the same family and have a high homology in their sequences [15,19,20], they could share functions. This prompted us to measure the mRNA levels of each of the PIM members when one of them was knocked down. Strikingly, we found an upregulation of *PIM2* and *PIM3* when *PIM1* was silenced. Likewise, an increase in *PIM1* and *PIM3* was observed when *PIM2* was inhibited (Figure 2C). Because the *PIM3* knockdown was less efficient than other PIM genes silencing, *PIM1* or *PIM2* upregulation after *PIM3* inhibition was less evident (data not shown). Again, very similar results were found in all cell lines, suggesting the existence of a compensatory mechanism among the PIM genes in PTCL.

This led us to exploit the simultaneous silencing of the 3 PIM genes: since the recommended maximum siRNA concentration is 100 nM and we aimed to inhibit 3 genes at the same time, the concentration of each siRNA was reduced to 33 nM. This meant that the knockdown efficiency was lower than for individual silencing: around 70% at the mRNA level on average for the 3 genes 24 h after the microporation (Figure 3A), and about 50% at

the protein level after 48 h (Figure 3B). Once more, however, cell survival was unaffected, producing no significant induction of apoptosis (Figure 3C) or cell cycle arrest (Figure S4) in any cell line under any of the studied conditions. These results could be due to the transient knockdown triggered by siRNAs.

Additionally, a more stable knockdown of PIM genes was approached using lentiviral particles containing shRNAs inserted into the pLKO.1-puro vector. Since infected cells should be selected with Puromycin, first we tested the sensitivity of several PTCL cell lines to this antibiotic. SU-DHL-1 and SR786 cell viability was rapidly impaired in the presence of Puromycin, while HH and MyLa cells showed a greater resistance (data not shown). Then, we checked the infection efficiency using lentiviral particles containing GFP, and observed a high proportion of green MyLa cells, while no green HH cells were found even after 15 days post-infection (data not shown). Thus, MyLa cell line was chosen to be infected with shPIM-lentiviral particles: 74% of cells were infected 8 days after lentiviral addition (Figure 4A). This efficiency was checked to be as high as possible, because in parallel, non-infected cells were cultured in the presence of Puromycin, and at this time point all these cells were dead (Figure 4A). However, under these conditions around 30% of PIM-mRNA was still detectable by RT-qPCR (data not shown). Even when the 3 shRNAs (shPIM1+ shPIM2+ shPIM3) were simultaneously added and cells selected for 15 days, we found a decrease of only 30%, on average, both at the mRNA (Figure 4B) and protein (Figure 4C) levels. Again, these conditions did not affect cell survival (Figures 4A and 4D).

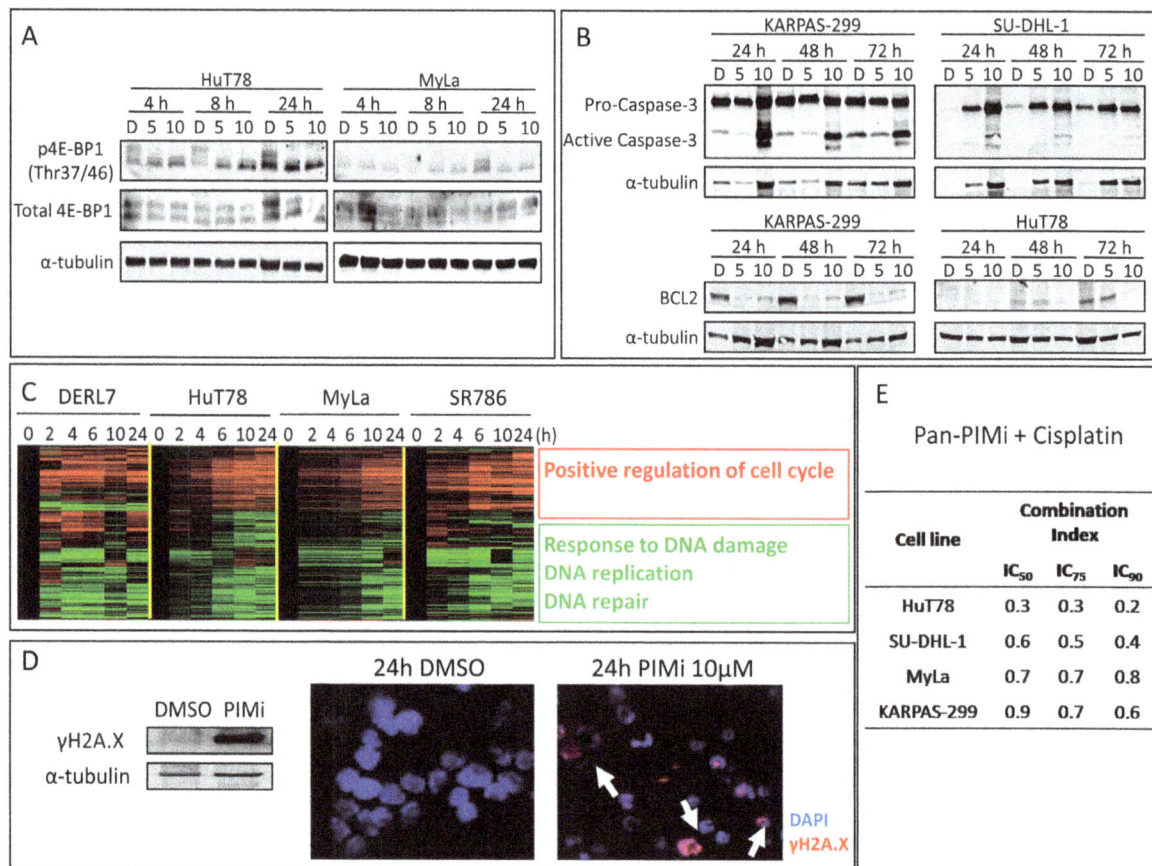

Figure 6. Molecular response to the pan-PIMi in PTCL. (A) The pan-PIMi ETP-39010 reduced phosphorylation of 4E-BP1 in PTCL cell lines. D: DMSO; 5: 5 μM pan-PIMi; 10: 10 μM pan-PIMi. (B) Key effectors of apoptosis, such as Caspase-3 and BCL2, were affected by the pan-PIMi in PTCL cell lines, in a time and dose-dependent manner. D: DMSO; 5: 5 μM pan-PIMi; 10: 10 μM pan-PIMi. (C) Heat-map showing the commonly differentially expressed genes (FDR<0.05) in all PIMi-treated cell lines (10 μM) compared with DMSO-treated cells at each time point. STEM program was used to identify significant genes, and FatiGO recognized the pathways in which they were involved (adjusted p-value<0.05). (D) Amount and pattern of distribution of γH2A.X was tested by Western blot and immunofluorescence, respectively, in MyLa cells treated with 10 μM pan-PIMi for 24 h. Arrows show γH2A.X foci (40X magnification). Images were obtained by a fluorescence microscope (Axio Imager Z1, Zeiss, Oberkochen, Germany). (E) PTCL cell lines were treated with a range of doses of the combination pan-PIMi + Cisplatin for 72 h. Combination Index (<1) showed synergism between both drugs in all studied PTCL cell lines.

These results could be due to the incomplete silencing of all 3 PIM kinases, with the remaining active protein still triggering enough survival signaling.

Pharmacological pan-PIM kinase inhibition in PTCL

In order to inhibit the catalytic activity of all PIM kinases more efficiently, the pharmacological pan-PIM inhibitor ETP-39010 [21] was used. We found that this drug reduced cell viability in all PTCL cell lines in the same low micromolar range of IC_{50} values (Figure 5A). This effect was mainly due to a strong dose- and time-dependent induction of apoptosis (Figure 5B and Figure S5A, S5B and S5C), without cell cycle arrest (Figure S5D). The subG0 population (reflecting dead cells) increased even with short-duration, low-dose treatments, especially in the KARPAS-299, SU-DHL-1 and SR786 cell lines, which are members of the ALCL subtype (Figure S5D).

These results indicated a direct and strong cytotoxic effect of the pharmacological pan-PIMi on PTCL cell lines.

Additionally, we tested the *ex vivo* efficiency of the pan-PIMi in PTCL. Primary T cells from 8 PTCL patients (Mycosis Fungoides and Sézary Syndrome) and 5 healthy donors were treated for 48 h, and we observed that tumoral T cell viability was slightly but significantly reduced, while normal T cells remained unaffected (Figure 5C).

Molecular response of PTCL to the pharmacological pan-PIMi

To confirm that the pharmacological pan-PIMi was really inhibiting PIM kinase activity, we measured the phosphorylation status of 4E-BP1, a well-established substrate of PIM kinases [13,14,15]. A decrease in p4E-BP1 was found in PTCL cell lines after short treatment with pan-PIMi (Figure 6A). Moreover, taking into account the dramatic proapoptotic effect of this drug, two key proteins involved in apoptosis were also examined: we found that the pan-PIMi induced cleavage and activation of Caspase-3 and decreased the levels of BCL2 (Figure 6B). These observations support and explain the strong apoptosis induced by the pan-PIMi in PTCL.

To understand the molecular response of PTCL cells to the pharmacological pan-PIMi, 4 PTCL cell lines were treated with 10 μM for varying periods, and changes in gene expression over time were examined. We found 390 genes that were differentially expressed (FDR<0.05) and commonly deregulated in all 4 cell

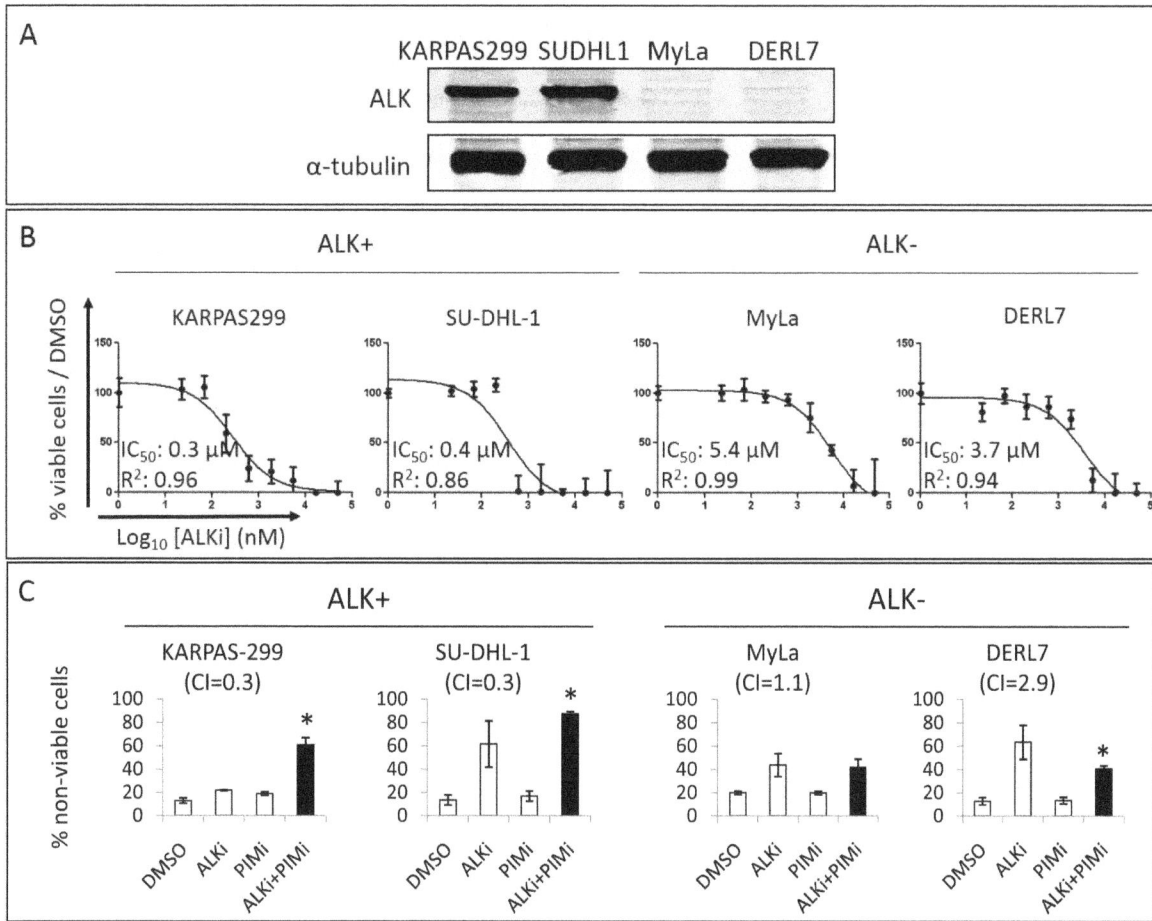

Figure 7. Synergism between ALK and PIM inhibition in ALCL. (A) ALK expression was explored by Western blot in 4 PTCL cell lines. (B) IC_{50} values were measured upon 72 h treatment with the ALKi Crizotinib: ALK+ ALCL cell lines were around 10 times as sensitive to the ALKi as the ALK− cells. (C) Cells were treated for 24 h with IC_{50} of ALKi and pan-PIMi, alone and combined. The combination of ALKi + PIMi was highly synergistic (Combination Index, CI<1) and strongly enhanced apoptosis in ALK+ ALCL cell lines after 24 h, while this combination was antagonistic in ALK− PTCL cell lines (CI>1) (*, p<0.05 in comparison with DMSO). Data represent Annexin V+/PI− and Annexin V+/PI+ cells in each treatment. Black columns highlight the combined treatment.

lines upon drug treatment (Figure 6C). On the basis of GO categories we found that the upregulated genes were those involved in the positive regulation of the cell cycle pathway, which could explain the aforementioned absence of cell cycle arrest, and that the downregulated genes were related to the response to DNA damage, repair and replication, which could be added and enhance the strong apoptosis induced by the pan-PIMi (Figure 6C). A more detailed list of genes and pathways deregulated in each PTCL cell line treated with the pan-PIMi can be found in the Tables S3 and S4, respectively.

To validate this result, the expression of several genes involved in DNA damage repair, such as *ERCC8*, *XRCC2* and *XRCC5* (Figure S6A) was measured by RT-qPCR. We found that treatment with the pan-PIMi downregulated the expression of these genes in a time- and dose-dependent manner (Figure S6B).

To functionally confirm that pharmacological PIM kinase inhibition impaired the DNA damage repair machinery, we measured the amount and distribution of γH2A.X protein, the classical hallmark for DNA damage [26,27], in MyLa cells. After treatment with the pan-PIMi increases in the amount and formation of γH2A.X foci corresponding to DNA damage foci were observed (Figure 6D).

These results indicated that the pharmacological pan-PIMi strongly induces DNA damage through the downregulation of genes involved in the DNA repair machinery.

Based on this, we hypothesized that the response to the pan-PIMi could be even improved by a DNA damaging agent, such as Cisplatin. Thus, 4 PTCL cell lines were treated with the drug combination pan-PIMi + Cisplatin for 72 h. In all tested cell lines, a synergistic effect between both drugs (Combination Index <1) was observed (Figure 6E), highlighting again the functional link between PIM kinases and DNA repair.

Synergism between PIM and ALK inhibition in ALCL

Since ALCL cell lines were the most sensitive to the pan-PIMi ETP-39010, and PIM2 expression was preliminarily associated with poor prognosis in our limited ALCL series, we decided to explore the therapeutic relevance of the PIM pathway in ALCL, especially in the ALK+ ALCL subtype, because ALK translocation is known to activate STAT3 [5,6], and STAT3 triggers PIM2 expression [13,14]. First, we treated 2 ALK+ ALCL cell lines (KARPAS-299 and SU-DHL-1) and 2 ALK− PTCL cell lines (MyLa and DERL7) with the ALKi Crizotinib (Figure 7A) and found, as expected, that the ALK+ cells were about 10 times as

A

Compound	IC$_{50}$ PIM1 (nM)	IC$_{50}$ PIM2 (nM)	IC$_{50}$ PIM3 (nM)	IC$_{50}$ FLT3 (nM)
ETP-39010	130	420	79	0.53
ETP-47652	0.3	22.7	4.8	9640
ETP-47551	0.5	2.5	5.4	9990
ETP-46638	7.8	178	229	30700

B % inhibition

	B-RAF-V600E	CK1	DYRK1A	EGFR	FAK	FGFR1	IGF1R	INSR	JAK2	JNK1	KIT	MST1	PAK1	PDGFR1	RPS6KA1	SGK1
ETP-39010	54	33	99	33	48	84	26	67	48	62	95	82	7	98	96	73
ETP-47551	0	41	5	0	0	0	7	0	0	11	0	17	4	0	17	8

C

Compound	72h - IC$_{50}$ (µM)							
	KARPAS299	SU-DHL-1	SR786	DERL7	HuT78	MyLa	HH	MJ
ETP-39010	4.1	4.7	4.8	5.4	6.1	6.5	7.8	16.4
ETP-47652	14.0	7.6	22.2	4.6	18.0	13.9	10.8	42.5
ETP-47551	9.0	8.7	8.2	5.8	6.4	7.4	5.3	18.5
ETP-46638	211.6	40.1	68.6	18.9	0.3	30.9	26.4	292.4

E Apoptosis induced by ETP-47551 (10 µM)

F ALKi + PIMi (ETP-39010)

ALK status	Cell line	Combination Index		
		IC$_{50}$	IC$_{75}$	IC$_{90}$
Positive	KARPAS299	0.3	0.4	0.5
Positive	SU-DHL-1	0.3	0.3	0.2
Negative	MyLa	1.1	0.8	0.5
Negative	DERL7	2.9	1.8	1.1

G ALKi + PIMi (ETP-47551)

ALK status	Cell line	Combination Index		
		IC$_{50}$	IC$_{75}$	IC$_{90}$
Positive	KARPAS299	0.3	0.2	0.1
Positive	SU-DHL-1	0.3	0.2	0.2
Negative	MyLa	1.2	1.0	0.8
Negative	DERL7	1.6	1.2	0.9

D % viable cells / DMSO — Log$_{10}$ [ETP-47551] (nM)

KARPAS-299: IC$_{50}$: 9.0 µM, R^2: 0.91
SU-DHL-1: IC$_{50}$: 8.7 µM, R^2: 0.86
HuT78: IC$_{50}$: 6.4 µM, R^2: 0.98
MyLa: IC$_{50}$: 7.4 µM, R^2: 0.90
HH: IC$_{50}$: 5.3 µM, R^2: 0.96

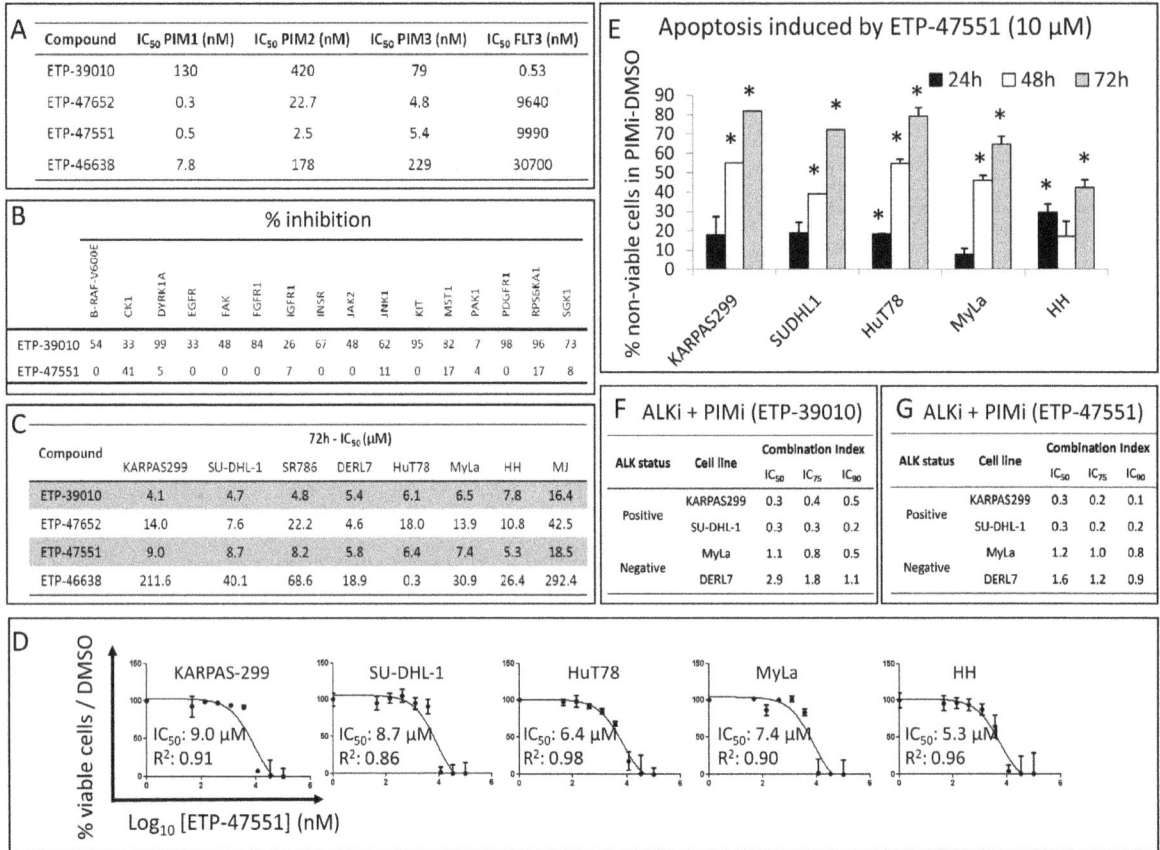

Figure 8. Comparison between the compound ETP-39010 and other pan-PIMi. (A) Selectivity profile showing the IC$_{50}$ values of each of the compounds for the kinase activity of the indicated enzymes. (B) Percentage of inhibition of a panel of unrelated kinases by ETP-39010 and ETP-47551. A similar profile was found for ETP-47551, ETP-47652 and ETP-46638 compounds. (C) Sensitivity of PTCL cell lines to all pan-PIMi. (D) The newly developed pan-PIMi ETP-47551 reduced cell viability in all studied PTCL cell lines (IC$_{50}$ values calculated after 72 h of treatment are shown). (E) The pan-PIMi ETP-47551 strongly induced apoptosis in a time-dependent manner in all studied PTCL cell lines (*, p<0.05, from comparison with DMSO-treated cells). The percentage of non-viable cells was calculated as Annexin V+/7AAD− plus Annexin V+/7AAD+ cells in the PIMi-treated condition minus the DMSO-treated control. (F) The combination of ALKi + ETP-39010 was highly synergistic only in ALK+ ALCL cell lines, as was (G) the combination of ALKi + ETP-47551 (Combination Index, CI, <1 indicates synergism between the two drugs; CI ≈1 indicates an additive effect; CI>1 indicates antagonism).

sensitive as the ALK− cells (Figure 7B). Next, we combined this ALKi with the pan-PIMi ETP-39010 to inhibit the same pathway at two sites, which produced a strong synergistic effect between these drugs only in ALK+ cells, but not in ALK − cells. Strikingly, 24 h of the combined treatment strongly enhanced apoptosis in KARPAS-299 and SU-DHL-1 cells (Combination Index <1), while a slight additive effect or even antagonism, was found in MyLa and DERL7 cells (Combination Index >1) (Figure 7C). The effects driven by the pan-PIMi shown here (24 h, 5 µM) were comparable with those in Figure S5A.

Finally, since the selectivity profile of the pan-PIMi ETP-39010 was not very specific, it was important to rule out the possibility that the effects we observed were due to off-target consequences. To this end, we confirmed the most significant results with newly developed and more specific pan-PIMi: ETP-47652, ETP-47551 and ETP-46638. Of these, ETP-47551 was the compound with the best selective profile (Figures 8A and 8B). We treated our panel of 8 PTCL cell lines with these new pan-PIMi, and found that all cell lines showed the highest sensitivity to the ETP-47551, with IC$_{50}$ values comparable to those obtained with ETP-39010 (Figure 8C). Additionally, we observed that the more specific ETP-47551 reduced cell viability (Figure 8D) and strongly

induced apoptosis in PTCL cell lines in a time-dependent manner (Figure 8E), similarly to the ETP-39010 compound. Lastly, the synergistic effect between the ALKi and the pan-PIMi ETP-39010 in ALK+ ALCL (Figure 8F) was confirmed using the combination ALKi plus the specific pan-PIMi ETP-47551 (Figure 8G). These results could help discard potential off-target effects driven by ETP-39010.

Discussion

We hypothesized that PIM kinase inhibition could be of therapeutic value in PTCL because: 1) PIM kinases have an important role in CD4+ T cell responses [28]; 2) *PIM1* and especially *PIM2* expression is increased in PTCL patients, cell lines and primary tumoral T cells of Sézary Syndrome patients; 3) they are significantly correlated with survival pathways, such as Jak/STAT, NF-κB and IL-2 signaling; and 4) pharmacological PIM inhibition is effective in other T cell-mediated malignancies, such as T cell acute lymphoblastic lymphoma [29].

PIM family members, especially *PIM2*, were found to be overexpressed in PTCL, as in many other tumor entities of hematological or epithelial origin, such as chronic lymphocytic leukemia, mantle cell lymphoma, diffuse large B cell lymphoma, acute myeloid leukemia, and prostate, pancreatic, gastric, colon and hepatocellular carcinomas [13,15]. This increased expression was found to be significantly correlated with Jak/STAT, NF-κB and IL-2 signalings in our PTCL patient series, suggesting that these pathways could be the responsible for PIM activation and could contribute to PTCL cell survival.

However, in spite of all of the supporting evidence, our results indicate that individual genetic silencing of *PIM1*, *PIM2* or *PIM3* genes does not affect PTCL cell survival, either at the level of apoptosis or the cell cycle. We found that this could be due, at least in part, to a compensatory mechanism among the 3 PIM genes, since *PIM1* knockdown was accompanied by the upregulation of both *PIM2* and *PIM3*, and vice versa. These redundant functions have also been described in *in vivo* models: mice lacking *PIM1* had a higher level of *PIM2* expression, while those deficient for *PIM1* and *PIM2* selectively activated *PIM3* [14,15]. These overlapping functions can be explained by the substantial homology (50–70%) of the PIM kinases at the amino acid level [15,19,20,30].

These observations suggested that in order to effectively treat PTCL an inhibition of all three PIMs would be required, as described for other hematological malignancies, such as multiple myeloma [31] and acute myeloid leukemia [32].

Unexpectedly, the simultaneous genetic inhibition of *PIM1+PIM2+PIM3* did not affect PTCL cell survival either. Nevertheless, it is important to note that the simultaneous use of 3 siRNAs makes them less efficient than when they are on their own; moreover, these cells are not easily transfected/infected, making the genetic inhibition approach less informative. The lack of effect could be due to incomplete PIM family inhibition (indeed, around 50% of each protein remained after triple-knockdown si/shRNA, in our case), or the dispensable effects that have been described for PIM (the triple-knockout mice were still viable and their mainly described phenotypic characteristics was a markedly reduced body size [13,14,15]). To address this possibility, we adopted a pharmacological inhibition approach to abolish all PIM kinase activity. Although it is conceivable that the different ATP-binding region of PIM kinases compared with other kinases would allow specific PIM inhibitors to develop, in practice this specificity does not seem to be reached, especially because they also inhibit FLT3, PDGFR and KIT [15,19,21]. Some pharmacological inhibitors are available that are selective for one of the PIM kinases [21], but consequently they will not avoid the compensatory mechanism among the other PIM kinases. We used the ETP-39010 compound, which is a pan-PIMi with a low specificity profile [21] for all the functional assays. Nevertheless, inhibition of PIM kinases by this drug was assessed, since it reduced 4E-BP1 phosphorylation, which is a very well established PIM kinase substrate [13,14,15,21], and could be a biomarker for PIM kinase inhibition in PTCL. In addition, the most significant effects observed with ETP-39010 were confirmed with a newly developed and much more selective compound (ETP-47551). Among our most striking findings was the potent cytotoxic effect in all PTCL cell lines upon pan-PIMi treatment, at doses similar to those used with other pan-PIMi, such as SGI-1776 in prostate cancer [33], acute myeloid leukemia [19], chronic lymphocytic leukemia [17] and mantle cell lymphoma [18]. Surprisingly, and in contrast to the findings of the great majority of these studies, apoptosis induction was not accompanied by cell cycle arrest in PTCL cell lines. An increase in the subG0 population was observed even at lower doses or with shorter-duration treatments, highlighting the potent efficiency of this pan-PIMi in PTCL, especially in ALCL cell lines. Moreover, this strong induction of apoptosis was in part

due to the cleavage of Caspase-3, the decrease in BCL2 protein levels (as extensively described in [13,14,15,32]), and the enhancement of the DNA damage, since we found that the pan-PIMi downregulated the expression of a number of genes involved in DNA damage repair signaling, leading to the formation of γH2A.X foci, the most well established surrogate biomarker for DNA damage [26,27]. Accordingly, there are several lines of evidence involving PIM kinases in the DNA repair machinery [34,35,36,37].

The cytotoxic effect found in pan-PIMi-treated PTCL cell lines was explored *ex vivo* in primary T cells from cutaneous T cell lymphoma patients. Interestingly, we found that although the effects on neoplastic cells was not very dramatic, normal T cells from healthy donors were not affected by the pan-PIMi, recalling the limited cytotoxicity observed in SGI-1776-treated normal lymphocytes [19]. These evidences could support the proof of concept that the PIM kinase inhibition strategy might be a preliminary safe therapeutic approach. Moreover, it has been reported that SGI-1776 treatment reduces tumor volume without causing significant changes in body weight [19]. These findings, along with the fact that the triple *PIM1+PIM2+PIM3* knockout mice had a mild phenotype [13,14], support the rationale of using pharmacological pan-PIMi as safe antitumoral agents.

A large fraction of the PTCL patients showed increased PIM2 protein expression, regardless of their subtype (although with a slight predominance in AITL, where a PIM2 increased expression has been already reported [38]). Importantly, PIM2 protein levels were significantly correlated with a worse outcome in ALCL patients, as described for the majority of malignancies [13]. It is important to note that in our limited ALCL series (n = 27), this association between PIM2 expression and a worse survival was found taking into account both ALK+ and ALK− ALCL patients. Although more samples are needed if more statistically significant conclusions are to be drawn, since in our series, the well-known prognostic marker ALK expression is almost significantly associated with outcome (p = 0.08).

This preliminary finding, along with the fact that ALCL cell lines are the most sensitive to the pan-PIMi ETP-39010, led us to hypothesize that the ALK - STAT3 - PIM2 pathway could be important for ALCL survival, at least in ALK+ ALCL, since ALK is a well-known STAT3 activator [5,6], and STAT3 has been extensively described to increase *PIM2* expression [13,14]. Thus, we aimed to target this axis at two different points using the ALKi Crizotinib plus pan-PIMi (i.e., the less specific ETP-39010 and the more selective ETP-47551). As expected, the simultaneous inhibition of ALK and PIM strongly affected cell survival in ALK+ ALCL but not in other PTCL cell lines, synergizing the apoptosis induced by each drug alone only in ALK+ ALCL cells. These results could highlight the potential therapeutic usefulness of this pathway in ALK+ ALCL.

Although ALK+ ALCL is the PTCL subtype with the most favorable outcome, frequently relapses have been reported in around 30% of patients treated with primary chemotherapy [39]. Some studies have recently described the efficacy of ALK inhibition in ALCL, both in murine models [40] and in preliminary clinical studies: in one trial 2 ALK+ ALCL patients reported complete remission of the disease within 1 month of treatment with Crizotinib, the response being sustained 5–6 months later [8]. A later clinical trial with 9 ALK+ ALCL patients treated with Crizotinib showed an objective response rate of 100%, a complete remission rate of 100%, a median duration of response of 10 months and 3-year progression-free survival of 63% with a plateau in the curve after 6 months [9]. In fact, Crizotinib has been approved by the FDA for the treatment of ALK+ non-small cell lung cancer [3]. Unfortunately, despite its initially impressive efficacy, resistance to Crizotinib has been found in patients carrying mutations in the fused ALK proteins [9,41]. For this reason, it might be worthwhile exploring drug combinations targeting downstream effectors of the oncogenic-driver ALK translocation. Additionally, PIMi are known to synergize strongly with other antitumoral agents, such as Cisplatin, as demonstrated here in PTCL, the MEK inhibitor UO126 in precursor T cell lymphoblastic leukemia [29], the PI3 K inhibitor GDC-0941 in acute myeloid leukemia [21], the HDAC inhibitor SAHA in classical Hodgkin lymphoma [42], Bendamustine in mantle cell lymphoma and splenic marginal zone lymphoma [43], the BCL2 inhibitor ABT-737 [44] and taxanes [45] in prostate cancer and the multi-kinase inhibitor Sunitinib in renal cell carcinoma [46].

In conclusion, our results suggest that the simultaneous inhibition of all PIM kinases could be an efficient therapeutic strategy in those PTCL with PIM upregulation. This strategy seems to be particularly relevant in the ALK+ ALCL subtype, whereby the increased expression of PIM2 is associated with shorter survival and the combinatory inhibition of ALK and all PIM kinases potently enhanced apoptosis.

Supporting Information

Figure S1   PIM2 protein in tumoral samples from PTCL patients. Representative immunohistochemical stainings for PIM2 (A) negative (<5% positive cells), (B) weakly positive (5–20% positive cells) and (C) strongly positive (>20% positive cells) samples from PTCL patients, specifically, a PTCL-NOS and two AITL, respectively (upper panels at 20X magnification and lower panels at 100X magnification).
(TIF)

Figure S2   Association between PIM2 protein expression and overall survival in PTCL patients. PIM2 protein (both weak and strong signal) was significantly associated with worse overall survival in ALCL (n = 27), but not in the PTCL-NOS (n = 42) + AITL (n = 39) subgroups.
(TIF)

Figure S3   Effects of single PIM genetic knockdown on cell cycle in PTCL cell lines. Individual PIM gene inhibition (100 nM siRNA) did not induce cell cycle changes over the time. (NTC: non-template control).
(TIF)

Figure S4   Effects of triple PIM genetic knockdown on cell cycle in PTCL cell lines. Simultaneous triple *PIM1+PIM2+PIM3* gene inhibition did not induce cell cycle changes over the time. (NTC: non-template control).
(TIF)

Figure S5   Effects of the pharmacological pan-PIMi on PTCL cell survival. (A) PTCL cell lines were treated with 5 µM of pan-PIMi for 24–72 h and effects on apoptosis were measured by flow cytometry. The percentage of non-viable cells was calculated as Annexin V+/PI− plus Annexin V+/PI+ cells in the PIMi-treated condition minus the DMSO-treated control. The pan-PIMi ETP-39010 strongly induced apoptosis in a time-dependent manner in all PTCL cell lines (*, p<0.05, from comparison with DMSO-treated cells). (B) Original scatter plots from FACS characterizing the effect of the pharmacological pan-PIMi on apoptosis in ALK+ ALCL cell lines: the X axis represents Annexin V staining and the Y axis represents PI staining. Representative plots from 3 independent experiments. (C) Original scatter plots from FACS characterizing the effect of the pharmacological pan-PIMi on apoptosis in other PTCL cell lines:

the X axis represents Annexin V staining and the Y axis represents PI staining. Representative plots from 3 independent experiments. (D) The pan-PIMi (24 h) did not promote cell cycle arrest at any phase, but a direct increase in the subG0 fraction, as indicated numerically (mean ± SEM), especially in ALK+ ALCL cell lines (KARPAS-299, SU-DHL-1 and SR786).
(PDF)

Figure S6   Downregulation of DNA damage repair signaling by the pharmacological pan-PIMi. (A) Heat-map showing an overall downregulation of genes involved in DNA damage repair machinery driven by the pharmacological pan-PIMi (10 µM at indicated times) in both MyLa and SR786 cell lines. These expression changes were significant (FDR<0.05), and extracted from Table S3. Some important genes, such as *ERCC8*, *XRCC2* and *XRCC5* (highlighted by arrows) were randomly selected to be validated. (B) Validation of microarray data by RT-qPCR. The expression of *ERCC8*, *XRCC2* and *XRCC5* genes was confirmed to be reduced in a time- and dose- dependent manner after pan-PIMi treatment in MyLa and SR786 cell lines. RQ, relative quantification, was calculated as described in the Methods section as $RQ = 2^{-\Delta Ct}$.
(TIF)

Table S1   Clinical characteristics of the series of PTCL patients used for immunohistochemical studies. PIM2 protein expression was explored in 136 PTCL patients. (PTCL-NOS: peripheral T cell lymphoma not otherwise specified; AITL: angioimmunoblastic T cell lymphoma; ALCL: anaplastic large cell lymphoma; NK-T: natural killer T cell lymphoma; IPI: international prognostic index; PIT: prognostic index for peripheral T-cell lymphoma, unspecified; ECOG: Eastern Cooperative Oncology Group; LDH: lactate dehydrogenase).
(TIF)

Table S2   Effects of single PIM genetic knockdown on apoptosis in PTCL cell lines. Individual PIM gene inhibition did not induce apoptosis over the time. The percentage of non-viable cells was calculated as Annexin V+/PI− plus Annexin V+/PI+ cells. (NTC: non-template control).
(TIF)

Table S3   Significantly PIMi-deregulated genes in PTCL cell lines. Differentially expressed genes in each cell line upon pan-PIMi treatment (10 µM) were identified using STEM program, which compared the expression profile in pan-PIMi-treated cells with DMSO-treated cells at each time point (0, 2, 4, 6, 10 and 24 h). Almost 400 genes were found significantly deregulated (FDR<0.05) upon pan-PIMi treatment. Expression values ($\log_2$ ratio) were normalized with the time point 0 h.
(XLS)

Table S4   Significantly PIMi-deregulated pathways in PTCL cell lines. Differentially expressed genes in each cell line upon pan-PIMi treatment identified by STEM (FDR<0.05) were applied to FatiGO to look for their functions. Significant biological processes at level 6 are shown (numbers indicate adjusted p-values). Red, green and white colors represent upregulation, downregulation and no significant deregulation, respectively. DNA-related processes are highlighted with arrows.
(TIF)

Methods S1   Additional detailed methodology.
(DOC)

Acknowledgments

The authors would like to thank the staff of the Spanish National Tumour Bank Network for their help in collecting and managing the samples from the hospitals. We also need to thank Flow Cytometry Unit from the Spanish National Cancer Research Centre (Madrid, Spain) and Dr Fidel Madrazo from the Microscopy Unit in the Research Institute Marqués de Valdecilla (IDIVAL, Santander, Spain) for their excellent technical help.

Author Contributions

Conceived and designed the experiments: MAP. Performed the experiments: EM-S LO BD-G GR SCdO HP RM CA. Analyzed the data: EM-S SMR-P MAP. Contributed reagents/materials/analysis tools: CB-A AMGC EGC JPF JRB MM FJA JM FG-P JLR-P PLO-R. Wrote the paper: EM-S. Manuscript revision: SMR-P MS-B MAP. Scientific discussion: FXR JFG.

References

1. de Leval L, Bisig B, Thielen C, Boniver J, Gaulard P (2009) Molecular classification of T-cell lymphomas. Crit Rev Oncol Hematol 72: 125–143.
2. Foss FM, Zinzani PL, Vose JM, Gascoyne RD, Rosen ST, et al. (2011) Peripheral T-cell lymphoma. Blood 117: 6756–6767.
3. Armitage JO (2012) The aggressive peripheral T-cell lymphomas: 2012 update on diagnosis, risk stratification, and management. Am J Hematol 87: 511–519.
4. Scarisbrick JJ, Kim YH, Whittaker SJ, Wood GS, Vermeer MH, et al. (2014) Prognostic Factors, Prognostic Indices and Staging in Mycosis Fungoides and Sezary Syndrome: Where are we now? Br J Dermatol Epub ahead of print.
5. Pearson JD, Lee JK, Bacani JT, Lai R, Ingham RJ (2012) NPM-ALK: The Prototypic Member of a Family of Oncogenic Fusion Tyrosine Kinases. J Signal Transduct 2012: 123253.
6. Barreca A, Lasorsa E, Riera L, Machiorlatti R, Piva R, et al. (2011) Anaplastic lymphoma kinase in human cancer. J Mol Endocrinol 47: R11–23.
7. O'Leary H, Savage KJ (2009) The spectrum of peripheral T-cell lymphomas. Curr Opin Hematol 16: 292–298.
8. Gambacorti-Passerini C, Messa C, Pogliani EM (2011) Crizotinib in anaplastic large-cell lymphoma. N Engl J Med 364: 775–776.
9. Intlekofer AM, Younes A (2014) From empiric to mechanism-based therapy for peripheral T cell lymphoma. Int J Hematol 99: 249–262.
10. Horwitz SM, Advani RH, Bartlett NL, Jacobsen ED, Sharman JP, et al. (2014) Objective responses in relapsed T-cell lymphomas with single agent brentuximab vedotin. Blood Epub ahead of print.
11. Dunleavy K, Piekarz RL, Zain J, Janik JE, Wilson WH, et al. (2010) New strategies in peripheral T-cell lymphoma: understanding tumor biology and developing novel therapies. Clin Cancer Res 16: 5608–5617.
12. Moskowitz AJ, Lunning M, Horwitz SM (2014) How I treat the peripheral T cell lymphomas. Blood Epub ahead of print.
13. Nawijn MC, Alendar A, Berns A (2011) For better or for worse: the role of Pim oncogenes in tumorigenesis. Nat Rev Cancer 11: 23–34.
14. Brault L, Gasser C, Bracher F, Huber K, Knapp S, et al. (2010) PIM serine/threonine kinases in the pathogenesis and therapy of hematologic malignancies and solid cancers. Haematologica 95: 1004–1015.
15. Alvarado Y, Giles FJ, Swords RT (2012) The PIM kinases in hematological cancers. Expert Rev Hematol 5: 81–96.
16. An N, Kraft AS, Kang Y (2013) Abnormal hematopoietic phenotypes in Pim kinase triple knockout mice. J Hematol Oncol 6: 12.
17. Chen LS, Redkar S, Bearss D, Wierda WG, Gandhi V (2009) Pim kinase inhibitor, SGI-1776, induces apoptosis in chronic lymphocytic leukemia cells. Blood 114: 4150–4157.
18. Yang Q, Chen LS, Neelapu SS, Miranda RN, Medeiros LJ, et al. (2012) Transcription and translation are primary targets of Pim kinase inhibitor SGI-1776 in mantle cell lymphoma. Blood 120: 3491–3500.
19. Chen LS, Redkar S, Taverna P, Cortes JE, Gandhi V (2011) Mechanisms of cytotoxicity to Pim kinase inhibitor, SGI-1776, in acute myeloid leukemia. Blood 118: 693–702.
20. Drygin D, Haddach M, Pierre F, Ryckman DM (2012) Potential use of selective and nonselective Pim kinase inhibitors for cancer therapy. J Med Chem 55: 8199–8208.
21. Blanco-Aparicio C, Collazo AM, Oyarzabal J, Leal JF, Albaran MI, et al. (2011) Pim 1 kinase inhibitor ETP-45299 suppresses cellular proliferation and synergizes with PI3 K inhibition. Cancer Lett 300: 145–153.
22. Pastor Fernández J (2011) Tricyclic compounds for use as kinase inhibitors. World International Property Organization.
23. Martin-Sanchez E, Rodriguez-Pinilla SM, Sanchez-Beato M, Lombardia L, Dominguez-Gonzalez B, et al. (2013) Simultaneous inhibition of pan-phosphatidylinositol-3-kinases and MEK as a potential therapeutic strategy in peripheral T-cell lymphomas. Haematologica 98: 57–64.
24. Chou TC, Talalay P (1984) Quantitative analysis of dose-effect relationships: the combined effects of multiple drugs or enzyme inhibitors. Adv Enzyme Regul 22: 27–55.
25. Ernst J, Bar-Joseph Z (2006) STEM: a tool for the analysis of short time series gene expression data. BMC Bioinformatics 7: 191.
26. Sak A, Stuschke M (2010) Use of gammaH2AX and other biomarkers of double-strand breaks during radiotherapy. Semin Radiat Oncol 20: 223–231.
27. Mah LJ, El-Osta A, Karagiannis TC (2010) gammaH2AX: a sensitive molecular marker of DNA damage and repair. Leukemia 24: 679–686.
28. Jackson IJ, Pheneger JA, Pheneger TJ, Davis G, Wright AD, et al. (2012) The role of PIM kinases in human and mouse CD4+ T cell activation and inflammatory bowel disease. Cell Immunol 272: 200–213.
29. Lin YW, Beharry ZM, Hill EG, Song JH, Wang W, et al. (2010) A small molecule inhibitor of Pim protein kinases blocks the growth of precursor T-cell lymphoblastic leukemia/lymphoma. Blood 115: 824–833.
30. Blanco-Aparicio C, Carnero A (2013) Pim kinases in cancer: diagnostic, prognostic and treatment opportunities. Biochem Pharmacol 85: 629–643.
31. Garcia PD, Langowski JL, Wang Y, Chen MY, Castillo J, et al. (2014) Pan-PIM Kinase Inhibition Provides a Novel Therapy for Treating Hematological Cancers. Clin Cancer Res (epub ahead of print).
32. Keeton EK, McEachern K, Dillman KS, Palakurthi S, Cao Y, et al. (2014) AZD1208, a potent and selective pan-Pim kinase inhibitor, demonstrates efficacy in preclinical models of acute myeloid leukemia. Blood 123: 905–913.
33. Siu A, Virtanen C, Jongstra J (2011) PIM kinase isoform specific regulation of MIG6 expression and EGFR signaling in prostate cancer cells. Oncotarget 2: 1134–1144.
34. Min X, Tang J, Wang Y, Yu M, Zhao L, et al. (2012) PI3 K-like kinases restrain Pim gene expression in endothelial cells. J Huazhong Univ Sci Technolog Med Sci 32: 17–23.
35. Hsu JL, Leong PK, Ho YF, Hsu LC, Lu PH, et al. (2012) Pim-1 knockdown potentiates paclitaxel-induced apoptosis in human hormone-refractory prostate cancers through inhibition of NHEJ DNA repair. Cancer Lett 319: 214–222.
36. Bednarski JJ, Nickless A, Bhattacharya D, Amin RH, Schlissel MS, et al. (2012) RAG-induced DNA double-strand breaks signal through Pim2 to promote pre-B cell survival and limit proliferation. J Exp Med 209: 11–17.
37. Zhang Y, Parsanejad M, Huang E, Qu D, Aleyasin H, et al. (2010) Pim-1 kinase as activator of the cell cycle pathway in neuronal death induced by DNA damage. J Neurochem 112: 497–510.
38. de Leval L, Rickman DS, Thielen C, Reynies A, Huang YL, et al. (2007) The gene expression profile of nodal peripheral T-cell lymphoma demonstrates a molecular link between angioimmunoblastic T-cell lymphoma (AITL) and follicular helper T (TFH) cells. Blood 109: 4952–4963.
39. Mak V, Hamm J, Chhanabhai M, Shenkier T, Klasa R, et al. (2013) Survival of patients with peripheral T-cell lymphoma after first relapse or progression: spectrum of disease and rare long-term survivors. J Clin Oncol 31: 1970–1976.
40. Laimer D, Dolznig H, Kollmann K, Vesely PW, Schlederer M, et al. (2012) PDGFR blockade is a rational and effective therapy for NPM-ALK-driven lymphomas. Nat Med 18: 1699–1704.
41. Mologni L (2012) Inhibitors of the anaplastic lymphoma kinase. Expert Opin Investig Drugs 21: 985–994.
42. Martin-Sanchez E, Sanchez-Beato M, Rodriguez ME, Sanchez-Espiridion B, Gomez-Abad C, et al. (2011) HDAC inhibitors induce cell cycle arrest, activate the apoptotic extrinsic pathway and synergize with a novel PIM inhibitor in Hodgkin lymphoma-derived cell lines. Br J Haematol 152: 352–356.
43. Yang Q, Chen LS, Neelapu SS, Gandhi V (2013) Combination of Pim kinase inhibitor SGI-1776 and bendamustine in B-cell lymphoma. Clin Lymphoma Myeloma Leuk 13 Suppl 2: S355–362.
44. Song JH, Kraft AS (2011) Pim kinase inhibitors sensitize prostate cancer cells to apoptosis triggered by Bcl-2 family inhibitor ABT-737. Cancer Res 72: 294–303.
45. Mumenthaler SM, Ng PY, Hodge A, Bearss D, Berk G, et al. (2009) Pharmacologic inhibition of Pim kinases alters prostate cancer cell growth and resensitizes chemoresistant cells to taxanes. Mol Cancer Ther 8: 2882–2893.
46. Mahalingam D, Espitia CM, Medina EC, Esquivel JA, 2nd, Kelly KR, et al. (2011) Targeting PIM kinase enhances the activity of sunitinib in renal cell carcinoma. Br J Cancer 105: 1563–1573.

18

Marine Hydroquinone Zonarol Prevents Inflammation and Apoptosis in Dextran Sulfate Sodium-Induced Mice Ulcerative Colitis

Sohsuke Yamada[1][*][9], Tomoyuki Koyama[2][9], Hirotsugu Noguchi[1], Yuki Ueda[2], Ryo Kitsuyama[3], Hiroya Shimizu[3], Akihide Tanimoto[4], Ke-Yong Wang[1,5], Aya Nawata[1], Toshiyuki Nakayama[1], Yasuyuki Sasaguri[1,6], Takumi Satoh[3,7]

1 Department of Pathology and Cell Biology, School of Medicine, University of Occupational and Environmental Health, Kitakyushu 807-8555, Japan, 2 Laboratory of Nutraceuticals and Functional Foods Science, Graduate School of Marine Science and Technology, Tokyo 108-8477, Japan, 3 Department of Welfare Engineering, Faculty of Engineering, Iwate University, Morioka 020-8551, Japan, 4 Department of Molecular and Cellular Pathology, Kagoshima University Graduate School of Medical and Dental Sciences, Kagoshima 890-8544, Japan, 5 Shared-Use Research Center, University of Occupational and Environmental Health, Kitakyushu 807-8555, Japan, 6 Laboratory of Pathology, Fukuoka Wajiro Hospital, Fukuoka 811-0213, Japan, 7 Department of Anti-Aging Food Research, School of Bioscience and Biotechnology, Tokyo University of Technology, Hachioji 192-0982, Japan

Abstract

Background and Aim: We previously identified an anti-inflammatory compound, zonarol, a hydroquinone isolated from the brown algae *Dictyopteris undulata* as a marine natural product. To ascertain the *in vivo* functions of zonarol, we examined the pharmacological effects of zonarol administration on dextran sulfate sodium (DSS)-induced inflammation in a mouse model of ulcerative colitis (UC). Our goal is to establish a safe and effective cure for inflammatory bowel disease (IBD) using zonarol.

Methods and Results: We subjected Slc:ICR mice to the administration of 2% DSS in drinking water for 14 days. At the same time, 5-aminosalicylic acid (5-ASA) at a dose of 50 mg/kg (positive control) and zonarol at doses of 10 and 20 mg/kg, were given orally once a day. DSS-treated animals developed symptoms similar to those of human UC, such as severe bloody diarrhea, which were evaluated by the disease activity index (DAI). Treatment with 20 mg/kg of zonarol, as well as 5-ASA, significantly suppressed the DAI score, and also led to a reduced colonic ulcer length and/or mucosal inflammatory infiltration by various immune cells, especially macrophages. Zonarol treatment significantly reduced the expression of pro-inflammatory signaling molecules, and prevented the apoptosis of intestinal epithelial cells. Finally, zonarol protected against *in vitro* lipopolysaccharide (LPS)-induced activation in the RAW264.7 mouse macrophage cell line.

Conclusions: This is the first report that a marine bioproduct protects against experimental UC via the inhibition of both inflammation and apoptosis, very similar to the standard-of-care sulfasalazine, a well-known prodrug that releases 5-ASA. We believe that the oral administration of zonarol might offer a better treatment for human IBDs than 5-ASA, or may be useful as an alternative/additive therapeutic strategy against UC, without any evidence of side effects.

Editor: Hossam M. M. Arafa, Future University in Egypt (FUE), Egypt

Funding: This work was supported in part by Grants-in-Aid for Scientific Research (21510223, 22500282, 24790394, 25350963 and 25350985) from the Ministry of Education, Culture, Sports, Science and Technology, Tokyo, Japan (to S.Y. T.K. and T.S.) and by A-STEP (Adaptable & Seamless Technology Transfer Program through Target-driven R&D) (AS251Z01987Q) from the JST (Japan Science and Technology Agency), Tokyo, Japan (to T.K. and T.S.). The funders had no role in study design, data collection and analysis, decision to publish, or preparation of the manuscript.

Competing Interests: The authors have declared that no competing interests exist.

* Email: sousuke@med.uoeh-u.ac.jp

9 These authors contributed equally to this work.

Introduction

Inflammatory bowel diseases (IBD), including ulcerative colitis (UC), are chronic autoimmune inflammatory disorders of the gastrointestinal tract [1,2]. UC causes bloody diarrhea, abdominal pain and weight loss. Although UC is a complex disease orchestrated by multiple factors, and its etiology/pathogenesis is poorly understood, it is likely that immune dysregulation, mucosal barrier dysfunction and/or a loss of immunological tolerance to commensal microbiota, lead to imbalanced and elevated inflammatory cells and aberrant cytokine production [1–6]. Inflammatory cytokines, such as tumor necrosis factor (TNF)-α or interleukin (IL)-1β, have been implicated in the pathogenesis of UC [3–6].

Sulfasalazine, a prodrug composed of 5-aminosalicylic acid (5-ASA) and sulfapyridine, has been used as a standard-of-care in UC for decades, but is a double edged sword because it generates excessive oxidative stress, resulting in severe adverse symptoms, such as blood disorders, hepatotoxicity, ulcerogenic potential and hypospermia and male infertility [7,8]. Other therapies or combinations of drugs, including novel molecular targeted drugs or antigen-specific immunotherapy, have been of no or very limited benefit, with potential severe side effects [1,2]. UC also predisposes patients to subsequent colorectal cancer and/or the need for intestinal surgeries [1,2,9].

In this context, promising safe and effective drugs are needed for these vulnerable UC patients. In fact, approximately 30–50% of IBD patients seek symptom relief and an improved quality of life, and complementary and alternative medicine (CAM) has often been administered in addition to their primary medications [10]. The variety of CAM therapies includes: (i) hypnosis, (ii) acupuncture, (iii) megadoses of vitamins and minerals, (iv) prebiotics, (v) probiotics and (vi) herbal therapies [10–12].

In the Asian-Pacific region, various types of seaweed have been used, particularly as foodstuff, and as folk medicine to maintain health throughout the ages. More recently, some species of seaweed and seaweed-containing ingredients have become a popular and easily recognized food around the world. In order to obtain a novel inhibitor of inflammation (carrageenan-induced edema in mice) from marine-derived biomass products, we screened the extracts of 150 marine species from around the shore of the Japanese mainland, and found that a crude extract of *Dictyopteris undulata* had the most potent inhibitory effects [13]. Our subsequent experiments showed that the active compound in this extract was zonarol, based on the nuclear magnetic resonance (NMR) data after bioassay-guided purification from the crude extract of *Dictyopteris undulata*. Originally, this sesquiterpene hydroquinone had been reported as a fungitoxic compound by Fenical and Cimino in the 1970's, and had been derived from *Dictyopteris zonarioides* (synonymous with *Dictyopteris undulata*) [14,15]. The absolute chemical structure of the sesquiterpene was elucidated in 1986 [16]. Other pharmacological actions of zonarol have been reported, such as antioxidant effects [17], phospholipase inhibition [18], feeding deterrents against abalone [19] and algicidal effects [20]. To the best of our knowledge, there are no data regarding the *in vivo* effects of the marine hydroquinone, zonarol, especially with regard to its anti-inflammatory effects.

In order to clarify the pharmacological actions of this compound, the present study examined the anti-inflammatory actions of zonarol purified from *Dictyopteris undulata* in both experimental animals and a cultured cell line. In particular, we examined the protective roles of zonarol in dextran sulfate sodium (DSS)-induced colon injury using young male Slc:ICR mice, since this model demonstrates the progression of inflamed mucosal lesions with erosion to ulcer formation, the infiltration of various inflammatory cells and accelerated production of multiple inflammatory and/or pro-inflammatory mediators, reminiscent of human UC. We examined the potential of using zonarol as an alternative/additive CAM treatment for UC.

Materials and Methods

Preparation of crude extract from the brown algae, *Dictyopteris undulata*

Brown algae (*Dictyopteris undulata*) was collected from the intertidal area in Shizuoka and Kanagawa prefectures, Japan, in 2013 (35.140612, 139.651754 or 34.709215, 138.984292 or 34.631562, 138.899008 by the GPS coordinates). For these locations/activities, no specific permissions were required. The fresh alga body (3.0 kg) was drained off on a paper towel, and then extracted with five volumes of methanol for five days at room temperature. The extract obtained by two times procedures was filtered, evaporated and freeze-dried to give dark green powder (108.0 g). The powder was stored at $-20°C$ until use for *in vivo* and *in vitro* experiments as a crude extract.

Purification and structural determination of zonarol

The active component of the crude extract was fractionated by partition and column chromatography techniques based on our preliminary data regarding the suppressive activity of the extract against carrageenin-induced paw edema in mice. The fraction with the activity was used for further fractionation until a single compound was detected based on high performance liquid chromatography (HPLC) data. The structure of the purified compound was then determined based on spectral data from NMR experiments. The NMR spectra in MeOD were obtained on a Bruker AV-400 spectrometer (Bruker, Tokyo, Japan). Liquid Chromatography–Mass Spectrometry (LC/MS) was performed using a GC-2010 instrument (SHIMADZU, Kyoto, Japan). Confirmation of the purity of the compound was based on the HPLC analysis and spectral data.

Animals and the ulcerative colitis (UC) model

Experiments were performed using five-week-old male Slc:ICR mice after a one-week acclimatization period. The mice weighed 30–35 g, were purchased from Japan SLC (Hamamatsu, Japan) and were maintained in a temperature and light-controlled facility with free access to standard rodent chow and water. In the current UC model, we subjected the five-week-old Slc:ICR mice in the DSS group to the administration of 2% DSS in drinking water for 14 days. The Slc:ICR mice in the positive control and zonarol groups were also allowed to drink 2% DSS water *ad libitum* for 14 days, and at the same time, were given 5-aminosalicylic acid (5-ASA; Sigma-Aldrich Chemical Co., Ltd.; St. Louis, MO, USA) at a dose of 50 mg/kg, and/or zonarol at doses of 10 and 20 mg/kg orally once a day for 14 days. Normal control ICR mice received a sham treatment. The body weight (BW) and food and water intake were assessed every day, and the organ weights and colon length were determined when the mice were killed. Food consumption was determined using metabolic cages obtained from SU-GIYAMA-GEN Co., Ltd. (Tokyo, Japan) [21]. Six weight-matched animals from each group were analyzed (n = 30 in total). The experimental procedure is summarized in Figure S1, as a schematic representation.

The disease activity index (DAI) was calculated by grading on a scale of 0 to 4 using the following parameters: loss of BW (0, normal; 1, 0–5%; 2, 5–10%; 3, 10–20%; 4, >20%), stool consistency (0, normal; 2, loose stools; 4, watery diarrhea) and the occurrence of gross blood in the stool (0, negative; 4, positive). The combined DAI scores were determined by two independent investigators (Sohsuke Yamada and Tomoyuki Koyama) blinded to the study results [21]. There were no cases of disagreement in this DAI score. On day 15 after the induction of UC or sham-treatment, the mice were euthanized by exsanguination under general anesthetization with spontaneous inhalation of isoflurane (Mylan Inc., Canonsburg, PA, USA). The peritoneal cavity was then opened, blood samples were taken from the inferior vena cava, and several tissues, including intestines and/or the spleen, were excised (n = 30 in total). In all animals, the colon from the ileocecal junction to the anus was excised, cut open lengthwise or cut into small pieces (n = 30 in total), and used for various experiments, as described below.

Ethics

The animal studies were conducted according to the 2006 guidelines entitled "Notification No. 88 of the Ministry of the Environment in Japan and Guidelines for Animal Experimentation of Tokyo University of Marine Science and Technology" with the approval of the Animal Care and Use Committee of Tokyo University of Marine Science and Technology. The investigation conformed to the Guide for the Care and Use of Laboratory Animals published by the US National Institutes of Health (NIH Publication No. 85-23, revised 1996).

Our field studies did not involve endangered or protected species, and no specific permissions for any locations/activities were required.

Histopathology

Colon specimens were stained with hematoxylin and eosin (H&E), Alcian blue or periodic acid-Schiff (PAS) stain, or were used for immunohistochemistry (IHC) preparations in sequential sections, after fixation in 15% neutral buffered formalin for 24 hr [22–26]. The analyses were performed in DSS-induced inflamed intestines in all experiments, whereas non-treated colons served as normal controls.

Colons embedded in paraffin for histological examinations were cut systematically in sequential longitudinal sections of 4-μm thickness using a sliding microtome (Leica SM2010R, Leica Microsystems, Wetzler, Germany). For the histological analyses of the large intestine, images of H&E (n = 30 in total) and specially stained sections or IHC sections (n = 18 in total) were captured and quantified using the NanoZoomer Digital Pathology Virtual Slide Viewer software program (Hamamatsu Photonics Corp., Hamamatsu, Japan). H&E-stained longitudinal sections were graded by two independent pathologists (Sohsuke Yamada and Hirotsugu Noguchi) blinded to the physical outcome and other biological and pathological data for each sample, using a scoring system to evaluate the neutrophil infiltration (0–3), lymphocyte infiltration (0–3), erosion to ulceration (0–4) and crypt destruction or loss (0–3) [21]. The maximum sum of the scores for a given section was 13. The DAI and histological scores were from the same mouse [21]. The mean number or average size of goblet cells per crypt was quantified by Alcian blue or PAS staining in 10 randomly selected fields per section (original magnification: ×400) [22–24].

Analyses of inflammatory responses to DSS-induced UC injury by immunohistochemistry (IHC) and double-immunofluorescence (IF) staining

One representative sequential section per mouse was prepared for IHC staining, and was captured and evaluated by a NanoZoomer Digital Pathology Virtual Slide Viewer (Hamamatsu Photonics Corp.) to avoid potential bias [22–25].

To evaluate the severity of DSS-induced UC on day 15, we determined the intensity of inflammation using a polyclonal rabbit anti-human CD3 antibody (1:1; Dako, Glostrup, Denmark), a rat anti-mouse Mac-2 monoclonal antibody (1:500; Cedarlane Laboratories Ltd., Burlington, Ontario, Canada) or a rat anti-mouse Ly-6G antibody (Gr-1; 1:500; Birmingham, AL, USA) [22–26]. We counted the number of positive T-lymphocytes, macrophages or neutrophils in 10 randomly selected fields of inflamed mucosal areas per section (original magnification: ×400) [22,23].

To assess the degree of infiltration of pro-inflammatory mucosal macrophages by double-immunofluorescence (IF), the injured colonic mucosa was labeled with a mouse monoclonal tumor necrosis factor (TNF)-α antibody (1:50; Abcam, Burlingame, CA, USA) and rat monoclonal Mac-2 antibody (1:500; Cedarlane Laboratories Ltd.), visualized with goat anti-mouse IgG antibodies conjugated with Alexa Fluor Dyes (red-stained) and goat anti-rat IgG and IgM antibodies conjugated with Alexa Fluor Dyes (green-stained) (Invitrogen Corp., Camarillo, CA, USA), respectively, and viewed by confocal laser scanning microscopy (LSM5 Pascal Exciter; Carl Zeiss, Oberkochen, Germany) (original magnification: ×400) [22,24]. We applied the HistoMouse Plus Kit (Invitrogen) to block endogenous mouse IgG [22–25]. Furthermore, in order to analyze the expression of inducible nitric oxide synthase (iNOS) in the inflamed mucosal lesions, an anti-iNOS rabbit polyclonal antibody (1:200; BD Biosciences, San Jose, CA, USA) was applied, and we quantified the positive areas in 10 randomly selected fields per section (original magnification: ×400) [22–26].

For IHC or IF studies, we examined one section from each of six mice per experimental group (n = 18 in total, respectively). All histological and IHC or IF slides were evaluated by two independent observers (certified pathologists: Sohsuke Yamada and Hirotsugu Noguchi) who were blinded to the physical outcome or other biological and pathological data for each sample. In case of disagreement, a consensus score was determined by a third board-certified pathologist (Yasuyuki Sasaguri). The agreement between observers was excellent (>0.9) for all sections investigated, as measured by interclass correlation coefficient.

Terminal deoxynucleotidyl transferase end-labeling (TUNEL)

TUNEL assays were performed using an In Situ Cell Death Detection Kit, POD (Roche Applied Science, Mannheim, Germany) [22–25]. Additionally, colon sections were stained with a rabbit polyclonal anti-mouse cytokeratin 20 (CK20) antibody (Abcam, Cambridge, England) to highlight the epithelial lining of the colonic mucosa. DSS-injured colons on day 15 were labeled with anti-fluorescein antibodies (brown-stained) (TUNEL POD; Roche Applied Science), or fluorescein-conjugated TUNEL reaction mixture (green-stained) (Roche Applied Science) and a rabbit polyclonal anti-CK20 antibody (1:200; Abcam). For the latter, the staining was visualized with donkey anti-rabbit IgG antibodies conjugated with Alexa Fluor Dyes (red-stained) (Invitrogen) by confocal laser scanning microscopy (LSM5 Pascal Exciter) (original magnification: ×400) [22,24]. For a quantitative analysis, we counted the TUNEL$^+$ lining epithelial cells (brown-stained) in 100 randomly selected crypts per section (original magnification: ×400) [22–25].

Enzyme-linked immunosorbent assay (ELISA) for TNF-α and interleukin (IL)-6

The levels of serum TNF-α and interleukin (IL)-6 in the DSS-induced UC model on day 15 were measured using an ELISA kit according to the manufacturer's instructions (R&D Systems, Minneapolis, MN, USA) [22,24].

Cell culture

RAW264.7 cells, obtained from the American Type Culture Collection (ATCC; Manassas, VA, USA) were grown in Dulbecco's modified Eagle's medium (DMEM) containing 10% fetal bovine serum (FBS), 100 μg/mL streptomycin and 100 U/ml penicillin (Life Technologies; Carlsbad, CA, USA) in 100-mm Petri dishes (BD Falcon; Franklin Lakes, NJ, USA). The final concentration of DMSO in the culture medium was 0.1%. These RAW264.7 cells are often used as an in vitro model of macrophage activation. The cells were seeded in 24-well plates at a density of 1×10^5 cells/cm^2 in normal DMEM medium. The next day, after washing the cells with PBS, the medium was replaced with 500 μL of serum-free DMEM containing 0.02% BSA and 10 μg/mL lipopolysaccharide (LPS) (L8274, *E. coli* 026:B6-derived) (Sigma-Aldrich Chemical Co. Ltd.) with or without zonarol at the indicated concentrations. After a 24-h incubation at 37°C, the cells were subjected to the following procedures: the 3-(4,5-dimethylthiazol-2-yl)-2,5-diphenyl tetrazolium bromide (MTT) assay to assess viability, nitric oxide (NO) assay and reverse transcription-polymerase chain reaction (RT-PCR), as described elsewhere [27–29].

MTT and NO assays

The viability and NO production of sister cultures of the cells were determined using the MTT assay (DOJINDO, Tokyo, Japan) and Griess reagent (Invitrogen; Carlsbad, CA, USA), respectively. The generation of NO was determined by measuring the nitrite accumulation in the medium with modified Griess reagent. The culture supernatant and Griess reagent were mixed and incubated for 5 min, and subsequently, the absorption was determined at 540 nm. Sodium nitrite (NaNO$_2$) was used to generate a standard curve for quantification [28,29].

Reverse transcriptase-polymerase chain reaction (RT-PCR)

Total RNAs were extracted with the Trizol reagent (Invitrogen) from the RAW264.7 mouse macrophage cell line after 24 h of treatment with zonarol (2 μM) and/or LPS. All procedures were performed as described previously [22–26]. RNase-free conditions were used to prevent mRNA degradation. First-strand cDNA was synthesized with Superscript II RT (Invitrogen) using random primers, according to the manufacturer's instructions. One one-hundredth of the cDNA was used for each PCR reaction. The cycling conditions were as follows: 50°C for 2 min, 95°C for 10 min followed by 45 cycles of 95°C for 15 s and 60°C for 1 min. The following mouse pairs of primers specific for β-actin, mIL-1β, mIL-6 and miNOS were used: 5′-ATC CGT AAA GAC CTC TAT GC-3′ (forward) and 5′-AAC GCA GCT CAG TAA CAG TC-3′ (reverse) for β-actin, 5′-CAA CCA ACA AGT GAT ATT CTC CAT-3 (forward) and 5′-GAT CCA CAC TCT CCA GCT GCA GGG-3′ (reverse) for mIL-1β, 5′-GGA GAC TTC ACA GAG GAT AC-3′ (forward) and 5′-CCA GTT TGG TAG CAT CCA TC-3′ (reverse) for mIL-6, and 5′-CAG CTG GGC TGT ACA AAC CTT-3′ (forward) and 5′-CAT TGG AAG TGA AGC GTT TCG-3′(reverse) for miNOS, resulting in 287-bp, 152-bp, 212-bp and 95-bp RT-PCR products, respectively. At the completion of the PCR, 10 μL of PCR products were mixed with 2 μL of loading buffer and electrophoresed in 1.5% agarose gel in the presence of 0.5 μg/mL of ethidium bromide, and were visualized with a UV transilluminator.

Statistical analysis

The results are expressed as the means ± SE (*in vivo*) or ± SD (*in vitro*). Significant differences were analyzed using Student's *t*-test, Welch's *t*-test or a one-way ANOVA (analysis of variance), where appropriate. In all cases when the ANOVA methodology was employed for non-parametric data (Figs. 1–8), except for results on a carrageenan-induced paw edema mouse model (Fig. S3), Tukey's multiple comparison *post-hoc* test was used [22–26]. Values of $P<0.05$ were considered to be statistically significant.

Results

Evaluation of the chemical properties of purified zonarol

Zonarol (Fig. 1A) was isolated from the crude extract of seaweed *Dictyopteris undulata* as one of the most potent inhibitors of inflammation in mice. To identify the fraction containing the inhibitor, a fractionation procedure was performed using the crude extract (Fig. S2). The final separation step on an Octadecyl Silyl (ODS) column (250×20 mm i.d.) by HPLC (85% aqueous MeOH, 10 mL/min) gave compound **1** (1.1% of yield) as a single peak at 17.0 min, which was detected by UV (280 nm). The purified compound showed significant effects in an assay in mice (Fig. S3). A LCMS analysis of **1** gave *m/z* 314 as a molecular ion [M+H]$^+$. Finally, the chemical structure of **1** was identified as zonarol based on these and the proton and carbon NMR data (Fig. S4).

Zonarol grossly suppresses DSS-induced UC in Slc:ICR mice

To determine the *in vivo* effects of the zonarol extract, Slc:ICR mice were exposed to 2% DSS in their drinking water for 14 days. Since gross bleeding in stool and diarrhea were early signs that occurred around day 9 after starting DSS administration, the BW loss compared to the group of normal control was clearly greater the DSS control group mice from day 11 of the present UC model, but the difference was less than 5%. Therefore, the DAI scores were significantly and dramatically increased in DSS-positive control mice during from day 9 to 15 in the UC model (day 15: DSS 3.83±0.28 vs. Normal 0±0; $P<0.0001$), compared with the other groups of mice treated with zonarol at 10 mg/kg (1.67±0.30) or 20 mg/kg (1.80±0.18) or with 5-ASA (1.67±0.30) ($P<0.001$, respectively) (Fig. 1B). We observed no apparent BW change in the mice treated with zonarol and 5-ASA.

In addition, there was no remarkable change in the food and drinking water intake between the groups of mice throughout the experimental period in the present UC model (Fig. 1C). However, the drinking water intake in the DSS groups tended to be gradually and slightly decreased after DSS administration (Fig. 1C). In contrast, the spleen/BW ratio (Fig. 1D) in the DSS control group was significantly elevated (DSS 8.45±0.80 mg/g vs. Normal 3.25±0.14 mg/g; $P<0.001$), whereas that in the zonarol 20 mg/kg (3.97±0.55 mg/g) and 5-ASA (4.98±0.65 mg/g) groups were significantly suppressed on day 15 after DSS injury ($P<0.05$, respectively) (Fig. 1D). However, the thymus/BW ratios did not change (data not shown). Correspondingly, the colon length was significantly shortened in the DSS group compared with the normal control mice on day 15 (DSS 8.87±0.26 cm vs. Normal 11.00±0.07 cm; $P<0.0001$), whereas the lengths in the zonarol 20 mg/kg (10.88±0.28 cm) and 5-ASA (10.28±0.33 cm) treatment groups exhibited significantly suppressed colon shortening ($P<0.001$ and $P<0.05$, respectively) (Fig. 1D).

On the other hand, there was no remarkable change in mortality between the normal control and the DSS-induced colitic mice within 15 days (data not shown), but each group of animals was also free of complications, and none of the mice died during the study period.

Zonarol decreases the DSS-induced UC-associated histological changes in Slc:ICR mice

Corresponding to the above gross findings, including the DAI scores, DSS administration significantly enhanced the inflammation of the colon compared to the normal control mice, as indicated by several parameters, such as a higher histological score, characterized by subacute to chronic inflammatory cell

A

B

C

D

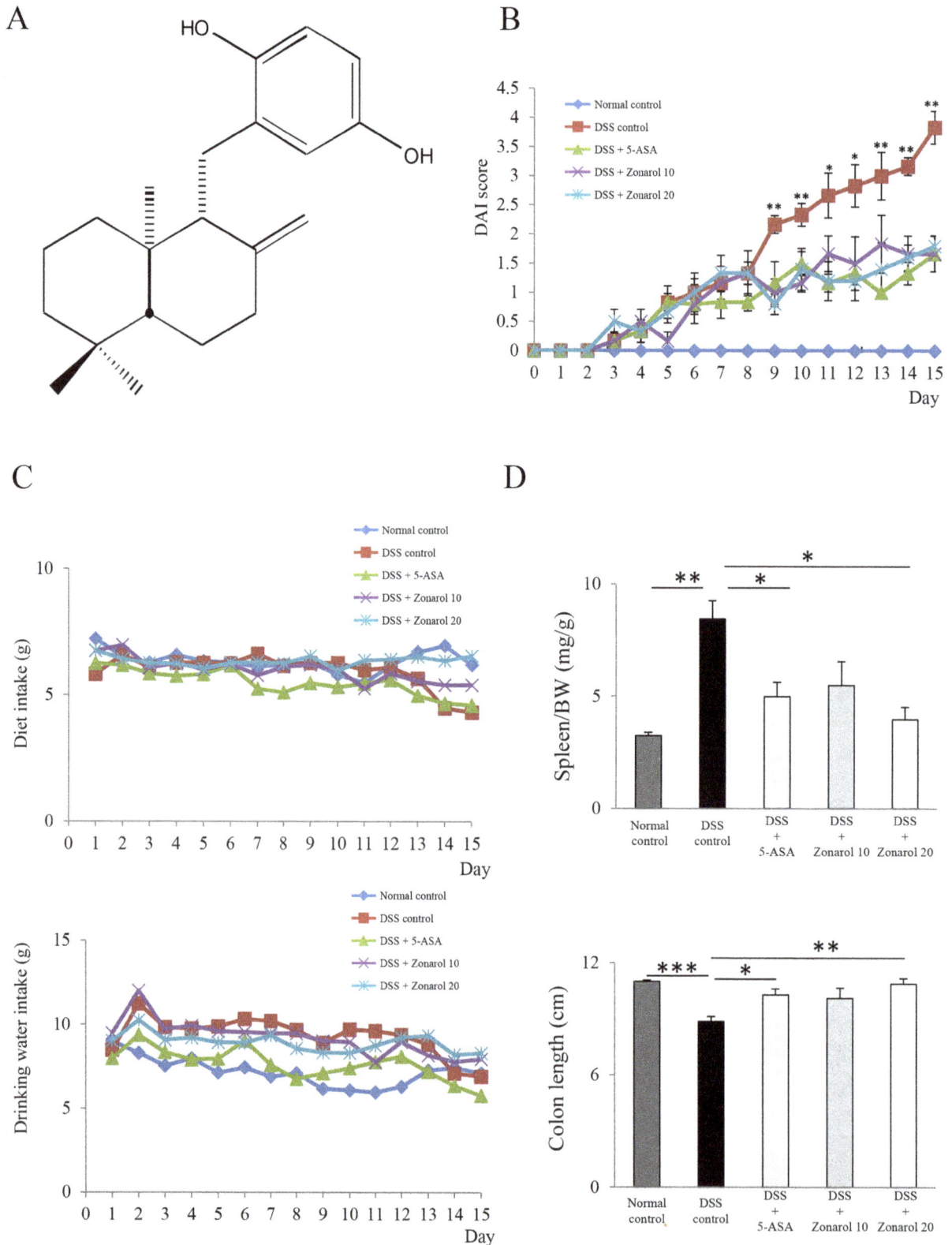

Figure 1. Zonarol suppresses DSS-induced UC in Slc:ICR mic. A) The chemical structure of zonarol, a sesquiterpene para-hydroquinone. **B**) The DAI scores were dramatically increased in DSS positive control mice compared with those in the other groups of mice treated with zonarol at 10 mg/kg or 20 mg/kg or 5-ASA 50 mg/kg from day 9 to 15. We observed no apparent difference in the DAI between the mice treated with zonarol and 5-ASA. **C**) There were no remarkable differences in the food and drinking water intake between the different groups of mice throughout the experimental period (n = 6 mice per group). However, the water intake in the DSS groups tended to be gradually and slightly decreased after DSS administration. **D**) On day 15 post-DSS administration (n = 6 mice per group), the spleen/BW ratio in the DSS control group was significantly elevated, whereas that in the zonarol 20 mg/kg and 5-ASA groups was not. Correspondingly, the colon length was significantly shortened in the DSS mice,

compared with the normal control mice on day 15 in the present UC model (n = 6 mice per group), whereas zonarol at 20 mg/kg and 5-ASA treatment both significantly suppressed the colon shortening. The values are the means ± SE. *P<0.05, **P<0.001, ***P<0.0001.

infiltration, erosion or occasional ulcer formation, and crypt loss (DSS 12.33±0.33 vs. Normal 0.67±0.21; P<0.0001) (Figs. 2A–C). Treatment with 5-ASA (7.17±0.65), as well as with zonarol at 10 mg/kg (7.33±0.95) and 20 mg/kg (5.40±1.36) significantly reduced the inflammatory histological score on day 15 (P<0.0001, P<0.05, and P<0.05, respectively) (Fig. 2A–C). Moreover, the sum of the histological ulcer length in the mice in the zonarol 20 mg/kg group (0.73±0.14 cm) was significantly longer than that in the normal control mice (0.00±0.00 cm) on day 15 post-DSS administration (P<0.05), but was significantly shorter than that in

the DSS positive control mice (3.68±1.25 cm) (P<0.05) (Fig. 2C). Indeed, the mice in the zonarol 20 mg/kg group had fewer and smaller colonic ulcers compared with the DSS positive control mice after DSS stimulation for 14 days (Fig. 2B). In contrast, the goblet cell number and size were not significantly between the untreated and each colitic group of mice, as confirmed by Alcian blue or PAS staining (data not shown).

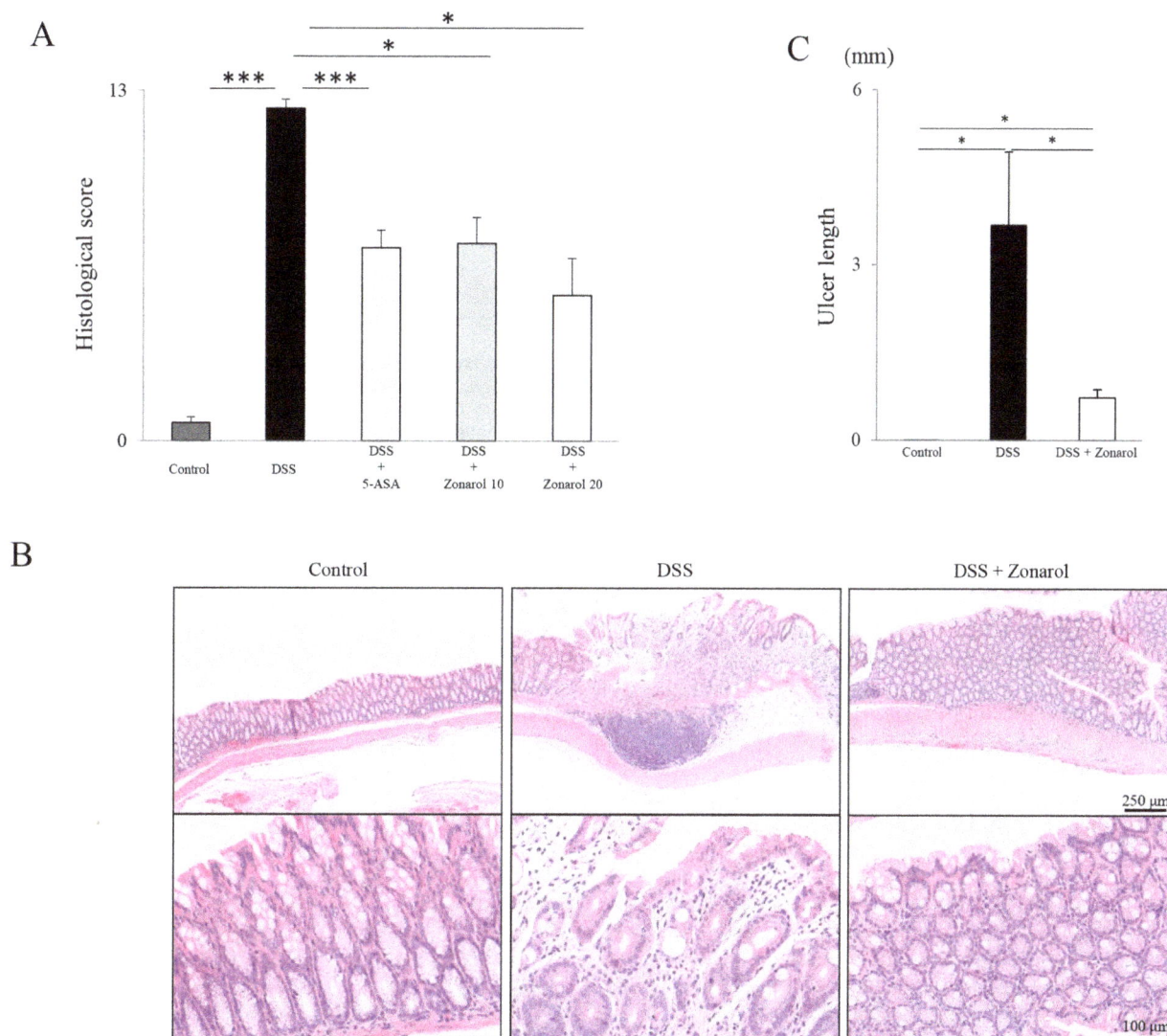

Figure 2. Zonarol histologically dampens DSS-induced UC in Slc:ICR mice. A) DSS administration resulted in a significantly higher histological score, characterized by acute and chronic inflammatory cell infiltration, erosion and/or occasional ulcer formation and crypt loss, compared to normal control mice (n = 6 mice per group). Both 5-ASA and zonarol at 10 and 20 mg/kg significantly reduced the inflammatory histological score on day 15. B) In the representative H&E-stained colon sections, fewer and smaller colonic ulcers were detected in the mice in the 20 mg/kg zonarol group, compared with the DSS positive control mice after DSS stimulation for 14 days (n = 6 mice per group). Normal control mice showed no remarkable changes in the colon on day 15. Upper panel: low-power view (Scale bar = 250 μm). Bottom panel: high-power view (Scale bar = 100 μm). C) The sum of the histological ulcer length in the mice in the 20 mg/kg zonarol was significantly larger than that in the normal control mice on day 15 post-DSS administration, but was smaller than that in the DSS positive control mice (n = 6 mice per group). The values are the means ± SE. *P<0.05, ***P<0.0001.

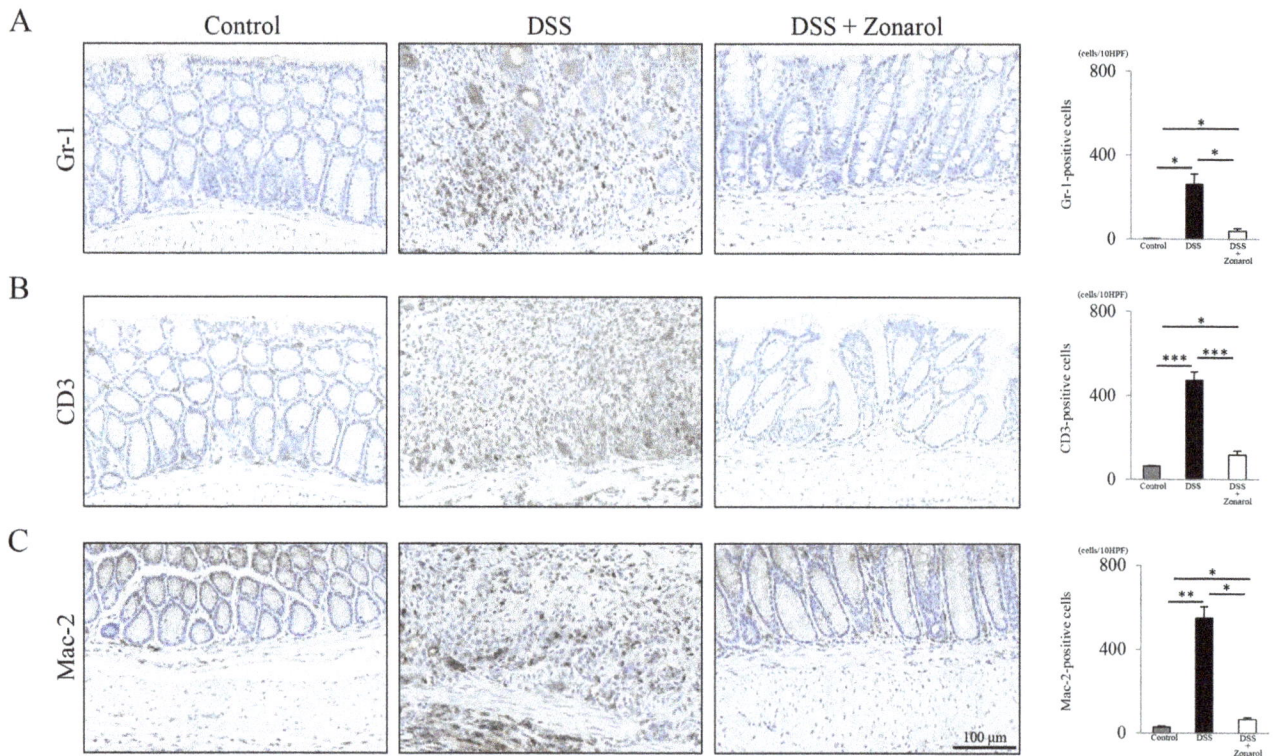

Figure 3. Zonarol represses the inflammatory responses in the subacute and chronic phases after DSS-administration in UC mice.
A) IHC for Gr-1 showed a significantly greater decrease in the numbers of accumulated neutrophils (i.e., subacute inflammatory cells) in the modestly injured colonic mucosa in the mice from the 20 mg/kg zonarol group compared to the positive control mouse colons on day 15 post-DSS administration (n = 6 mice per group). Fewer than 10 neutrophils per 100 crypts were noted in sham-treated normal control mice. **B, C**) IHC for CD3 revealed that the modestly-injured colons in mice from the 20 mg/kg zonarol group had significantly fewer infiltrating T-lymphocytes, especially around the crypts in the lamina propria, compared with the DSS positive control mice on day 15. In addition, Mac-2 staining showed that there were significantly fewer macrophages per mucosa in the mice in the 20 mg/kg zonarol group than in the mice in the positive control group. In contrast, untreated normal control animals had markedly fewer chronic inflammatory cells (T-lymphocytes and macrophages) compared to the mice in the 20 mg/kg zonarol group. Scale bar = 100 μm. Values are the means ± SE. *$P<0.05$, **$P<0.001$, ***$P<0.0001$.

Zonarol represses inflammatory responses in the both subacute and chronic phases after DSS administration

The Gr-1-positive cells (accumulated neutrophils) in the mice in the zonarol 20 mg/kg group were significantly more decreased than in the positive control mice colons on day 15 post-DSS administration (DSS 259.7±48.7 per 10 fields vs. Zonarol 36.6±12.8 per 10 fields; $P<0.05$) (Fig. 3A). No, or fewer than five, neutrophils per 10 high-power fields were noted in sham-treated normal control mice (Normal 2.5±0.4 per 10 fields) (Fig. 3A).

IHC for CD3 demonstrated that the modestly-injured colons in mice in the zonarol 20 mg/kg group contained significantly fewer infiltrating T-lymphocytes, especially around the crypts in the lamina propria, compared with the DSS positive control mice on day 15 (DSS 473.8±39.3 per 10 fields vs. Zonarol 116.6±18.6 per 10 fields; $P<0.0001$) (Fig. 3B). Mac-2-staining also revealed significantly fewer macrophages per areas of mucosa in the mice in the zonarol 20 mg/kg group than in the mice in the positive control group in the present UC model (DSS 549.5±53.8 per 10 fields vs. Zonarol 65.4±9.1 per 10 fields; $P<0.001$) (Fig. 3C). Untreated normal control animals had markedly fewer chronic inflammatory cells (Figs. 3B–C), such as CD3+ T lymphocytes (64.0±3.0 per 10 fields) and Mac-2+ macrophages (28.8±4.2 per 10 fields) compared to the mice treated with zonarol at 20 mg/kg ($P<0.05$, respectively).

Zonarol suppresses the expression of pro-inflammatory signaling molecules during DSS-induced UC

By performing an IF study, the TNF-α+ (red-stained) mucosal cells of the injured colons of the DSS-positive control mice were found to be much more common than those in the colons of the zonarol 20 mg/kg group (Fig. 4A). In addition, the numbers of both TNF-α+ (red-stained) and Mac-2+ (green-stained) macrophages in the lamina propria of the positive control mice were higher than those of the zonarol-treated mice 15 days after the DSS administration (Fig. 4A).

Next, we determined the levels of TNF-α and IL-6 in the serum by ELISA. Control mice had very low levels of expression, whereas TNF-α and IL-6 were significantly induced in the DSS-positive control mice. Zonarol significantly reduced the induction of TNF-α and IL-6 (TNF-α: Normal 3.85±0.67 pg/mL vs. DSS 8.23±1.21 pg/mL vs. Zonarol 3.66±1.24 pg/mL, $P<0.05$, respectively) (IL-6: Normal 5.85±2.08 pg/mL vs. DSS 36.54±8.98 pg/mL vs. Zonarol 5.57±2.23 pg/mL, $P<0.05$, respectively) (Fig. 4B).

Furthermore, IHC for iNOS revealed that, in mice with established DSS-induced UC, the iNOS expression level was overtly and substantially upregulated, especially in the surface colonic epithelium (Fig. 5A), but this was suppressed by zonarol treatments (Normal 0±0% vs. DSS 10.59±3.04% vs. Zonarol 2.28±1.20%, $P<0.05$, respectively) (Figs. 5A–B). No apparent

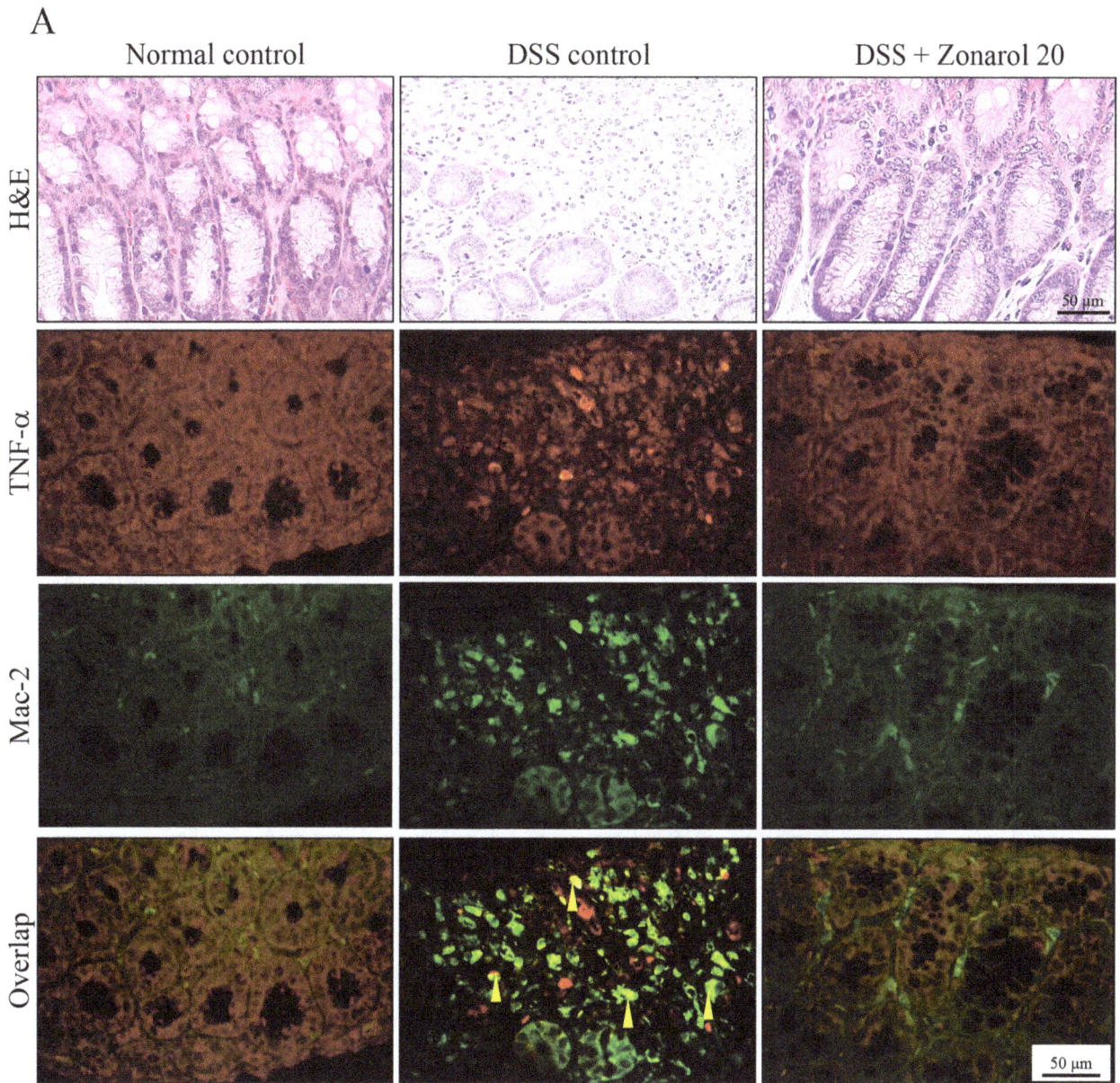

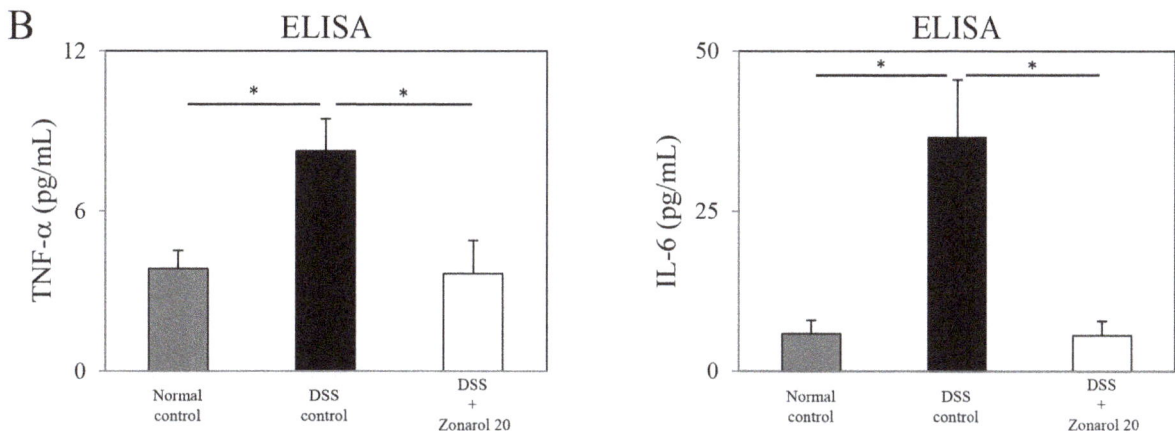

Figure 4. Zonarol suppresses the expression of pro-inflammatory signaling factors, such as TNF-α and IL-6, in mice with DSS-induced UC. A) The IF study revealed that the number of TNF-α[+] (*red-stained*) mucosal cells was obviously higher in the injured colons (H&E stain) of the DSS positive control mice than in the modestly inflamed colons (H&E stain) of the 20 mg/kg zonarol group (n = 6 mice per group). Additionally,

the number (overlap) of both TNF-α⁺ (red-stained) and Mac-2⁺ (green-stained) macrophages in the inflamed lamina propria was also significantly more increased in the positive control mice than in the zonarol-treated mice 15 days after the DSS administration based on the IF results. Sham-treated normal control animals showed no remarkable changes, and carried no or very few cells with overlapping staining. **B**) Corresponding to these IHC and IF data, an ELISA demonstrated that the serum levels of not only TNF-α, but also IL-6, were significantly higher in the DSS positive control mice than in both the zonarol-treated mice and the normal control mice (n = 6 mice per group). Scale bar = 50 μm. The values are the means ± SE. *P< 0.05.

iNOS-positive areas were seen in the untreated normal control mice.

Zonarol decreases the apoptotic activity of the colonic epithelium in the DSS-induced UC model

Although a small, but substantial, number of apoptotic epithelial cells in crypts was observed in each group of mice 15 days after the DSS administration, the number of TUNEL⁺ large intestinal epithelial cells in the zonarol-treated mice was significantly higher than that in the normal control mice on day 15 post-DSS administration ($P<0.05$), but was significantly smaller than that in the DSS positive control mice ($P<0.05$) (Fig. 6A) (Normal 4.67±0.88 per 100 crypts vs. DSS 27.00±4.16 per 100 crypts vs. Zonarol 7.60±1.21 per 100 crypts; $P<0.05$, respectively). Double-IF staining (Fig. 6B) confirmed that these apoptotic cells (green-stained in the nuclei) were CK20⁺ colonic epithelial cells in the crypts (red-stained in the cytoplasm).

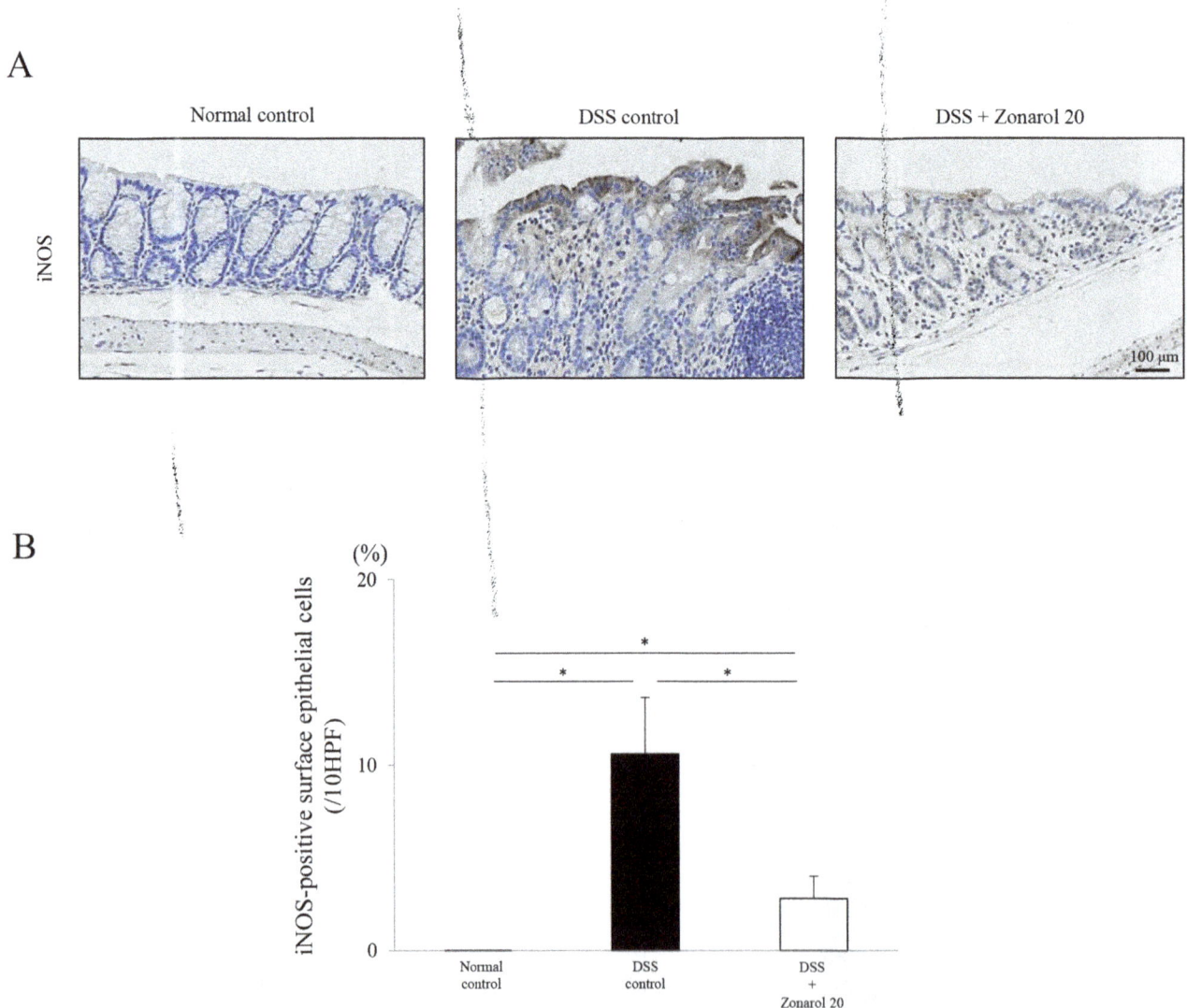

Figure 5. Zonarol suppresses the expression of pro-inflammatory signaling molecules, such as iNOS, in mice with DSS-induced UC.
A, B) IHC of iNOS showed that, in established DSS-induced UC, the iNOS expression level (i.e., the iNOS-positive area) was substantially upregulated, especially in the surface colonic epithelium of the DSS positive control mice, but not in the mice treated with zonarol, on day 15 post-DSS administration (n = 6 mice per group). No apparent iNOS-positive areas were seen in the sham-treated normal control mice. Scale bar = 100 μm. The values are the means ± SE. *P<0.05.

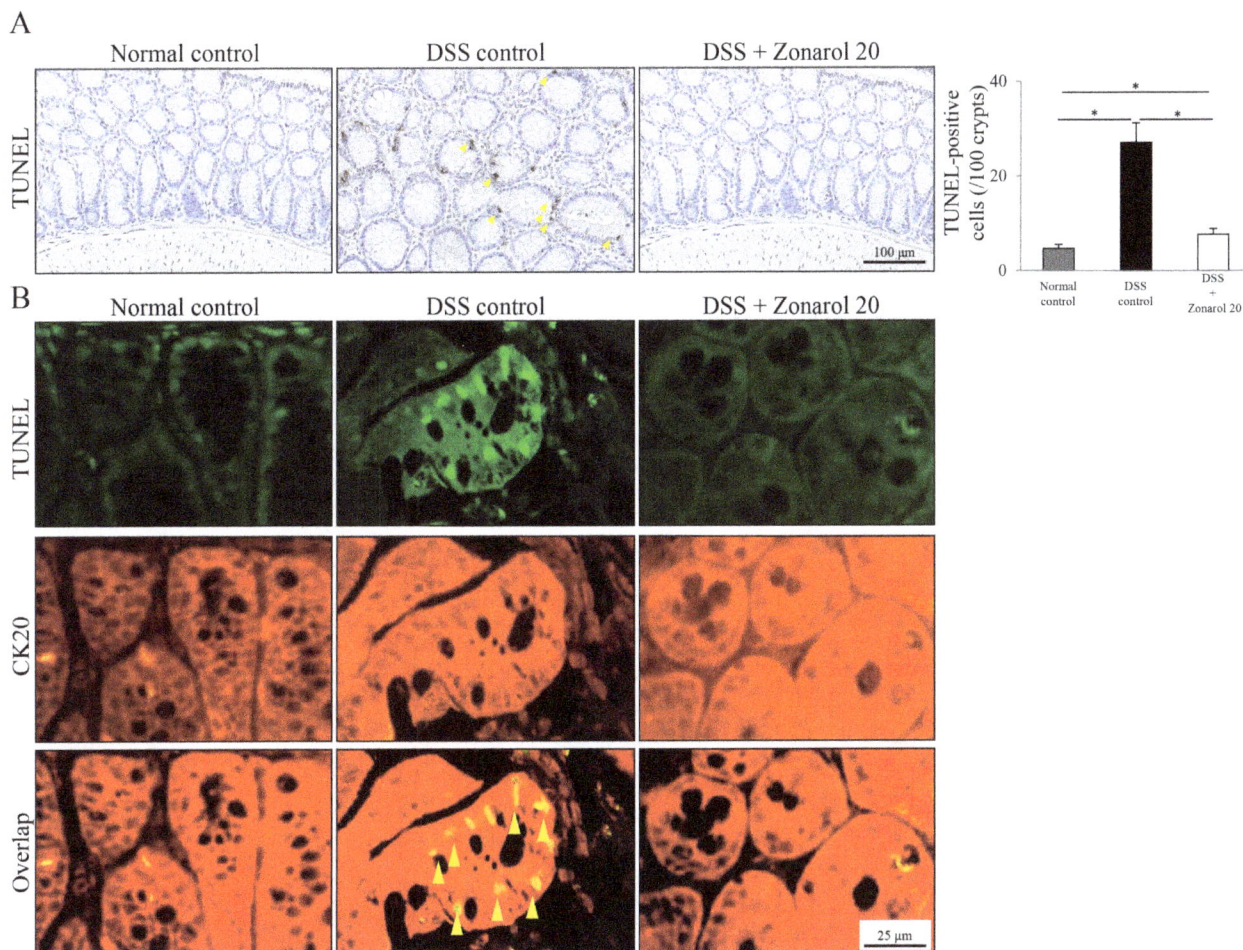

Figure 6. Zonarol reduces the apoptotic activity of the colonic epithelium in mice with DSS-induced UC. A) A small but substantial number of apoptotic epithelial cells (TUNEL staining) in crypts were identified in each group of mice 15 days after the administration of DSS (n = 6 mice per group). The number of TUNEL+ (*green-stained* in nuclei) large intestinal epithelial cells in the zonarol-treated mice was significantly larger than that in the normal control mice on day 15 post-DSS administration, but was smaller than that in the DSS positive control mice. **B)** Double-IF staining confirmed that these TUNEL+ apoptotic cells (*green-stained* in nuclei) were CK20+ colonic epithelial cells in the crypts (*red-stained* in cytoplasm). Scale bars = 100 μm (medium-power view); and 25 μm (high-power view). The values are the means ± SE. *$P<0.05$.

Zonarol inhibits NO production without any effects on the survival of cultured RAW264.7 cells after LPS-stimulation

In order to confirm the absence of cytotoxicity at the concentrations used in the present *in vitro* study, we exposed RAW264.7 cells to different concentrations of zonarol and LPS (applied alone or in combination). After a 24 h incubation with different concentrations (0, 1, 2 and 5 μM) or zonarol, the viability of the cells was determined by performing a standard MTT assay. As shown in Figure 7A, the application of zonarol for 24 h at the indicated concentrations did not affect the viability of the cells, as indicated by the stable metabolic activity. Furthermore, the application of LPS (10 μg/mL), alone or together with different concentrations of zonarol, did not significantly affect the cell viability (Fig. 7A). Thus, none of the conditions used in the present study affected cell survival.

A hallmark of macrophage activation is the production of NO in response to LPS. Therefore, we determined whether or not zonarol could modulate the NO production in LPS-activated RAW264.7 cells by using the sister cultures used in the MTT assay. As shown in Figure 7B, LPS induced a strong increase in NO production in the RAW264.7 cells 24 h after LPS stimulation compared with the control level. Zonarol significantly suppressed the LPS-induced increase in NO in a concentration-dependent manner (Fig. 7B).

Zonarol downregulates the expression of immune system mediators in cultured RAW264.7 cells after LPS stimulation

In order to confirm the inhibition of the hyperactivation of macrophages by zonarol, we examined the effects of the compound on other pro-inflammatory factors (IL-1β, IL-6 and iNOS) by performing RT-PCR (Fig. 8A–C, respectively). In the absence of LPS, the cells had very low expression levels of these genes; but in its presence, there was a significant increase in their expression levels. Zonarol at 2 μM modestly decreased the mRNA levels of IL-1β, IL-6 and iNOS (Fig. 8A–C, respectively).

Discussion

The present study revealed, for the first time, a protective role for zonarol, a marine natural product isolated from *Dictyopteris*

A

MTT assay

B

NO production assay

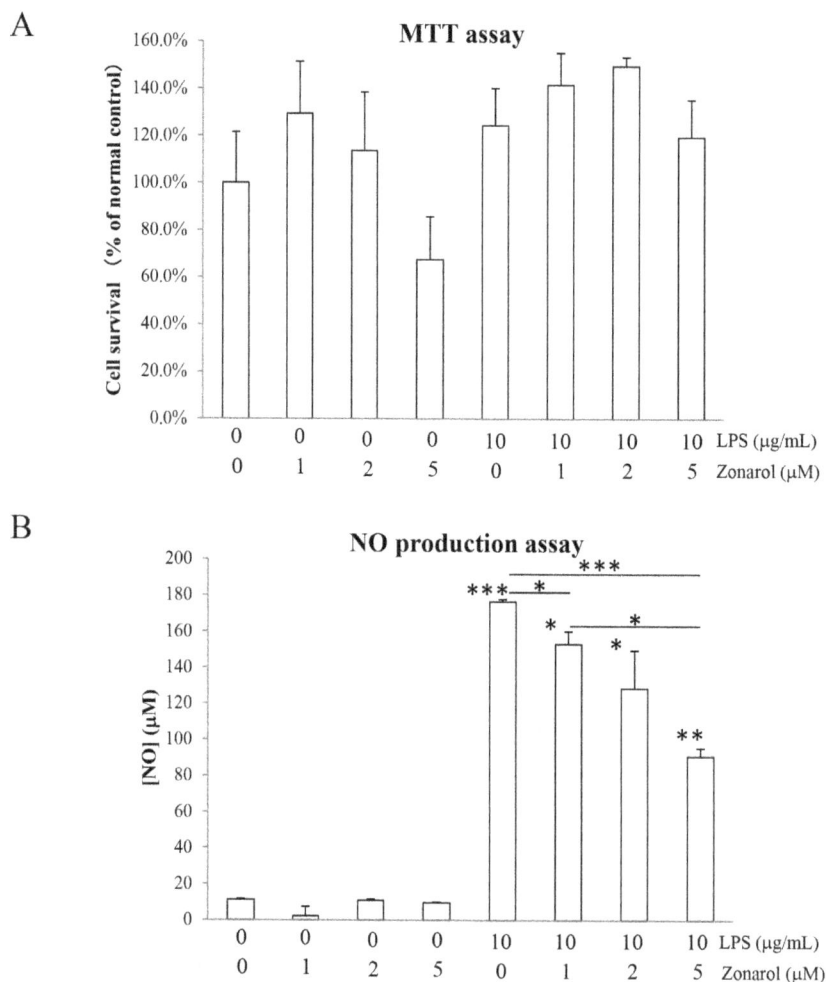

Figure 7. Zonarol inhibits NO production without any effects on the survival of cultured RAW264.7 cells after LPS stimulation. A) Cell survival. RAW264.7 cells were incubated for 24 h with the various combinations of zonarol and LPS, as indicated in the figure. The cell viability was determined using the MTT assay. Note that there were no significant differences in the viability of any of the treated cells compared to the normal or positive control cells. **B) NO production.** The LPS-induced NO production was inhibited by zonarol in a dose-dependent manner in RAW264.7 cells. The RAW264.7 cells were treated with combinations of LPS and zonarol for 24 h, and the NO concentrations were determined using the Griess reagent. The values are the means ± SD from four separate measurements. * and ** Significant differences ($P<0.05$ and 0.001, respectively) compared with the 0 μg/mL LPS- and 0 μM zonarol-treated cells (normal control) or the 10 μg/mL LPS- and zonarol 0 (positive control) or 1 μM-treated cells.

undulata, in a mouse model of UC. Seaweed zonarol significantly reduced the DSS-induced inflammation and apoptosis in Slc:ICR mice, very similar to 5-ASA treatments. Zonarol administration led to anti-inflammatory effects, including reduced bloody diarrhea, a decreased spleen/BW and less shortening of the colon length, a suppression of the extensive inflammatory and pro-inflammatory reactions and decreased apoptotic activity of the colonic epithelium in the large intestine. These pharmacological effects improved the DAI score, especially in the second half of day 9 to 15-post-DSS injury. Since UC is a chronic and idiopathic IBD mediated by various types of immune dysfuction [1,2], zonarol might offer a promising therapeutic strategy and/or an alternative/additive therapy without any apparent adverse effects. We can also propose that DSS-induced apoptosis closely correlates with the potency of the inflammatory responses. Furthermore, we confirmed that the marine hydroquinone, zonarol, had anti-inflammatory actions in the RAW264.7 mouse macrophage cell line under *in vitro* LPS stimulation. However, our study has two limitations in its interpretation: the absence of a prevention

administration of zonarol, as should be the case with nutraceuticals; and the model of colitis, which is a chemical but not immune model, even though it is an accepted one.

Polyphenols have received a great deal of attention, and are a category of compounds commonly used to treat various diseases, because they are present in teas, fruits and vegetables, and these play a pivotal role in anti-inflammatory responses due to their potent antioxidant effects [10,12,30–32]. Other groups have reported the protective roles of green tea and apple polyphenols against the same model of UC in mice [31,32]. The administration of polyphenols significantly suppressed the DAI score, along with reducing the histological severity of colitis and downregulating the expression of pro-inflammatory signaling factors, such as TNF-α, IL-1β and IL-6 [31,32]. Since our data regarding zonarol are novel in terms of the inhibition of UC by a marine bioproduct, zonarol may be useful as an alternative/additive herbal therapy (i.e., a complementary and alternative medicine (CAM)) for human UC. It is also conceivable that treatment with a marine natural product, zonarol, would have no severe side effects.

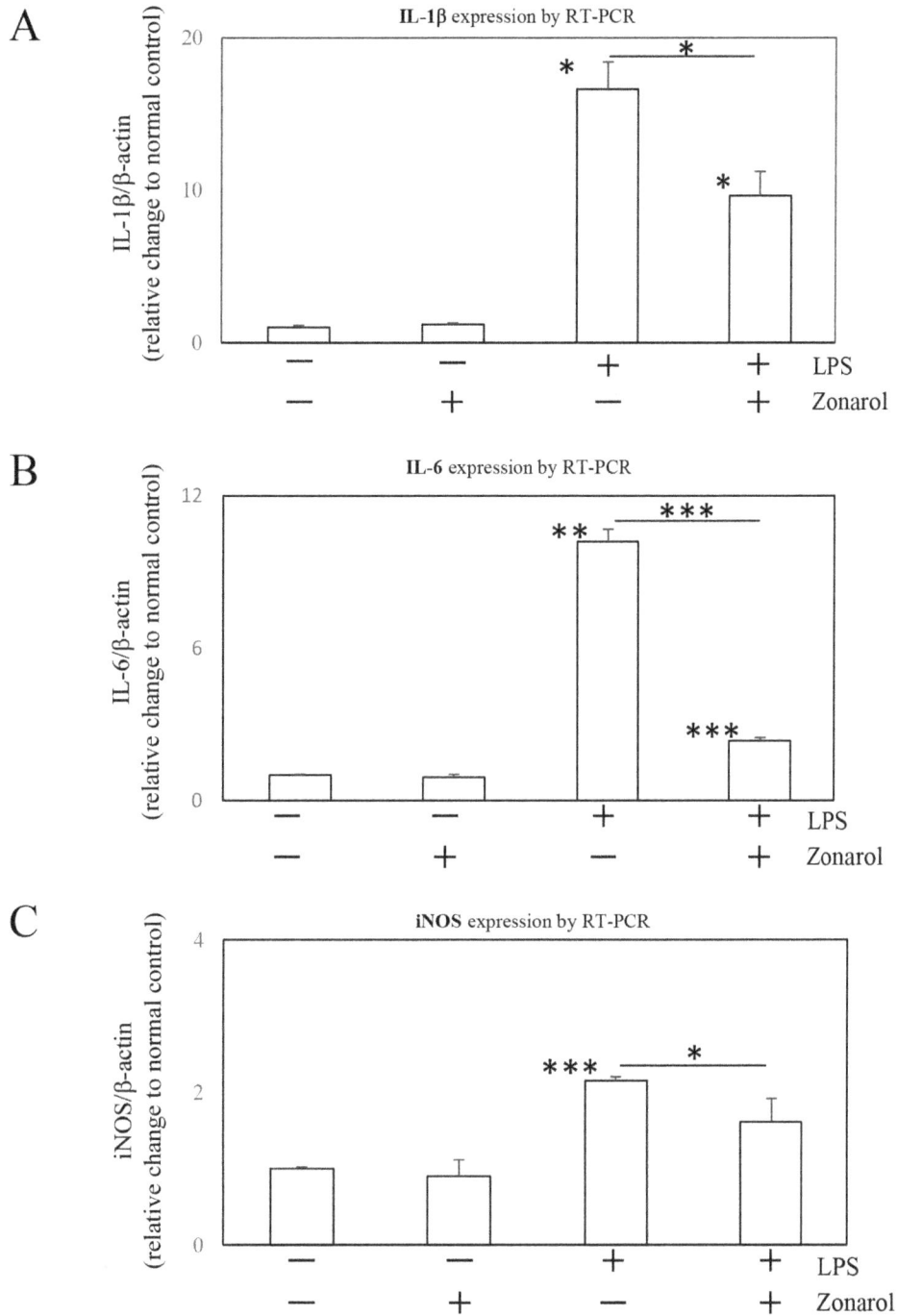

Figure 8. Zonarol downregulates the expression of immune system mediators in cultured RAW264.7 cells after LPS stimulation. A, B, C) RAW264.7 cells were left untreated or were treated with zonarol (10 µM), LPS (10 µg/ml) or both for 24 h. The levels of IL-1β, IL-6 and iNOS mRNA were determined by RT-PCR. In the absence of LPS, the cells had very low expression levels of these genes; whereas in the presence of LPS, there was a significant increase in their expression. Zonarol at a concentration of 2 µM significantly decreased the mRNA levels of IL-1β (A), IL-6 (B) and iNOS (C). The values are the means ± SD from four separate measurements and were normalized to the β-actin expression (RT-PCR). *, **, and *** Significant differences (P<0.05, 0.001, and 0.0001, respectively) compared with the 0 µg/mL LPS- and 0 µM zonarol-treated cells (normal control).

Further follow-up investigations of the safety and efficacy of zonarol will be necessary before it can be considered for use against human IBDs.

Macrophages may play a key role in the DSS-induced UC via their expression of TNF-α. The current *in vivo* model showed chronic, but not acute, inflammatory cells-rich damaged mucosa consisting of a larger number of macrophages, rather than neutrophils and T-lymphocytes. Furthermore, TNF-α is the major and central key cytokine involved in initiating and perpetuating the colonic inflammatory responses in UC, and in fact, it has been recently reported that the most successful treatments for human IBDs are therapeutics targeting TNF-α [33,34]. We herein used both an *in vivo* UC model and an *in vitro* macrophage cell line to assess the anti-inflammatory effects. Zonarol significantly suppressed the inflammatory reactions of the mouse macrophage cell line, RAW264.7, after stimulation by LPS, by downregulating the expression of various immune system mediators, including ILs and/or iNOS, and subsequently reducing the NO production. Consistent with these findings, the *in vivo* administration of the zonarol extract significantly decreased the levels of iNOS expression in the injured colonic surface epithelium, in addition to repressing various inflammatory and pro-inflammatory cytokines, such as TNF-α or IL-6. The NO system is an important signaling pathway associated with colonic inflammation, and is involved in strengthening the mucus barrier and potentially reducing the risk of subsequent tumorigenesis [35,36]. Therefore, zonarol might reduce the risk of UC-associated cancer, even though zonarol treatments did not significantly affect the number or size of mucus-producing goblet cells in the present study. Further molecular and morphological studies are needed to clarify this possibility.

We herein demonstrated that zonarol inhibited the apoptosis of the colonic epithelium, possibly by interfering with a TNF-α-mediated signaling pathway. A smaller number of TUNEL$^+$ colonic epithelial cells in the zonarol-treated mice was found compared to that in the DSS positive control mice. These results are also in line with findings of other groups, such as the finding that p53-upregulated modulator of apoptosis (PUMA) induction by TNF-α contributed to activating inflammation and epithelial apoptosis in the large intestine of a DSS-induced animal model of UC, and conversely, its suppression by anti-TNF-α antibody treatments prevented colitis and repressed the apoptotic activity of the colonic epithelium [37]. In fact, anti-TNF-α therapies for treating human IBD patients have been revealed to inhibit not only the inflammatory responses, but also epithelial cell apoptosis [37,38]. Apoptosis has been considered to be one of major hallmarks in strongly regulating homeostatic and pathogenic mechanisms of intestinal epithelium in IBDs, even though the molecular basis of epithelial apoptosis in response to aberrant intestinal inflammation is unclear [39]. On the other hand, apoptosis in the colonic epithelium is responsible for disrupting the mucosal integrity and barrier function to bacterial invasion [37–39]. In these senses, it remains to be elucidated whether apoptosis or inflammation comes first in the development of UC, reminiscent of the chicken-and-egg problem. Taken together, our present data showed, for the first time, that a marine hydroquinone can play a pivotal role in protecting against both colitis and apoptosis, decreasing the activity of UC, at least partially by inhibiting the TNF-α signaling pathway.

In conclusion, based on our collected data, we believe that zonarol plays critical and broad functional roles in ameliorating DSS-induced colonic injury (i.e., improves the DAI score), together with (i) reducing the accumulation and recruitment of various inflammatory cells into the modestly damaged mucosa, accompanied by downregulation of the expression of various inflammatory and pro-inflammatory mediators; (ii) in particular,

by decreasing the number of mucosal TNF-α-expressing macrophages; (iii) suppressing the apoptosis of the intestinal epithelium. This was strongly supported by (iv) the *in vitro* experiments, showing that zonarol alleviated the inflammatory responses of the mouse RAW264.7 cells after stimulation by LPS. Hence, we can conclude that zonarol prevents the development of subacute (induced by macrophages, T-lymphocytes, and to a lesser extent neutrophils) to chronic (predominantly induced by macrophages and T-lymphocytes) inflammatory responses and the subsequent apoptotic activity, exerting various beneficial effects in the DSS-induced mouse model of UC. All of these features indicate that the oral administration of the marine hydroquinone, zonarol, from *Dictyopteris undulata* might offer an alternative/additive therapeutic strategy (i.e., CAM) against human IBDs, including UC.

Supporting Information

Figure S1 A schematic presentation of the experimental procedure in DSS-induced mice UC model. DSS: dextran sulfate sodium, 5-ASA: 5-aminosalicylic acid, DAI: disease activity index, H&E: hematoxylin and eosin, IHC: immunohistochemistry, IF: immunofluorescence.
(PPTX)

Figure S2 The separation scheme for compound 1. The MeOH extract from the seaweed *Dictyopteris undulate* showed anti-edematous activity in mice. Bioassay-guided fractionation of the crude extract (108.0 g as 100%) gave compound 1 (1.1% of yield), which had the activity. MeOH: methanol, HPLC: high performance liquid chromatography, ODS: Octadecyl Silyl.
(PPTX)

Figure S3 Inhibitory effects of purified zonarol in a carrageenan-induced paw edema mouse model. A) An increased paw edema volume. **B**) The increase in paw edema thickness. Open circles: control. Closed circles: zonarol (62.5 mg/kg) administration. Each value represents the mean ± SE. (n = 5 mice per group). *$P < 0.05$ vs control.
(PPTX)

Figure S4 The NMR spectral data of purified zonarol. A) The proton NMR data (400 MHz, MeOD). **B**) The carbon NMR data (100 MHz, MeOD). NMR: nuclear magnetic resonance.
(PPTX)

Acknowledgments

We would like to thank Hana Nishimura and Naoko Une for their expert technical assistance.

Author Contributions

Conceived and designed the experiments: SY TK TS. Performed the experiments: SY TK YU RK HS TS. Analyzed the data: SY TK HN YS TS. Contributed reagents/materials/analysis tools: AT KYW AN TN. Wrote the paper: SY TK TS. Contributed excellent technical assistance and helpful comments: AT TN YS.

References

1. Podolsky DK (2002) Inflammatory bowel disease. N Engl J Med 347: 417–429.
2. Xavier RJ, Podolsky DK (2007) Unravelling the pathogenesis of inflammatory bowel disease. Nature 448: 427–434.
3. Sanchez-Munoz F, Dominguez-Lopez A, Yamamoto-Furusho JK (2008) Role of cytokines in inflammatory bower disease. World J Gastroenterol 14: 4280–4288.
4. Olsen T, Goll R, Cui G, Husebekk A, Vonen B, et al. (2007) Tissue levels of tumor necrosis factor-alpha correlates with grade of inflammation in untreated ulcerative colitis. Scand J Gastroenterol 42: 1312–1320.

5. Kwon KH, Murakami A, Hayashi R, Ohigashi H (2005) Interleukin-1beta targets interleukin-6 in progressing dextran sulfate sodium-induced experimental colitis. Biochem Biophys Res Commun 337: 647–654.
6. Obermeier F, Kojouharoff G, Hans W, Schölmerich J, Gross V, et al. (1999) Interferon-gamma (IFN-gamma)- and tumour necrosis factor (TNF)-induced nitric oxide as toxic effector molecule in chronic dextran sulphate sodium (DSS)-induced colitis in mice. Clin Exp Immunol 116: 238–245.
7. Katsanos KH, Voulgari PV, Tsianos EV (2012) Inflammatory bowel disease and lupus: a systematic review of the literature. J Crohns Colitis 6: 735–742.

8. Linares V, Alonso V, Domingo JL (2011) Oxidative stress as a mechanism underlying sulfasalazine-induced toxicity. Expert Opin Drug Saf 10: 253–263.

9. Montrose DC, Horelik NA, Madigan JP, Stoner GD, Wang LS, et al. (2011) Anti-inflammatory effects of freeze-dried black raspberry powder in ulcerative colitis. Carcinogenesis 32: 343–350.

10. Opheim R, Bernklev T, Fagermoen MS, Cvancarova M, Moum B (2012) Use of complementary and alternative medicine in patients with inflammatory bowel disease: results of a cross-sectional study in Norway. Scand J Gastroenterol 47: 1436–1447.

11. Szigethy E, McLafferty L, Goyal A (2011) Inflammatory bowel disease. Pediatr Clin North Am 58: 903–920.

12. Geerling BJ, Badart-Smook A, Stockbrügger RW, Brummer RJ (2000) Comprehensive nutritional status in recently diagnosed patients with inflammatory bowel disease compared with population controls. Eur J Clin Nutr 54: 514–521.

13. Koyama T, Shirosaki M, Ishii M, Hirose T, Yazawa K (2010) New value and functionality found in undeveloped food materials. J Jpn Soc Med Use Func Foods (In Japanese) 6: 109–114.

14. Fenical W, Sims JJ, Squatrito D, Wing RM, Radlick P (1973) Zonarol and isozonarol, fungitoxic hydroquinones from the brown seaweed *Dictyopteris zonarioides*. J Org Chem 38: 2383–2386.

15. Cimino G, de Stefano S, Fenical W, Minale L, Sims JJ (1975) Zonaroic acid from the brown seaweed *Dictyopteris undulate* (which is the same as zonarioides). Experientia 31: 1250–1251.

16. Mori K, Komatsu M (1986) Synthesis and absolute configuration of zonarol, a fungitoxic hydroquinone from the brown seaweed *Dictyopteris zonarioides*. Bulletin des Societes Chimiques Belges 95: 771–781.

17. Lee JH, Kim GH (2013) Evaluation of antioxidant activity of marine algae-extracts from Korea. J Aquatic Food Product Technol. (online: 11 Oct, 2013). DOI:10.1080/10498850.2013.770809.

18. Mayer AMS, Paul VJ, Fenical W, Norris JN, de Carvalho MS, et al. (1993) Phospholipase A$_2$ inhibitors from marine algae. Hydrobiologia 260/261: 521–529.

19. Taniguchi K, Yamada J, Kurata K, Suzuki M (1993) Feeding-deterrents from the brown alga *Dictyopteris undulata* against the abalone Haliotis discus hannai. Nippon Suisan Gakkaishi (in Japanese) 59: 339–343.

20. Ishibashi F, Sato S, Sakai K, Hirao S, Kuwano K (2013) Algicidal sesquiterpene hydroquinones from the brown alga *Dictyopteris undulata*. Biosci Biotech Biochem 77: 1120–1122.

21. Sha T, Igaki K, Yamasaki M, Watanabe T, Tsuchimori N (2013) Establishment and validation of a new semi-chronic dextran sulfate sodium-induced model of colitis in mice. Int Immunopharmacol 15: 23–29.

22. Noguchi H, Yamada S, Nabeshima A, Guo X, Tanimoto A, et al. (2014) Depletion of apoptosis signal-regulating kinase 1 prevents bile duct ligation-induced necro-inflammation and subsequent peribiliary fibrosis. Am J Pathol 184: 644–661.

23. Nabeshima A, Yamada S, Guo X, Tanimoto A, Wang KY, et al. (2013) Peroxiredoxin 4 protects against nonalcoholic steatohepatitis and type 2 diabetes in a nongenetic mouse model. Antioxid Redox Signal 19: 1983–1998.

24. Tasaki T, Yamada S, Guo X, Tanimoto A, Wang KY, et al. (2013) Apoptosis signal-regulating kinase 1 deficiency attenuates vascular injury-induced neoin-timal hyperplasia by suppressing apoptosis in smooth muscle cells. Am J Pathol 182: 597–609.

25. Yamada S, Ding Y, Tanimoto A, Wang KY, Guo X, et al. (2011) Apoptosis signal-regulating kinase 1 deficiency accelerates hyperlipidemia-induced atheromatous plaques via suppression of macrophage apoptosis. Arterioscler Thromb Vasc Biol 31: 1555–1564.

26. Yamada S, Wang KY, Tanimoto A, Fan J, Shimajiri S, et al. (2008) Matrix metalloproteinase 12 accelerates the initiation of atherosclerosis and stimulates the progression of fatty streaks to fibrous plaques in transgenic rabbits. Am J Pathol 172: 1419–1429.

27. Satoh T, Kosaka K, Itoh K, Kobayashi A, Yamamoto M, et al. (2008) Carnosic acid, a catechol-type electrophilic compound, protects neurons both in vitro and in vivo through activation of the Keap1/Nrf2 pathway via S-alkylation of targeted cysteines on Keap1. J Neurochem 104: 1116–1131.

28. Takenouchi T, Ogihara K, Sato M, Kitani H (2005) Inhibitory effects of U73122 and U73343 on Ca^{2+} influx and pore formation induced by the activation of P2X7 nucleotide receptors in mouse microglial cell line. Biochim Biophys Acta 1726: 177–186.

29. Yanagitai M, Kitagawa T, Takenouchi T, Kitani H, Satoh T (2012) Carnosic acid, a pro-electrophilic compound, inhibits LPS-induced activation of microglia. Biochem Biophys Res Commun 418: 22–26.

30. Larrosa M, Luceri C, Vivoli E, Pagliuca C, Lodovici M, et al. (2009) Polyphenol metabolites from colonic microbiota exert anti-inflammatory activity on different inflammation models. Mol Nutr Food Res 53: 1044–1054.

31. Oz HS, Chen T, de Villiers WJ (2013) Green Tea Polyphenols and Sulfasalazine have Parallel Anti-Inflammatory Properties in Colitis Models. Front Immunol 4: e132.

32. Skyberg JA, Robison A, Golden S, Rollins MF, Callis G, et al. (2011) Apple polyphenols require T cells to ameliorate dextran sulfate sodium-induced colitis and dampen proinflammatory cytokine expression. J Leukoc Biol 90: 1043–1054.

33. Reinisch W, Sandborn WJ, Rutgeerts P, Feagan BG, Rachmilewitz D, et al. (2012) Long-term infliximab maintenance therapy for ulcerative colitis: the ACT-1 and -2 extension studies. Inflamm Bowel Dis 18: 201–211.

34. Rutgeerts P, Sandborn WJ, Feagan BG, Reinisch W, Olson A, et al. (2005) Infliximab for induction and maintenance therapy for ulcerative colitis. N Engl J Med 353: 2462–2476.

35. Schreiber O, Petersson J, Waldén T, Ahl D, Sandler S, et al. (2013) iNOS-dependent increase in colonic mucus thickness in DSS-colitic rats. PLoS One 8: e71843.

36. Kubes P, McCafferty DM (2000) Nitric oxide and intestinal inflammation. Am J Med 109: 150–158.

37. Qiu W, Wu B, Wang X, Buchanan ME, Regueiro MD, et al. (2011) PUMA-mediated intestinal epithelial apoptosis contributes to ulcerative colitis in humans and mice. J Clin Invest 121: 1722–1732.

38. Zeissig S, Bojarski C, Buergel N, Mankertz J, Zeitz M, et al. (2004) Downregulation of epithelial apoptosis and barrier repair in active Crohn's disease by tumour necrosis factor alpha antibody treatment. Gut 53: 1295–1302.

39. Edelblum KL, Yan F, Yamaoka T, Polk DB (2006) Regulation of apoptosis during homeostasis and disease in the intestinal epithelium. Inflamm Bowel Dis 12: 413–424.

19

Live Imaging and Gene Expression Analysis in Zebrafish Identifies a Link between Neutrophils and Epithelial to Mesenchymal Transition

Christina M. Freisinger, Anna Huttenlocher*

Departments of Pediatrics and Medical Microbiology and Immunology, University of Wisconsin-Madison, Madison, Wisconsin, United States of America

Abstract

Chronic inflammation is associated with epithelial to mesenchymal transition (EMT) and cancer progression however the relationship between inflammation and EMT remains unclear. Here, we have exploited zebrafish to visualize and quantify the earliest events during epithelial cell transformation induced by oncogenic HRas^{V12}. Live imaging revealed that expression of HRas^{V12} in the epidermis results in EMT and chronic neutrophil and macrophage infiltration. We have developed an *in vivo* system to probe and quantify gene expression changes specifically in transformed cells from chimeric zebrafish expressing oncogenic HRas^{V12} using translating ribosomal affinity purification (TRAP). We found that the expression of genes associated with EMT, including *slug*, *vimentin* and *mmp9*, are enriched in HRas^{V12} transformed epithelial cells and that this enrichment requires the presence of neutrophils. An early signal induced by HRas^{V12} in epithelial cells is the expression of *il-8* (*cxcl8*) and we found that the chemokine receptor, Cxcr2, mediates neutrophil but not macrophage recruitment to the transformed cells. Surprisingly, we also found a cell autonomous role for Cxcr2 signaling in transformed cells for both neutrophil recruitment and EMT related gene expression associated with Ras transformation. Taken together, these findings implicate both autocrine and paracrine signaling through Cxcr2 in the regulation of inflammation and gene expression in transformed epithelial cells.

Editor: Olivier de Wever, Ghent University, Belgium

Funding: This work was supported by the National Institutes of Health (NIH) Grant R01 GM074827 (A. Huttenlocher), NCI Grant NIH R01 GM102924-01 (A. Huttenlocher), National Institute of Environmental Health Sciences grant ES007015 (to C.M. Freisinger) and National Cancer Institute grant CA157322 (to C.M. Freisinger). The funders had no role in study design, data collection and analysis, decision to publish, or preparation of the manuscript.

Competing Interests: The authors have declared that no competing interests exist.

* Email: huttenlocher@wisc.edu

Introduction

Epithelial to mesenchymal transition (EMT) is essential for normal embryonic development, but also occurs during wound healing and the invasion of transformed cells during cancer progression [1,2]. One main difference between the activation of programmed EMT during early development and EMT associated with pathology is the presence of inflammation [3]. Chronic inflammation associated with diseases like Rheumatoid Arthritis, Crohns disease, Chronic obstructive pulmonary disease (COPD) and pancreatitis is known to increase cancer risk [4,5] and neutrophil depletion has been shown to reduce tumor burden in a mouse model of lung cancer [6]. The connection between inflammation and cancer risk is further supported by studies that suggest that treatment with anti-inflammatory agents can decrease the incidence of some cancers [7–9]. Although chronic inflammation has been linked to EMT and cancer invasion [10–12], it is not clear how innate immune inflammation is associated with EMT and participates in cancer progression.

Understanding how transformed cells induce chronic innate immune inflammation in tissues and if this inflammation plays a role in EMT progression has been limited due to the difficulty visualizing the early tissue microenvironment around small clusters of transformed epithelial cells in live animals. Zebrafish is therefore an ideal model system to study these questions since zebrafish larvae are transparent allowing for real time imaging of EMT in live animals. Indeed, zebrafish have emerged as a powerful model system to study the pathogenesis of cancer since many of the signaling pathways and mechanisms are conserved [13,14]. In fact, recent progress in zebrafish has identified signaling pathways that mediate leukocyte recruitment to wounds [15–17], infection [18] and transformed melanocytes [19]. Additionally, chronic inflammation of the epidermis in zebrafish has been associated with the activation of EMT programs and developmental defects in epidermal homeostasis, further supporting the use of zebrafish to study the relationship between inflammation and EMT [10,20].

Chemokine-dependent signaling in immune cells is an important mechanism that mediates leukocyte recruitment to bacterial infections and wounds. A large body of work has explored the role of the chemokine (C-X-C motif) receptor 2 (CXCR2) during leukocyte recruitment to sites of inflammation [6,15–19,21–23]. Previous studies, utilizing the zebrafish model system, have shown that Cxcr2 receptor signaling axis is involved in both long-range systemic neutrophil mobilization from hematopoietic tissue as well as local recruitment to infection or purified Cxcl8 (IL-8, a potent Cxcr2 ligand) [17,18]. Previous studies have also implicated

CXCR2 signaling in tumor progression [21,22,24–29]. CXCR2 expression is increased in some tumor types [26,30–32] and pharmacological inhibition of CXCR1 and CXCR2 inhibits neutrophil recruitment into A547 lung tumor spheroids resulting in slower tumor growth [33]. Mouse models have also been instrumental in demonstrating that CXCR2 signaling is involved in the recruitment of myeloid-derived suppressor cells into the tumor microenvironment. For instance, expression of human CXCL8 in mice results in increased mobilization of immature myeloid cells, which exacerbates inflammation and accelerates colon carcinogenesis [34]. Tumor trafficking of myeloid-derived suppressor cells is inhibited by CXCR2 deficiency in a mouse model of rhabdomyosarcoma [35] and data from a mouse model of colitis-associated cancer suggests that CXCR2 is required for recruitment of myeloid-derived suppressor cells [24,36]. Moreover, activation of CXCR2 on Ras-transformed keratinocytes contributes to tumor progression in a mouse model of skin cancer [23]. These findings support a role for CXCR2 signaling in inflammation and cancer progression; however the connection between CXCR2-mediated neutrophil recruitment and EMT remains unclear.

In this study we have exploited advances in real time imaging and analysis of tissue-specific gene expression in zebrafish to interrogate the role of Cxcr2 and neutrophil recruitment in $HRas^{V12}$-induced EMT. We found that signaling through Cxcr2 is required for neutrophil, but not macrophage, recruitment to transformed epithelial cells. We further show that both Cxcr2 in transformed cells and the presence of neutrophils, but not macrophages, in the microenvironment are required for expression of EMT-related genes. These findings establish an essential role for Cxcr2 in regulating chronic neutrophil inflammation and EMT-related gene expression via both autocrine and paracrine mechanisms.

Results

$HRas^{V12}$ expression in epithelial cells induces EMT and inflammation

Tissue damage or oncogenic signals induce EMT [37]. To visualize EMT in zebrafish, we used the *krt4* promoter to drive gene expression in epidermal cells (*krt4*; previously termed *krt8*) [38]. We found that the *krt4* promoter drives GFP expression in the developing epidermis during early gastrulation and by 12 hours post fertilization (hpf) uniform expression is observed throughout the epidermis (Figure 1A). To express $HRas^{V12}$ in the zebrafish epidermis, RFP-$HRas^{V12}$ was cloned into a Tol2 containing plasmid and co-injected with transposase RNA into one-cell stage embryos (Figure 1B). Active Ras signaling promotes cell transformation [39–43] and has been shown to drive chemokine and cytokine expression [44–46]. Early expression of $HRas^{V12}$ using the *krt4* promoter induced cell extrusion in developing embryos (Figure 1C), as has previously been reported for apoptotic epithelial cells in zebrafish [47] or in response to activating Src [48]. To reduce early transgene expression, we designed an antisense morpholino oligonucleotide (MO) targeting the 3′ end of the *krt4* promoter 25 bases directly 5′ to the AUG translational start site of RFP-$HRas^{V12}$ (Figure 1B). Microinjection of the *krt4* MO inhibited GFP expression in *krt4*:GFP transgenic larvae (Figure 1D) and reduced transgene expression in 24 hpf embryos injected with Tol2 flanked:*krt4*: RFP-$HRas^{V12}$ (Figure 1E). By reducing early $HRas^{V12}$ transgene expression, we were able to significantly reduce the early apical extrusion of $HRas^{V12}$ expressing cells (Figure 1F).

High resolution confocal imaging revealed that chimeric embryos expressing wild type $HRas^{WT}$ had membrane localization of the transgene and displayed a cuboidal morphology typical of epithelial cells at 3.5 days post fertilization (dpf) (Figure 2B). Cells expressing constitutively active $HRas^{V12}$ also had membrane localization of the transgene but displayed altered cell morphology (Figure 2C). Live imaging, of chimeric 3.5 dpf embryos, revealed that $HRas^{WT}$ cells maintained their shape over a four hour time period (Figure 1D, Movie S1) while, $HRas^{V12}$ cells displayed an abnormal morphology with dynamic protrusions (Figure 2E, Movie S2), quantified by reduced 2D cell area and roundness (Figure 2F–G).

To determine if $HRas^{V12}$ expression in epithelial cells resulted in changes in gene expression consistent with EMT, we investigated the expression of a transcriptional activator of EMT, Slug (also known as Snail2) which has been identified as a driving factor of EMT in keratinocytes during wound healing [37] and is increased during cancer progression [49]. We also tested expression of a matrix metalloproteinase (Mmp9) that has been linked to EMT, and a type III intermediate filament protein (Vimentin) that is expressed in mesenchymal cells and has been previously shown to be a reliable marker of EMT [50–52]. Double label Whole Mount *In Situ* Hybridization (WMISH) revealed that the EMT associated genes *mmp9*, *slug* and *vimentin* were enriched in $HRas^{V12}$ transformed epithelial cells, compared to control $HRas^{WT}$ expressing cells (Figure 2H–I). To better quantify these changes in gene expression we used translating ribosome affinity purification (TRAP) [53] to isolate RNA specifically from the transformed epithelial cells followed by Quantitative Reverse Transcriptase Polymerase Chain Reaction (qRT-PCR). We found that transforming $HRas^{V12}$ induced EMT gene expression specifically in the transformed epithelial cells, including increased *slug* and *mmp9*, compared to $HRas^{WT}$ control at 3.5 dpf (Figure 2J).

To characterize the host innate immune responses to transformed epithelial cells, we used the transgenic zebrafish lines Tg(*mpx*:GFP) and Tg(*mpeg*:Dendra) to visualize neutrophils and macrophages respectively *in vivo* [20,54–56]. In zebrafish larvae, neutrophils are generally localized to the caudal hematopoietic tissue (CHT) [57], which has a hematopoietic function similar to the fetal liver in mammals [58]. Live high resolution spinning disk confocal microscopy revealed that neutrophils (Figure 3B, Movie S4) and macrophages (Figure 3E, Movie S6) are recruited to $HRas^{V12}$ but not control $HRas^{WT}$ expressing epithelial cells (Figure 3A and D, Movie S3 and S5). Quantification of leukocytes as a ratio of transformed cell number revealed a significant increase in neutrophils (Figure 3C) and macrophages (Figure 3F) per $HRas^{V12}$ transformed cell compared to control $HRas^{WT}$ cells. These findings indicate that chimeric $HRas^{V12}$ expression in the zebrafish epidermis is sufficient to stimulate neutrophil and macrophage recruitment, similar to the effects reported with oncogene-transformed melanoblasts in zebrafish [19].

Neutrophils, but not macrophages, are necessary for *mmp9* and *slug* expression in transformed epithelial cells

To determine if there is a cell autonomous role for neutrophils in regulating EMT, we characterized EMT related gene expression in larvae with impaired neutrophil function. We took advantage of a zebrafish model of primary immunodeficiency (zf307Tg, Tg(mpx:mCherry,rac2^{D57N})), where neutrophil recruitment to tissue damage is impaired. In this model, expression of the human inhibitory Rac2^{D57N} mutation in neutrophils results in reduced neutrophil migration and recruitment to wounds and infection [57]. We found a significant decrease in neutrophil

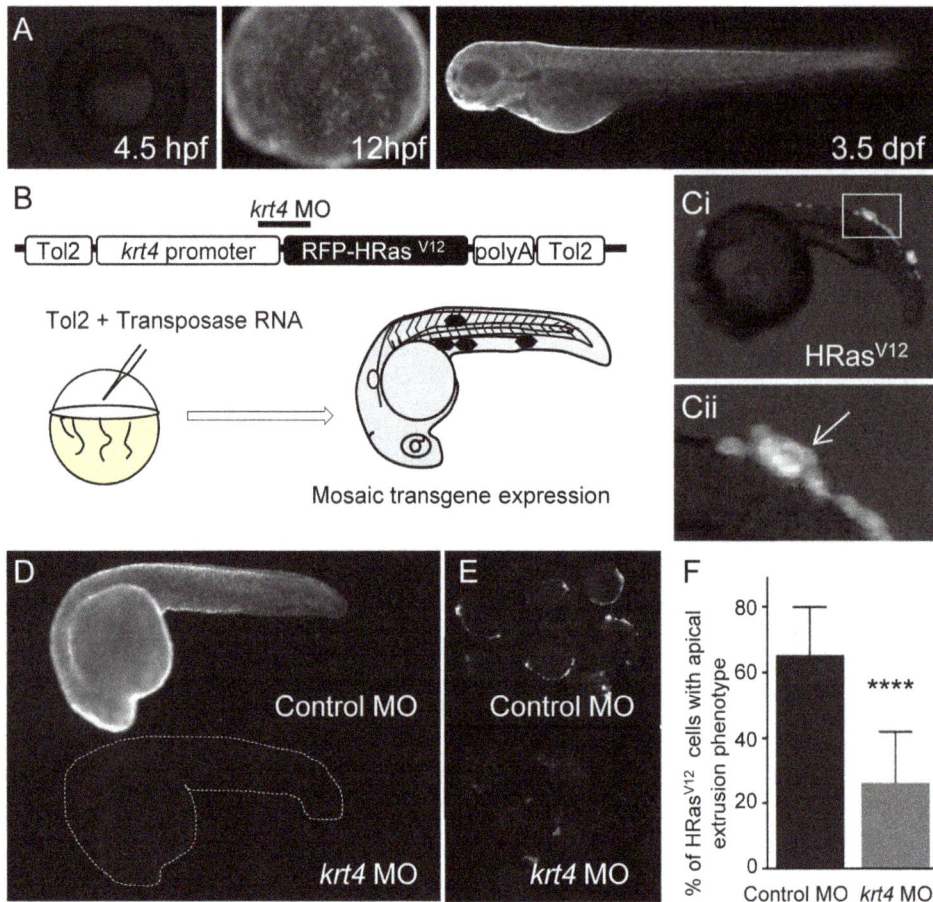

Figure 1. Early HRas^{V12} expression in epithelial cells induces cell extrusion. (A) Lateral fluorescent images of transgenic krt4-GFP embryos at 4.5 hpf, 12 hpf and 3 dpf. (B) Schematic of the Tol2 flanked:krt4:RFP-HRas^{V12} construct+transposase one-cell stage injection resulting in mosaic RFP-HRas expression by 24 hpf (black hexagons). (C) (i) Lateral fluorescent image of a 24 hpf live H-Ras^{V12} expressing embryo. (ii) High-magnification view of the inset in (i) indicating the apical cell extrusion phenotype (white arrow). (D) Fluorescent images of live 24 hpf krt4:GFP transgenic embryos injected with either control MO (Top) or Krt4 MO (bottom dashed outline) at 24 hpf illustrating that the krt4 MO reduces transgene levels in a stable transgenic line. (E) Fluorescent images of live 24 hpf embryos transiently expressing HRas^{V12} injected with either control MO or krt4 MO illustrating that the krt4 MO reduces transgene levels in embryos with mosaic transgene expression. (F) Quantification of cell extrusion (one representative graph shown n = 3) of HRas^{V12} expressing cells from control MO and Krt4 MO injected embryos shows a significant decrease in the cell extrusion in embryos injected with the Krt4 MO. **** = p<.0001.

recruitment to HRas^{V12} expressing cells in Rac2^{D57N} larvae compared to control (Figure 4B and D). To ensure that macrophages were still recruited to transformed cells in the absence of neutrophil recruitment we quantified macrophage numbers at transformed cells in Rac2^{D57N} larvae and found that macrophage recruitment was not affected (Figure 4G and I). Surprisingly, we found that EMT associated gene expression is impaired in neutrophil-deficient larvae (Figure 4K) indicating that neutrophils are necessary for the expression of EMT associated genes in transformed epithelial cells.

To determine if there is a cell autonomous role for macrophages in regulating EMT associated gene expression, we utilized a previously published MO targeting interferon regulatory factor 8 (Irf8), which is essential for directing macrophage but not neutrophil differentiation [59]. We found a significant decrease in macrophage recruitment to HRas^{V12} expressing cells in irf8 morphants compared to control (Figure 4 H and J). To determine if neutrophils were still recruited to transformed cells in irf8 morphants we quantified neutrophil numbers at transformed cells and found that neutrophil recruitment was not affected (Figure 4C

and E). Moreover, mmp9 and slug transcripts were not reduced in irf8 morphants compared to control (Figure 4K), suggesting that macrophages do not induce EMT gene expression in transformed cells. Interestingly, mmp9 expression was increased in irf8 morphants, likely due to the increase in total numbers of neutrophils in irf8 morphants. Taken together, these findings suggest that neutrophils but not macrophages influence EMT associated gene expression in transformed epithelial cells in vivo.

Cxcr2 is required for neutrophil recruitment to transformed cells

Previous work has predominantly focused on the role of macrophages in cancer progression and few studies have characterized the role of neutrophils within the tumor microenvironment [60–65]. Our findings suggest that neutrophils play a critical role in influencing gene expression in transformed epithelial cells. To identify the signals that mediate neutrophil recruitment to transformed epithelial cells, we targeted specific pathways that have been implicated in neutrophil wound attraction, including Cxcl8 signaling [66]. Indeed, human liver

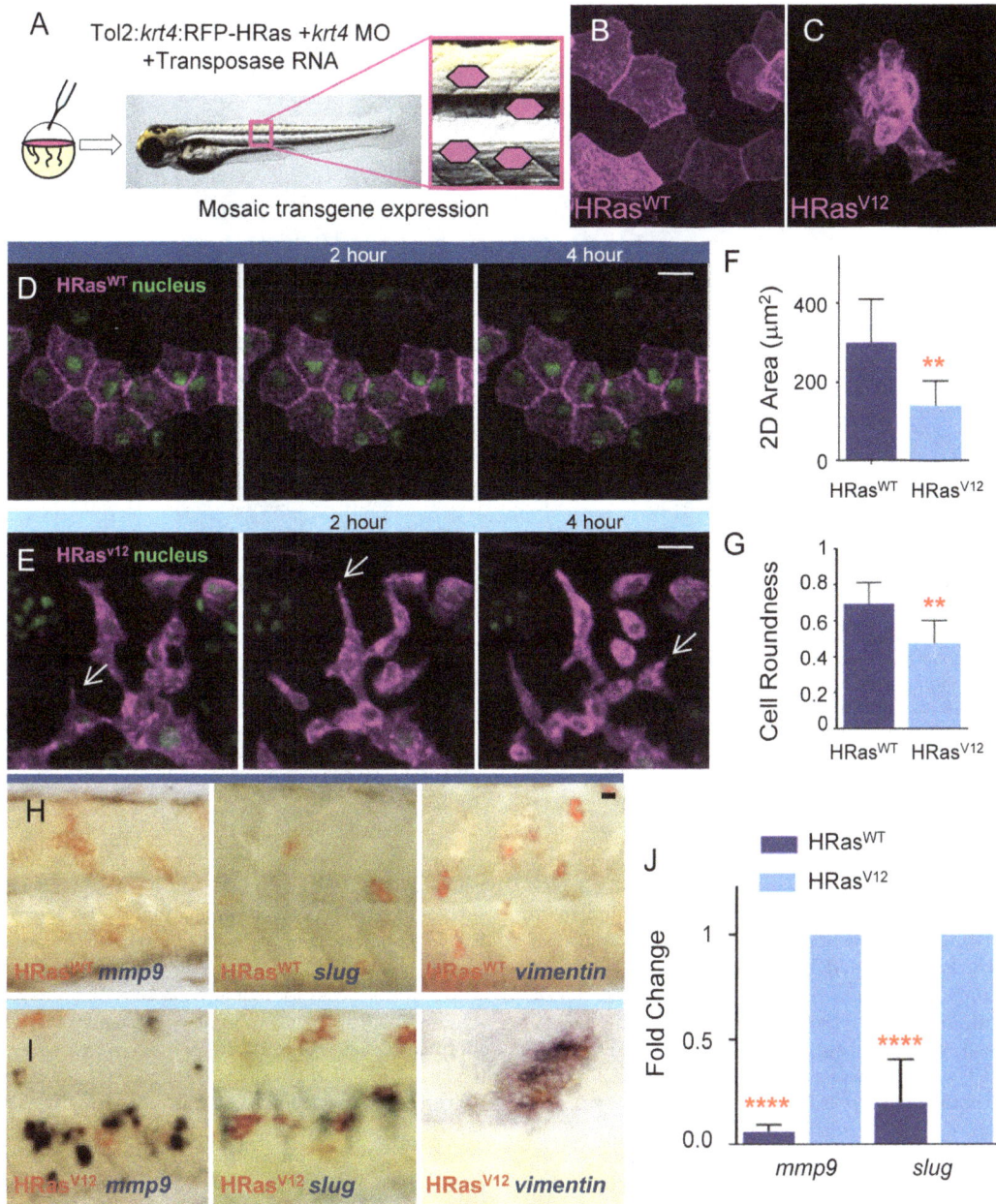

Figure 2. HRas^{V12} expression in epithelial cells induces cell shape and genetic changes associated with EMT *in vivo*. (A) Schematic of Tol2 flanked:*krt4*:RFP-HRas+transposase one-cell stage injection resulting in mosaic expression. (B–C) Fluorescent Z stack projections of HRas^{WT} and HRas^{V12} expressing epithelial cells (magenta) in the trunk region of 3.5 dpf larvae (illustrated in A). (D–E) Lateral fluorescent images, from live imaging, of 3.5 dpf embryos co-expressing GFP-H2B to label the nuclei and either HRas^{WT} (D) or HRas^{V12} (E) at 0, 2 hr and 4 hr time points. Arrows in E indicate cell extensions. (F) Quantification of the 2D area of H-Ras^{WT} and H-Ras^{V12} expressing cells shows a significant decrease in the 2D area of HRas^{V12} expressing cells compared to controls. (G) Quantification of the cell roundness of HRas^{WT} and HRas^{V12} expressing cells shows a significant decrease in the cell roundness of HRas^{V12} expressing cells compared to controls. (H–I) Double label WMISH with HRas^{WT} (H) and HRas^{V12} (I) transcript labeled in red and *mmp9*, *slug*, and *vimentin* transcript label in blue illustrating that *mmp9*, *slug*, and *vimentin* expression are induced in RFP-HRas^{V12} compared to control RFP-HRas^{WT} expressing larvae. (J) Quantitative RT-PCR (one representative graph shown n = 5) indicates a statistically significant increase in *mmp9* and *slug* transcripts in HRas^{V12} transformed cells compared to control HRas^{WT} expressing cells. hr = hour, dpf = days post fertilization, ** = p< .005, **** = p<.0001 scale bars = 20 microns.

epithelial cells from hepatocellular carcinoma have been shown to produce the CXC chemokine CXCL8 and promote neutrophil infiltration [67]. To determine if Cxcl8 is up-regulated by epithelial cell transformation we performed double label WMISH and found an increase in Cxcl8 in regions with HRas^{V12}

expressing cells (Figure 4M), compared to HRas^{WT} control (Figure 4L).

We recently reported that Cxcr2, but not Cxcr1, is necessary for neutrophil recruitment to exogenous purified Cxcl8, suggesting that Cxcr2 may mediate neutrophil recruitment to transformed epithelial cells that produce Cxcl8 [18]. To determine if Cxcr2

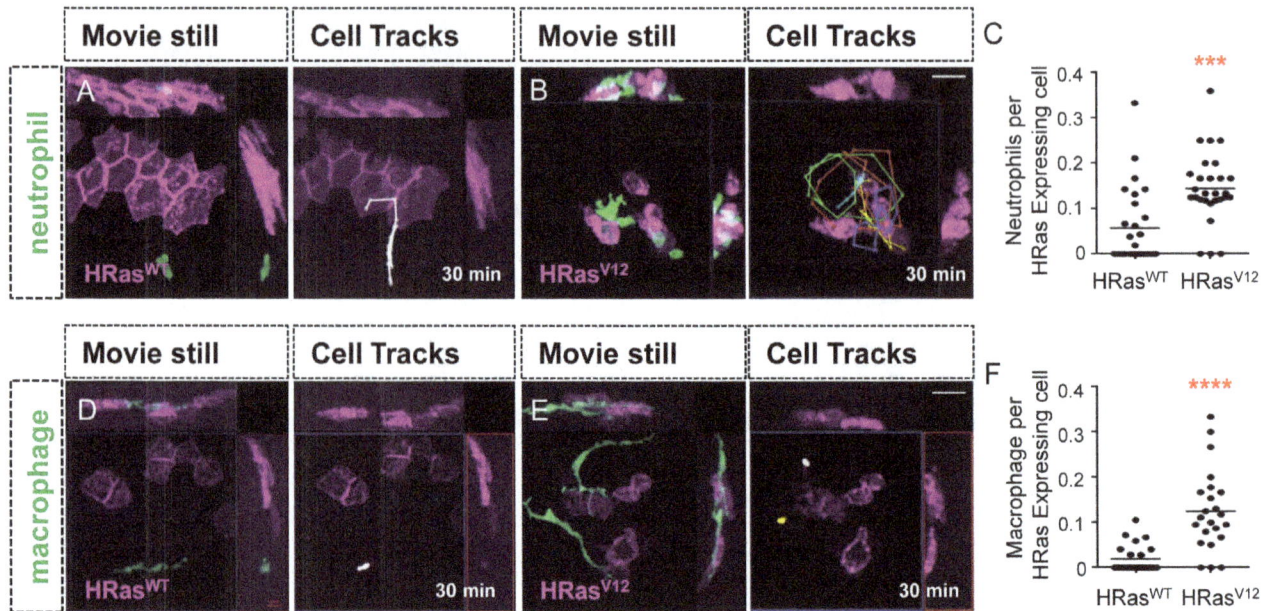

Figure 3. Leukocytes are recruited to HRas^{V12} expressing epithelial cells. (A–B) Analysis of time-lapse movies of control HRas^{WT} expressing epithelial cells (A and D) and HRas^{V12} expressing epithelial cells (B and E) in 3.5 dpf transgenic *mpx*:GFP (green neutrophils) larvae (A–B) and 3.5 dpf transgenic *mpeg*:Dendra (green macrophage) larvae (D–E). For cell tracks leukocyte migration was tracked every 2 minutes for 30 minutes. (C) Quantification of A–B (as a ratio of neutrophils per transformed cell) confirms a statistically significant increase in neutrophil recruitment to HRas^{V12} expressing cells compared to HRas^{WT} expressing cells. (F) Quantification of D–E (as a ratio of macrophages per transformed cell) confirms a statistically significant increase in macrophage recruitment to HRas^{V12} expressing cells when compared to macrophages recruited to HRas^{WT} expressing cells. dpf = days post fertilization, scale bar = 20 microns, *** = p < .001 **** = p < .0001.

mediates neutrophil recruitment we depleted *cxcr2* using a previously published MO [18]. We found that depletion of *cxcr2* resulted in a significant decrease in neutrophil recruitment to HRas^{V12} expressing cells, quantified as a ratio of neutrophils per transformed cell (Figure 5B and E). To determine if Cxcr2 also mediates macrophage recruitment we quantified macrophage infiltration, and found that, *cxcr2* depletion did not have a significant impact on macrophage recruitment (Figure 5D and F), suggesting that Cxcr2 mediates neutrophil but not macrophage recruitment to transformed epithelial cells.

To determine if Cxcr2 mediates the invasive progression of transformed cells we characterized the effect of *cxcr2* depletion on the HRas^{V12}-induced expression of *mmp9* and *slug*. We found that depletion of *cxcr2* blocked the HRAS^{V12}-induced expression of EMT related genes (Figure 5G). It is important to note that, although neutrophil recruitment required Cxcr2, the early morphological changes induced by HRas^{V12} were not affected by *cxcr2* depletion. These findings indicate the Cxcr2 is necessary for HRAS^{V12}-induced expression of EMT associated genes.

Cxcr2 signaling in transformed epithelial cells is necessary for neutrophil recruitment and HRas^{V12} induced expression of vimentin, mmp9 and slug in epithelial cells

Previous studies have shown that Cxcr2 expression is necessary for neutrophil recruitment to exogenous Cxcl8, indicating that neutrophil Cxcr2 mediates chemotaxis to Cxcl8 *in vivo*. It is possible that Cxcr2 mediates EMT gene expression in transformed epithelial cells indirectly through its effects on neutrophil recruitment. However, Cxcr2 is also expressed in tumor cells, suggesting that Cxcr2 may play cell autonomous roles in epithelial cells. Indeed, we found that zebrafish epithelial cells express *cxcr2*

(Figure 6A), suggesting that Cxcr2 in epithelial cells may affect gene expression changes induced by cell transformation independent of the effects of Cxcr2 in neutrophils. To determine if there is a cell autonomous role for Cxcr2 in transformed epithelial cells we utilized a cell transplantation strategy to deplete Cxcr2 specifically in transformed cells without altering Cxcr2 signaling in neutrophils (Figure 6B). Cells from embryos expressing RFP-HRas^{V12} in *cxcr2* morphants or control morphants were transplanted into Tg(mpx:GFP) embryos. Interestingly, we found a significant decrease in neutrophil recruitment toward Cxcr2-deficient HRas^{V12} expressing cells even though the neutrophils expressed Cxcr2 (Figure 6D and E), suggesting that Cxcr2 signaling in transformed cells is necessary for neutrophil recruitment. To determine if Cxcr2-deficient epithelial cells that express HRas^{V12} induce EMT associated genes, we tested the expression of *vimentin*, *mmp9* and *slug* in the Cxcr2-deficient and control transformed epithelial cells. Surprisingly, expression of *vimentin*, *slug* and *mmp9* were reduced in Cxcr2-deficient transformed epithelial cells compared to control (Figure 6F); indicating a cell autonomous role for Cxcr2 signaling in epithelial cells in the induction of EMT related gene expression.

Discussion

Here, we uncovered roles for Cxcr2 and neutrophils in oncogene induced EMT gene expression in epithelial cells in zebrafish. By exploiting the transparency of zebrafish we showed that expression of oncogenic HRas^{V12} induced EMT and invasive growth. Interestingly, early expression of HRas^{V12} induced cell extrusion, suggesting that depending on the developmental stage of the epithelium the fate of the transformed cell may be either extrusion or EMT. This provides a powerful model system to understand how early EMT is regulated within a live host, and

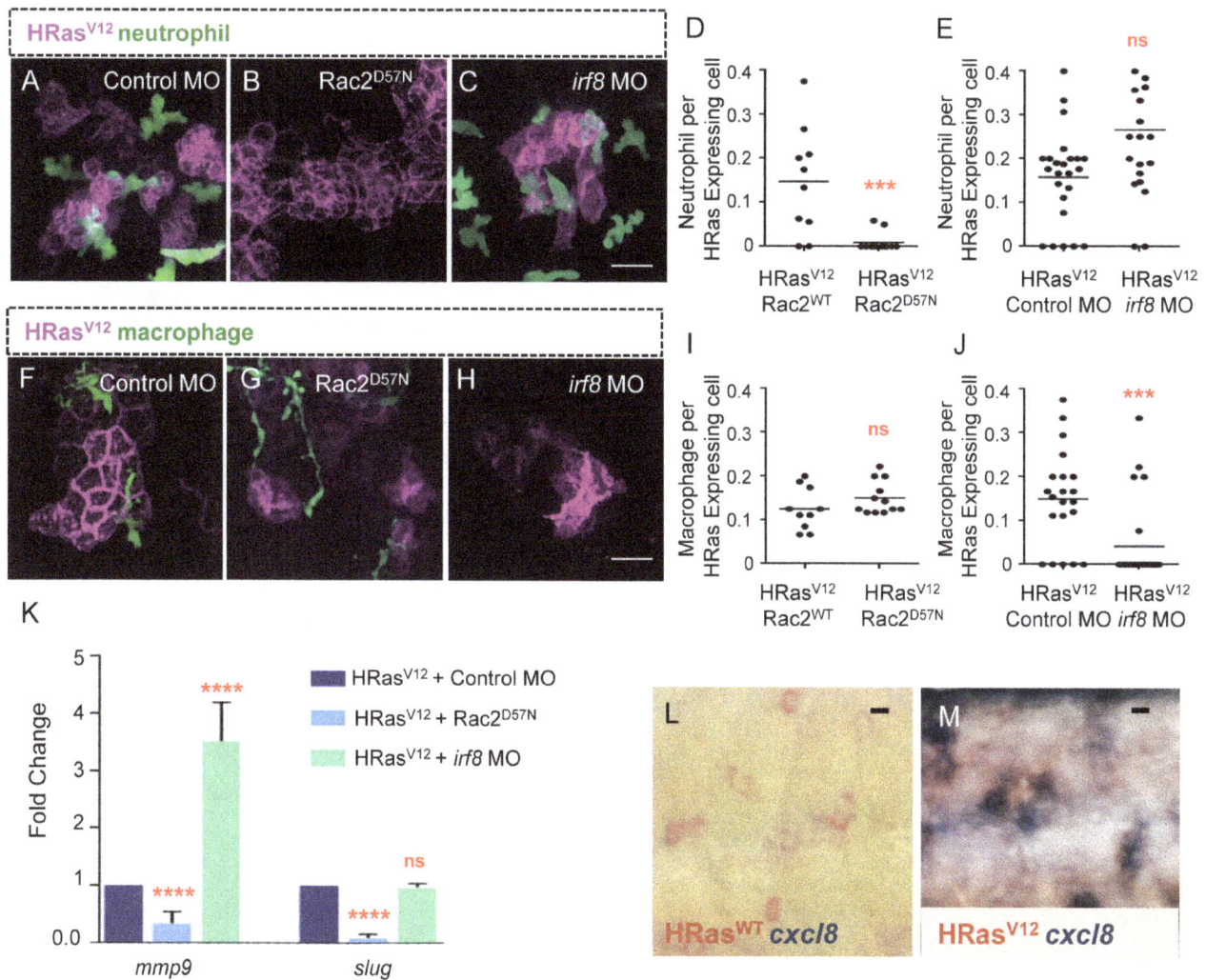

Figure 4. Neutrophils, but not macrophages, mediate EMT related gene expression in HRas^V12 expressing epithelial cells. (A–C) Fluorescent Z stack projections of live 3.5 dpf transgenic *mpx*:GFP (green neutrophils) control MO injected (A), Rac2^D57N (B) and *irf8* MO (C) larvae expressing HRas^V12. (D–E) Quantification of neutrophil recruitment (as a ratio of neutrophils per transformed cell) shows a significant decrease in neutrophil recruitment to HRas^V12 expressing cells in Rac^D57N embryos when compared to controls (D), no significant change was observed in neutrophil recruitment in *irf8* morphant larvae compared to control (E). (F–H) Fluorescent Z stack projections of live 3.5 dpf of transgenic *mpeg*:Dendra (green macrophages) control MO injected (F), Rac2^D57N (G) and *irf8* MO (H) larvae expressing HRas^V12. (I–J) Quantification of macrophage recruitment (as a ratio of macrophages per transformed cell) shows a significant decrease in macrophage recruitment to HRas^V12 expressing cells in irf8 morphants compared to controls (D). No significant change was observed in macrophage recruitment in Rac2^D57N larvae compared to control (E). (K) Quantitative RT-PCR (one representative graph shown n = 4) indicates a statistically significant decrease in *mmp9* and *slug* transcripts in transformed cells from Rac2^D57N larvae compared to control MO injected larvae while no significant decrease was seen in *mmp9* and *slug* transcripts in transformed cells from *irf8* Mo injected larvae compared to controls. (L–M) Double label WMISH with HRas^WT (A) and HRas^V12 (B) transcript labeled in red and *cxcl8* transcript label in blue. *cxcl8* expression is induced in HRas^V12 expressing larvae compared to control HRas^WT expressing larvae. *** = P<.001, **** = P<.0001, ns = not significant. Scale bar = 20 microns.

how different triggers for EMT during development, cell transformation or wounding induce distinct EMT programs.

Previous studies have identified roles for both macrophages [60–65] and neutrophils [6,33,68] during cancer progression. For example, neutrophil activation is associated with the progression of head and neck cancers [68] supporting the idea that neutrophils influence tumor progression. CXCR2 has a known role in the recruitment of neutrophils to cancer cells. Of interest CXCR2 expressing ovarian cancers are aggressive with poor outcomes [69]. However, the mechanisms of these effects remain poorly understood.

Here we show directly that depletion of Cxcr2 in transformed cells results in decreased neutrophil recruitment and impairs the early expression of EMT genes in transformed epithelial cells. Our findings reveal a pro-inflammatory role for Cxcr2 in Ras transformed keratinocytes and provides direct evidence that neutrophils impact the progression of transformed cells in a live animal. It is likely that chronic neutrophil infiltration results in increased amounts of neutrophil derived elastase which has been previously shown to support the progression of pancreatic tumor cells [70] and lung cancer in mice [6]. To test this possibility we exposed zebrafish larvae transiently expressing HRas^V12 in the epidermis to a specific inhibitor of human neutrophil elastase

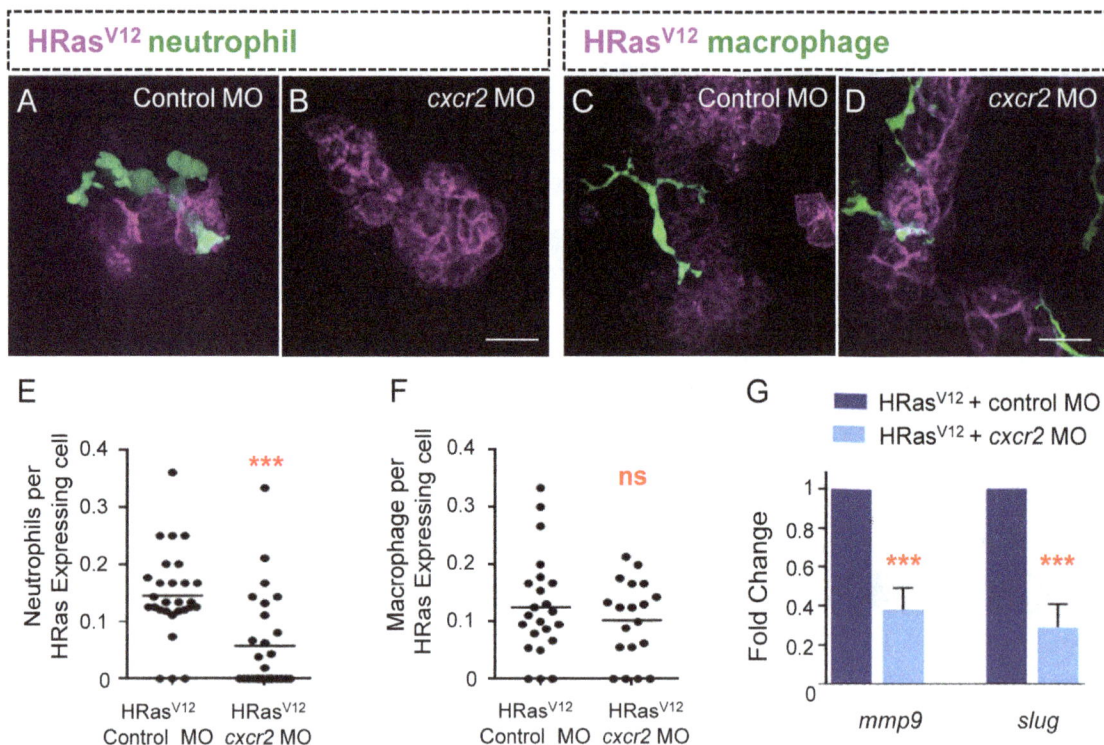

Figure 5. Cxcr2 is required for EMT related gene expression in HRas^{V12} expressing epithelial cells. (A–B) Fluorescent Z stack projections of live 3.5 dpf transgenic *mpx*:GFP (green neutrophils) control MO injected (A) and *cxcr2* morphant (B). (C–D) Fluorescent Z stack projections of live 3.5 dpf transgenic *mpeg*:Dendra (green macrophages), control MO injected (C) and *cxcr2* morphant (D). (E) Quantification of A–B (as a ratio of neutrophils per transformed cell) reveals a significant decrease in neutrophil recruitment to HRas^{V12} expressing cells in *cxcr2* MO injected larvae compared to control. (F) Quantification of C–D (as a ratio of macrophages per transformed cell) shows that macrophage numbers at HRas^{V12} expressing cells in *cxcr2* MO injected larvae is similar to macrophage numbers at HRas^{V12} expressing cells in control larvae. (G) Quantitative RT-PCR (one representative graph shown n = 4) indicates a statistically significant decrease in *mmp9* and *slug* transcripts in transformed cells from cxcr2 MO injected larvae when compared to control MO injected larvae. *** = P<.001, ns = not significant. Scale bar = 20 microns.

(Sivelestat) from 1–3.5 dpf, however we did not observe any difference in either neutrophil recruitment or the transcription of EMT related genes. It is possible that Sivelestat may not be effective in inhibiting zebrafish neutrophil elastase and future experiments are needed to determine the role of neutrophil derived elastase in the transcription of EMT related genes. Additionally, it is also possible that a positive feedback loop between neutrophil derived Cxcl8 and Cxcr2 signaling in the transformed cells may contribute to these changes. This is especially interesting since recent evidence suggests that CXCL8 is associated with progression of some cancers [45].

The zebrafish model is particularly powerful since the transparency allows for the real time visualization of the earliest events that occur after an oncogene turns on. We found that early after HRas^{V12} was first expressed in epithelial cells both neutrophils and macrophages are recruited to small foci of transformed cells. A previous report showed that transformed melanoblasts in zebrafish also induces early leukocyte recruitment [19]. The previous study showed that hydrogen peroxide generated by the transformed cells mediates leukocyte recruitment. We found that reactive oxygen species inhibition with DPI did not impair neutrophil recruitment to the transformed epithelial cells, but this may have been due to the short time of inhibitor treatment as longer treatments resulted in lethality. It is also possible that different signals mediate neutrophil recruitment to transformed melanocytes versus epithelial cells. Our findings support an essential role for Cxcr2 signaling in chronic tumor associated inflammation.

In summary, here we report a new *in vivo* model of epithelial cell transformation that is amenable to live imaging and probing the microenvironment. We have identified a pathway that specifically mediates neutrophil but not macrophage recruitment to transformed epithelial cells. We have also provided evidence that Cxcr2 and neutrophils are both necessary for HRas^{V12}-induced changes in gene expression in epithelial cells (Figure 6G). This study highlights a novel cell autonomous role for Cxcr2 signaling in transformed cells in both influencing neutrophil infiltration and EMT-related gene expression, suggesting that both autocrine and paracrine signaling contribute to Cxcr2 effects on EMT. Future studies will be necessary to identify the specific neutrophil factors that influence gene expression induced by oncogenic HRas. It is possible that neutrophils regulate gene expression in transformed epithelial cells at least in part through the release of Cxcl8 that signals to epithelial cell Cxcr2 in a positive feedback loop. The zebrafish model is poised to contribute to a better understanding of the trophic factors involved in the reactivation of EMT programs *in vivo*, which will likely aid in identifying novel therapeutic targets that modulate EMT with implications to both wound and cancer biology.

Materials and Methods

Zebrafish maintenance and general procedures

University of Wisconsin - Madison (A3368-01) Institutional review board specifically approved this study. Adult AB fish, including Transgenic (Tg) zebrafish lines Tg(*mpx*:GFP), Tg(*mpeg*:-

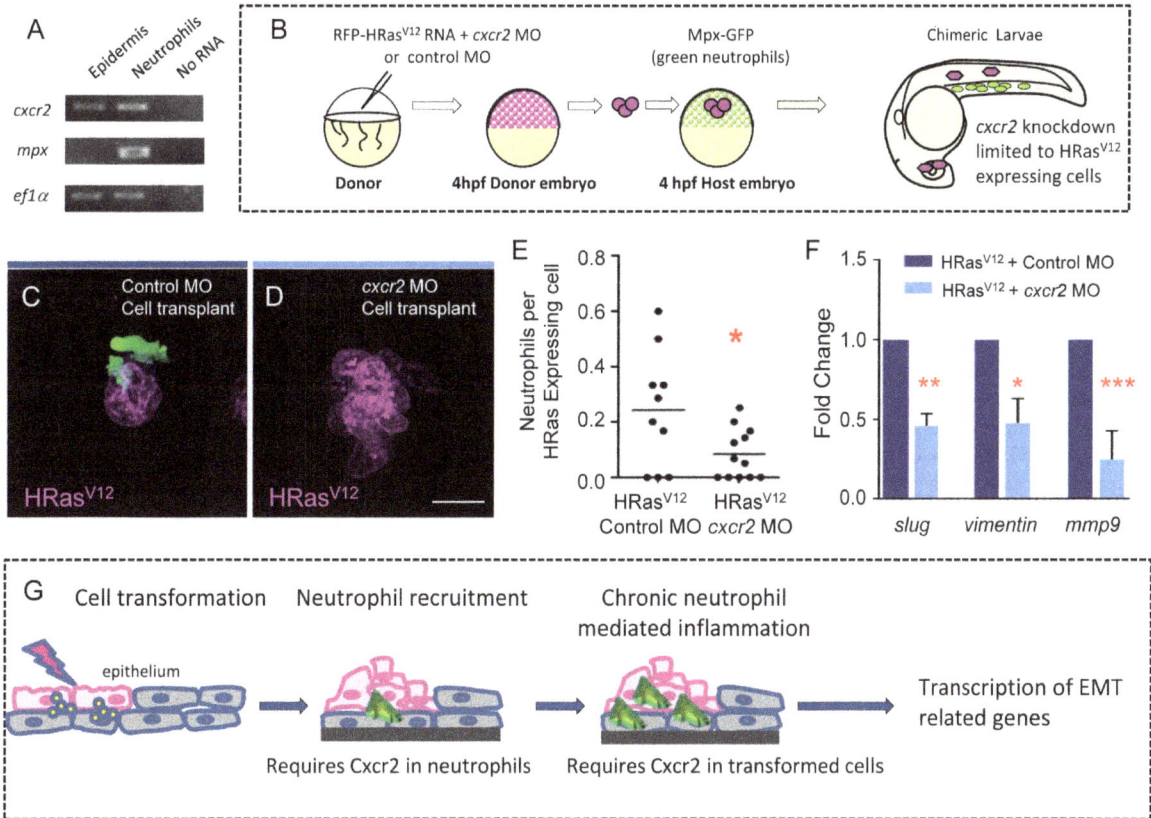

Figure 6. Cxcr2 signaling in HRas^{V12} transformed epithelial cells is required for neutrophil recruitment and EMT related gene expression. (A) For analysis of tissue specific Cxcr2 expression TRAP was performed on 3.5 dpf transgenic krt4-EGFP-L10a and mpx-EGFP-L10a larvae and one-step RT-PCR was performed. *cxcr2* expression is observed in the epidermis and in neutrophils. *mpx* expression is only observed in neutrophils supporting that there is not neutrophil contamination in the epidermal samples. (B) Schematic diagram to illustrate the cell transplantation used to generate chimeric HRas^{V12} expressing larvae in which the transformed cells express either control MO or Cxcr2 MO. (C–D) Fluorescent Z stack projections of live 3.5 dpf of transgenic *mpx*:GFP (green neutrophils) larvae with control MO in the HRas^{V12} expressing cells (C) or with *cxcr2* MO within the HRas^{V12} expressing cells (D). (E) Quantification of C–D (as a ratio of neutrophils per transformed cell) shows a statistically significant decrease in neutrophil recruitment to HRas^{V12} expressing cells that have *cxcr2* MO compared to HRas^{V12} expressing cells that have control MO. (F) Quantitative RT-PCR (one representative graph shown n = 3) indicates a statistically significant decrease in *slug*, vimentin and *mmp9* transcripts in HRas^{V12} expressing cells that have *cxcr2* MO compared to HRas^{V12} expressing cells with control MO. (G) Schematic illustrating the requirement for Cxcr2 in neutrophils for initial neutrophil recruitment to transformed cells as well as a cell autonomous function of Cxcr2 in transformed cells to mediate changes associated with EMT. * = P<.05, ** = P<.01, *** = P<.001. Scale bar = 20 microns.

Dendra), Tg(*mpx*: EGFP-L10a [53]), Tg(*krt4*: EGFP-L10a [53]) and Tg(mpx:mCherry,rac2^{D57N}, zf307Tg [57]) were maintained at 28°C in a 14-hour light/10-hour dark cycle in the Research Animal facilities at the University of Wisconsin, which are fully accredited by the American Association for the Accreditation of Laboratory Animal Care. Embryos were staged by both hours post fertilization (hpf) at 28.5°C and by using morphological criteria [71]. To prevent pigment formation, larvae were maintained in E3 containing 0.2 mM N-phenylthiourea (PTU, Sigma Aldrich). For live imaging, 1–3.5 dpf larvae were anesthetized in E3 containing 0.2 mg/mL Tricaine (ethyl 3-aminobenzoate, Sigma Aldrich) and mounted in in 1% low melting point agarose and/or corresponding culture medium. Zebrafish that needed to be euthanized were placed into.05% Tricaine (diluted in E3 water) for 10–15 minutes. After this time the fish were checked to ensure they are not moving or breathing and are then placed into a latex glove for disposal. Alternative way to euthanize: Larval forms between 4 and 10 dpf were maintained in an ice water bath for a minimum of 20 minutes. Death was confirmed when heart and gill movements have ceased.

Tol2 plasmid injections

Zebrafish embryos were microinjected with a pressure injector with approximately 3 nano-liter volumes at the 1-cell stage. All DNA expression vectors contained the *krt4* promoter for epithelial cell expression [72,73]. All expression vectors contain minimal Tol2 elements flanking the promoter and gene of interest for efficient integration [74] and an SV40 polyadenylation sequence (Clontech Laboratories, Inc). The following constructs were generated: *krt4*-RFP-HRAS^{WT}, *krt4*-RFP-HRAS^{V12}, *krt4*-EGFP-L10a and *krt4*-GFP-H2B. Mosaic expression of transgenes was obtained by injecting 3 nano-liter of solution containing 12.5 ng/μL of Tol2 DNA plasmid and 17.5 ng/μL *in vitro* transcribed (Ambion) transposase mRNA into the cytoplasm of one-cell stage embryo.

Live imaging

For figure 1A, C, D and E, fluorescence images were acquired using Nikon SMZ-1500 zoom microscope equipped with epifluorescence and a CoolSnap ES camera (Roper Scientific, Duluth, GA). For all confocal imaging 1–3.5 dpf larvae were mounted in 1% low melting point agarose and/or corresponding culture medium. For figure 2B–E fluorescence images were acquired using a line scanning confocal microscope (FluoView FV1000, Olympus) using a NA 0.75/20× objective. For figure 3A–B and D–E, Figure 4A–C and F–H, Figure 5A–D and Figure 6C–D fluorescence images were acquired using a spinning disk confocal microscope (Yokogawa CSU-X) with confocal scanhead on a Zeiss Observer Z.1 inverted microscope (NA1.3/63× water immersion objective). Maximum intensity projection images were made using the Zen 2012 (blue edition) software (Carl Zeiss). Neutrophils and macrophages were tracked and analyzed by using plugins MTrackj (3D tracking) and Chemotaxis and Migration tool (ibidi) for ImageJ (NIH, Bethesda, MD). Transformed cell 2D area and cell roundness was measured using the analyze function of ImageJ. Data of time-lapse images represent at least three separate movies. For Figure 2H–I and Figure 4L–M WMISH images were acquired using Nikon SMZ-1500 zoom microscope equipped with a color camera.

MO mediated Gene knockdown

Morpholino oligonucleotides (Gene Tools) were suspended in distilled water, and stored at room temperature at a concentration of 1 mM. Zebrafish embryos were microinjected with a pressure injector with approximately 3 nano-liter volumes at the 1-cell stage. For cxcr2 knockdown, a cxcr2 MO targeting the ATG region (5′- ACTCTGTAGTAGCAGTTTCCATGTT-3′) [18], was used at 100 µM.

For irf8 knockdown, a previously published splice blocking irf8 MO [59] (5′-AATGTTTCGCTTACTTTGAAAATGG-3′) [18], was used at 100 µM. For knockdown of exogenous Krt4 driven genes, a krt4 MO targeting the region directly upstream of the ATG of targets cloned downstream of Krt4 using the BamHI cloning site (krt4 MO: 5′-GCTGCTGAGAGACACGCAGAGG-GAT-3′) was used at 20 µM (knockdown through 15 hpf). As a control, Gene Tools standard control morpholino (5′-CCTCTTACCTCAGTTACAATTTATA-3′) was used at 100 µM. Gene knockdown was obtained by injecting 3 nano-liter of solution into the cytoplasm of one-cell stage embryo.

Whole Mount In situ Hybridization

For in whole mount in situ hybridization, Larvae were fixed in 4% paraformaldehyde in PBS and mRNA was labelled by in situ hybridization as previously described [75]. In short, both Dig and fluorescein-labeled antisense probes were hybridized using a 55° hybridization temperature. Purple color was developed with AP-conjugated anti-Dig and BM purple (Roche Applied Science), and red color was developed with AP-conjugated anti-fluorescence and fast red (Roche Applied Science). Reactions were stopped in PBS. Imaging was performed with a Nikon SMZ-1500 stereomicroscope.

The T7 promoter was attached 3′ of the coding sequence of primers to make the DNA templates for the probes. After sequence confirmation of the DNA templates, labelled RNA probes were transcribed with the use of T7 RNA polymerase (Ambion).

Oligo sequences used for PCR were as follows:

Cxcl8 F: 5′-ATGACCAGCAAAATCATTTCAGTGTGTG-TTATTG-3′
T7 Cxcl8 R: 5′-TAATACGACTCACTATAGGGAGATCA-TGGTTTTCTGTTGACAA
TGATCCTATCAATGATC-3′
Mmp9 F: 5′-AAGGAGTTTGACGCCATCAC-3′
T7 Mmp9 R: 5′TAATACGACTCACTATAGGGGAATGG-GGTCAATGCAGAAT 3′
Vimentin F: 5′- CTTCAACAATAACCCGCAAA- 3′

T7 Vimentin R: 5′- TAATACGACTCACTATAGGGGGT-CAGGTTTGGTCACTTCC -3′
Slug F: 5′-GCATGCCTCGTTCATTCCTA- 3′
T7 Slug R: 5′- TAATACGACTCACTATAGGGGAGGCAC-TTGTTGAATGCAG -3′
RFP F: 5′-CTTCATGTACGGCAGCAGAA-3′
T7 RFP R: 5′-TAATACGACTCACTATAGGGTGCTAGG-GAGGTCGCAGTAT-3′

Translating ribosome affinity purification (TRAP)

To enrich for transcripts present in RFP-HRas expressing epithelial cells, Tol2 flanked-krt4- EGFP-L10a plasmids were co-injected with either Tol2 flanked-Krt4:RFP-HRas[WT] or Tol2 flanked -Krt4:RFP-HRas[V12] into one cell zebrafish embryos. We find that co-injection of Tol2 constructs results in their overlapping expression (Figure 2D and E) therefore allowing us to enrich for actively translating RNA from HRas expressing keratinocytes. TRAP was performed as previously published for mRNA purification from zebrafish tissue [53]. In short, 50 3.5 dpf larvae co-expressing L10-EGFP with either HRas[WT] or HRas[V12] were homogenized and rabbit anti-GFP antibody (Invitrogen A11122) was used for immunoprecipitation. After immunoprecipitation and high-salt polysome buffer washing steps, RNA was isolated using an RNeasy Mini Kit (Qiagen, Valencia, CA, USA) with in-column DNase digestion. RNA was eluted in 40 µl RNase free water.

One Step RT PCR

For analysis of tissue specific Cxcr2 expression TRAP was performed on 3.5 dpf transgenic krt4-EGFP-L10a and mpx-EGFP-L10a larvae and one-step RT-PCR (QIAGEN) was performed using 2 ul of purified RNA as template. Primers used to amplify ef1α and mpx [76] have been described previously. Primers for cxcr2 were as follows; cxcr2 42 forward, 5′-TC-CTTGCCCGGAGACCGTGA -3′; cxcr2 284 reverse, 5′-AT-GGTGCCGAACGGCCAGTG-3′. PCR products were analyzed using 1% agarose electrophoresis.

Quantitative PCR

All quantitative PCR was performed using 2 µl purified TRAP RNA as template. Following RNA isolation, one step qPCR was performed using superscript 3 one step qPCR kit (Invitrogen). All experiments had at least two identical samples and were done in three biological replicates with the reference gene ef1α [77] and gene specific primers, which were checked to have produced clean melt curves with one sharp peak indicating specific amplification of the target genes. Fold change was determined using the efficiency-corrected delta comparative quantification method and students t-test (unpaired, two tailed) were performed to determine significance.

Oligo sequences used for qPCR were as follows:
ef1α qFw   5′-TGCCTTCGTCCCAATTTCAG- 3′
ef1α qRv   5′-TACCCTCCTTGCGCTCAATC- 3′
vimentin qFw   5′-GCAGGAGTCTGAGGATTGGT- 3′
vimentin qRv   5′-AATCATTGGCCTCCTGTTTG- 3′
slug qFw   5′-TTATAGTGAACTGGAGAGTCCAACA- 3′
slug qRv   5′-TCCATACTGTTATGGGATTGTACG- 3′
mmp9 qFw   5′-TGATGTGCTTGGACCACGTAA- 3′
mmp9 qRv   5′-ACAGGAGCACCTTGCCTTTTC- 3′

Cell transplants

One cell stage donor embryos were microinjected with approximately 3 nano-liter volumes of injection mixes containing 45 ng/µL in vitro transcribed (Ambion) RFP-HRas[V12] mRNA mixed with either 100 µM cxcr2 or control MO. During the blastula period, 10–20 cells were transplanted from donor embryos into transgenic Mpx:GFP hosts. Cell transplants resulted in ~45% success rate of incorporation of RFP labeled donor cells into host embryos. To generate chimeric embryos for TRAP experiments and qPCR analysis one cell stage transgenic *krt4*-EGFP-L10a donor embryos were injected with 3 nano-liter volumes of injection mixes containing 45 ng/µL in vitro transcribed RFP-HRas^{V12} mRNA mixed with either 100 µM cxcr2 MO or control MO and during the blastula period 10–20 cells were transplanted into AB host embryos. Of the chimeric embryos generated ~60% had RFP expression in epithelial cells in the trunk region and not in the surrounding tissues. These chimeric zebrafish were used for analysis.

Statistical Analysis

Each *in vivo* experiment was done at least three times. Dot plots contain data from one representative experiment from at least three biological replicates. Each dot is from one foci of HRas labeled cells in the trunk region of an individual embryo and each embryo is represented by one dot. Assuming Gaussian distribution of overall population of values, P values were derived by the following analyses. One-way ANOVA with Dunnett post-test: Figure 3C and F, Figure 4 D–E and I–J, Figure 5E–F, and Figure 6E. Students T-test (unpaired, two tailed) was used in: Figure 1G, Figure 2F–G and J, Figure 4K, Figure 5 G and Figure 6 F. Experimental results were analyzed with Prism version 6 (GraphPad Software) statistical software and standard error is displayed. The resulting P values are included in the figure legends for each experiment.

Supporting Information

Movie S1 Live imaging of HRas^{WT} expressing epithelial cells. Live imaging of epidermal cells in the trunk region of a 3.5 dpf chimeric zebrafish expressing GFP-H2B (green-nucleus) and HRas^{WT} (magenta) in the epidermis. Images were collected at 10 minute intervals for 4 hours. Movie shows the stationary phenotype of HRas^{WT} expressing cells.
(AVI)

Movie S2 Live imaging of HRas^{V12} expressing epithelial cells. Live imaging of epidermal cells in the trunk region of a 3.5 dpf chimeric zebrafish expressing GFP-H2B (green-nucleus) and HRas^{V12} (magenta) in the epidermis. Images were collected in 10 minute intervals for 4 hours. Movie shows the dynamic phenotype of HRas^{V12} expressing cells characterized by cell division and active protrusions.
(AVI)

Movie S3 Neutrophil recruitment to HRas^{WT} expressing cells. Live imaging of epidermal cells in the trunk region of a 3.5 dpf transgenic *mpx*:GFP (green-neutrophils) chimeric zebrafish expressing HRas^{WT} (magenta). Images were collected for 30 minutes with 2 minute intervals. Movie shows that neutrophils are not recruited to HRas^{WT} expressing cells.
(AVI)

Movie S4 Neutrophil recruitment to HRas^{V12} expressing cells. Live imaging of epidermal cells in the trunk region of a 3.5 dpf transgenic *mpx*:GFP (green-neutrophils) chimeric zebrafish expressing HRas^{V12} (magenta). Images were collected for 30 minutes with 2 minute intervals. Movie shows that neutrophils are recruited to HRas^{V12} expressing cells.
(AVI)

Movie S5 Macrophage recruitment to HRas^{WT} expressing cells. Live imaging of epidermal cells in the trunk region of a 3.5 dpf transgenic *mpeg*:Dendra (green-macrophages) chimeric zebrafish expressing HRas^{WT} (magenta). Images were collected for 30 minutes with 2 minute intervals. Movie shows that macrophages are not recruited to HRas^{WT} expressing cells.
(AVI)

Movie S6 Macrophage recruitment to HRas^{V12} expressing cells. Live imaging of epidermal cells in the trunk region of a 3.5 dpf transgenic *mpeg*:Dendra (green-macrophages) chimeric zebrafish expressing HRas^{V12} (magenta). Images were collected for 30 minutes with 2 minute intervals. Movie shows that macrophages are recruited to HRas^{V12} expressing cells.
(AVI)

Acknowledgments

We thank lab members for discussions and critical reading of the manuscript.

Author Contributions

Conceived and designed the experiments: CF AH. Performed the experiments: CF. Analyzed the data: CF AH. Contributed reagents/materials/analysis tools: CF AH. Wrote the paper: CF AH.

References

1. Kalluri R (2009) EMT: when epithelial cells decide to become mesenchymal-like cells. J Clin Invest 119: 1417–1419.
2. Lim J, Thiery JP (2012) Epithelial-mesenchymal transitions: insights from development. Development 139: 3471–3486.
3. Lopez-Novoa JM, Nieto MA (2009) Inflammation and EMT: an alliance towards organ fibrosis and cancer progression. EMBO Mol Med 1: 303–314.
4. Mariani F, Sena P, Roncucci L (2014) Inflammatory pathways in the early steps of colorectal cancer development. World J Gastroenterol 20: 9716–9731.
5. Moghaddam SJ, Li H, Cho SN, Dishop MK, Wistuba, II, et al. (2009) Promotion of lung carcinogenesis by chronic obstructive pulmonary disease-like airway inflammation in a K-ras-induced mouse model. Am J Respir Cell Mol Biol 40: 443–453.
6. Gong L, Cumpian AM, Caetano MS, Ochoa CE, De la Garza MM, et al. (2013) Promoting effect of neutrophils on lung tumorigenesis is mediated by CXCR2 and neutrophil elastase. Mol Cancer 12: 154.
7. Chan AT, Lippman SM (2011) Aspirin and colorectal cancer prevention in Lynch syndrome. Lancet 378: 2051–2052.
8. Shen X, Han L, Ma Z, Chen C, Duan W, et al. (2013) Aspirin: A Potential Therapeutic Approach in Pancreatic Cancer. Curr Med Chem.
9. Cossack M, Ghaffary C, Watson P, Snyder C, Lynch H (2013) Aspirin Use is Associated with Lower Prostate Cancer Risk in Male Carriers of BRCA Mutations. J Genet Couns.
10. Kalluri R, Weinberg RA (2009) The basics of epithelial-mesenchymal transition. J Clin Invest 119: 1420–1428.
11. Tanaka T, Kohno H, Suzuki R, Yamada Y, Sugie S, et al. (2003) A novel inflammation-related mouse colon carcinogenesis model induced by azoxymethane and dextran sodium sulfate. Cancer Sci 94: 965–973.
12. Guerra C, Collado M, Navas C, Schuhmacher AJ, Hernandez-Porras I, et al. (2011) Pancreatitis-induced inflammation contributes to pancreatic cancer by inhibiting oncogene-induced senescence. Cancer Cell 19: 728–739.
13. Blackburn JS, Langenau DM (2014) Zebrafish as a model to assess cancer heterogeneity, progression and relapse. Dis Model Mech 7: 755–762.
14. Yen J, White RM, Stemple DL (2014) Zebrafish models of cancer: progress and future challenges. Curr Opin Genet Dev 24: 38–45.
15. Niethammer P, Grabher C, Look AT, Mitchison TJ (2009) A tissue-scale gradient of hydrogen peroxide mediates rapid wound detection in zebrafish. Nature 459: 996–999.
16. Yoo SK, Starnes TW, Deng Q, Huttenlocher A (2011) Lyn is a redox sensor that mediates leukocyte wound attraction in vivo. Nature 480: 109–112.
17. de Oliveira S, Reyes-Aldasoro CC, Candel S, Renshaw SA, Mulero V, et al. (2013) Cxcl8 (IL-8) mediates neutrophil recruitment and behavior in the zebrafish inflammatory response. J Immunol 190: 4349–4359.

18. Deng Q, Sarris M, Bennin DA, Green JM, Herbomel P, et al. (2013) Localized bacterial infection induces systemic activation of neutrophils through Cxcr2 signaling in zebrafish. J Leukoc Biol 93: 761–769.

19. Feng Y, Santoriello C, Mione M, Hurlstone A, Martin P (2010) Live imaging of innate immune cell sensing of transformed cells in zebrafish larvae: parallels between tumor initiation and wound inflammation. PLoS Biol 8: e1000562.

20. Dodd ME, Hatzold J, Mathias JR, Walters KB, Bennin DA, et al. (2009) The ENTH domain protein Clint1 is required for epidermal homeostasis in zebrafish. Development 136: 2591–2600.

21. Boppana NB, Devarajan A, Gopal K, Barathan M, Bakar SA, et al. (2014) Blockade of CXCR2 signalling: a potential therapeutic target for preventing neutrophil-mediated inflammatory diseases. Exp Biol Med (Maywood) 239: 509–518.

22. Verbeke H, Geboes K, Van Damme J, Struyf S (2012) The role of CXC chemokines in the transition of chronic inflammation to esophageal and gastric cancer. Biochim Biophys Acta 1825: 117–129.

23. Cataisson C, Ohman R, Patel G, Pearson A, Tsien M, et al. (2009) Inducible cutaneous inflammation reveals a protumorigenic role for keratinocyte CXCR2 in skin carcinogenesis. Cancer Res 69: 319–328.

24. Wang D, DuBois RN (2014) Myeloid-derived suppressor cells link inflammation to cancer. Oncoimmunology 3: e28581.

25. Vandercappellen J, Van Damme J, Struyf S (2008) The role of CXC chemokines and their receptors in cancer. Cancer Lett 267: 226–244.

26. Jamieson T, Clarke M, Steele CW, Samuel MS, Neumann J, et al. (2012) Inhibition of CXCR2 profoundly suppresses inflammation-driven and spontaneous tumorigenesis. J Clin Invest 122: 3127–3144.

27. Brat DJ, Bellail AC, Van Meir EG (2005) The role of interleukin-8 and its receptors in gliomagenesis and tumoral angiogenesis. Neuro Oncol 7: 122–133.

28. Kline M, Donovan K, Wellik L, Lust C, Jin W, et al. (2007) Cytokine and chemokine profiles in multiple myeloma; significance of stromal interaction and correlation of IL-8 production with disease progression. Leuk Res 31: 591–598.

29. Varney ML, Li A, Dave BJ, Bucana CD, Johansson SL, et al. (2003) Expression of CXCR1 and CXCR2 receptors in malignant melanoma with different metastatic potential and their role in interleukin-8 (CXCL-8)-mediated modulation of metastatic phenotype. Clin Exp Metastasis 20: 723–731.

30. Hertzer KM, Donald GW, Hines OJ (2013) CXCR2: a target for pancreatic cancer treatment? Expert Opin Ther Targets 17: 667–680.

31. Lee YS, Choi I, Ning Y, Kim NY, Khatchadourian V, et al. (2012) Interleukin-8 and its receptor CXCR2 in the tumour microenvironment promote colon cancer growth, progression and metastasis. Br J Cancer 106: 1833–1841.

32. Yang G, Rosen DG, Liu G, Yang F, Guo X, et al. (2010) CXCR2 promotes ovarian cancer growth through dysregulated cell cycle, diminished apoptosis, and enhanced angiogenesis. Clin Cancer Res 16: 3875–3886.

33. Tazzyman S, Barry ST, Ashton S, Wood P, Blakey D, et al. (2011) Inhibition of neutrophil infiltration into A549 lung tumors in vitro and in vivo using a CXCR2-specific antagonist is associated with reduced tumor growth. Int J Cancer 129: 847–858.

34. Asfaha S, Dubeykovskiy AN, Tomita H, Yang X, Stokes S, et al. (2013) Mice that express human interleukin-8 have increased mobilization of immature myeloid cells, which exacerbates inflammation and accelerates colon carcinogenesis. Gastroenterology 144: 155–166.

35. Highfill SL, Cui Y, Giles AJ, Smith JP, Zhang H, et al. (2014) Disruption of CXCR2-mediated MDSC tumor trafficking enhances anti-PD1 efficacy. Sci Transl Med 6: 237ra267.

36. Katoh H, Wang D, Daikoku T, Sun H, Dey SK, et al. (2013) CXCR2-expressing myeloid-derived suppressor cells are essential to promote colitis-associated tumorigenesis. Cancer Cell 24: 631–644.

37. Arnoux V, Nassour M, L'Helgoualc'h A, Hipskind RA, Savagner P (2008) Erk5 controls Slug expression and keratinocyte activation during wound healing. Mol Biol Cell 19: 4738–4749.

38. Gong Z, Ju B, Wang X, He J, Wan H, et al. (2002) Green fluorescent protein expression in germ-line transmitted transgenic zebrafish under a stratified epithelial promoter from keratin8. Dev Dyn 223: 204–215.

39. McKenna WG, Weiss MC, Bakanauskas VJ, Sandler H, Kelsten ML, et al. (1990) The role of the H-ras oncogene in radiation resistance and metastasis. Int J Radiat Oncol Biol Phys 18: 849–859.

40. Downward J (1996) Control of ras activation. Cancer Surv 27: 87–100.

41. Zachos G, Varras M, Koffa M, Ergazaki M, Spandidos DA (1996) The association of the H-ras oncogene and steroid hormone receptors in gynecological cancer. J Exp Ther Oncol 1: 335–341.

42. Wittinghofer A, Franken SM, Scheidig AJ, Rensland H, Lautwein A, et al. (1993) Three-dimensional structure and properties of wild-type and mutant H-ras-encoded p21. Ciba Found Symp 176: 6–21; discussion 21–27.

43. Downward J (2003) Targeting RAS signalling pathways in cancer therapy. Nat Rev Cancer 3: 11–22.

44. Ancrile BB, O'Hayer KM, Counter CM (2008) Oncogenic ras-induced expression of cytokines: a new target of anti-cancer therapeutics. Mol Interv 8: 22–27.

45. Sparmann A, Bar-Sagi D (2004) Ras-induced interleukin-8 expression plays a critical role in tumor growth and angiogenesis. Cancer Cell 6: 447–458.

46. Wislez M, Fujimoto N, Izzo JG, Hanna AE, Cody DD, et al. (2006) High expression of ligands for chemokine receptor CXCR2 in alveolar epithelial neoplasia induced by oncogenic kras. Cancer Res 66: 4198–4207.

47. Eisenhoffer GT, Rosenblatt J (2011) Live imaging of cell extrusion from the epidermis of developing zebrafish. J Vis Exp.

48. Kajita M, Hogan C, Harris AR, Dupre-Crochet S, Itasaki N, et al. (2010) Interaction with surrounding normal epithelial cells influences signalling pathways and behaviour of Src-transformed cells. J Cell Sci 123: 171–180.

49. Casas E, Kim J, Bendesky A, Ohno-Machado L, Wolfe CJ, et al. (2011) Snail2 is an essential mediator of Twist1-induced epithelial mesenchymal transition and metastasis. Cancer Res 71: 245–254.

50. Peinado H, Olmeda D, Cano A (2007) Snail, Zeb and bHLH factors in tumour progression: an alliance against the epithelial phenotype? Nat Rev Cancer 7: 415–428.

51. Thiery JP (2002) Epithelial-mesenchymal transitions in tumour progression. Nat Rev Cancer 2: 442–454.

52. Sato H, Kida Y, Mai M, Endo Y, Sasaki T, et al. (1992) Expression of genes encoding type IV collagen-degrading metalloproteinases and tissue inhibitors of metalloproteinases in various human tumor cells. Oncogene 7: 77–83.

53. Lam PY, Harvie EA, Huttenlocher A (2013) Heat shock modulates neutrophil motility in zebrafish. PLoS One 8: e84436.

54. Renshaw SA, Loynes CA, Trushell DM, Elworthy S, Ingham PW, et al. (2006) A transgenic zebrafish model of neutrophilic inflammation. Blood 108: 3976–3978.

55. Mathias JR, Perrin BJ, Liu TX, Kanki J, Look AT, et al. (2006) Resolution of inflammation by retrograde chemotaxis of neutrophils in transgenic zebrafish. J Leukoc Biol 80: 1281–1288.

56. Hall C, Flores MV, Storm T, Crosier K, Crosier P (2007) The zebrafish lysozyme C promoter drives myeloid-specific expression in transgenic fish. BMC Dev Biol 7: 42.

57. Deng Q, Yoo SK, Cavnar PJ, Green JM, Huttenlocher A (2011) Dual roles for Rac2 in neutrophil motility and active retention in zebrafish hematopoietic tissue. Dev Cell 21: 735–745.

58. Murayama E, Kissa K, Zapata A, Mordelet E, Briolat V, et al. (2006) Tracing hematopoietic precursor migration to successive hematopoietic organs during zebrafish development. Immunity 25: 963–975.

59. Li L, Jin H, Xu J, Shi Y, Wen Z (2011) Irf8 regulates macrophage versus neutrophil fate during zebrafish primitive myelopoiesis. Blood 117: 1359–1369.

60. Becker M, Muller CB, De Bastiani MA, Klamt F (2013) The prognostic impact of tumor-associated macrophages and intra-tumoral apoptosis in non-small cell lung cancer. Histol Histopathol.

61. Rogers TL, Holen I (2011) Tumour macrophages as potential targets of bisphosphonates. J Transl Med 9: 177.

62. Cieslewicz M, Tang J, Yu JL, Cao H, Zavaljevski M, et al. (2013) Targeted delivery of proapoptotic peptides to tumor-associated macrophages improves survival. Proc Natl Acad Sci U S A.

63. Rodriguez D, Silvera R, Carrio R, Nadji M, Caso R, et al. (2013) Tumor microenvironment profoundly modifies functional status of macrophages: Peritoneal and tumor-associated macrophages are two very different subpopulations. Cell Immunol 283: 51–60.

64. Burke RM, Madden KS, Perry SW, Zettel ML, Brown EB (2013) Tumor-associated macrophages and stromal TNF-alpha regulate collagen structure in a breast tumor model as visualized by second harmonic generation. J Biomed Opt 18: 86003.

65. Kennedy BC, Showers CR, Anderson DE, Anderson L, Canoll P, et al. (2013) Tumor-associated macrophages in glioma: friend or foe? J Oncol 2013: 486912.

66. Baggiolini M, Clark-Lewis I (1992) Interleukin-8, a chemotactic and inflammatory cytokine. FEBS Lett 307: 97–101.

67. Kuang DM, Zhao Q, Wu Y, Peng C, Wang J, et al. (2011) Peritumoral neutrophils link inflammatory response to disease progression by fostering angiogenesis in hepatocellular carcinoma. J Hepatol 54: 948–955.

68. Dumitru CA, Gholaman H, Trellakis S, Bruderek K, Dominas N, et al. (2011) Tumor-derived macrophage migration inhibitory factor modulates the biology of head and neck cancer cells via neutrophil activation. Int J Cancer.

69. Dong YL, Kabir SM, Lee ES, Son DS (2013) CXCR2-driven ovarian cancer progression involves upregulation of proinflammatory chemokines by potentiating NF-kappaB activation via EGFR-transactivated Akt signaling. PLoS One 8: e83789.

70. Grosse-Steffen T, Giese T, Giese N, Longerich T, Schirmacher P, et al. (2012) Epithelial-to-mesenchymal transition in pancreatic ductal adenocarcinoma and pancreatic tumor cell lines: the role of neutrophils and neutrophil-derived elastase. Clin Dev Immunol 2012: 720768.

71. Kimmel CB, Ballard WW, Kimmel SR, Ullmann B, Schilling TF (1995) Stages of embryonic development of the zebrafish. Dev Dyn 203: 253–310.

72. Chen CF, Chu CY, Chen TH, Lee SJ, Shen CN, et al. (2011) Establishment of a transgenic zebrafish line for superficial skin ablation and functional validation of apoptosis modulators in vivo. PLoS One 6: e20654.

73. Yoo SK, Freisinger CM, LeBert DC, Huttenlocher A (2012) Early redox, Src family kinase, and calcium signaling integrate wound responses and tissue regeneration in zebrafish. J Cell Biol 199: 225–234.

74. Urasaki A, Morvan G, Kawakami K (2006) Functional dissection of the Tol2 transposable element identified the minimal cis-sequence and a highly repetitive sequence in the subterminal region essential for transposition. Genetics 174: 639–649.

75. Long S, Rebagliati M (2002) Sensitive two-color whole-mount in situ hybridizations using digoxigenin- and dinitrophenol-labeled RNA probes. Biotechniques 32: 494, 496, 498 passim.

76. Mathias JR, Dodd ME, Walters KB, Yoo SK, Ranheim EA, et al. (2009) Characterization of zebrafish larval inflammatory macrophages. Dev Comp Immunol 33: 1212–1217.

77. Oehlers SH, Flores MV, Hall CJ, O'Toole R, Swift S, et al. (2010) Expression of zebrafish cxcl8 (interleukin-8) and its receptors during development and in response to immune stimulation. Dev Comp Immunol 34: 352–359.

20

Mosaicism of Podocyte Involvement Is Related to Podocyte Injury in Females with Fabry Disease

Michael Mauer[1,2], Emily Glynn[3], Einar Svarstad[4,5], Camilla Tøndel[5,6], Marie-Claire Gubler[7], Michael West[8], Alexey Sokolovskiy[3], Chester Whitley[1], Behzad Najafian[3]*

1 Department of Pediatrics, University of Minnesota, Minneapolis, United States of America, 2 Department of Medicine, University of Minnesota, Minneapolis, United States of America, 3 Department of Pathology, University of Washington, Seattle, United States of America, 4 Department of Medicine, Haukeland University Hospital, Bergen, Norway, 5 Department of Clinical Medicine, University of Bergen, Bergen, Norway, 6 Department of Pediatrics, Haukeland University Hospital, Bergen, Norway, 7 U983, Université René Descartes, Hôpital Necker-Enfants Malades AP-HP, Paris, France, 8 Division of Nephrology, Department of Medicine, Dalhousie University, Halifax, Nova Scotia, Canada

Abstract

Background: Fabry disease. an X-linked deficiency of α-galactosidase A coded by the GLA gene, leads to intracellular globotriaosylceramide (GL-3) accumulation. Although less common than in males, chronic kidney disease, occurs in ~15% of females. Recent studies highlight the importance of podocyte injury in Fabry nephropathy development and progression. We hypothesized that the greater the % of podocytes with active wild-type GLA gene (due to X-inactivation of the mutant copy) the less is the overall podocyte injury.

Methods: Kidney biopsies from 12 treatment-naive females with Fabry disease, ages 15 (8–63), median [range], years were studied by electron microscopy and compared with 4 treatment-naive male patients.

Results: In females, 51 (13–100)% of podocytes (PC) per glomerulus had no GL-3 inclusions, this consistent with a non-Fabry podocyte phenotype (NFPC). In PC with GL-3 inclusions [Fabry podocyte phenotype (FPC)], GL-3 volume density per podocyte was virtually identical in females and males, consistent with little or no cross-correction between FPC and NFPC. %NFPC per glomerulus (%NFPC/glom) correlated with age in females ($r = 0.65$, $p = 0.02$), suggesting a survival disadvantage for FPC over time. Age-adjusted %NFPC/glom was inversely related to foot process width (FPW) ($r = -0.75$, $p = 0.007$), an indicator of PC injury. GL-3 volume density in FPC in females correlated directly with FPW.

Conclusions: These findings support important relationships between podocyte mosaicism and podocyte injury in female Fabry patients. Kidney biopsy, by providing information about podocyte mosaicism, may help to stratify females with Fabry disease for kidney disease risk and to guide treatment decisions.

Editor: Stuart E. Dryer, University of Houston, United States of America

Funding: This work was supported by an NIH RDCRN U54 grant (5U54NS065768-04) and an investigator initiated grant from Genzyme, a Sanofi Company. The funder provided support in the form of research grants for authors [BN, MM, and MLW], and travel support and honoraria for authors [BN, MM, CT, and MLW] but did not have any additional role in the study design, data collection and analysis, decision to publish, or preparation of the manuscript. The specific roles of these authors are articulated in the 'author contributions' section.

Competing Interests: BN is a consultant to Genzyme and Amicus Therapeutics, receives investigator initiated research support from Genzyme and Roche, and honoraria and travel support from Genzyme. BN is also a member of the Medical Advisory Board of Amicus Therapeutics. MM is a consultant to Genzyme, and receives investigator initiated research support, honoraria, and travel support from Genzyme. MM is also a member of the Genzyme funded FDA mandated Fabry Registry Board. This interest for MM has been reviewed and managed by the University of Minnesota in accordance with its conflict of interest policies. MM is also a consultant to Amicus. CT and ES received travel support and speakers honoraria from Shire and Genzyme. MLW has received research support, honoraria, and/or travel support from Actelion, Amicus, Excelsior Pharmaceuticals, Genzyme, Glaxo SmithKline, Shire, and Sumitomo Pharma.

* Email: najafian@u.washington.edu

Introduction

Fabry disease is a storage disease caused by deficiency of the α-galactosidase A (αGal A) enzyme that hydrolyzes the terminal α-galactosyl moieties from glycolipids and glycoproteins. This leads to the accumulation of its substrates, predominately globotriaosylceramide (GL-3) in various cell types and organs, causing a constellation of complications including skin lesions, strokes, cardiac arrhythmias and cardiomyopathy, neuropathies and renal failure. [1] αGal A is encoded by the GLA gene located on the X chromosome locus Xq21.3-q22. Similar to other X-linked diseases, the complications are typically less frequent and more variable in severity in females, [2,3,4] although they can be as severe as in male patients. [5,6] A significant proportion of female patients suffer from important complications, including 40% with clinical renal disease (mainly proteinuria) [7] and about 15% with serious renal events. [2] Fabry disease is associated with significant life expectancy reductions in both sexes. [8] It is of great importance to understand the factors associated with disease severity in females. Currently, there are no reliable tests to identify females at greater risk to develop kidney failure, thus justifying earlier treatment with enzyme replacement therapy (ERT). Podocytes are terminally differentiated cells with pivotal role in preserving glomerular structure and function. [9] Recent studies suggest that GL-3 accumulation in podocytes plays an important role in the pathophysiology of Fabry nephropathy. [10] These cells are also much more resistant to ERT than most other kidney cell types. [11,12] Similar to other "terminally differentiated cells" podocytes do not easily regenerate following injury [13]. Continuous podocyte loss leads to progressive reduction of these cells in the glomeruli, this eventually reaching critical levels causing irreversible glomerular scarring [14]. Despite recent evidence that higher doses of ERT during childhood may result in partial to almost complete clearance of podocytes from GL-3 inclusions, [15] there is no consensus as to when to initiate ERT, especially in females, and the relative clinical effectiveness of the different licensed ERT doses remain unsettled. [16,17,18] We hypothesized that podocytes, due to random X-inactivation, are heterogeneously involved by Fabry disease in female patients and that this heterogeneity could influence podocyte injury. Herein we describe a method to quantify the % of podocytes with the Fabry phenotype and report an inverse relationship in females between age-adjusted % podocytes with no GL-3 inclusions in glomeruli and foot process width, a sensitive indicator of podocyte injury [19], supporting a relationship between X-inactivation and podocyte injury in females with Fabry disease. We also found no evidence of cross-correction between podocytes without and with the Fabry phenotype in females with Fabry disease.

Methods

These studies were performed in accordance with principles of the Declaration of Helsinki and were reviewed and approved by the Institutional Review Board of the University of Minnesota, Comité. de Protection des Personnes "Ile-De-France II." and the Regional Ethics Committee of Western Norway. Informed consents approved by the institutional board review committees were obtained prior to these studies.

Subjects and Clinical Parameters

Kidney biopsies from 12 ERT-naive females with Fabry disease, age 15 (8–63) years were studied by electron microscopy for distribution of podocyte involvement by the Fabry phenotype. Biopsies were obtained for assessment of the severity of the lesions of Fabry nephropathy in order to aid clinical decision-making regarding ERT initiation and/or as a baseline biopsy prior to ERT initiation. Biopsies from 4 ERT-naive males with Fabry disease, age 14 (7–18), were studied for comparison; 7/16 patients presented here were included in our previous publications. [10,15] The demographic and clinical data of all patients are presented in Table 1.

9/12 female and 3/4 male patients had results of GLA mutation analysis in their medical records confirming the diagnosis of Fabry disease (Table 1). The diagnosis of Fabry disease in the other patients was based on family history or clinical findings with or without reduced leukocyte αGal A activity and confirmed by the kidney biopsy findings. Protein excretion per gram creatinine (UPCR) was based on urine samples obtained close to the date of biopsy. GFR was estimated by the plasma clearance of iohexol where available or by creatinine clearance. Except for one of the patients where we were not able to find information about the use

of renin-angiotensin system blockers, none of the patients were receiving these drugs.

Biopsies from 6 healthy living kidney donors, age 37 (16–52) were used to estimate normal control values for podocyte foot process with (FPW), as described below.

Biopsy Tissue Preparation and Electron Microscopy

Electron microscopy specimens were fixed in 2.5% glutaraldehyde, and embedded in PolyBed. Random glomerular sections were prepared as previously described. [20] Thin sections were mounted on formvar coated copper slot grids. Overlapping digital low magnification (~10,000 x) images of the entire glomerular profiles were obtained using a JEOL CX100 electron microscope for the podocyte mosaicism studies. High magnification (~30,000 x) images were obtained according a systematic uniform random sampling protocol for estimation of fraction of the volume (Vv) of PC cytoplasm occupied by GL-3 inclusions [Vv(Inc/PC)], Vv of inclusions/glomerular mesangial cell [Vv(Inc/Mes)], Vv of inclusions/glomerular endothelial cell [Vv(Inc/Endo)], and podocyte average FPW as previously described [10,20].

Identification of Podocytes with and without the Fabry Phenotype

Observers were masked to any of the patient characteristics. Montages of complete glomerular profiles were prepared from the above images in Adobe Photoshop software (Adobe Photoshop CS5 Extended, version 12.0×32). Twice digital magnification was applied to the images. Podocyte nuclei were identified and glomerular profiles with less than 10 podocyte nuclei (n = 3) were excluded from these studies. The cytoplasmic profiles surrounding each podocyte nucleus were carefully examined for presence of GL-3 inclusions. Podocyte nuclear profiles with cytoplasmic GL-3 inclusions, consistent with Fabry phenotype podocytes (FPC) or without cytoplasmic GL-3 inclusions, consistent with non-Fabry phnotype podocytes (NFPC) cytoplasmic GL-3 inclusions were counted in each glomerulus and %NFPC/glom was calculated. The maximum number of immediately adjacent podocytes, including podocytes on the other side of the same capillary loop, which were NFPC was recorded as an estimate of the size of podocyte mosaic patches on the section.

Electron Microscopy Stereology

Based on the best quality of tissue preservation and images, one glomerulus per biopsy was arbitrarily selected for detailed GL-3 volume density measurement in podocytes with visible nuclei on the section. Boundaries of nuclei and cell membranes, excluding the tertiary foot processes were traced using the magnetic lasso tool in separate layers in Adobe Photoshop (Figure 1). Similarly, the most convex points of cytoplasmic GL-3 inclusions were connected using the magnetic lasso tool to draw a polygon around the GL-3 inclusion aggregates in a separate layer. The tracings were colored differentially for nuclei, cytoplasm and inclusions (Figure 1). The observed magnification was calculated from the average of 10 horizontal and 10 vertical random measurements performed on images from a SPI grating carbon replica #02902-AB (Structure Probe, Inc., West Chester, PA, USA) with horizontal and vertical lines 0.463 μm apart obtained at the same magnification as for the montage images. Subsequently, the measurement tool of the software was calibrated. The area of cell, nucleus and inclusion aggregate profiles were obtained separately for each podocyte profile with a visible nucleus from the Adobe Photoshop measurement log. The fractional volume of GL-3 inclusions per each nucleated podocyte profile with GL-3 inclusions [Vv(Inc/

Table 1. Clinical characteristics of subjects.

Case	Sex	Age (year)	UPCR (mg/g)	UACR (mg/g)	GFR (ml/min/1.73 m²)	GLA Mutation	Mutation Type	Aangiokeratoma	Corneal Opacity
1	F	8	40	NA	NA*	NA	NA	+	+
2	F	11	0.02	53	105	c.800T>G (p.M267R)	Missense	+	+
3	F	12	29	NA	109	W236X	Nonsense	–	–
4	F	13	0	NA	97	Y216D	Missense	–	+
5	F	13	60	5	100	NA	NA	+	–
6	F	14	62	11	90	c.800T>G (p.M267R)	Missense	NA	NA
7	F	16	30	12	127	NA	NA	–	–
8	F	34	150	NA	118	R301Q	Missense	+	–
9	F	34	100	5	99	R112C	Missense	–	+
10	F	39	100	NA	78	I270T	Missense	+	+
11	F	39	40	ND	99	N215S	Missense	+	–
12	F	63	1150	NA	46	C.427G>C p.Ala143Pro	Missense	+	–
13	M	7	0	NA	183	Y216D	Missense	+	+
14	M	16	92	12	112	c.1212_1214delAAG	Deletion	+	+
15	M	18	251	135	96	c.800T>G(p. M267R)	Missense	+	+
16	M	23	102	NA	111	NA	NA	NA	NA

Abbreviations: UPCR = urine protein/creatinine ratio; UACR = urine albumin/creatinine ratio; GFR = glomerular filtration rate; NA = data not available; *Serum creatinine within the normal range; F = female; M = male; ND = Not detectable.

FPC)] was estimated as follows: $V_V(Inc/FPC) = \dfrac{A_{inclusions} \times 100}{A_{cell} - A_{nucleus}}$.
The overall average glomerular volume fraction of GL-3 inclusions per podocytes [Vv(Inc/PC)], endothelial cells [Vv(Inc/Endo)] and mesangial cells [Vv(Inc/Mes)] were estimated using unbiased stereology methods as previously detailed. [10] For clarity, we emphasize that Vv(Inc/FPC) is an estimate of GL-3 inclusion density in nucleated podocyte profiles with GL-3 inclusions, while Vv(Inc/PC) is an estimate of the same parameter in all visible podocyte profiles regardless of GL-3 content and including the podocytes with and without visible nuclei over 3 (1–3), median (range), glomeruli per biopsy. Average foot process width (FPW) was also estimated using unbiased stereology methods as detailed elsewhere. [10,20,21] In order to compare podocyte injury in FPC vs. NFPC in female patients with Fabry disease, FPW was separately estimated in systematically and uniformly obtained electron micrographs with and without FPC.

Statistical Analyses

Statistica 8.0 (Statsoft, Inc.) was used for statistical analysis. Comparison between groups was made by student t-test after confirming homogeneity of variances. Relationships between variables were evaluated using Pearson correlation. Partial correlations were performed to control for confounding variables. Random effects model variance component analysis was performed to estimate % contribution of biopsies (inter-subject) and glomeruli (intra-subject) variations to total variance of %NFPC per glomerulus (%NFPC/glom). $p < 0.05$ was considered statistically significant.

Results

Electron Microscopy Examination of Kidney Biopsies

Examination of electron micrographs from all biopsies allowed easy and reliable distinction between male and female patients by the identification in females of podocytes with visible nuclei without GL-3 cytoplasmic inclusions, termed non-Fabry podocytes (NFPC) (Figure 1) in contrast with podocytes containing GL-3 inclusions, termed Fabry phenotype podocytes (FPC). However, mosaicism of the Fabry phenotype was not easily identifiable in the other glomerular or extra-glomerular cells, perhaps, at least in part, due to uncertainty about cellular boundaries (e.g., mesangial or endothelial cells). In 4 female patient biopsies, no GL-3 inclusions were identified in endothelial and/or mesangial cells, thus, comments about mosaicism could not be made in those cell types. In 7/12 female patient biopsies, parietal epithelial cell profiles with no GL-3 inclusions were identified while occasional parietal epithelial cells with enlarged cytoplasm had abundant GL-3 inclusions. Characteristic lamellar GL-3 inclusions were not easily identified in proximal tubular epithelial cells. Distal tubular epithelial cells showed variable GL-3 inclusions in both males and females. Thus, this variability could not be accounted for X-inactivation mosaicism in those cells.

Distribution of GL3 Inclusions among Podocytes in Males and Females

54 (27–87) podocytes per biopsy were examined for presence of GL-3 inclusions in female patients. 51 (13–100)% of podocyte profiles per biopsy with visible nuclei and no GL-3 inclusions, were classified as NFPC in these females. NFPC were distributed as

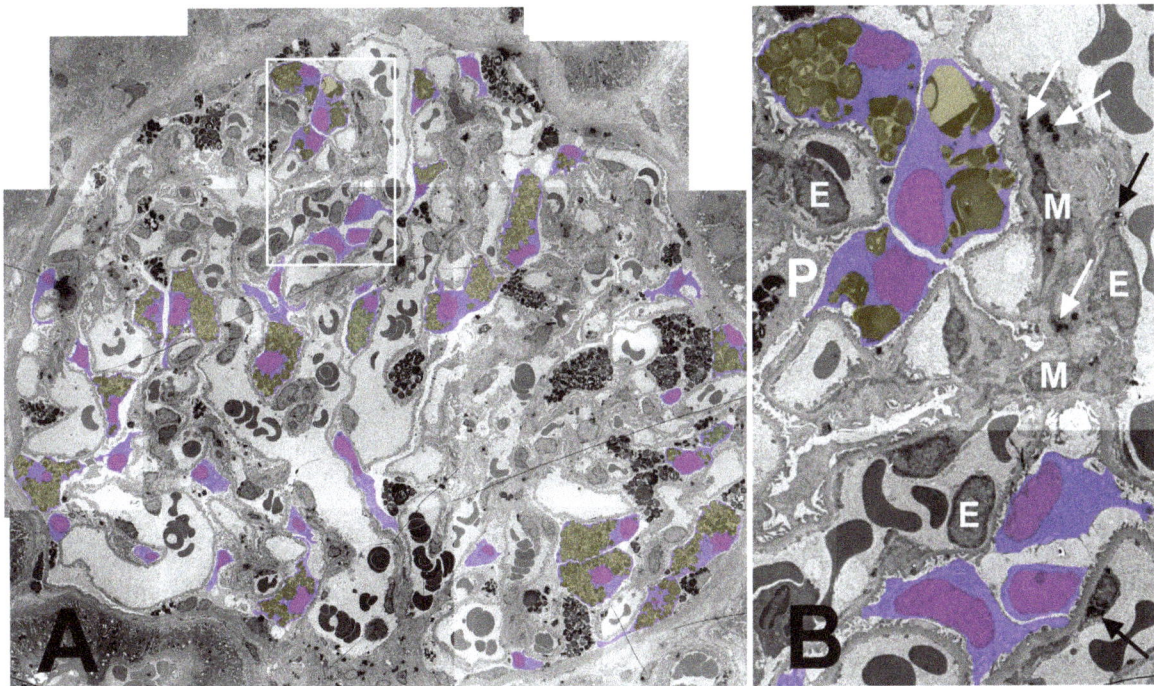

Figure 1. Mosaicism of podocyte Fabry phenotype in a glomerulus from a female patient with Fabry disease. (**A**) Montage image of a glomerulus (~3,000×). Podocyte bodies with visible nuclei are colored blue, podocyte nuclei purple, and GL-3 inclusions yellow. The white rectangle is magnified in B. (**B**) Magnified view of three podocyte profiles without (at the bottom) and three other podocyte profiles with GL-3 inclusions (on the top). Arrows show GL-3 inclusions in mesangial (M) cells (black) and endothelial (E) cells. P is a podocyte profile with no visible nucleus on this section.

single cells among FPC or in patches composed of 2–6 podocytes (Figure 1).

Two biopsies from female patients (one with 3 and another with 2 glomeruli) had no GL-3 inclusions in podocytes with visible nuclei (cases #9 and #11, Table 1). Case #9 showed rare podocyte profiles that were filled with GL-3. However, because these GL-3 containing podocytes had no visible nuclei they were not included in calculation of %NFPC per glomerulus. This case had a missense mutation (R112C) with GFR, UPCR and UACR values all within the normal range (Table 1). Clinical examination revealed corneal opacities, but no angiokeratoma. Echocardiograms showed normal left ventricular size and function with an estimated ejection fraction of 55–60% and normal right ventricular size and systolic function. Case #11 had distal tubular cells with GL-3 inclusions. This case had a cardiac variant mutation (N215S) with normal GFR and UPCR values and no detectable albumin in the urine (Table 1). The diagnosis of Fabry disease was made based on known family history. Clinical examination revealed angiokeratoma, but no corneal opacities. Clinically, she was asymptomatic. No echocardiograms were available from this case. None of these two subjects had a history of stroke. In order to determine whether random sectioning through podocytes may have obscured the observation of GL-3 inclusions in podocyte profiles 4 male patients with Fabry disease were similarly studied, 1–3 (median 2.5) glomeruli, containing 18–36 (median 22) podocyte profiles per glomerulus with visible nuclei were examined (Table 1). All podocyte profiles from these glomeruli contained abundant GL-3 inclusions, consistent with FPC, except for two very small profiles in a 7-year-old boy. The volume fraction of GL-3 inclusions per FPC [Vv(Inc/FPC)] was nearly identical in males (0.56 ± 0.11) and females (0.53 ± 0.13; $p = 0.54$).

Inter- and Intra-subject Variations of Podocyte Phenotype Mosaicism

Biopsies from 9 female patients with more than one glomerulus (3 (2–5), median (range)) available for electron microscopy were used to compare inter- and intra- subject variability of podocytes with the Fabry the phenotype. The %NFPC/glom in 2–4 glomeruli per biopsy in female patients is shown in Figure 2. Variance component analysis showed that only 9.6% of total variance in podocyte Fabry phenotype mosaicism originated from inter-glomerular (intra-subject) variation, while the vast majority of variance lay in differences in this parameter among the subjects.

Relationships Between % Podocytes with no GL-3 Inclusions and Female Patient Characteristics, Renal Function and Other Glomerular Structural Parameters

Values of %NFPC/glom, Vv(Inc/PC), volume fraction of GL-3 inclusions per mesangial cells [Vv(Inc/Mes)], volume fraction of inclusions per endothelial cells [Vv(Inc/Endo)], and foot process width (FPW) are provided in Table 2. The average %NFPC/glom was calculated in biopsies from female patients with more than one available glomerulus. There was a direct relationship between age and %NFPC/glom ($r = 0.65$; $p = 0.02$, Figure 3). No statistically significant relationship was found between %NFPC/glom and urine albumin/creatinine ratio (UACR) (available in 6/12 patients), urine protein creatinine ratio (UPCR) or glomerular filtration rate (GFR). As expected, %NFPC/glom was inversely related to Vv(Inc/PC) ($r = -0.70$, $p = 0.02$) for all podocytes. Simple linear regression analysis revealed no statistically significant relationships between %NFPC/glom and foot process width, Vv(Inc/Endo), Vv(Inc/Mes). However, adjusted for age, significant inverse relationships were found between %NFPC/glom and

FPW ($r = -0.75$, $p = 0.007$), and Vv(Inc/Mes) ($r = 0.70$, $p = 0.02$), but not with Vv(Inc/Endo).

To better visualize the relationships between %NFPC/glom and FPW and UPCR, 10 female patients were grouped into 5 age-matched pairs, 3 pairs with identical ages and the 2 other pairs with ages no more than 2 years apart. Except for one pair, in each pair, the subject with lower %NFPC/glom had greater FPW value, suggestive of an inverse relationship between the extent of podocyte injury and the number of NFPC in age-matched Fabry females (Figure 4). Even an 8 year old female with 20% NFPC/glom (case #1) had greater FPW than an 11 year old (case #2) with 50% NFPC/glom. The one exception was a pair with greater FPW in a 14 year old girl with 22% NFPC/glom (case #6) compared to a 16 years old with 13% %NFPC/glom (case #7) (Figure 4). The relationships between %NFPC/glom and UPCR among the above pairs paralleled the relationships between %NFPC/glom and FPW, except for cases #2 and #3 with almost identical %NFPC/glom (50 and 52%, respectively) and slightly (~15%) greater UPCR for case#2 (Figure 4). However, the relationship between %NFPC and UPCR remained not statistically significant after age adjustment. Also, when adjusted for age, Vv(Inc/FPC) in females correlated with FPW ($r = 0.64$, $p = 0.03$). In females with Fabry disease, FPW in electron micrographs where glomerular basement membranes were covered by FPC (562 ± 160 nm) was not statistically different from those where glomerular basement membranes were covered by NFPC (663 ± 283 nm). On the other hand, FPW in either of these areas were greater than FPW in normal control biopsies (406 ± 34 nm, $p = 0.037$ for FPC and $p = 0.048$ for NFPC).

Discussion

We recently demonstrated that the fraction of the volume of podocytes occupied by GL-3 [Vv(Inc/PC)] increases with age in children with Fabry disease and is directly correlated with FPW and to proteinuria,[9] the latter a strong predictor of renal disease risk among Fabry disease patients.[23] Increased FPW is a common concomitant of injury in podocytes and is seen in a variety of conditions known to be associated with injury in these cells. [21,22], [23] Thus careful examination of this cell in Fabry disease is important. This is the first study to provide unbiased electron microscopic morphometric measures of the heterogeneity of podocyte involvement in females with Fabry disease, almost certainly as a result of X-inactivation. Gubler et al first described the heterogeneous distribution of GL-3 inclusions in podocytes in 3 females with Fabry disease. [24] Valbuena et al also described variable podocyte GL-3 accumulation in 4 females with Fabry disease. [25] However, no quantitative assessment of podocyte GL-3 or statistical analyses was provided in these reports. Similar to these studies, [24,25] we found that a distinction between Fabry and non-Fabry phenotype, consistent with cells carrying active mutant or wild-type GLA, respectively, could be easily made in podocytes but not in other renal cells of female patients. This could be due to distinct borders of podocyte cell bodies from their neighbor cells, or because podocytes are apparently very long lived [26] and may thus retain GL-3 inclusions for years while other cell types are more frequently replaced.

Importantly, we documented, through unbiased morphometric measurements, that the average fraction of podocyte cytoplasm occupied by GL-3 was virtually identical in male and female patients, suggesting that FPC do not benefit from the enzymatic activity of the adjacent NFPC or from the generally higher residual plasma αGal A in females than on males. [27] [28,29].

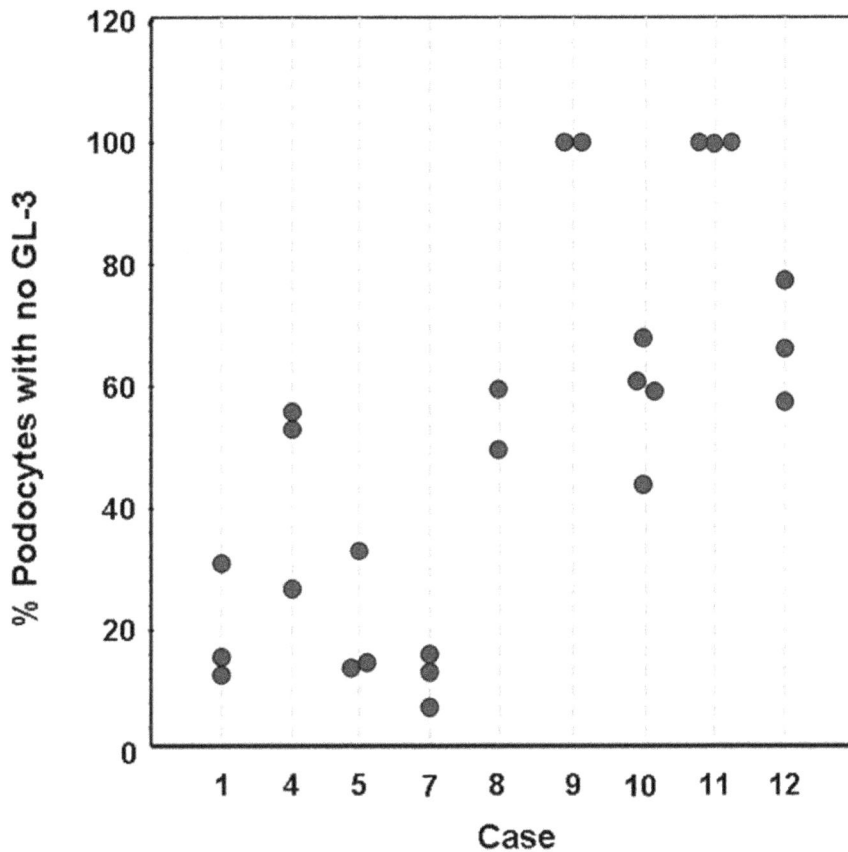

Figure 2. Intra- and inter-subject variability of podocyte mosaicism for Fabry phenotype in females. X axis shows case numbers (see Table 1). Each vertical dashed line represents a biopsy and each circle represents % podocytes with no GL-3 inclusions in one glomerulus.

Also important, we found that inter-glomerular variation in podocyte phenotype mosaicism in a given female Fabry patient's renal biopsy is much smaller than inter-patient variation. This suggests that estimation of podocyte phenotypic mosaicism even in a single glomerulus is representative of this phenomenon in the biopsy and validates the study of podocyte phenotype mosaicism in a few glomeruli. It also suggests that podocyte mosaicism in females is established relatively early in embryogenesis. It should be noted that in these studies we used random profiles of glomeruli. Although we observed NFPC in patches of up to 5 cells in these two-dimensional glomerular cross-sections, these patches are likely larger in three dimensions. Nonetheless we posit that these patches are not very large, otherwise we might have expected greater inter-glomerular variability as a result of random sectioning through glomeruli.

This study is the first to show a quantitative relationship in females with Fabry disease between the X-inactivation phenomenon and podocyte injury manifest as increased FPW. Although X-inactivation may play a role in the clinical phenotypic expression of X-linked diseases, a direct link between skewed X-inactivation and severity of the Fabry phenotype has been controversial. Dobrovolny et al. reported that the trend line between the age and the Mainz severity score index (MSSI) [30] was steeper in 10 Fabry females with vs. 28 without unfavorably skewed X-inactivation in leukocytes, urinary and salivary cells. This suggested that random X-inactivation could influence the severity of the Fabry phenotype in female patients. [31] In contrast, Maier et al. found that in 46% of the 28 Fabry females

studied, skewed X-inactivation did not correlate with phenotype severity. [4] Similarly, in a more recent study, while confirming random X-inactivation in leukocytes in ~82% of 77 female Fabry patients, there was no relationship between X-inactivation ratios and age, αGal A activity, MSSI scores, cardiac involvement, neuropathic pain or proteinuria. [32] We did not find a statistically significant relationship between % NFPC/glom and UPCR. However, in regression models including UPCR among the predictor variables, UPCR accounted for much less of the variance for rates of GFR decline in women than in men with Fabry disease. [33] Also, increased UPCR can reflect parameters other than podocyte injury, such as impaired tubular reabsorption reabsorption of filtered protein. However, after adjusting for age, we documented a significant inverse relationship between %NFPC/glom and FPW, a widely accepted indicator of podocyte injury. Thus, having more NFPC in glomeruli was associated with less podocyte injury. However, having a greater proportion of NFPC in older females with Fabry disease is not necessarily indicative of less podocyte injury. In fact, the observed increase in the %NFPC/glom with age in female patients in the current study is suggestive of progressive FPC loss with aging due to a survival disadvantage caused by the Fabry phenotype. Thus, glomeruli of older female patients may have fewer total podocytes than those of younger females with lesser %NFPC/glom, a hypothesis that remains to be tested in future studies. On the other hand, our side-by-side comparisons of age-matched female pairs revealed a robust inverse relationship between %NFPC/glom and FPW. However, given that Fabry disease is genetically heterogeneous, with more

Current Progress in Hematology

Table 2. Glomerular Structural Parameters.

Case	Sex	Age (year)	%NFPC/glom	Vv(Inc/PC)	Vv(Inc/Mes)	Vv(Inc/Endo)	Vv(Inc/FPC)	FPW* (nm)
1	F	8	20	0.28	0.03	0.08	0.50	524
2	F	11	50	0.43	0.02	0	0.62	426
3	F	12	52	0.21	0	0	0.42	372
4	F	13	45	0.20	0	0.03	0.42	464
5	F	13	21	0.26	0.03	0.03	0.68	663
6	F	14	22	0.38	0.07	0.02	0.53	602
7	F	16	13	0.51	0.03	0.02	0.67	461
8	F	34	55	0.43	0.01	0.01	0.70	620
9	F	34	100	0	0	0.01	0	427
10	F	39	58	0.21	0.01	0	0.35	654
11	F	39	100	0.02	0.01	0	0	441
12	F	63	68	0.16	0.04	0.06	0.48	673
13	M	7	8**	0.21	0.01	0.09	0.58	369
14	M	16	0	0.44	0.10	0.37	0.56	551
15	M	18	0	0.50	0.16	0.21	0.61	823
16	M	23	0	0.34	0.56	0.27	0.65	714

Abbreviations: %NFPC/glom = % non-Fabry podocytes per glomerulus; Vv(Inc/PC) = volume fraction of GL3 inclusions per podocyte; Vv(Inc/Mes) = volume fraction of GL3 inclusions per mesangial cell; Vv(Inc/Endo) = volume fraction of GL3 inclusions per endothelial cell; Vv(Inc/FPC) = volume fraction of GL3 inclusions per Fabry podocytes; FPW = foot process width; F = female; M = male; *Normal values for FPW obtained from biopsies from 6 healthy living donors was 406÷34 nm. **The biopsy contained two very small podocyte profiles with no GL3 inclusions, most likely due to random sectioning.

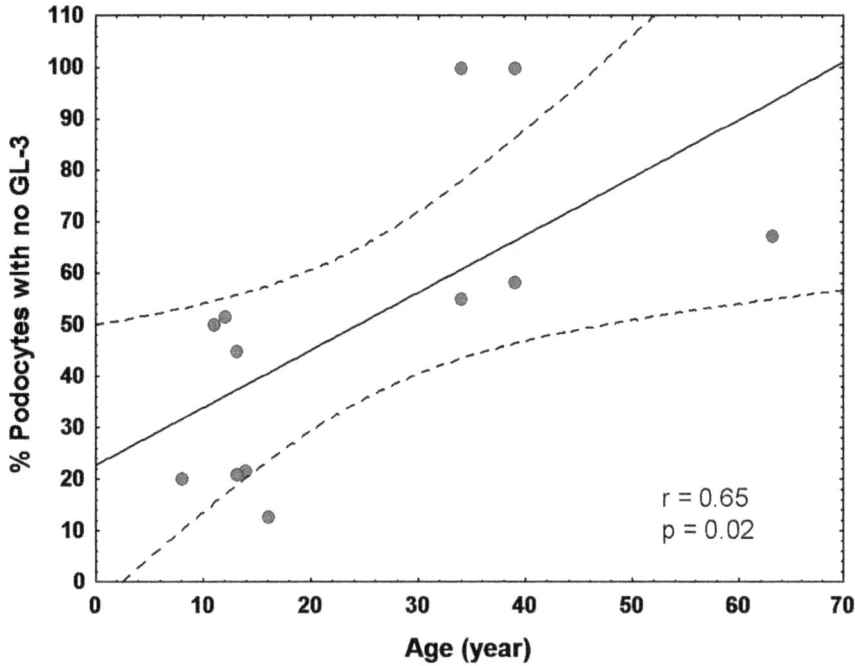

Figure 3. Relationship between age and % podocytes with no GL-3 in females. Dashed lines represent 0.95 confidence interval.

than registered 600 mutations, [34] it should be expected that attempts to explain all phenotype variation by a single parameter such as mosaicism will necessarily be overambitious. [35,36] Nevertheless, it will be interesting to examine if a relationship can be found between podocyte mosaicism status in the kidney and skewed X-inactivation in other organs or cell types, especially that of leukocytes. However, some of the cases presented in this study were from historical archived material and no simultaneous blood samples or skin biopsies had been obtained for x-inactivation studies at the time other biopsies were performed.

The relationship between podocyte mosaicism and podocyte injury in female Fabry patients suggests that the status of podocyte

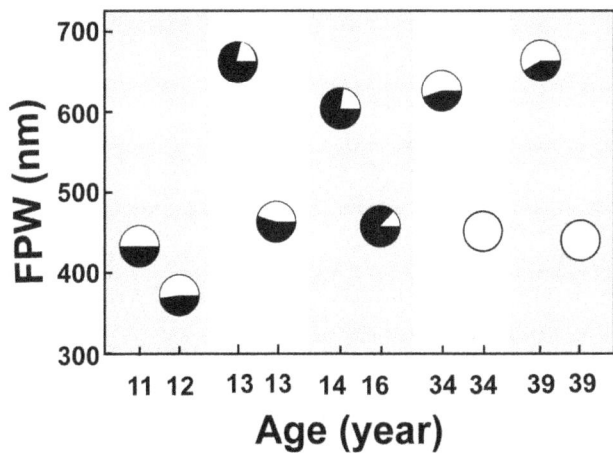

Figure 4. Relationships between podocyte mosaicism and foot process width in age-matched paired females. Each vertical grey or white band represents an age-matched pair. Each pie chart represents %NFPC/glom as white and %FPC/glom as black area. Abbreviation: FPW: foot process width.

X-inactivation, after making adjustment for the age of the patient, could help to identify females with greater risk of progression of Fabry nephropathy. Although it would be desirable to use less invasive methods to obtain information about the proportion of cells with active mutant GLA, the status of mosaicism may be cell type and organ specific. Moreover, as outlined above, studies attempting to link X-inactivation in peripheral blood leukocytes and clinical manifestations of Fabry females have produced contradictory results. [4,31] Thus far, renal biopsy may be the only reliable way to obtain information about podocyte mosaicism in these patients.

Importantly, the present study showed that not only podocyte mosaicism for Fabry phenotype and podocyte injury are linked in female patients, but also podocyte injury in these patients is not limited to FPC and extends to NFPC, evidenced by increased FPW in GBM areas covered by NFPC compared with normal control biopsies. This is consistent with experimental studies performed by Matsusaka et al. where following administration of the immunotoxin LMB2 to the mice chimeric for hCD25 (LMB2 receptor), not only hCD25+ podocytes, but also hCD25- podocytes were injured and showed foot process widening, suggesting that specific injury to some podocytes can induce non-specific injury to other podocytes, [14] a phenomenon that if severe enough could lead to a vicious cycle of podocyte loss and glomerulosclerosis.

To our knowledge, this is the first report of the finding of rare cells with GL-3 inclusions in kidney biopsies from female Fabry patients. We encountered two females, ages 34 (case #9) and 39 years (case #11), with known Fabry disease by mutation analysis with very rare kidney cells with GL-3 inclusions. One (case #11), had a cardiac variant GLA mutation (N215S) [37] and the other (case #9) had a missense mutation (R112C). Thus, in contrast to males, the finding of even rare cells with GL3 inclusions in kidney biopsies from females should raise strong suspicion for Fabry disease. Notably, both of these subjects had very mild phenotypes, raising suspicion that the favorable skewed X-inactivation (predominantly affecting the mutant copy of GLA) observed in kidney biopsies may have also been present in other organs, especially since R112C mutation has been associated with classical Fabry disease causing ESRD [38], while case #9 in the present study had normal renal function and no history of cardiac disease or strokes. We did not have access to blood samples or other biopsies from these subjects to do correlative studies with our findings in kidney biopsies.

This study has some limitations. Although, it is the largest kidney biopsy study of females with Fabry disease, given the heterogeneity of Fabry mutations and clinical manifestations, additional studies are needed to confirm our results. We did not examine the status of X-inactivation in podocytes directly, rather we studied their apparent phenotype as to presence/absence of GL-3 inclusions in cell body profiles as a surrogate for X-inactivation. However, the easy discrimination between males and females on biopsies based on podocyte mosaicism supports validity of this surrogate. We cannot exclude the possibility of overestimation of %NFPC/glom in this study due to missing GL-3 inclusions in a single section through podocyte cell bodies. However, among 4 biopsies examined from male patients, only 2 of 98 podocyte nucleated profiles, both of very small size, had no GL-3 inclusions. Thus, we believe the extent of %NFPC/glom overestimation due to random sectioning is trivial.

In summary, this is the first study showing that mosaicism of podocytes in females with Fabry disease is related to podocyte injury. The extent of podocyte mosaicism for the Fabry phenotype is quite uniform among the glomeruli. The fraction of the cell body occupied by GL-3 in affected podocytes in females is the same as in males, indicating the absence of significant cross-correction. The relative number of podocytes without the Fabry phenotype increases with age in female patients, suggesting either a disproportionate loss of Fabry-affected podocytes over time and/or selection bias. Information about podocyte mosaicism in kidney biopsies may be useful to identify females with Fabry disease with increased risk of developing progressive podocyte and nephron loss. The methodology we introduced is applicable to future longitudinal biopsy studies to test this hypothesis.

Acknowledgments

Special thanks to Frieda Maiers, Ann Palmer and Paul Murry for their help with electron microscopy images and histologic measurements, Cathy Bagne for clinical coordinator assistance, and Kristina Chayet for secretarial assistance.

Author Contributions

Conceived and designed the experiments: MM BN. Performed the experiments: MM EG AS BN. Analyzed the data: AS BN. Contributed reagents/materials/analysis tools: MM ES CT MG MW CW. Contributed to the writing of the manuscript: MM BN EG ES CT MG AS MW CW.

References

1. Zarate YA, Hopkin RJ (2008) Fabry's disease. Lancet 372: 1427–1435.
2. Wilcox WR, Oliveira JP, Hopkin RJ, Ortiz A, Banikazemi M, et al. (2008) Females with Fabry disease frequently have major organ involvement: lessons from the Fabry Registry. Mol Genet Metab 93: 112–128.
3. MacDermot KD, Holmes A, Miners AH (2001) Anderson-Fabry disease: clinical manifestations and impact of disease in a cohort of 60 obligate carrier females. J Med Genet 38: 769–775.
4. Maier EM, Osterrieder S, Whybra C, Ries M, Gal A, et al. (2006) Disease manifestations and X inactivation in heterozygous females with Fabry disease. Acta Paediatr Suppl 95: 30–38.
5. Wang RY, Lelis A, Mirocha J, Wilcox WR (2007) Heterozygous Fabry women are not just carriers, but have a significant burden of disease and impaired quality of life. Genet Med 9: 34–45.
6. Gibas AL, Klatt R, Johnson J, Clarke JT, Katz J (2008) Disease rarity, carrier status, and gender: a triple disadvantage for women with Fabry disease. J Genet Couns 17: 528–537.
7. Deegan PB, Baehner AF, Barba Romero MA, Hughes DA, Kampmann C, et al. (2006) Natural history of Fabry disease in females in the Fabry Outcome Survey. J Med Genet 43: 347–352.
8. Mehta A, Ricci R, Widmer U, Dehout F, Garcia de Lorenzo A, et al. (2004) Fabry disease defined: baseline clinical manifestations of 366 patients in the Fabry Outcome Survey. Eur J Clin Invest 34: 236–242.
9. Reiser J, Sever S (2013) Podocyte biology and pathogenesis of kidney disease. Annu Rev Med 64: 357–366.
10. Najafian B, Svarstad E, Bostad L, Gubler MC, Tondel C, et al. (2011) Progressive podocyte injury and globotriaosylceramide (GL-3) accumulation in young patients with Fabry disease. Kidney Int 79: 663–670.
11. Thurberg BL, Rennke H, Colvin RB, Dikman S, Gordon RE, et al. (2002) Globotriaosylceramide accumulation in the Fabry kidney is cleared from multiple cell types after enzyme replacement therapy. Kidney Int 62: 1933–1946.
12. Germain DP, Waldek S, Banikazemi M, Bushinsky DA, Charrow J, et al. (2007) Sustained, long-term renal stabilization after 54 months of agalsidase beta therapy in patients with Fabry disease. J Am Soc Nephrol 18: 1547–1557.
13. Kriz W, LeHir M (2005) Pathways to nephron loss starting from glomerular diseases-insights from animal models. Kidney Int 67: 404–419.
14. Matsusaka T, Sandgren E, Shintani A, Kon V, Pastan I, et al. (2011) Podocyte injury damages other podocytes. J Am Soc Nephrol 22: 1275–1285.
15. Tondel C, Bostad L, Larsen KK, Hirth A, Vikse BE, et al. (2013) Agalsidase benefits renal histology in young patients with Fabry disease. J Am Soc Nephrol 24: 137–148.
16. Terryn W, Cochat P, Froissart R, Ortiz A, Pirson Y, et al. (2013) Fabry nephropathy: indications for screening and guidance for diagnosis and treatment by the European Renal Best Practice. Nephrol Dial Transplant 28: 505–517.
17. Najafian B, Mauer M, Hopkin RJ, Svarstad E (2013) Renal complications of Fabry disease in children. Pediatr Nephrol 28: 679–687.
18. Warnock DG, Mauer M (2014) Fabry Disease: Dose Matters. J Am Soc Nephrol.
19. Kriz W, Shirato I, Nagata M, LeHir M, Lemley KV (2013) The podocyte's response to stress: the enigma of foot process effacement. Am J Physiol Renal Physiol 304: F333–347.
20. Najafian B, Mauer M (2011) Quantitating glomerular endothelial fenestration: an unbiased stereological approach. Am J Nephrol 33 Suppl 1: 34–39.
21. Toyoda M, Najafian B, Kim Y, Caramori ML, Mauer M (2007) Podocyte detachment and reduced glomerular capillary endothelial fenestration in human type 1 diabetic nephropathy. Diabetes 56: 2155–2160.
22. Deegens JK, Dijkman HB, Borm GF, Steenbergen EJ, van den Berg JG, et al. (2008) Podocyte foot process effacement as a diagnostic tool in focal segmental glomerulosclerosis. Kidney Int 74: 1568–1576.
23. Topham PS, Haydar SA, Kuphal R, Lightfoot JD, Salant DJ (1999) Complement-mediated injury reversibly disrupts glomerular epithelial cell actin microfilaments and focal adhesions. Kidney Int 55: 1763–1775.
24. Gubler MC, Lenoir G, Grunfeld JP, Ulmann A, Droz D, et al. (1978) Early renal changes in hemizygous and heterozygous patients with Fabry's disease. Kidney Int 13: 223–235.
25. Valbuena C, Carvalho E, Bustorff M, Ganhao M, Relvas S, et al. (2008) Kidney biopsy findings in heterozygous Fabry disease females with early nephropathy. Virchows Arch 453: 329–338.
26. Wolf G, Chen S, Ziyadeh FN (2005) From the periphery of the glomerular capillary wall toward the center of disease: podocyte injury comes of age in diabetic nephropathy. Diabetes 54: 1626–1634.
27. Pinto LL, Vieira TA, Giugliani R, Schwartz IV (2010) Expression of the disease on female carriers of X-linked lysosomal disorders: a brief review. Orphanet J - Rare Dis 5: 14.
28. Migeon BR (2006) The role of X inactivation and cellular mosaicism in women's health and sex-specific diseases. JAMA 295: 1428–1433.
29. Aerts JM, Groener JE, Kuiper S, Donker-Koopman WE, Strijland A, et al. (2008) Elevated globotriaosylsphingosine is a hallmark of Fabry disease. Proc Natl Acad Sci U S A 105: 2812–2817.
30. Whybra C, Kampmann C, Krummenauer F, Ries M, Mengel E, et al. (2004) The Mainz Severity Score Index: a new instrument for quantifying the Anderson-Fabry disease phenotype, and the response of patients to enzyme replacement therapy. Clin Genet 65: 299–307.
31. Dobrovolny R, Dvorakova L, Ledvinova J, Magage S, Bultas J, et al. (2005) Relationship between X-inactivation and clinical involvement in Fabry heterozygotes. Eleven novel mutations in the alpha-galactosidase A gene in the Czech and Slovak population. J Mol Med (Berl) 83: 647–654.
32. Elstein D, Schachamorov E, Beeri R, Altarescu G (2012) X-inactivation in Fabry disease. Gene 505: 266–268.
33. Warnock DG, Ortiz A, Mauer M, Linthorst GE, Oliveira JP, et al. (2012) Renal outcomes of agalsidase beta treatment for Fabry disease: role of proteinuria and timing of treatment initiation. Nephrol Dial Transplant 27: 1042–1049.

34. (2013) The Human Gene Mutation Database at the Institute of Medical Genetics in Cardiff.
35. Ashton-Prolla P, Tong B, Shabbeer J, Astrin KH, Eng CM, et al. (2000) Fabry disease: twenty-two novel mutations in the alpha-galactosidase A gene and genotype/phenotype correlations in severely and mildly affected hemizygotes and heterozygotes. J Investig Med 48: 227–235.
36. Eng CM, Ashley GA, Burgert TS, Enriquez AL, D'Souza M, et al. (1997) Fabry disease: thirty-five mutations in the alpha-galactosidase A gene in patients with classic and variant phenotypes. Mol Med 3: 174–182.
37. Bekri S, Enica A, Ghafari T, Plaza G, Champenois I, et al. (2005) Fabry disease in patients with end-stage renal failure: the potential benefits of screening. Nephron Clin Pract 101: c33–38.
38. Wang C, Wang Y, Zhu F, Xiong J (2013) A Missense Mutation of the alpha-Galactosidase A Gene in a Chinese Family of Fabry Disease with Renal Failure. Kidney Blood Press Res 37: 221–228.

Permissions

All chapters in this book were first published in PLOS ONE, by The Public Library of Science; hereby published with permission under the Creative Commons Attribution License or equivalent. Every chapter published in this book has been scrutinized by our experts. Their significance has been extensively debated. The topics covered herein carry significant findings which will fuel the growth of the discipline. They may even be implemented as practical applications or may be referred to as a beginning point for another development.

The contributors of this book come from diverse backgrounds, making this book a truly international effort. This book will bring forth new frontiers with its revolutionizing research information and detailed analysis of the nascent developments around the world.

We would like to thank all the contributing authors for lending their expertise to make the book truly unique. They have played a crucial role in the development of this book. Without their invaluable contributions this book wouldn't have been possible. They have made vital efforts to compile up to date information on the varied aspects of this subject to make this book a valuable addition to the collection of many professionals and students.

This book was conceptualized with the vision of imparting up-to-date information and advanced data in this field. To ensure the same, a matchless editorial board was set up. Every individual on the board went through rigorous rounds of assessment to prove their worth. After which they invested a large part of their time researching and compiling the most relevant data for our readers.

The editorial board has been involved in producing this book since its inception. They have spent rigorous hours researching and exploring the diverse topics which have resulted in the successful publishing of this book. They have passed on their knowledge of decades through this book. To expedite this challenging task, the publisher supported the team at every step. A small team of assistant editors was also appointed to further simplify the editing procedure and attain best results for the readers.

Apart from the editorial board, the designing team has also invested a significant amount of their time in understanding the subject and creating the most relevant covers. They scrutinized every image to scout for the most suitable representation of the subject and create an appropriate cover for the book.

The publishing team has been an ardent support to the editorial, designing and production team. Their endless efforts to recruit the best for this project, has resulted in the accomplishment of this book. They are a veteran in the field of academics and their pool of knowledge is as vast as their experience in printing. Their expertise and guidance has proved useful at every step. Their uncompromising quality standards have made this book an exceptional effort. Their encouragement from time to time has been an inspiration for everyone.

The publisher and the editorial board hope that this book will prove to be a valuable piece of knowledge for researchers, students, practitioners and scholars across the globe.

List of Contributors

Xiao-Lin Li, Shubha P. Kale, Harris McFerrin, Madhusoodanan Mottamal, Xin Yao, Fengkun Du, Baihan Gu, Kim Hoang, Yen H. Nguyen, Nichelle Taylor, Chelsea R. Stephens and Qian-Jin Zhang
Department of Biology, Xavier University of Louisiana, New Orleans, Louisiana, United States of America

Marjolein Sluijter, Elien M. Doorduijn and Thorbald van Hall
Clinical Oncology, K1-P, Leiden University Medical Center, Leiden, the Netherlands

Yong-Yu Liu
Department of Basic Pharmaceutical Sciences, University of Louisiana at Monroe, Monroe, Louisiana, United States of America
Yan Li
Department of Biology, Xavier University of Louisiana, New Orleans, Louisiana, United States of America
College of Chemistry & Environmental Science, Hebei University, Hebei Province, Baoding, China

Menelaos N. Manoussakis
Department of Pathophysiology, School of Medicine, University of Athens, Athens, Greece
Hellenic Pasteur Institute, Athens, Greece

George E. Fragoulis, Aigli G. Vakrakou and Haralampos M. Moutsopoulos
Department of Pathophysiology, School of Medicine, University of Athens, Athens, Greece

Bo Yang
Department of Food Science and Nutrition, Zhejiang University, Hangzhou, China
Department of Preventive Medicine, Wenzhou Medical University, Wenzhou, China

Feng-Lei Wang
Department of Food Science and Nutrition, Zhejiang University, Hangzhou, China

Xiao-Li Ren
Medical Laboratory Animal Center, Wenzhou Medical University, Wenzhou, China

Duo Li
Department of Food Science and Nutrition, Zhejiang University, Hangzhou, China

Chiaki Ono, Zhiqian Yu, Yoshiyuki Kasahara, Yoshie Kikuchi
Department of Disaster Psychiatry, Internal Research Institute of Disaster Science, Tohoku University, Sendai, Japan
Department of Biological Psychiatry, Tohoku University Graduate School of Medicine, Sendai, Japan

Naoto Ishii
Department of Microbiology and Immunology, Tohoku University Graduate School of Medicine, Sendai, Japan
Tohoku Medical Megabank Organization, Tohoku University, Sendai, Japan

Hiroaki Tomita
Department of Disaster Psychiatry, Internal Research Institute of Disaster Science, Tohoku University, Sendai, Japan
Department of Biological Psychiatry, Tohoku University Graduate School of Medicine, Sendai, Japan
Tohoku Medical Megabank Organization, Tohoku University, Sendai, Japan

Nan lan, Xiaoqiong Yang, Yuanyuan Cheng, Yun zhang, Xiaoyun Wang, Xing Wang and Tao Xie
Inflammations & Allergic Diseases Research Unit, Affiliated Hospital of Luzhou Medical College, Luzhou, 646000, Sichuan, China

Guangyan Luo
Hygiene Section, Luzhou Medical College, Luzhou, 646000, Sichuan, China

Guoping Li
Inflammations & Allergic Diseases Research Unit, Affiliated Hospital of Luzhou Medical College, Luzhou, 646000, Sichuan, China

Zhigang Liu
State Key Laboratory of Respiratory Disease for Allergy at Shengzhen University, School of Medicine, Shenzhen University, Nanhai Ave 3688, Shenzhen, Guangdong, 518060, PR China

Nanshan Zhong
State Key Laboratory of Respiratory Disease, Guangzhou Medical University, Guangdong, 510120, PR China

Saptak Banerjee, Tithi Ghosh, Subhasis Barik, Arnab Das, Sarbari Ghosh, Avishek Bhuniya, Anamika Bose and Rathindranath Baral
Department of Immunoregulation and Immunodiagnostics, Chittaranjan National Cancer Institute (CNCI), Kolkata, India

Fanhua Wei
Department of Orthopaedic Surgery, New York University Medical Center, New York, New York, United States of America
Institute of Pathogenic Biology, Shandong University School of Medicine, Jinan, China

Yuying Zhang
Department of Orthopaedic Surgery, New York University Medical Center, New York, New York, United States of America

Weiming Zhao and Xiuping Yu
Institute of Pathogenic Biology, Shandong University School of Medicine, Jinan, China

Chuan-ju Liu
Department of Orthopaedic Surgery, New York University Medical Center, New York, New York, United States of America
Department of Cell Biology, New York University School of Medicine, New York, New York, United States of America

Deborah H. Strickland, Vanessa Fear, Alexander N. Larcombe and Mathew E. Wikstrom
Telethon Institute for Child Health Research and Centre for Child Health Research, University of Western Australia, Perth, W.A., Australia

Graeme Zosky
Telethon Institute for Child Health Research and Centre for Child Health Research, University of Western Australia, Perth, W.A., Australia
School of Medicine, University of Tasmania, Hobart, Tasmania, Australia

Seth Shenton and Philip A. Stumbles
Telethon Institute for Child Health Research and Centre for Child Health Research, University of Western Australia, Perth, W.A., Australia
School of Veterinary and Life Sciences, Murdoch University, Perth, W.A., Australia

Patrick G. Holt
Telethon Institute for Child Health Research and Centre for Child Health Research, University of Western Australia, Perth, W.A., Australia
Queensland Children's Medical Research Institute, University of Queensland, Brisbane, Qld., Australia

Cassandra Berry
School of Veterinary and Life Sciences, Murdoch University, Perth, W.A., Australia

Christophe von Garnier
Telethon Institute for Child Health Research and Centre for Child Health Research, University of Western Australia, Perth, W.A., Australia
Pulmonary Medicine, Bern University Hospital and Department of Clinical Research, Berne University, Berne, Switzerland

Sara M. Reed
Department of Pharmacology, University of Iowa, Iowa City, Iowa, United States of America
Medical Scientist Training Program, University of Iowa, Iowa City, Iowa, United States of America

Jussara Hagen
Department of Pharmacology, University of Iowa, Iowa City, Iowa, United States of America

Viviane P. Muniz
Department of Pharmacology, University of Iowa, Iowa City, Iowa, United States of America
Molecular and Cellular Biology Program, University of Iowa, Iowa City, Iowa, United States of America,

Timothy R. Rosean
Interdisciplinary Program in Immunology, University of Iowa, Iowa City, Iowa, United States of America

Nick Borcherding, J. Adam Goeken, Paul W. Naumann, Van S. Tompkins and David K. Meyerholz
Department of Pathology, University of Iowa, Iowa City, Iowa, United States of America

Sebastian Sciegienka
Department of Pharmacology, University of Iowa, Iowa City, Iowa, United States of America

Weizhou Zhang
Interdisciplinary Program in Immunology, University of Iowa, Iowa City, Iowa, United States of America
Department of Pathology, University of Iowa, Iowa City, Iowa, United States of America

Siegfried Janz
Interdisciplinary Program in Immunology, University of Iowa, Iowa City, Iowa, United States of America
Department of Pathology, University of Iowa, Iowa City, Iowa, United States of America

Dawn E. Quelle
Department of Pharmacology, University of Iowa, Iowa City, Iowa, United States of America
Medical Scientist Training Program, University of Iowa, Iowa City, Iowa, United States of America
Molecular and Cellular Biology Program, University of Iowa, Iowa City, Iowa, United States of America
Department of Pathology, University of Iowa, Iowa City, Iowa, United States of America

Hsin-Hou Chang
Department of Molecular Biology and Human Genetics, Tzu-Chi University, Hualien, Taiwan
Institute of Medical Sciences, Tzu-Chi University, Hualien, Taiwan

Ya-Wen Chiang and Ting-Kai Lin
Department of Molecular Biology and Human Genetics, Tzu-Chi University, Hualien, Taiwan

Guan-Ling Lin and You-Yen Lin
Institute of Medical Sciences, Tzu-Chi University, Hualien, Taiwan

Jyh-Hwa Kau
Department of Microbiology and Immunology, National Defense Medical Center, Taipei, Taiwan

Hsin-Hsien Huang and Hui-Ling Hsu
Institute of Preventive Medicine, National Defense Medical Center, Taipei, Taiwan

Jen-Hung Wang
Department of Medical Research, Tzu Chi General Hospital, Hualien, Taiwan

Der-Shan Sun
Department of Molecular Biology and Human Genetics, Tzu-Chi University, Hualien, Taiwan
Institute of Medical Sciences, Tzu-Chi University, Hualien, Taiwan

Iain J. T. Thompson
Biomedical Sciences Department, Defence Science and Technology Laboratory, Porton Down, Salisbury, Wiltshire, SP4 0JQ, United Kingdom

Elizabeth R. Mann
Antigen Presentation Research Group, Imperial College London, Northwick Park and St. Mark's Campus, Watford Road, Harrow, HA1 3UJ, United Kingdom

Margaret G. Stokes
Biomedical Sciences Department, Defence Science and Technology Laboratory, Porton Down, Salisbury, Wiltshire, SP4 0JQ, United Kingdom

Nicholas R. English
Antigen Presentation Research Group, Imperial College London, Northwick Park and St. Mark's Campus, Watford Road, Harrow, HA1 3UJ, United Kingdom

Stella C. Knight
Antigen Presentation Research Group, Imperial College London, Northwick Park and St. Mark's Campus, Watford Road, Harrow, HA1 3UJ, United Kingdom

Diane Williamson
Biomedical Sciences Department, Defence Science and Technology Laboratory, Porton Down, Salisbury, Wiltshire, SP4 0JQ, United Kingdom

Junning Wang
Department of Infectious Diseases, Tangdu Hospital, Fourth Military Medical University, Xi'an, Shaanxi Province, China

Weijuan Guo
Department of Obstetrics and Gynecology, Chang An Hospital, Xi'an, Shaanxi Province, China

Hong Du, Haitao Yu, Wei Jiang, Ting Zhu, Xuefan Bai and Pingzhong Wang
Department of Infectious Diseases, Tangdu Hospital, Fourth Military Medical University, Xi'an, Shaanxi Province, China

Stefania Loffredo, Rosaria I. Staiano and Francescopaolo Granata
Department of Translational Medical Sciences and Center for Basic and Clinical Immunology Research (CISI), University of Naples Federico II, Naples, Italy

Valeria Costantino and Alfonso Mangoni
The NeaNAT group - Department of Pharmacy, University of Naples Federico II, Naples, Italy

Francesco Borriello, Annunziata Frattini, Maria Teresa Lepore and Gianni Marone
Department of Translational Medical Sciences and Center for Basic and Clinical Immunology Research (CISI), University of Naples Federico II, Naples, Italy

Massimo Triggiani
Division of Allergy and Clinical Immunology, University of Salerno, Salerno, Italy

Ravi P. Sahu, Samin Rezania, Justin D. Richey, Simon J. Warren, Badri Rashid and Joshua R. Bradish
Departments of Pathology & Laboratory Medicine, Indiana University School of Medicine, Indianapolis, IN, 46202, United States of America

Jesus A. Ocana
Department of Dermatology, Indiana University School of Medicine, Indianapolis, IN, 46202, United States of America

Sonia C. DaSilva-Arnold and Raymond L. Konger
Departments of Pathology & Laboratory Medicine, Indiana University School of Medicine, Indianapolis, IN, 46202, United States of America
Department of Dermatology, Indiana University School of Medicine, Indianapolis, IN, 46202, United States of America

Jeffrey B. Travers
Department of Dermatology, Indiana University School of Medicine, Indianapolis, IN, 46202, United States of America
Richard L. Roudebush Veterans Administration Medical Center, Indianapolis, IN, 46202, United States of America

Karen Staines, Lawrence G. Hunt, John R. Young and Colin Butter
The Pirbright Institute, Compton, United Kingdom

Sohsuke Yamada, Hirotsugu Noguchi, Aya Nawata and Nakayama
Department of Pathology and Cell Biology, School of Medicine, University of Occupational and Environmental Health, Kitakyushu 807-8555, Japan

Tomoyuki Koyama
Laboratory of Nutraceuticals and Functional Foods Science, Graduate School of Marine Science and Technology, Tokyo 108-8477, Japan

Yuki Ueda
Laboratory of Nutraceuticals and Functional Foods Science, Graduate School of Marine Science and Technology, Tokyo 108-8477, Japan

Ryo Kitsuyama and Hiroya Shimizu
Department of Welfare Engineering, Faculty of Engineering, Iwate University, Morioka 020-8551, Japan

Akihide Tanimoto
Department of Molecular and Cellular Pathology, Kagoshima University Graduate School of Medical and Dental Sciences, Kagoshima 890-8544, Japan

Ke-Yong Wang
Department of Pathology and Cell Biology, School of Medicine, University of Occupational and Environmental Health, Kitakyushu 807-8555, Japan
Shared-Use Research Center, University of Occupational and Environmental Health, Kitakyushu 807-8555, Japan

Toshiyuki Yasuyuki Sasaguri
Department of Pathology and Cell Biology, School of Medicine, University of Occupational and Environmental Health, Kitakyushu 807-8555, Japan
Laboratory of Pathology, Fukuoka Wajiro Hospital, Fukuoka 811-0213, Japan

Takumi Satoh
Department of Welfare Engineering, Faculty of Engineering, Iwate University, Morioka 020-8551, Japan
Department of Anti-Aging Food Research, School of Bioscience and Biotechnology, Tokyo University of Technology, Hachioji 192-0982, Japan

Christina M. Freisinger and Anna Huttenlocher
Departments of Pediatrics and Medical Microbiology and Immunology, University of Wisconsin-Madison, Madison, Wisconsin, United States of America

Michael Mauer
Department of Pediatrics, University of Minnesota, Minneapolis, United States of America
Department of Medicine, University of Minnesota, Minneapolis, United States of America

Emily Glynn
Department of Pathology, University of Washington, Seattle, United States of America

Einar Svarstad
Department of Medicine, Haukeland University Hospital, Bergen, Norway
Department of Clinical Medicine, University of Bergen, Bergen, Norway

Camilla Tøndel
Department of Clinical Medicine, University of Bergen, Bergen, Norway
Department of Pediatrics, Haukeland University Hospital, Bergen, Norway

Marie-Claire Gubler
U983, Université René Descartes, Hô pital Necker-Enfants Malades AP-HP, Paris, France

Michael West
Division of Nephrology, Department of Medicine, Dalhousie University, Halifax, Nova Scotia, Canada

Alexey Sokolovskiy
Department of Pathology, University of Washington, Seattle, United States of America

Chester Whitley
Department of Pediatrics, University of Minnesota, Minneapolis, United States of America

Behzad Najafian
Department of Pathology, University of Washington, Seattle, United States of America

Index

www.ingramcontent.com/pod-product-compliance
Lightning Source LLC
Chambersburg PA
CBHW061252190326
41458CB00011B/3653